CONSERVATIVE CARE OF LOW BACK PAIN

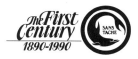

CONSERVATIVE CARE OF LOW BACK PAIN

EDITED BY

ARTHUR H. WHITE, M.D.

Medical Director
San Francisco Spine Institute at Seton Medical Center
Medical Director
SpineCare Medical Group
Daly City, California

ROBERT ANDERSON, M.D., Ph.D., D.C.

Director of Manual Medicine
San Francisco Spine Institute at Seton Medical Center
Daly City, California

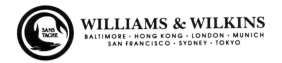

WILLIAMS & WILKINS
BALTIMORE · HONG KONG · LONDON · MUNICH
SAN FRANCISCO · SYDNEY · TOKYO

Editor: Jonathan W. Pine
Associate Editor: Linda Napora
Copy Editor: Barbara Werner
Design: Dan Pfisterer
Illustration Planning: Ray Lowman
Production: Raymond E. Reter

Copyright © 1991
Williams & Wilkins
428 East Preston Street
Baltimore, Maryland 21202, USA

Accurate indications, adverse reactions, and dosage schedules for drugs are provided
in this book, but it is possible that they may change. The reader is urged to review
the package information data of the manufacturers of the medications mentioned.

Printed in the United States of America

Library of Congress Cataloging in Publication Data

Conservative care of low back pain / edited by Arthur H. White, Robert
  Anderson.
    p. cm.
  Includes bibliographical references.
  ISBN 0-683-09007-0
  1. Backache.—Chiropractic treatment.   I. White, Arthur H., 1938–
II. Anderson, Robert Thomas, 1926–
  [DNLM: 1. Backache—therapy. WE 755 C755]
RZ265.S64C66 1991
617.5′64—dc20
DNLM/DLC

for Library of Congress   90-12041
                                                CIP

90 91 92 93
1 2 3 4 5 6 7 8 9 10

PREFACE

Nearly all people suffering from low back pain require some nonsurgical, conservative form of treatment. Such patients have a wide variety of treatment options. While doctors and/or therapists have much to offer, not all of the options may be effective. Often, what clinicians offer is out-of-date or inappropriate.

Recent years have witnessed the development of vastly improved methods that are still known for the most part only to specialists and through journal articles and papers read at professional meetings. In this book we present between two covers the current status of each of the many fields of conservative treatment and prevention. To do that, we have as collaborators outstanding specialists, each contributing in his or her field of expertise. These authors come from diverse fields. A few have no medical training, but write as scientists, teachers, or administrators; the rest are clinicians. They include physical therapists, physicians, surgeons, chiropractors, and osteopathic physicians; several possess dual qualifications as trained scientists. In addition, the work of nonmainstream health care providers is presented by a physical therapist who possesses qualifications in the practice of these techniques.

In collaboration with these eminent practitioners, we hope that this book will be of value to both specialist and nonspecialist physicians and surgeons, physical therapists, osteopathic physicians, and chiropractors. The book is meant for all clinicians who encounter back pain patients. Our hope is that these chapters will provide at least introductory instructions to those who want to try out methods with which they are unfamiliar. More advanced, hands-on training will usually be required as a follow-up. Equally, it is our hope that those who practice their specialty effectively will find in this book the resources and information on additional care that can enhance their own effectiveness in providing patient care. These chapters should be thought of as a reference book as well as an instructional manual.

We believe in the importance of interprofessional collaboration and the need to integrate research exploration with clinical treatment. To that end, the editors and authors have agreed to contribute whatever royalties may accrue from sales of this book to the research program of the San Francisco Spine Institute at Seton Medical Center, which is a nonprofit organization devoted solely and entirely to research and education.

As editors, this has been a labor of love as well as an expression of our dedication to an important field of health care. We take advantage of an editor's prerogative and dedicate our work on this book not only to those who struggle with us in this noble enterprise, but also to Jennifer White and to Robin, Dylan, and Kyle Anderson.

Arthur H. White
Robert Anderson

CONTRIBUTORS

David J. Anderson, M.D.
Department of Psychiatry
SpineCare Medical Group
Daly City, California

Robert Anderson, M.D., Ph.D., D.C.
Professor of Anthropology
Mills College
Director of Manual Medicine
San Francisco Spine Institute
   at Seton Medical Center
Daly City, California

Nikki L. Burrous
Manager, Loss Control Department
Risk Management Division
Safeway Stores, Inc.
Oakland, California

James M. Cox, D.C., D.A.C.B.R.
Director
Low Back Pain Clinic
Chiropractic Associates Diagnostic and
   Treatment Center
Fort Wayne, Indiana

Gregory Cramer, D.C., Ph.D.
Assistant Professor
Research and Anatomy
National College of Chiropractic
Lombard, Illinois

Tammy de Koekkoek, D.C.
Los Angeles College of Chiropractic
Whittier, California

Richard Derby, M.D.
Anesthesiology
SpineCare Medical Group
Daly City, California

Ronald B. Donelson, M.D.
Assistant Professor
Orthopedic Surgery
SUNY College of Medicine
Syracuse, New York

Thomas A. Dorman, M.D., Ch.B.,
   M.R.C.P. (U.K.), F.R.C.P. (C.)
Private Practice
Internal Medicine and Orthopedic Medicine
San Luis Obispo, California

Sandy Dutro, D.C.
Palo Alto, California

W. Harry Fahrni, M.D.
Orthopedic Surgery
Vancouver, British Columbia, Canada

Ross E. Goldstein, Ph.D.
President
Summit Psychological Associates
San Francisco, California

Philip E. Greenman, D.O., F.A.A.O.
Professor of Biomechanics
College of Osteopathic Medicine
Michigan State University
MSU-College of Osteopathic Medicine
East Lansing, Michigan

Scott Haldeman, M.D., Ph.D., D.C.
Assistant Clinical Professor
Department of Neurology
University of California, Irvine
Santa Ana, California

Richard E. Hunt, Ph.D.
Holiday, Utah

Gregory S. Johnson, P.T.
Co-Owner
Marin Spine and Orthopedic Center
The Institute of Physical Art
San Anselmo, California

Gerald Keane, M.D.
Clinical Instructor
Stanford University School of Medicine
Physical Medicine and Rehabilitation
SpineCare Medical Group
Daly City, California

Elizabeth Kirkaldy-Willis
Coordinator for Volunteers
Low Back School
University Hospital
Saskatoon, Saskatchewan, Canada

Patricia V. Kunse, P.T.
Peninsula Spine Education and Treatment
    Center
San Mateo, California

Rowlin L. Lichter, M.D.
Clinical Assistant Professor
John A. Burns School of Medicine—
    University of Hawaii
Orthopedic Surgery Inc.
Honolulu, Hawaii

Michael Moskowitz, M.D.
Psychiatry
SpineCare Medical Group
Daly City, California

Brian Miller, P.T.
Sommerset, New Jersey

Sigmund Miller, D.C.
San Francisco, California

Robert D. Mootz, D.C.
Associate Professor of Clinical Sciences
Palmer College of Chiropractic West
Sunnyvale, California

Stanley V. Paris, Ph.D., P.T.
President
Institute of Graduate Health Sciences
St. Augustine, Florida

Kelli Pearson, D.C., D.A.B.C.O.
Postgraduate Faculty
Los Angeles College of Chiropractic
Director, Department of Chiropractic
Group Health Northwest
Spokane, Washington

Peter B. Polatin, M.D.
Associate Clinical Professor of Psychiatry
University of Texas, Southwestern Medical
    School
Dallas, Texas

Jeffrey A. Saal, M.D.
Director of Research and Education
San Francisco Spine Institute
Chief of Physical Medicine and Rehabilitation
SpineCare Medical Group
Daly City, California

Joel S. Saal, M.D.
Attending Physician/Consultant
San Francisco Spine Institute
Physical Medicine and Rehabilitation
SpineCare Medical Group
Daly City, California

Vicky Saliba, P.T.
Director
Marin Spine and Orthopedic Center
The Institute of Physical Art
San Anselmo, California

H. Duane Saunders, M.S., P.T.
Educational Opportunities
Bloomington, Minnesota

Jerome Schofferman, M.D.
Director
Internal Medicine/Pain Management
SpineCare Medical Group
Daly City, California

Nancy C. Selby
Director
Spine Education Center
Dallas, Texas

Roy A. Slack, M.D.
Back-In-Action, Inc.
Beaverton, Oregon

Mark Sontag, M.D.
Team Physician
San Mateo Junior College
Physical Medicine and Rehabilitation
SpineCare Medical Group
Redwood City, California

David A. Thompson, Ph.D.
Professor Emeritus
Industrial Engineering and Engineering
    Management
Stanford University
Stanford, California

John Triano, D.C., Ph.D.
Director
Spinal Ergonomics Research Laboratory
National College of Chiropractic
Lombard, Illinois

Patrick P. Venditti, D.C.
Director
The Ergonomics Center
Logan College of Chiropractic
Chesterfield, Missouri

Lindsay Wheeler, D.C.
Oakbay Chiropractic Center
Oakland, California

Arthur H. White, M.D.
Medical Director
San Francisco Spine Institute
    at Seton Medical Center
Medical Director
SpineCare Medical Group
Daly City, California

CONTENTS

SECTION VI: PSYCHOLOGICAL AND MEDICAL DIMENSIONS

SECTION VII: PREVENTION IN THE WORK PLACE

SECTION VIII: RECONDITIONING THE INJURED WORKER

SECTION IX: CHALLENGE OF LOW BACK PAIN

Section I

APPROACHES TO PATIENT CARE

1

INTRODUCTION TO CONSERVATIVE CARE

Arthur H. White

You may be a physician, a physical therapist, a chiropractor, an osteopathic physician or a specialist in some other field of health care. Whatever your field, if it includes the conservative care of low back pain disorders, your primary interest and concern is the well-being of your patient. To have helped that patient become well and happy is your highest reward. What a wonderful feeling of accomplishment! And what an excellent way to keep busy, because others in pain will be referred to you by satisfied patients.

Conservative care commends itself as the first resort for all but the very rare patient who comes to you as a surgical emergency. Conservative care commends itself, when properly carried out, as the only kind of treatment that will be needed for 99% of your back pain patients. But what do we mean by this characterization of our approach to treatment?

Surprisingly, although commonly spoken of and written about, conservative care is nowhere adequately defined. Perhaps the most common implication is that conservative therapy is meant to preserve and restore health to the musculoskeletal system by nonradical methods. But with this definition we have merely shifted the uncertainty. What is meant by radical?

In some cases, conservative versus radical refers to nonsurgical versus surgical intervention. Although not explicitly defined, this is the way the concept is used by Bernard E. Finneson (1). William H. Kirkaldy-Willis notes that some refer to "nonoperative measures" as an alternative designation (2). On the whole, we too think of nonsurgical methods. Yet sometimes, surgery is the conservative approach. This would be consistent with Kirkaldy-Willis' observation that the term conservative "is not altogether accurate because more aggressive methods sometimes prove more conservative in the sense of conserving, that is of restoring, normal function quickly" (2).

Often, conservative is taken to mean noninvasive. Surgery is invasive, but massage and stretching are not. However, acupuncture is invasive to the extent that a thin needle breaks the skin, and epidural or facet blocks penetrate deeply with large-gauge needles, yet they are conservative to my way of thinking.

Medicating patients rather than operating on them is part of what some seem to have in mind. Yet one of the most difficult problems we face with chronic back pain patients is their addiction to prescribed narcotic drugs. All drugs have side effects. Even aspirin can cause gastritis and ulcers. A successful surgery such as a percutaneous nuclectomy might seem relatively conservative in contrast with some kinds of pharmacologic intervention. The most conservative treatment of all, then, is nonpharmacologic as well as nonsurgical.

Conservative sometimes refers to traditional methods or views. In other words, it refers to treatment that is in the mainstream of health culture rather than on the margin. Certainly, much that we do is highly traditional. Massage, counter-irritation, heat, and other modalities are sanctioned by history. Yet history alone does not make all of the approaches used here acceptable as mainstream. Spinal manipulative therapy (SMT) and acupuncture, in particular, are very ancient and yet remain topics of emotional controversy for many. On the other hand, new approaches such as back school are not traditional and yet have rather good acceptance in mainstream health care. So, conservative may mean an accepted part of contemporary health care culture, but not all that is covered in this book is accepted in that sense.

Finally, cost appears to be a part of people's thinking on this issue. Conservative can mean relatively inexpensive. Again, there is ambiguity; surgery is sometimes cheaper than a long-term rehabilitation program.

Conservative care, then, is a multifaceted concept. On the whole, in what follows we will cover methods that are nonsurgical, noninvasive, nonpharmacologic, mainstream, and relatively inexpensive. The reader may find, however, that any one form of conservative care will deviate to some extent from this overall characterization and yet fit with the philosophical orientation of the book. A treatment may be considered conservative even if it is surgical, invasive, pharmacologic, unorthodox, or expensive. It is conservative nonetheless if in other ways it does meet the above criteria and thus allows us to help patients in pain in effective, acceptable ways. Perhaps this is what Gregory P. Grieve means in saying, "In clinical practice, the classical division between conservative and radical treatment becomes less important as the combined skills of the medical, surgical and paramedical team are applied to help the patient" (3).

We all have a common goal. It is interesting that we approach that common goal in quite varied ways, most of which are at least partially successful. The physician classically works by prescribing medication, bed rest, corsets, and physical therapy. The osteopathic physician relies upon many of the same methods, but frequently adds an osteopathic version of spinal manipulative therapy. The chiropractor depends chiefly upon chiropractic forms of SMT, but may add additional interventions, including diet and exercise. The physical therapist, who leaves medications and injections to the prescribing physician, depends classically on modalities such as traction, heat, ultrasound, and manual therapy. Manual therapy has extended increasingly in the hands of some therapists into a version of SMT that tends to emphasize mobilization but may, in some cases, include manipulation.

Many other specialities in the treatment of back pain are also on the scene. Some limit themselves to unique and very precise methods. In the posture and movement realm, these include Feldenkreis, Aston Patterning, Alexander Technique, and Rolfing. For the relief of pain, acupuncture has been used successfully for centuries. More recently, other pain-relieving techniques have evolved, including the use of various electrical stimulators, localized manual pressure techniques, and psychotherapy.

Every one of these techniques and many more appear to be successful in the hands of the practitioners who continue to use and teach them. These practitioners obviously are convinced of the usefulness of their approaches. It must be noted, however, that little or no verification of the efficacy of any of the above techniques is to be found in the scientific literature, whether the practitioner is a medical doctor or a tribal shaman.

Why is this? Part of the explanation lies in the fact that time alone will heal most back patients. While nature unobtrusively mends an aching back, the treating clinician understandably assumes that a valued methodology was responsible. A patient who is much improved reinforces the practitioner's belief in what was taught in clinical training. Handed-down skills in that way get validated in the practitioner's mind as beneficial techniques that should continue to be taught and applied.

At the same time, it is certainly possible that many of the hundreds of conservative methods available do have significant value in altering certain low back pain conditions. We have all encountered the patient who has migrated from one practitioner to the next, searching for a cure. That patient may eventually happen upon a practitioner who offers the most appropriate tool for that condition. Success in such a case results in a high level of patient satisfaction, to be followed by recommendations to friends and acquaintances who also suffer from low back pain. Usually patients refer fellow sufferers with very little awareness of how one back pain may differ from another in terms of cause and potentially effective treatment. With enough successful responses, however, the practitioner may develop a good reputation and a successful practice.

It seems probable, then, that value resides in every specialty of spinal practice. To take advantage of this potential, however, practitioners need to identify precisely the disease process taking place in each individual in order to make it possible to select or recommend the most appropriate specialist or combination of specialists. Leaving a patient to go blindly from one practitioner to another in search of the one with the needed methods is extremely inefficient and very costly. The whole field of spine care, whatever the specialty, gets tarnished in the eyes of other health care providers when patients are left to drift about painfully in need of appropriate treatment.

Who are we, the specialists in spine care, to whom patients turn? We are skilled. We are confident. But we are unorganized, with inadequate means of interprofessional communication. We know too little about the expertise of those outside our own practice. We tend to feel competitive, even jealous, of one another. Patients do not benefit from these attitudes. Society does not benefit. It is clear that we as practitioners also do not benefit.

It is essential to recognize that, although we are diverse, each of us offers a potentially useful approach to the amelioration of back pain. This simple observation suffices to provide a guideline for improvement. We must take steps immediately to learn about each other. We must determine where and how each of us can fit in to provide the total spectrum of skilled methods back patients require. Multidisciplinary conferences in which all specialties are represented can contribute to our mutual education. We need to collaborate on books and scientific papers as we explore and describe alternative methods of care. We need to tear away the blinders of interprofessional prejudice and closed-mindedness and look, instead, to each other to learn and to contribute.

As of now, unfortunately, the blinders are largely still in place. Much of the competition among various members of the conservative care network is unhealthy even though it is understandable. Fear is probably the greatest impediment to openness. One fear is that of inadequacy. Any practitioner is subject to the fear that someone else actually possesses better answers to the low back problem. Some may fear that they will be discovered not to be as all-knowing and successful as their reputation

might suggest. Another fear is financial. Each practitioner must face the challenge of survival in a competitive marketplace for conservative care.

Competition, suspicion, fear, and distrust are probably greatest between chiropractors and medical practitioners. Unfortunately, I know from my own side of that political barrier that the relationship can elicit extraordinary negative energy. At times I have experienced the personal and professional rewards that come to a surgeon who has invited chiropractors to speak at meetings or has collaborated with chiropractors in the care of mutually interesting patients. But in those same episodes, I have felt the anger and listened to the irrational fears of my medical and surgical colleagues who fail to see mutuality of benefit in such encounters. Some would believe, even in our time, that chiropractors are diabolical in character and greedy in purpose in contrast to an angelic persona they would claim for themselves.

Opponents of openness among professions can usually identify a nonmedical practitioner who warrants disdain. They inevitably fail to remember those they know well from their own ranks who are known to be unethical or incompetent. In a calm moment, we all realize that there are good and bad in any profession. Chiropractic doctors do not have an exclusive claim to therapeutic badness. Medical doctors do not have sole rights to goodness.

In calm moments one can recall practices, including spine centers, in which chiropractors and physician-surgeons work together closely. In collaborative settings, each learns to recognize that the one can do what the other cannot, and that each has limitations in responding to the enormously complex needs of back pain patients. The physician who denies patients the advantages of spinal adjusting is just as shortsighted as the chiropractor who denies access to appropriate medical interventions. They suffer the darkness of ignorance but, worse, their patients suffer treatable pain and dysfunction.

Another chasm that separates professionals who ought to be collaborating in the treatment of back problems is that which separates physical therapists from occupational therapists. It always comes as a shock to me when I attempt to join practitioners from these two related professions in the common enterprise of a spine center and encounter mutual hostility and a resistance to working together. I am sure it has to do with belief systems that are engendered in training. Therapists of either kind leave school with a belief in the strong delineation of responsibilities and capabilities that allocates what the one should treat and what should be left to the other. This strikes me as artificial, and quite lacking in scientific justification.

But physical and occupational therapists did not invent professional isolationism. However realistic in political terms, science and the needs of patients cannot justify a delimiting of the chiropractic turf that would exclude physical therapists from practicing SMT, or of identifying an osteopathic educational domain that would close its doors to other practitioners of SMT who would sit in on instructional courses. No room can be found, to my way of thinking, for jealousies and failure to cooperate. It is short-sighted because it harms those who get caught up in these restrictive postures, both patients and the clinicians themselves. A refusal to train, communicate, or share patient care between any two specialties of spinal care is, in my opinion, as inexcusable and immoral as book burning in a fascist dictatorship or reserving sumptuary prerogatives for the born rich in an hereditary aristocracy.

I argue for the importance of professional mutuality not only because I believe that we all grow wiser and succeed better in an open system, but also because I believe it is essential if we are to survive the political and economic changes in place or on the horizon for health care providers in the United States. In the past, we have been able to bill and be paid for any services that we rendered if they were reasonable. In recent years, reimbursement has become increasingly problematic. Preventive care has suffered especially. For a time it was difficult to get paid for "back school" but, by identifying the proper codes, most of us have been paid for patient education, which clearly is highly beneficial even though it does not sound sufficiently medical to some third-party payers.

The difficulties in assuring reimbursement have increased in the last couple of years. With each new HMO and PPO, we find still new restrictions on what we are permitted to provide for our patients. Operations that we can justify on surgical grounds as necessary are currently being denied in case after case. We can expect to see increasingly tighter restrictions on the provision of conservative care as well.

Who is making the decisions as to what treatments will be reimbursed? What is the standard of care to which we are to be held? Is the standard of care the same for a chiropractor, a physician or an osteopath? To what extent is the physical therapist permitted to provide entry care?

As we develop newer and better techniques for treating spinal problems, will our patients be denied their use until the "old standard of care" catches up with the forms of treatment? We have reason to worry. The computed tomography (CT) scan was available for years before it was authorized for reimbursement by the U.S. Government. Back school has not been paid for under the designation of "back school" by any insurance company for the past 15 years. In our center we are still fighting with the State of California for acceptance of back school as part of the standard of best possible care for low back problems.

To protect ourselves against having patient care dictated to us by insurance companies, we as a spinal medical community need to arrive at decisions regarding standards of care, including time frames for treatment and protocols for advancement from one kind of treatment to another. Insurance companies and government agencies will be more likely to acknowledge our expertise if we can attain a level of agreement among ourselves. Our present divisiveness is harmful to each of us and to those we serve.

I propose that we abandon clinical isolationism and educational exclusionism. We must get out of the separatist mode. We need to cross-fertilize in order to achieve a hybrid vigor of clinical expansiveness and efficacy. Medical schools need to have chiropractors on their teaching staffs, just as chiropractic colleges often already include medical doctors on their staffs. We each need to recognize that we came out of our training limited to some degree by philosophical blind areas. Each of us was taught to believe that the only "right" way to treat patients is that of our own profession.

As a way of contributing to the breakdown of this nonproductive and detrimental separatism, let us open our minds, shift our attitudes, and take a good look at what others do as alternative specialists in spinal care. Let us recognize limitations in what each of us does. Let us look for successes in what others do in ways that are different from what we learned. Let us do this and then note something that struck me with the force of a thunderbolt when I broke away from my own medical provincialism. Some patients get better faster by going to what we benightedly think of as "the opposition."

We must learn to think of other specialists as collaborators. We need to develop guidelines for identifying patients who need alternative care in addition to our own or instead of our own. To enjoy your practice, you need to experience success. Success comes with referring or sharing those patients who can profit from additional or different care. You will also get patients that way. Above all, you have more fun,

because your patients will do better. You will experience the excitement of a practice that increases your access to the highest reward a clinician can hope for: to help your patients become well and happy.

References

1. Finneson BE. Low back pain. 2nd ed. Philadelphia: JB Lippincott, 1980.
2. Kirkaldy-Willis WH. ed. Managing low back pain. 2nd ed. London: Churchill Livingstone, 1988, 250.
3. Grieve GP. Common vertebral joint problems. London: Churchill Livingstone, 1981, 376.

2

DIAGNOSIS AND TREATMENT OF LOW BACK PAIN SINCE 1850

Robert Anderson

MEDICAL PRACTICE AROUND 1850

In order better to evaluate the quality of current methods utilized in the diagnosis and treatment of low back pain, let us look back to those physicians and surgeons who practiced around the middle of the last century. Information from that time can serve as a baseline against which to evaluate the state of the art in our own time. For heuristic purposes, reference will be made to medicine and surgery as practiced around 1850, but the documentation includes some sources from earlier in the century. Most date from 1840 to 1860.

Our attention will be directed to the particular kind of low back pain that derives either from biomechanical defects in lumbar vertebrae or from painful and incapacitating changes in soft tissue around the spine, including muscles, nerves, tendons, and ligaments. The pain may be limited to the lumbosacral area or it may extend into more distal areas, particularly into the buttock and leg. Whatever the details, musculoskeletal disorders of the lumbar spine constitute our medical battlefield (1).

In 1850, Sir Benjamin C. Brodie, M.D. described a "Mr. Jones" who came to his office complaining of restricted spinal flexion associated with back, buttock, and leg pain that was exacerbated by sneezing. His clinical notes read as follows (verbatim but with deletions which are not indicated):

A gentleman, thirty-one years of age, consulted me under the following circumstances: He complained of pain referred to the spine. When he attempted to stoop, he experienced a sense of stiffness, the stooping being apparently confined to the motion of the pelvis on the thigh. A sudden motion had often occasioned an aggravation of the pain in the spine, and on all occasions pain was induced by the act of sneezing. He also experienced at times pains in the pelvis and lower extremities. I could not find that there was anything like paralysis of the limbs, and there was no difficulty of micturition (2).

Differential Diagnosis around 1850

Mr. Jones of 1850 was diagnosed as having ankylosis of the vertebrae subsequent to a long-continued chronic inflammation (2). Based upon the assumed presence of inflammation of the spine, his case fell into the diagnostic category of rheumatism.

Mid-nineteenth century physicians commended themselves in the belief that medicine had made enormous progress since 1800 (3). In the differential diagnosis, it was thought, physicians had advanced significantly beyond the ancients who simply called every disease of the joints arthritis (4). It was still true in 1850, however, that low back pain fell into a residual category only somewhat less sweepingly inclusive and vague than was the category of arthritis in earlier times.

The symptoms of rheumatism, "generally called by the people Rheumatiz," included pain and swelling affecting the joints and muscles (4–6). Acute rheumatism was distinguished by pain of recent onset combined with pyrexia. It might shift suddenly from one "muscular or articular structure" to another with a special penchant for ligaments, tendons, and bursae (6). Chronic rheumatism was described as a lingering, painful disease in which fever was absent, or nearly so. It attacked the same parts of the body as acute rheumatism; however, chronic rheumatism frequently affected "some distinct nerve, or branches of nerves," in which cases it was known as rheumatism of the nerve or neuralgia (6). Neuralgia in the spine sometimes presented as rheumatism of the sciatic nerve or sciatica. When the pain occured in the low back, it was identified as lumbago. Neuralgia, as a rheumatism of the nerve, was sometimes differentiated from muscular rheumatism, in which the pain was somehow different (4, 6).

These diagnostic categories confuse as much as they help. Was neuralgia a synonym for rheumatism, a subcategory of rheumatism, or a disorder sui generis that sometimes overlapped rheumatism in signs and symptoms? From the authorities available for this study, one cannot be sure. Again, it is not clear what the physician concluded who encountered a patient with low back pain of recent onset but without an elevated temperature. Was the case acute or chronic? Recall that most practitioners did not use thermometers, so identifying an elevated temperature constituted a highly subjective judgment call (7). No doubt the individual with a recent onset of back pain always seemed feverish to the doctor's hand, while some fever did not preclude a diagnosis of chronicity.

Again, how did one respond to a patient complaining of severe buttock or leg pain if it was of recent onset? Was it sciatica, which was assumed always to be chronic? One's sense of time can be rather subjective, so perhaps any sciatica seemed comparatively lingering to the sympathetic physician and the suffering patient. Given the impressionistic approach that characterized the physicial examination at that time, it would also seem arbitrary to differentiate pain in nerves from pain in muscles. Was the difference between lumbago and sciatica one of muscle versus nerve or merely one of back versus leg pain? The answer is not clear.

GOUT

To some extent, the nineteeth century practitioner did succeed in arriving at a differential diagnosis. Diagnosticians in 1850 made it a point to distinguish rheumatism from gout, a dichotomy that had been recognized for the preceding two centuries, although some doctors still con-

fuse the two. "Gout . . . is a disease of a certain part, and periodical; rheumatism, of the whole body, and uncertain in its time of coming" (4). "You may distinguish Gout from Rheumatism by the fact that it attacks the smaller joints, and nearly always those of the toes and fingers; while Rheumatim attacks the larger ones" (6). Since gout was not known to cause low back pain, it was not a consideration in making spinal diagnoses (8).

RICKETS

In the presence of a spinal curve that was "distinguished by the alteration of shape in the other bones with which it is accompanied, especially in those of the lower limbs and the chest," one could make the diagnosis of rickets or rachitis (2). Rickets, a widespread disorder, was sometimes referred to as the "disease of the spine" (6).

STOOPED POSTURE

A "hoop-like curvature" could occur in rheumatism. However, a smoothly rounded anterior curvature could also be congenital or developmental. "Some persons, either from their original conformation, or from an early habit of stooping, present the appearance of a very considerable gradual or hoop-like curvature" (2). In the absence of pain, a kyphosis was not identified either as rheumatism, rickets, or any other disease entity. It was simply a stooped posture.

TUBERCULOSIS

It was especially important to differentiate rheumatism, rickets, and mere postural deformities from bony tuberculosis, known as caries of the spine, an infection frequently encountered in those days. Tuberculosis, referred to as scrofula or white swelling, was identified in the spine on the basis of a kyphosis that, instead of being smoothly rounded, was interrupted by "an angle projecting posteriorly. . . . Such an angular curvature can be produced in no other way, and can never be mistaken" (2). One physician, writing in 1833, described with pride observed advances in understanding, because, as he noted, "from the time of Pott until very recently, caries of the bones was almost universally considered, as causing all varieties of spinal deformity" (2). From such past limitations, he felt that the beginning of the nineteenth century marked a new era in medicine (3, 6).

SYPHILIS

The other infectious disease one had to keep in mind was syphilis, although not as a common cause of back pain. It was usually encountered in the skull, tibia, or ulna. Pain cases showing nonrachitic skeletal deformities, especially those presenting with a deformed and painful shin bone, were diagnosed as muscular rheumatism resulting either from a syphilitic cause or from the aggressive treatment of syphilis with mercurial drugs, in which case it was known as mercurial rheumatism. The chronic pain of bony syphilis was thought to result from tenderness in the periosteum (4).

SCOLIOSIS

Known as lateral curvature of the spine, scoliosis was often encountered, especially in girls. The direction of the curve made the diagnosis easy. No doctor would confuse the lateral curve of scoliosis with the anterior curve of rheumatism or rickets or with the angular kyphotic curve that was pathognomonic of caries (9).

RHEUMATISM

With nearly all patients, it was fairly straightforward for the nineteenth century physician to identify those suffering from the relatively well-characterized diseases of caries of the spine, lateral curvature of the spine, and rickets of the spine. Syphilis and gout were rare in the axial skeleton. Every other spinal disorder, a salmagundi of common and uncommon diseases, fell into a giant residual category known as rheumatism.

Subcategories might designate differences between muscular rheumatism and neuralgia. Sciatica was distinguished from lumbago. Acute was differentiated from chronic. But all were soaked up in that spongelike entity known as rheumatism. Rheumatism, then, is the disease in 1850 that frequently presented as low back pain.

Pathophysiology around 1850

Exposure to changeable weather, and especially cold and wet exposure, were frequently cited as causes of rheumatism (8).

> Rheumatism is brought on by exposure to the cold and wet; by sleeping in damp places; by remaining too long on the damp ground; by sleeping in a current of air at night, immediately under an open window; by exposure to the night dews; by taking off a warm dress and putting on a thin one; by being greatly heated, and becoming suddenly cool, thereby checking the perspiration or sweat (10).

Other "causes of rheumatism" were thought to include a hereditary tendency, intemperance in eating and drinking, being a man (for the acute form) or a woman (for the chronic form), being young (for the acute) or older (for the chronic), suffering from disorders of the stomach, liver and bowels (especially for the chronic), abuse of mercurial medications (rheumatic mercurialis), and infections with gonorrhea, syphilis, or malaria (8, 10).

The underlying pathophysiologic cause of the pain and dysfunction of rheumatism was thought of as a general tendency to inflammation that settled in the spine and cord or marrow in response to indiscretions of habit or to misfortunes of birth and lifestyle. It was conceptualized as a systemic disease. As one author put it, "under the general inflammatory diathesis of the system, one part will scarcely be affected by rheumatism without other parts participating" (4).

Irritation was thought to begin in internal organs such as the liver, the intestines, or the bladder from which it "metastacized" to cause inflammation and pain in the spine. The viscera, therefore, might require treatment even though the case manifested primarily as an inflammation in the locomotor system. The digestive system, above all, was thought to cause general inflammation in the locomotor system. (1, 4, 6). Some physicians described the same sequence of events, but in reverse, believing that inflammation began in the spine and then spread to the viscera (8).

Individual case histories might note instances in which the onset of low back pain was subsequent to a stressful movement, as in the case of the young man who fell while carrying a basket of vegetables on his head (1). A biomechanical mechanism was not accorded priority in discussions of etiology, however. Curvatures of the spine, which were "very commonly" attributed to rheumatism (i.e., inflammation), although not originating in trauma could be exacerbated by it.

> In subjects predisposed to rheumatism, the slightest twist of the spine will often produce a return of the disease: the writer of this, experienced an attack of lumbago and sciatica, which lasted for months, by suddenly jumping out of bed and giving the back a jar.

This he attributed in part to a common defect in rheumatism, namely weakness in the extensor muscles of the back (3).

Treatment in 1850

SURGERY

Curvatures of the spine constituted the primary focus of nineteenth century biomechanical or anatomic reasoning. Surgeons at times operated on severe cases of scoliosis that had proven unresponsive to conservative care, even though some authorities believed that surgery was ineffective for this purpose. The technique was to perform a dorsal myotomy, in which large back muscles were sectioned. Even when done without anesthesia, it was said that the operation was "attended with little pain, or chance of subsequent accident. . . ." (11). More extensive surgery was never considered for rheumatism, however, so in one sense, all surgical treatment for the category of spinal disorder that concerns us here was conservative.

Because rheumatism was thought primarily to constitute a medical problem relating to a "general inflammatory diathesis of the system," constitutional remedies were the first line of attack for the doctor. Bleeding, "being the most sure and speedy depletive we possess, demands our first attention" (8). In the treatment of acute rheumatism, "general bleeding is a remedy of great importance" (4). In this sense, minor surgery, that is, venesection, was common in the treatment of acute back pain.

Because bleeding could debilitate a patient, one might well question whether it was truly conservative. The patient had to be robust to withstand it. Indeed, "If the patient be of a delicate constitution, blood letting by leeches will be sufficient," but even in these patients, blood

is removed until one can note "a reduced force and frequency of the heart's action; *The Pulse should feel it*" (8).

In 1849, Dr. Edward Stanley reported on a patient:

> A man, aged twenty-one, whilst carrying a basket of vegetables on his head, was knocked down and fell on his back. . . . The motor power in the [lower] limbs was wholly lost, but the sensation in them was preternaturally acute . . . , and there was, besides, retention of the urine.

This unfortunate young man was diagnosed as suffering from inflammation of the spine and cord from injury, i.e., rheumatism (1).

Dr. Stanley, in treating him, entered the following note in his records: "Ten ounces of blood were removed by cupping from the spine, and afterwards twelve ounces of blood were taken from the arm" (1).

INTERNAL MEDICINE

Various kinds of medicine were prescribed for back pain. The harshness of these medications eliminates all of them as part of a conservative methodology, quite aside from the observation that they were probably completely ineffective for the treatment of the diseases known as rheumatism (12).

The stomach and bowels needed to be cleansed. For this purpose, emetics and purgatives were prescribed (8). "When Rheumatism is connected with a disordered state of the Liver, Emetics are particularly useful, followed by a dose of Cathartic Pills" (6). To induce vomiting in Dr. Stanley's patient, "Saline medicine, with antimony and hydrargyrum cum crêta, was freely administered." The bladder was "daily washed out with tepid water, by means of a double-tubed catheter." To evacuate the lower digestive system, mercury was administered until the patient's teeth loosened and the gums became inflamed. "The gums became sore, and they were kept so by the continued administration of mercury" (1).

Mr. Jones was not given an emetic, but his treatment included calomel for the digestive tract. After one or two months of treatment it was noted that ". . . the mercury had not affected the gums, but his symptoms were much relieved." In chronic cases, it was common to prescribe iodide of potassium, which was tried with Mr. Jones when the calomel was discontinued. It disagreed with him and had to be stopped (2).

Narcotics, referred to as sedatives, were found helpful in many patients. The calomel given to patient Mr. Jones included "one-third of a grain of opium, to be taken three times daily" (4, 2).

Purification of the body could also be accomplished with sudorifics. To make a patient sweat, one might prescribe ". . . antimony in conjunction with calomel and purgatives, or of antimony or ipecacuanha with opium in moderate doses" (4).

PHYSICAL MEDICINE

Rest assumed prominence as a major therapeutic recommendation. From the second half of the nineteenth century through the first half of the twentieth, it was orthodox medical practice to prescribe extensive rest for all cases of severe pain (13, 14). Specifically as concerns diseases of the spine, rest in the recumbent position was highly recommended (1, 24, 10).

Stabilization or bracing was attempted solely by means of corsets and braces, and then only in efforts to correct scoliosis, and not in the treatment of rheumatism (9, 15).

Exercise was much talked of as a preventive measure, including some exercises reputed to strengthen the back (16). Only an occasional author recommended exercise in the treatment of rheumatism, however, and by exercise was meant generic active movement, including walking (4). No writer described treatment exercises for developing stability, strength, or flexibility.

Local topical applications at the site of the pain were also available to low back pain patients. For acute rheumatism, heat was thought beneficial. Heat might be applied in the form of a hot water bottle or a poltice of hot bran or salt in a flannel bag (4, 10). Warm bathing was also recommended (5, 8). Exposure of the sore area to the heat of a steam bath was not unknown (10).

Cold douches or baths were recommended for robust patients who had recovered from rheumatism, but never for the person still suffering from the disease. In acute rheumatism, direct cold applications were to be strictly avoided. They were thought dangerous because they could drive the disease inward to affect important internal structures (4, 8).

Local treatment usually included the application of a counterirritant. Bleeding was not only undertaken as a general medical measure, but was applied directly at the site of pain as well. Local bleeding might take the form of leeching or cupping. Cupping was especially recommended for lumbago and sciatica. Blistering was also performed. Irritating liniments and plasters were frequently recommended (1, 2, 4, 8, 11). Electric irritation (galvanism) was described by some authorities (4, 6, 8).

Acupuncture or acupuncturation, "once so extensively employed for almost every painful affection, has also been used for the cure of Rheumatism, and especially chronic Rheumatism. . . . I applied it in one instance to the Spine, and the result was the same as from cupping, or other counter irritation; it gave immediate relief"(8). *Electro Puncturation* has succeeded in cases," it was reported, "after ordinary acupuncturation repeatedly performed had failed." Moxa as a counterirritant was also known (8).

MANUAL MEDICINE

Friction, kneading, and massage were thought useful for rheumatism (6, 8, 11). Spinal manipulative therapy (SMT) for conditions diagnosed as rheumatism had apparently not been carried out by physicians and surgeons for a couple of centuries (17). Because spinal disorders frequently were associated with curvatures of the spine, earlier medical attention often focused upon the anatomic deformity. "Before the time of Mr. Pott, these diseases were only considered with respect to their external characters; the distortions were mechanically treated without any regard to their causes" (3). Some authorities still considered spinal manipulation under traction an acceptable option for the treatment of scoliosis, but they acknowledged that it was dangerous and caution was advised (3). Others refused to condone it for any purpose (15). Simple traction was described for scoliosis, but not for rheumatism (9, 10).

Because physicians did not practice spinal manipulation, individuals who wanted it sought out folk practitioners. In England, bonesetters kept quite busy for this reason (18–20). Those afflicted with low back pain in the

United States were rarely able to locate a bone-setter and therefore had almost no opportunity to seek SMT as an alternative to medical treatment (21).

State of the Art around 1850

Although the diagnosis of lumbago or sciatica has a contemporary sound, in 1850 these designations only meant that pain could be localized to the low back or to the leg. Lumbago and sciatica were medical lost causes at that time. Diagnostically, they fell into the broad, ill-defined category of rheumatism. The ultimate cause of rheumatism was believed to reside in nonmechanical, nonergonomic factors in the environment and in lifestyle. A cold draft of air rather than a way of lifting or of sitting was regarded as the chief culprit. Beliefs about underlying pathophysiology bogged down in the concept of constitutional inflammation, with no more than minimal recognition of possible biomechanical contributions to the disease.

Consistently with these ways of thinking, lumbago and sciatica were treated as constitutional diseases for which surgery was not appropriate (except the minor surgery of venesection). Internal medicine provided the main battery of the physician, and an assault on the body is a good way to characterize their approach. Emetics, purgatives, sudorifics, and narcotics liberally poured down the throats of low back patients helped spinal pain largely to the extent that these drugs made patients so sick or bewildered that the mere excruciating pain of lumbago or sciatica might be momentarily forgotten.

A topical approach to painful areas modulated these otherwise misdirected efforts at obtaining a cure. Yet, although doctors made extensive use of heat, patients were denied the benefits of cold because mid-nineteenth century concepts of etiology targeted cold exposure as a frequent villain in the onset of rheumatism. Counterirritants remained as the major topical treatment. Cupping, bleeding, blistering, burning, and puncturing on the whole were applied in a far harsher manner than was necessary to achieve the pain relief of counterirritation as such. The side effects were substantial even though some benefit no doubt was achieved. Finally, rest was overused while manual therapy was underused.

To what extent, then, did a mid-nineteenth century patient profit from conservative measures in the hands of a physician? From a psychological perspective, perhaps it was comforting to place one's health problem in the hands of a doctor. Palliation from rest, heat and mild counterirritation was offered. On balance, these benefits were rather minimal, and were achieved at a high cost in pain and debility. Patients suffering from low back pain who avoided physicians probably did better than did those who sought profesional care, because only a small part of a doctor's treatment was conservative enough to fit the dictum, "first, do no harm".

MEDICINE AROUND THE TURN OF THE CENTURY

By 1899, a major figure in academic medicine could write of "phenomenal strides in every branch of scientific medicine"(22). Certainly, some advances had been achieved in the treatment of low back pain, but did they constitute phenomenal strides? Pronounced but modest would better characterize developments in this area (23). Physicians in major urban centers no longer utilized heroic measures that caused severe iatrogenic disease. However, while they no longer did severe harm, they also did not achieve notable cures. The most striking medical advance was the discovery of aspirin.

To evaluate the branch of scientific medicine relevant to low back pain, we will rely primarily upon the textbook that set standards in medical education for a decade on either side of the century mark. William Osler published the first edition of *The Principles and Practice of Medicine* in 1892 and the seventh edition in 1909 (24, 25). What differences do we detect when the turn of the century is compared with the middle of the nineteenth century as we examine the textbook that shaped a transformation in medical education in the United States and the English-speaking world (26)?

Differential Diagnosis around 1900

What might have been the diagnosis of Mr. Jones had he come to a physician in 1900 instead of 1850? He probably would still have been diagnosed as suffering from rheumatism. Most likely, his condition would also have been characterized as sciatica or lumbago secondary to an inflammatory diathesis. However, by this time, he might have suffered from a recently discovered entity, arthritis deformans due to a bacterial infection. A mechanical diagnosis would still not have been thought of.

One clear-cut entity got chipped away from the many other diseases that formerly were incorporated into the global concept of rheumatism. Rheumatic fever was recognized as a distinctive infectious disease that could include acute arthritis in the spine as one of its manifestations. Much confusion continued to cloud diagnostic reasoning, however, in part because rheumatoid arthritis was still not differentiated from osteoarthritis (8, 24, 25).

The concept of rheumatism persisted as a generic term, but was divided for teaching purposes into four disease entities: arthritis deformans, chronic rheumatism, muscular rheumatism, and neuritis. Low back pain cut across these four categories (24, 25).

Sciatica in part perpetuated its earlier identity as neuralgia or rheumatism of the sciatic nerve. It could be categorized as neuritis, localized neuritis, or rheumatic neuritis. "The most important symptom is pain of a boring or stabbing character, usually felt in the course of the nerve and in the parts to which it is distributed" (24, 25).

Although sciatica could be considered a neuritis, in Osler's text it simultaneously belonged to the diagnostic category of arthritis deformans, which in part included traits we would now identify as degenerative joint disease or osteoarthritis: Heberden's nodes, atrophic changes in bone and cartilage, and hypertrophy and overgrowth of bone, including osteophytes. These osteoarthritic changes were especially well described in the 1909 edition, based upon x-ray studies, which had become available only after the first edition was published. The differential diagnosis was obscured, however, because osteoarthritic forms of degeneration were not separated from the inflammatory and degenerative changes characteristic of rheumatoid arthritis, Still's disease, and anchylosing spondylitis (27).

Arthritis deformans was too broad a category because it merged osteoarthritis with rheumatoid arthritis. It was also too narrowly defined, because it failed to include a frequent manifestation of osteoarthritis, namely lumbago.

Lumbago was diagnosed as muscular rheumatism or myalgia, "A painful affection of the voluntary muscles and of the fasciae and periosteum to which they are attached" (24, 25). Thus, according to Osler, sciatica could result from either osteoarthritic changes or inflammation of the sciatic nerve, but lumbago was thought to be the product of an inflammation of muscle and other soft tissue. To add to this confusion, some authors distinguished rheumatism of the joints from rheumatism of the muscles, and considered both lumbago and sciatic neuritis to be expressions of muscular rheumatism (28).

Residually, chronic rheumatism persisted as a reduced version of the mid-nineteenth century catch-all category of rheumatism. It survived as an inflammatory disease of capsules, ligaments and tendons, with very little involvement of the joints, although, "In long-standing cases the cartilages also undergo changes, and may show erosions" (24, 25). No clear criteria assisted the diagnostician in differentiating arthritis deformans from acute rheumatism in the early stages, from rheumatism as such in the "advanced stage," or from chronic rheumatism in late cases, when it might be "difficult or impossible to distinguish" the one from the other (24, 25). Diagnosis, in short, continued to lead clinicians treacherously into muddied waters and unplumbed depths.

Pathophysiology around 1900

By the turn of the century, assisted by the imaging capabilities of an emergent x-ray technology, medicine added some thinking about osteoarthritic degeneration. It did so, however, without full appreciation of the role degenerative joint disease could play in the etiology of low back pain. Rheumatism as an inflammatory condition continued to dominate diagnostic thinking and to divert inquiry.

Uncertainties allowed some in the profession to advocate more sweeping monocausal theories of the cause of back pain. "I shall," one author argued, "take the position that gout, rheumatism and arthritis deformans are kindred conditions in that they spring from a common cause ... uric acid diathesis" (28a). Infection, however, was the favored concept of the time.

An enormous change took place in medical thinking during the last decades of the nineteenth century when it was realized that many major diseases were caused by infectious microorganisms. It is hardly surprising that these discoveries influenced thinking about how back pain might occur. Osler rather cautiously suggested that arthritis deformans might result from a chronic infection, although he thought that attacks of muscular rheumatism "follow cold and exposure." In his section on arthritis deformans, he reports, "A number of the very best students of the disease ... have accepted the infective theory of origin, which is gaining adherents, though it still lacks demonstration" (24, 25).

Arthritism, an arthritic diathesis or special vulnerability, one author argued, makes certain individuals subject to "acute articular rheumatism, the various chronic rheumatisms (including rheumatoid arthritis), and gout, allied affections originating in a same morbid cause, differing only in their external manifestations." The specific disease may be set off by "sudden changes of temperature," but the underlying cause is germs, which "have here found a favorable soil in which to develop" (29). Back pain, in short, was an infectious disease in the thinking of many practicing physicians.

Treatment around 1900

The notion that lumbago, sciatica and other forms of rheumatism or arthritis were systemic diseases that ought to respond to appropriate oral medications persisted at the turn of the century, but with the thought that in some cases infection was involved.

SURGERY

Major surgery, increasingly done to correct deformities of the extremities, was also used in the treatment of severe spinal disorders, but not for the type of low back pain under discussion here. Osler did at times refer spinal patients to surgeons for immobilization in plaster jackets during the acute phase (24, 25).

The Age of Heroic Medicine came to an end. Venesection was "completely abandoned" (29). This abandonment of systemic bleeding was part of an enormous change that occurred in the practice of medicine. Harsh emetics and cathartics also went out of vogue. Milder forms of treatment were recommended.

INTERNAL MEDICINE

In place of the worst of the old harsh remedies, physicians now treated rheumatism with salicylates. The wonder drug of the year 1900 was aspirin (30). The salicylates were thought by some to cure joint disease through an hypothesized bactericidal effect that was felt to be far more important than any slight pain-relieving capability it might also possess (29). Dr. George Dock, Osler's counterpart at the University of Michigan medical school, usually prescribed a modest 10 grains in 24 hours. Harsh, heroic medicine was obsolete, but in severe cases Dock recommended as much as 30 grains per hour, which unquestionably caused salicylate poisoning. "In such a case you can't get the medicine in too fast, and you can't give too much" (31).

Osler, for his part, recommended that arthritis deformans patients could be strengthened with a general tonic. "Arsenic in full doses is helpful in some cases" (24, 25). Milder medication, it would seem, is a relative concept.

PHYSICAL MEDICINE

Bed rest measured in weeks was liberally recommended, along with a temperate diet (31).

In topical treatment, liniments and poltices that did not blister or burn were favored. Dock frequently treated with a poltice or wrap of cotton drenched in oil of wintergreen (31). Osler saw some benefit in hot baths, hot compresses, and hot-air treatment. He also noted that thermocautery could relieve pain and reduce ligamentous thickening. "Repeated applications are helpful along the spine in the spondylitis deformans." Acupuncture was also part of Osler's approach to rheumatism, a hat pin serving as a suitable needle despite its formidable diameter and bluntness (24, 25).

MANUAL MEDICINE

Osler urged the benefits of appropriate exercise and of hands-on treatment. "Massage, carefully given, reduces the periarticular infiltrations, increases the mobility of stiffened joints, and most important of all, prevents the atrophy of the muscles adjacent to the affected joints" (24, 25). Spinal manipulation, however, was not an option for orthodox practitioners. In the United States, turn-of-the-century physicians turned their backs on chiropractors who had recently come onto the scene, and they disparaged osteopaths who by then had been around for a bit longer (31). In England, physician practitioners of spinal manipulative therapy were still almost nonexistent (31a). Bonesetters continued to earn endorsements from a multitude of patients who were not satisfied with medical treatment. Bonesetters, however, were attacked in medical journals (32).

State of the Art around 1900

Conservative care by the turn of the century had become more attractive to back pain sufferers, mainly because it was no longer dominated by harsh medications, although an element of harshness persisted. In addition to prolonged rest, doctors offered analgesics, heat, and counterirritants—all of which could palliate but did not cure. Under these conditions, many patients bypassed the physician in favor of a bonesetter, an osteopath, or a chiropractor (33).

MEDICINE AT MID-TWENTIETH CENTURY

At mid-century, one historian of medicine noted that "medicine has matured as a science and medical practice has, as a result, become more effective" (34). One cannot fault that judgment as it concerns many fields of medicine. In the treatment of back pain, however, it was only partially true. In the approach to spinal disorders, emphasis shifted to new forms of aggressive treatment that frequently left a patient worse off than if no treatment had been offered. In that sense, medical change constituted a step backwards toward 1850. In its twentieth century form, the overly aggressive culprit was surgery, which achieved near supremacy in the treatment of low back pain between 1910 and 1950. Conservative care was thought important, but most physicians merely perpetuated old forms, sometimes in the guise of new technology.

Diagnosis around 1950

What might a diagnostician have concluded of Mr. Jones, had he been seen in 1950 rather than a full century earlier? Well, his diagnosis would probably have been arthritis rather than rheumatism. Most likely the orthopedic surgeon, a specialty by then on the scene, would have decided that his pain was caused by a herniated nucleus pulposus. However, a rheumatologist, by then also on the scene, might have insisted that first you would need to rule out arthritis of the spine secondary to pyorrhea or some other occult focus of infection. Spinal manipulation by medical practitioners was almost unknown in the United States and still relatively unknown in Great Britain and Europe. Osteopaths and chiropractors were beyond the pale. A biomechanical lesion would probably not have been considered in orthodox medical circles.

More refinement in diagnostic precision took place between the two world wars. Rheumatoid arthritis was acknowledged as a disease different from osteoarthritis and other kinds of back pain.

For many, the term arthritis replaced rheumatism as the catch-all designation within which lumbago and sciatica now found their typological home. The old term, rheumatism, was relegated, on the whole, to colloquial and archaic usage (35). Rheumatologists remained loyal to the term, including it in the larger category of rheumatic diseases, "those conditions in which pain and stiffness of some portion of the musculo-skeletal system are prominent" (36). The overall tendency to abandon the term rheumatism was made clear, however, in the 16th and last edition of Osler's text, written in 1947. Writing of chronic rheumatism, which constituted Osler's residual category in his first edition, the editor of the 16th edition notes that, "this term deserves mention because it is so commonly used, but its retention is not justified" (37).

Within the category of arthritis, back pain was differentiated according to whether it was an infective arthritis, a myositis (inflammation of the voluntary muscles), a fibrositis (inflammation of fibrous tissue, including ligaments and tendons), degenerative joint disease (also known as hypertrophic arthritis or osteoarthritis), or a protruded intervertebral disc (also called a herniation of the nucleus pulposus) (37). Facet syndrome and discogenic syndrome were also recognized at that time (36).

Pathophysiology around 1950

As early as 1911, Goldthwait explored potential mechanical causes of back pain (38). In the late 1920s, Bucy and Dandy showed that the pressure of disc herniations could produce neurological symptoms (39). Schmorl and Junghanns published their anatomic descriptions of the spine in 1932. Based upon the autopsies of 10,000 spines, this work demonstrated a growing understanding of the morphology of the spine and its relevance to the etiology of low back pain (40). By 1934, Mixter and Barr had begun to operate on herniated discs as a way to treat back and leg pain (41). Increasingly, disc pathology was scrutinized as a cause of pain.

The concept of arthritic pain as a product of infection was also to survive, however. Bacteria versus vertebral disc degeneration became the choices diagnosticians had to make. Infective arthritis won the most converts at first. At times, it was found in the form of a frank infection of a joint from which an offending bacterium could be cultured. In the spine, tuberculosis was sometimes the culprit, as had been recognized more than a hundred years earlier.

However, a divergent concept of infective arthritis emerged early in the twentieth century, the idea that a local pocket of smoldering, low-grade, often asymptomatic infection could seed germs or toxins into the bloodstream that ultimately found their way to joints where they resulted in arthritic pain and degeneration. This kind of thinking led physicians increasingly to attribute most forms of arthritis, including degenerative joint disease, to this form of autointoxication.

Theorizing that unidentified bacteria were the ultimate cause of low back pain, one physician writing in 1910 saw the process as fundamentally a matter of faulty digestion. Above all, sagging of the intestines, demonstrated by means of contrast radiological studies, was believed to result in constipation. Delayed motility in the bowels, in turn, was thought to lead to the formation of bacteria and bacterial toxins (28). It took decades for the concept of visceroptosis to be eliminated as a gastroenterologic diagnosis relevant to arthritis (42).

From the intestines, or whatever other point of entrance they used, bacteria were postulated to migrate to joints, or to good breeding grounds in the prostate gland, tonsils, teeth, or other hidden places where they could persist as a low-grade infection that spread to articular tissues. To find the disease, the "focus of infection must be sought," it was argued (28). A 1912 article

published by Frank Billings popularized the phrase "focal infection," and stressed the need to search for the hidden places where it might originate or lodge. The concept was to dominate pathologic thinking for almost half a century (43).

The idea of focal infection as the culprit in back pain demonstrated remarkable staying powers. Focal infection was regarded as an etiologic factor in joint pain by at least one well-known back specialist writing in the mid-1960s (44) and is still found in at least one current textbook in medical anthropology (45). Yet, its scientific validity at mid-century was clear: the concept was bankrupt. In 1947, the 7th edition of Cecil's *Textbook of Medicine* distanced itself from an earlier enthusiasm of the concept. "Many students today question seriously its validity and some are quite willing to throw it completely overboard" (46). Henry Christian, who edited the last edition of Osler's text in 1947, also distanced himself: "The earlier belief in the great frequency and importance of focal infection as an explanation of many subacute and chronic diseases now is on the wane; many are skeptical of this relationship except in relatively few patients; with this view the present author is in agreement" (37). The 1949 edition of Comroe's *Arthritis and Allied Conditions* similarly takes note of a lost faith. "Some ... have gone so far as to say that [the] whole concept [of focal infection] is false" (36).

It is striking how every one of these authorities acknowledged the failure of clinical research to validate the theory, and yet continued to mention it in their texts. Cecil, Christian, and Comroe each recommended that, in arthritis, one should look for a focus of infection in the tonsils, the teeth, the nasal sinuses, the genitourinary tract, the gallbladder and according to Cecil and Christian, the intestines as well.

However, fewer and fewer cases of back pain were thought to be infectious. Most were ascribed to physical changes in and around the joints. Above all, disc disease was believed to be the culprit in most cases of lumbago and sciatica, although myositis, fibrositis, and neuritis were still frequently postulated. "Ideas on backache have wholly altered since it became apparent that by far the commonest cause is fragmentation of a low lumbar intervertebral disc, and that 'lumbar fibrositis' ... is an imaginary disorder" (35). Some thought that disc disease was responsible for 90% or more of all backaches, although it should be noted that others tended to identify muscular strain as the culprit in the majority of cases of backache (36). By mid-century, the concept that won out was that a herniated nucleus pulposus (HNP) most commonly was the villain in back and leg pain.

Treatment around 1950

SURGERY

Two dominant theories of arthritis contended during the first half of the twentieth century to explain the ultimate etiology of low back pain. If a back pain was not the product of a focal infection, it probably was caused by an HNP. Surgery was the treatment of choice in either case if symptoms were severe.

Arthritis patients with back pain diagnosed as caused by a focal infection routinely went to surgery for tooth extractions, tonsillectomies and adenoidectomies, appendectomies, cholecystectomies, hysterectomies, oöphorectomies and salpingectomies, prostatectomies, and Lane's operation for removal of the colon. "Many physicians routinely removed teeth, tonsils, and appendices from their arthritis patients" (47). By 1950, however, it was clear to medical scientists that this treatment was useless for back pain.

About 10% of low back pain patients who were diagnosed as disc cases also were sent to surgery. Whatever the identified cause, many patients received surgery that would not be considered appropriate in our time.

INTERNAL MEDICINE

Systemic treatment was now limited. Some physicians prescribed vaccine therapy for the treatment of focal infections, even though the treatment was never shown to work. Most recommended dietary changes, mainly to control obesity. It was still common to recommend the avoidance of dampness, cold, and drafts. But systemic medications were only recommended for the disorders that concern us here in the form of analgesics and sedatives.

Analgesics were liberally prescribed. Aspirin and phenacetin were widely used survivals of an earlier period. Codeine was prescribed in many cases and morphine in some. Nerve blocks were also provided. Sedatives were prescribed (36).

PHYSICAL MEDICINE

Rest continued to have its advocates, even though an early voice urged that rest should be prescribed selectively and in a limited manner (35).

Stabilization by means of corsets, strapping, belts, molded casts, and binders was prescribed to limit motion (36).

Exercises were recommended for strength and postural correction. William's flexion exercises became a vogue. Good body mechanics were recommended, but it was not clear what that should mean (36).

Heat and massage applied by physical therapists were mainstays of treatment.

MANUAL MEDICINE

Spinal manipulation had become more available in England. Bonesetters were nearly extinct, but physicians specializing in SMT were being trained, as were physical therapists. On the fringes of medicine, osteopaths practiced their version of manual therapy. Very few chiropractors had set up in England.

In the United States, although widely appreciated by many who sought care at their hands, osteopaths and chiropractors were much criticized by official representatives of medicine. Osteopaths were on the verge of getting licensed for a full scope of medical and surgical practice. As that took place, the practice of SMT was left largely in the hands of chiropractors. Gradually, after World War II, physicians and physical therapists skilled in SMT began to be found in North America.

Curiously, SMT in this period gained some prominent medical advocates. This was especially so in Great Britain (35). In the United States it was less common, and yet, Comroe's Arthritis recommended manipulative treatment for some cases of backache. Comroe even spoke of cases which respond "miraculously" to manipulation. "Unfortunately," Comroe's successor concluded, "the average surgeon considers any form of manipulation beneath his dignity. Manipulative methods of therapy in this disorder have been ignored by most of the medical profession" (36).

State of the Art around 1950

By 1950, the once popular theory that arthritis was the product of an occult low-grade focal infection was moribund. Surgeries to remove foci of infection were obsolete. Spinal surgery to correct disc herniations gained in popularity (48). By the 1970s, however, a high incidence of failed surgeries dampened enthusiasm for lumbar spine surgery. It became apparent that probably 99% of back pain patients would not benefit from surgery of any kind (49). What, then, could one do for people in pain?

By the 1970s, it was clear that nearly all back patients needed conservative care. Yet, nonsurgical methods were still bogged down in old, largely unexamined practices. Most clinicians did little more than offer palliation and play a waiting game. Eventually, most back pain patients would get better, a natural history of disease that obscured the inadequacy of the most popular treatments. Patients who did not get well, however, began the "pain game" of going from one doctor to another, seeking help in vain.

But the 1970s also marked an upturn in the techniques of conservative care. The last quarter of this century witnessed a proliferation of innovative achievements, and that is what this book is about. Were Mr. Jones alive today, reliance upon approaches described in the chapters that follow would offer him a vastly improved likelihood to achieve pain relief and regain function, and the world is full of back pain sufferers just like Mr. Jones.

Acknowledgments

The contributions of librarians Eda Regan and Carol Jarvis at Mills College and Betty Vadenboncoeur and Steve Urbano of Lane Medical Library, Stanford University are gratefully acknowledged. From her personal library, Loretta M. Costedoat of Mills College generously made available a copy of *Gunn's New Family Physician*.

References

1. Stanley E. Treatise on diseases of the bones. London: Longman, Brown, Green, and Longmans, 1849.
2. Brodie C. Pathological and surgical observations on the diseases of the joints. London: Longman, Brown, Green, and Longmans, 1850.
3. Beale J. A treatise on the distortions and deformities of the human body. Exhibiting a concise view of the nature and treatment to the principal malformations and distortions of the chest, spine, and limbs. London: John Churchill, 1833.
4. Scudamore C. Treatise on the nature and cure of gout and rheumatism, including general considerations on morbid states of the digestive organs; some remarks on regimen; and practical observations on gravel. London: Printed for the Author, 1819.
5. Haygarth J. I. Clinical history of the acute rheumatism, or rheumatick fever. II. A clinical history of the nodosity of the joints. rev. ed. London: Cadell and Davies, 1813.
6. Gunn C. Gunn's new family physician: or, home book of health. New York: Moore, Wilstach & Moore, 1868.
7. Reiser SJ. Medicine and the reign of technology. Cambridge: Cambridge UP, 1978, 115–116.
8. Monell GC. Rheumatism, acute and chronic: A prize essay. New York: HG Langley, 1845.
9. Lonsdale EF. Observations on the treatment of lateral curvature of the spine. Pointing out the advantages to be gained by placing the body in a position to produce lateral flexion of the vertebral column, combined with the after application of firm mechanical support. London: John Churchill, 1847.
10. Gunn JC. Gunn's domestic medicine or poor man's friend, in the hours of affliction, pain, and sickness. rev. ed. (original ed, 1853.) New York: CM Saxton, Barker & Co, 1860.
11. Bigelow HJ. Manual of orthopedic surgery, being a dissertation which obtained the Boylston Prize for 1844, on the following question: "In what cases and to what extent is the division of muscles, tendons, or other parts proper for the relief of deformity or lameness?" Boston: William D. Ticknor, 1845.
12. Haller JS Jr. American medicine in transition: 1840–1910. Urbana: University of Illinois Press, 1981: 67–99.
13. Hilton J. On the influence of mechanical and physiological rest in the treatment of accidents and surgical diseases. London: Bell & Dalby, 1863.
14. Cyriax J. Textbook of orthopaedic medicine. Vol. 1. London: Baillière Tindall, 1978: 19.
15. Tuson EW. The cause and treatment of curvature of the spine, and diseases of the vertebral column. London: John Churchill, 1841.
16. Taylor GH. An exposition of the swedish movement-cure. New York: Fowler and Wells, 1860.
17. Anderson R. On doctors and bonesetters in the 16th and 17th centuries. Chiropractic History 3 (1), 1983: 11–15.
18. Paget, J. Cases that bone-setters cure. Br Med J 1, 1867: 1–4.
19. Schiotz EH, Cyriax J. Manipulation: Past and present. London: William Heinemann, 1975: 29.
20. Hood W. On the so-called 'bone-setting', its nature and results. Lancet, 1, 1871: 336–338, 372–341, 441–443, 449–501, 631.
21. Lomax E. Manipulative therapy: A historical perspective from ancient times to the modern

era. In Goldstein M. ed. The research status of spinal manipulative therapy. NINCDS Monograph No. 15. DHEW Publication No. (NIH) 76-998. Washington, DC: US Department of Health, Education, and Welfare, 1975: 11–17.

22. Osler W. After Twenty-Five Years. In Osler W. Aequanimitas with other addresses to medical students, nurses and practitioners of medicine. 3rd ed. Philadelphia: Blakiston, 1932; 199.

23. Harvey A McG, McKusick VA. Osler's textbook revisited. New York: Appleton-Century-Crofts, 1967: 9–10.

24. Osler W. The principles and practice of medicine. Edinburgh & London: Young J. Pentlane, 1892.

25. Osler W. The principles and practice of medicine. 7th ed. New York and London: D. Appleton, 1909.

26. Ludmerer, Kenneth M. Learning to heal: The development of American medical education. New York: Basic Books, 1985; 134–135.

27. Robinson WD. Rheumatoid Arthritis. In Harvey A McG, McKusick VA. Osler's textbook revisited. New York: Appleton-Century-Crofts, 1967; 159–162.

28. Peckham FE. The classification and treatment of diseases commonly known as rheumatism. Fiske Fund Prize Dissertation No. LIII. Providence, RI: Snow and Farnham Co., 1910.

28a. Conklin, AB. Gout, rheumatism and arthritis deformans. Ambler, PA: Published by the Author, 1904.

29. Gros EL. A modern pathological and therapeutical study of rheumatism, gout, rheumatoid arthritis and allied affections. London: Hubert H. Mason, 1897.

30. Drinkwater H. Fifty years of medical progress: 1873–1922. New York: Macmillan, 1924.

31. Davenport HW. Doctor Dock: Teaching and learning medicine at the turn of the century. New Brunswick, NJ: Rutgers U P, 1987.

31a. Anderson, R. Wharton Hood, MD, the rejected father of manual medicine. Archives of the California Chiropractic Association 1981; 5(2): 59–63.

32. Anderson R. Medical prejudice: The case of bonesetting. European J Chiropractic, 31, 1983: 5–12.

33. McCorkle T. Chiropractic: A deviant theory of disease and treatment in contemporary western culture. Human Organization, 20 (1), 1961: 20–22.

34. Stern BS. American medical practice in the perspectives of a century. New York: The Commonwealth Fund, 1945.

35. Cyriax J. Rheumatism and soft tissue injuries. London: Paul B. Hoeber, 1946.

36. Comroe BI. Arthritis and allied conditions. 4th ed. Hollander JL. ed. Philadelphia: Lea & Febiger, 1949.

37. Christian HA. The principles and practice of medicine. 16th ed. New York: D. Appleton-Century, 1947.

38. Goldthwaite JE. The lumbosacral articulation. Boston Med Surg J 1911: 164: 365.

39. Bucy PC. Sixty years of neurological surgery. JAMA 1988: 260: 2264–2266.

40. Schmorl G, Junghanns H. The human spine in health and disease. Wilk SP, Goin GS, translators. New York: Grune & Stratton, 1959.

41. Mixter WJ, Barr JS, Rupture of the intervertebral disc with involvement of the spinal canal. N Engl J Med, 211, 1934: 210–215.

42. Kirsner JB. Gastroenterology comes of age. JAMA 1988: 260 (2): 244–246.

43. Billings F. Chronic focal infections and their etiologic relations to arthritis and nephritis. Arch Internal Med 9, 1912: 484–490.

44. Mennell JMcM. Joint pain: Diagnosis and treatment using manipulative techniques. Boston: Little, Brown, 1964; 166.

45. Wood CS. Human sickness and health. Palo Alto, CA: Mayfield, 1979: 14, 22, 26.

46. Cecil RL, McDermott W. A textbook of medicine. 7th ed. Philadelphia: WB Saunders, 1947.

47. Lambert EC. Modern medical mistakes. Bloomington: Indiana UP, 1978; 27–32.

48. Wiltse LL. A history of lumbar spine surgery. In White AH, Rothman RH, Ray CD. eds. Lumbar spine surgery: Techniques & complications. St. Louis: CV Mosby, 1987.

49. White AH. Introduction and Purpose. In White AH, Rothman RH, Ray CD eds. Lumbar spine surgery: Techniques & complications. St. Louis: CV Mosby, 1987.

3

REHABILITATION OF THE PATIENT

Jeffrey A. Saal
Joel S. Saal

Rehabilitation of the low back pain patient is a comprehensive process. An accurate diagnosis followed by early intervention is necessary. A rehabilitation plan can be divided into a pain-control phase and a training phase. The pain-control phase may include a variety of passive modalities, flexion or extension exercises, lumbar mobilization, traction, and selective injection procedures. The key element of the rehabilitation program is the training phase, which emphasizes back school, movement training, and specific dynamic muscular lumbar stabilization exercises. The scientific rationale and components of this rehabilitation program are presented below.

WHAT PAIN ARE WE TREATING?

The first and most important task a clinician has when faced with a patient suffering from low back pain is to establish a diagnosis. Without an accurate and timely diagnosis, it is virtually impossible to plan a specific treatment and rehabilitation program to enable patients to return to their normal active lifestyles. Localization of a pain generator is paramount in spinal pain diagnostics. Indeed, the structure that appears to be most involved on a computed tomography (CT) scan or other imaging study may not be the structure that is generating the disabling pain. Therefore, a careful correlation of the patient's history, mechanism of injury, physical exam, and diagnostic studies is important for establishing the location of the pain generator(s). An adequate understanding of spinal biomechanics, referral pain, and potential pain generators is therefore necessary for

this undertaking (1). Repetitive flexion and torsional loads to the lumbar spine have been noted to cause annular injury that leads to disc degenerative changes (2, 3). Lifting is a major cause of intervertebral disc injuries, especially when twisting or when lateral bending is combined with flexion. Recently, these same torsional stresses have been noted to cause leakage of synovial fluid from the lumbar facet joints, which may lead to early advancement of facet arthropathy (4). Motion segments at risk for torsional injury lie above the intercristal line, i.e., usually the L4–5 interspace coupled with the L3–4 interspace. The L5–S1 motion segment would seem to be protected from torsion, but is exposed to repetitive flexion and axial loading (5, 6). In the skeletally immature patient, the vertebral endplate is at risk from intraosseous disc herniation. This is probably a direct consequence of an axial loading injury (7). Schmorl's node formation is caused by intraosseous disc herniation of nuclear material into the relatively soft vertebral endplate (8). Patients with Schmorl's nodes develop early degenerative changes probably due to interruption of disc nutrition secondary to vertebral endplate damage (9).

The lumbar facet joints are exposed to increased articular cartilage loading pressures in extension as well as in torsional maneuvers (5, 10). Repetitive extension maneuvers can cause facet synovitis and potentially lead to facet arthropathy. Additionally, a degenerative segment has, by nature, decreased resistance to torsional stress (11). Changes in foraminal size have been noted in the degenerative segment with postural movement (12). An appreciation of this phenomenon is important for understanding the potential cause of foraminal nerve root injury when only a mildly narrowed neuroforamen is found. Facet tropism will lead to asymmetric loads being transferred to the facet articular surfaces as well as to the anulus (13). Facet tropism may be a predisposing factor for the development of facet pain syndromes in athletes, but this will need to be demonstrated in controlled research studies. The hallmark work of Kirkaldy-Willis outlining the stages of the degenerative process forms the foundation for understanding lumbar spine injuries (14).

DOES NONOPERATIVE TREATMENT WORK?

In a recent study, we reported on the nonoperative treatment of a group of patients suffering from a herniated nucleus pulposus with radiculopathy who were followed for three years (14a). Inclusion criteria for the study were as follows: a CT or magnetic resonance imaging (MRI) scan that demonstrated a herniated nucleus pulposus, a primary complaint of leg pain, straight-leg raising that reproduced the leg pain at less than 60° and an EMG that demonstrated electrophysiologic evidence of radiculopathy. All of the patients underwent an aggressive physical rehabilitation program. Included in the study group were a subset of patients who were seen for a second opinion regarding lumbar disc surgery. All of these patients had been advised by the previous examining surgeon to undergo disc excision. The results were analyzed for this group and the study population as a whole. Additionally, a group of patients with extruded nuclear fragments was analyzed separately.

The results are quite startling. Fifty of the 52 patients, i.e., 96%, who were treated nonoperatively, achieved successful outcomes. A successful outcome was based on a patient self-rating in the good or excellent category as defined by the study's outcome criteria. When the study population was analyzed as a whole, including the patients who did not respond to the questionnaires, the success rate was 85%. Eighty-three per cent of the second opinion cases also had successful nonoperative outcomes. Patients with extruded nuclear fragments achieved an 86% success rate. The return to work rate for the entire study population was 92% as compared to previously reported surgical studies that ranged from a low of 75% (15) to a high of 85% (16). The sick leave time for patients in our study was a median of 3.9 months, which compares favorably with the surgical series that have been presented. Neurologic weakness of the lower extremity musculature did not adversely affect the outcome.

Functional restoration of chronic patients successfully returned them to work (17). Patients who successfully completed the program had strength and range of motion gains which correlated with their improved functional capacity. Therefore, nonoperative care is efficacious for patients with herniated nucleus pulposus, and functional restoration programs can resolve chronic low back disability. The nonoperative program used in the herniated disc outcome study is presented as an appendix to this chapter.

TREATMENT PROGRAM

Pain Control Phase

Pain control treatment should be instituted as early and efficiently as possible. It is important not to get stuck in the pain control phase, but rather to advance as rapidly as possible to the training phases of treatment. The initial stage of pain control, back first aid, treats the pain and teaches the patient to control pain and muscle spasm. The treatment includes the application of ice (18), rest in a position of comfort, and basic instruction in body mechanics to facilitate pain-free movement using chairs, cars, bathtubs, and toilet seats. Medications can then be kept to a minimum. Depending on the type of injury sustained, anterior structures (the discovertebral joints) or posterior structures (the facet joints and neural arch) will determine the position of comfort. During this initial phase, rest is also specifically prescribed.

Bedrest is the most abused and overprescribed treatment in lumbar spine care. Bedrest need only be prescribed to control pain in the early days following the injury. There is absolutely no evidence to support total and absolute bedrest after any injury to the lumbar spine (19). Excessive bedrest will lead to hypomobile lumbar motion segments, tightened soft tissues, loss of muscle strength, blunting of motivation, and loss of mineral matrix from bone (19).

Pain-relieving modalities such as transcutaneous nerve stimulation (20) and pulsed alternating electrical muscle stimulation coupled with ice can also be useful to reduce the acute pain (20, 21). Extension exercises are valuable for pain reduction in discogenic injury subsets (22). The principle of extension exercises may very well be explained by a reduction in neural tension rather than by nuclear migration as initially proposed (23). When extension exercises cause centralization, that is, a movement of the low back pain medially, without exacerbating it and without peripheralizing it toward the lower extremity, i.e., causing radicular pain, they can be prescribed. Peripheralization of the pain, i.e., an increase in radicular referral pain into the buttock or lower extremity, is a contraindication to the use of extension exercises and may indicate the presence of significant stenosis, posterior element abnormality, or disc herniation in the subarticular, foraminal or extraforaminal zones. The correction of a list is necessary before beginning extension exercises. If the exercises are attempted while the patient is still listed, exacerbation of pain may occur that may lead to an erroneous decision to abandon the extension exercises. Overuse of extension exercises can lead to facet pain, which may delay the treatment program.

As will be discussed further below, no one should remain on one particular type of exercise regime during the entire treatment phase. The patient should progress through all treatment phases and not be solely left with, for example, an extension exercise program as the only component. Flexion exercises are most useful for patients suffering from facet pain or symptomatic neural compromise from a stenotic canal. Flexion has been noted to cause a reduction in articular weight-bearing stress to the facet joints (10). Flexion exercises have the additional benefit of stretching the dorso-lumbar fascia (2).

Spinal immobilization with a corset or semi-rigid brace may be useful for patients who are not yet strong enough for their own musculature to stabilize the spine. Studies of these devices demonstrate the corset's inability to immobilize the lower lumbar spinal segments (24). Caution must be exercised when prescribing these appliances because they will lead to trunk flexor and extensor muscle weakness if overused. Patients must be instructed to remove the orthotic device at least once daily to exercise the trunk musculature. Patients who

have become dependent upon the appliance must be weaned slowly while the supporting musculature is progressively strengthened. Immobilization may be useful as a diagnostic tool for patients suspected of having symptomatic segmental instability, but the inability of lumbar spinal orthotic devices truly to immobilize the lower lumbar segments makes this diagnostic intervention questionable. Lumbar bracing may be useful in the treatment of acute spondylolysis (25).

Mobilization techniques can be extraordinarily useful for attaining articular as well as soft tissue range of motion (26). Stiffened segments should be mobilized and tight soft tissues should be adequately stretched. Ultrasound application can facilitate soft tissue extensibility in order to allow adequate articular as well as soft tissue mobilization to occur (27). Caution should be taken when ultrasound is used in the presence of an acute radiculopathy. Possible posttreatment exacerbation of radicular symptoms, which may be related to neural swelling, may occur. Mobilization treatment is appropriate for thoracolumbar junctional segments, which may often become hypomobile and indeed may be pain generators often masquerading as a lumbar pain syndrome (28). Overvigorous mobilization may be harmful in all types of injuries, and should be carefully graded and timed in the treatment program.

Traction may be useful for obtaining symptomatic relief in the treatment of discogenic injury subtypes. There are proponents of gravity inversion (29), gravity lumbar reduction (30), autotraction (31, 32), and pelvic traction (33). Depending on the size of the patient, the type of equipment available, and the type of disc abnormality, all of these traction modalities may provide symptomatic relief. Although many studies report subjective symptom improvement, there is no scientific evidence to support the contention that any of the traction techniques actually facilitate nuclear migration. There is also no direct correlation with disc contour changes before and after traction (31). A recent study reports a disc contour change following 45 kg of pelvic traction noted on pre- and posttreatment CT scans. The study does not indicate how long these contour changes remained, and the precise control of lumbar lordosis and CT image cut is suspect (34).

Autotraction possesses some unique advantages in its ability to be polyaxial and patient controlled (32), while gravity inversion traction can be used appropriately at home and on an ongoing basis as long as hypertension or retinal problems are not contraindicative (35, 36). A force equal to approximately 26% of the body's weight is required to overcome the surface resistance of the lower half of the body (37). Bed traction is unable to overcome this enormous resistance and does not facilitate any separation of the vertebral elements. Bed traction only serves to restrain the patient. With a split table to reduce frictional forces, 50 pounds of intermittent force for 15 minutes has been reported to cause posterior interbody separation, but no residual separation has been noted 30 minutes after traction (38, 39). It is, therefore, unclear by what mechanism traction reduces symptoms. Theoretically, the pain relief may be mediated by a neurophysiological mechanism that reduces the transmission of the pain message rather than by direct mechanical forces on the disc.

One of the most powerful tools during the pain control phase is selective injections, including epidural cortisone injections from the translumbar or sacral approach, intraarticular facet injections, and lumbar selective nerve root blocks. These procedures can also be used for precise diagnostic localization of spinal pain generators. This can be accomplished by coupling injection procedures with an accurate history and physical exam, and confirming the diagnosis with appropriate imaging and/or electrophysiological studies prior to operative intervention. A full discussion of differential diagnosis is beyond the scope of this chapter. However, the reader is referred to existing comprehensive literature on the subject (40).

It is counterproductive to prolong the pain control phase of treatment. The use of an epidural cortisone injection in the face of a disabling lumbar radiculopathy caused by disc injury or stenosis can provide dramatic relief (41, 42). The rationale for using corticosteroid anti-inflammatory agents is well established (43). Epidural cortisone is most beneficial for patients with more leg pain than back pain, and for those who manifest signs of dural tension on physical examination. Early aggressive use of epidural cortisone injections in this clinical setting can be of tremendous benefit to the rehabilitation program. However, these injections are purely facilitators and not treatment by

themselves. Intraarticular lumbar facet injections under fluoroscopic guidance are useful to place corticosteroids into inflamed facet capsules (44). Actual injection of spondylitic defects has also been noted to give symptomatic relief, probably due to the spreading of the medication onto an inflamed exiting nerve root subjacent to the lytic defect. Lumbar selective nerve root blocks instill medication around an inflamed nerve root that is principally entrapped within the foramen or is entrapped by a large lateral disc fragment that has migrated foraminally (45). Extraforaminal nerve entrapments by either herniated disc material or by a large transverse process (as may occur at the L5–S1 level) is another context for this technique. Coupling epidural injection with selective nerve root block is often necessary in the face of a very large disc herniation with or without foraminal stenosis.

Trigger point injections with local anesthetic can only reduce painful muscle spasm associated with persistent trigger zones identified in the offending muscles (46). There is no physiologic basis for the addition of corticosteroids in this type of injection (47). Although attempts have been made to explain these trigger points on the basis of inflammatory focus, they have never been satisfactory.

Trigger point injections followed by soft tissue stretching and joint mobilization can improve range of motion and pain reduction. Often the soft tissue component of pain is the principal disabling factor even in the face of a structural diagnosis of discogenic pathology. It has been reported that dry needling a trigger point is just as effective as injecting the trigger point with local anesthetic solution alone, saline alone, or local anesthetic solution plus corticosteroid (47, 48). It has also been noted that every known trigger point injection reported in the medical literature in the West corresponds to a known acupuncture point (49). Endorphin release following acupuncture treatment has also been scientifically demonstrated (50–52). Naloxone can block the endorphin release and can blunt acupuncture analgesia (17).

There are numerous well-controlled scientific studies demonstrating the usefulness of acupuncture as a pain relieving modality (53). Acupuncture may break a pain cycle and facilitate an active exercise program. It must be kept in mind that acupuncture as well as the other injection procedures described above are purely facilitators of treatment and should be considered as adjunctive therapy only. They are useful in the pain control phase and should be utilized in a framework and clinical context that enhances rehabilitation. They are not treatment ends in themselves.

Anti-inflammatory medication in the early phases of treatment may be appropriate. The recent report of high levels of phospholipase A2 activity in herniated discs supports the contention that inflammation plays a role in symptomatic disc herniation (54). The analgesic effect of the nonsteroidal anti-inflammatory agents and their ability to act as prostaglandin synthetase inhibitors play a significant role in the treatment of lumbar pain syndromes. Oral corticosteroids can be useful in the treatment of acute radiculopathy. The exact dosage and optimal time frame are questionable, but their efficacy has been established (43).

The prescribing of so-called muscle relaxants has no physiologic basis. All of the currently marketed muscle relaxants are indeed central nervous system depressants and not peripherally acting muscle relaxants. Caution should, therefore, be exercised when prescribing them, and their potential depressive and addictive nature should be kept in mind (55). Opiate analgesics are occasionally necessary during the initial week of treatment of lumbar pain syndromes, but rarely need to be prolonged any further once the specific treatment program has begun. The proper use of positioning, rest, ice, transcutaneous nerve stimulation, extension and/or flexion exercises and the selective injection procedures described above will usually handle the pain satisfactorily, thus precluding a need for opiate analgesics.

TRAINING PHASE

Principles of Training Phase

After having successfully completed the pain control phase of the rehabilitation program, the patient should begin the training phase. The goal of the training phase is to attain adequate musculoligamentous control of lumbar spine forces in order to eliminate repetitive injury to the intervertebral discs, facet joints, and related structures. Without progressing beyond the pain control phase, patients would continue to be at risk of suffering a repeat injury, further limiting their activity. It is very important to try to identify why they injured themselves, and what risk factors for further injury they face. Patients must be made aware of these principles so preventive measures can be taught.

A lumbar motion segment once having been injured is at risk for repetitive injury. Numerous studies point out recidivism in low back pain patients (55). Studies have demonstrated the benefits of prevention programs in the industrial work place (56). These prevention techniques can be taught in a back school setting. Studies have demonstrated the effect of fatigue on the lumbar intervertebral disc and the progressive development of gradual disc prolapse (57). These findings illustrate the biomechanical construct of repetitive injuries to the intervertebral disc leading to progressive pathology. It also should make us aware of how a "simple" anular tear can, with subsequent anular injury, develop into a full-blown disc protrusion or herniation.

Therefore, the early identification of an individual with an anular tear can facilitate the immediate institution of a back school program in an attempt to prevent future injury and disability. Our role in spine care delivery should not simply be to provide band-aid treatment. Our mandate should be to prevent back pain before it starts. Society can ill afford for the health care profession to ignore prevention and only endeavor to treat pain.

Dynamic Muscular Lumbar Stabilization Concepts

Repetitive flexion and torsional stress to the lumbar intervertebral discs and facet joints will lead to advanced degenerative changes (3, 6). In addition, gradual disc prolapse secondary to fatiguing of the anular fibers is also important for understanding repetitive microtrauma applied to the lumbar segments (57). Stabilization involves elimination of this repetitive microtrauma to the lumbar motion segments, thereby limiting the injury and allowing healing to occur. It can also potentially alter the natural history of degenerative processes.

Muscle fusion is the implementation of the musculature to brace the spine and protect motion segments against repetitive microtrauma and excessively high, single-occurrence loads. The abdominal mechanism, which consists of the midline ligament and the dorsolumbar fascia, when combined with a slight reduction in lumbar lordosis, can eliminate shear stress to the lumbar intervertebral segments. The abdominal musculature has a unique ability to flex the lumbar spine by acting upon the superficial portion of the dorsolumbar fascia. It can also extend the lumbar spine by acting on the deep portions of the fascia that form the alar interspinal ligaments. This coupled action allows the abdominal muscles to corset the lumbar region when they function in concert with the latissimus dorsi, a muscle that also acts upon the dorsolumbar fascia. Lowering the center of gravity with the use of slight knee flexion facilitated by adequately strong quadriceps is another important part of the formula for bracing the spine.

The hypothesis underlying this biomechanical and pathophysiological construct is that for its own protection, the intervertebral joint reacts to its internal stress controlling the force exerted on it by an applied load. Furthermore, the hypothesis contends that a feedback mechanism monitoring the stress at the intervertebral joint can modify muscular activity in such a way as to minimize stress at the joint and, therefore, reduce the risk of injury. Because muscular activity, in turn, modifies spinal geometry, the feedback system also controls stress and ligaments. The stress induced by the activity of these muscles may also be monitored and controlled by a potential feedback mechanism. Through this mechanism, which lowers the level of equalized stress to a minimum, the potential of risk of injury to the lumbar spine is reduced. The existence of an extensively distributed, well-developed network of nerve fibers connecting receptor systems located in places such as the periosteum has been identified. This system is not only important in pain transmission but may also be important in kinesthetic feedback for joint positioning (58).

Because of the changes in axial rotation at the intervertebral segments at different degrees of lordosis, control of lordosis in flexion and extension is extremely important. Once these relations are clear, it is easy to understand how balanced muscular function and flexibility and control of the stresses applied to the lumbar intervertebral segments work together. It should be pointed out that the anulus of the intervertebral disc appears to be entirely responsible for load transmission of the intervertebral segment. Removal of the nucleus reportedly does not greatly affect the joint response. Therefore, repetitive loads applied to the lumbar interver-

tebral joint will by necessity fall upon the outer fibers of the anulus, leading to progressive tearing, progressive fatigue, and potentially progressive disc prolapse. It is simpler to understand load transmission to the facet joints by repetitive extension maneuvers. It has been well demonstrated that narrowing of the intervertebral disc will also increase load transmission to the facet joints (59). The combination of a degenerative segment combined with repetitive extension and rotation loads to the lumbar intervertebral joints can lead to joint failure. Once again, the principle of neutral spine positioning may be applied to this portion of the motion segment as well.

Muscle fusion, therefore, involves the cocontraction of the abdominal muscles to maintain a "corseting" effect to the lumbar spine using the midline ligament and thoracolumbar fascia, coupled with proper pelvic positioning to accomplish the task. The use of the spinal extensor muscles to reduce translational stress to the intervertebral segments is important during activity as well, for balancing shear stress to the intervertebral segments. The multifidus muscle appears to be the most active during this activity. It is also the most difficult to strengthen because of its short segmental nature. The gluteus maximus may indeed be the most important extensor muscle controlling the lumbar spine's lifting power (2).

Obviously abdominal muscles play a key role in dynamic muscular lumbar spine stabilization. Many exercises to strengthen the abdominal muscles have been advocated, and a careful review of the scientific literature on this subject is quite revealing. The iliacus is the major muscle involved in the phase of the sit-up exercise from 45° to vertical sitting (60). The exercises that require the least effort of the abdominal muscles are full sit-ups and abdominal curl-ups after the initial 30% of motion (61). The total concentric phase of the sit-up exercise is accompanied by a greater percentage of activity in the abdominal muscles than during the total eccentric phase (62). The oblique musculature and the rectus abdominis are the most active during the initial head and shoulder phases of abdominal sit-ups. The force of abdominal muscle contraction can be increased by adding resistance, either by slantboard inversion, manual resistance, or cross-chest weight holding (62).

The magnitude of muscle recruitment for the lower section of the rectus abdominis is greatly increased when the feet are supported in a lying position (62). Nonsupported feet during this exercise favor greater contraction of the upper section of the rectus abdominis. Raising both legs while supporting the trunk, as in an elevated chair position, or hanging from a bar or rings, causes a greater degree of muscle recruitment than any other exercise (62). The trunk curl, raising only the head and scapula off the surface with the knees flexed at 45°, with or without the feet supported, accompanied by a body twist causes greater muscle recruitment in all portions of the rectus abdominis and oblique musculature than symmetrical exercises (62). This curl-up position, with only the scapula and head raised off the surface, has also been demonstrated to cause the least amount of movement of the lumbar spine (63).

The internal oblique muscles participate in any activity involving pelvic tilt (64). Trunk rotation is performed largely by the internal obliques coupled with the dorsolumbar fascia and latissimus dorsi. The rectus adominis does not really function as a trunk flexor, but rather only maximally contracts during flexion when the spine has attained almost full flexion by the action of gravity (62, 64).

It would appear that the curl-up exercise with the feet either supported or unsupported while raising only the head and scapula off the ground using both a symmetrical contraction pattern as well as a rotated diagonal pattern is the appropriate beginning exercise for abdominal strengthening. There is no need to do complete sit-ups. The abdominal muscles do not work in the second 45° of the motion. Instead, the iliacus and rectus femoris muscles are doing all the work. Additionally, this complete type of sit-up places greater stress on the lumbar spine. Therefore, from the point of view of exercise physiology and biomechanics, the full sit-up exercise should not be undertaken even by an individual without a lumbar spine problem. Many lumbar spine injuries are caused by an improper abdominal strengthening technique.

Combining fast repetitions with isometric repetitions will involve all the muscle fibers and will train both the endurance as well as absolute isometric strength of the abdominal musculature. It would seem prudent to use the foot-supported position for the sit-ups with the knees bent at 45° to allow for maximal contraction of the lower rectus abdominis and oblique muscles because of their importance in pelvic tilting, although performing some repetitions unsupported will develop more isolated upper rectus abdominis strength. Advanced abdominal exercises can be carried out with bilateral straight-leg raising and lowering while in an elevated chair or while lying on the floor. Slowly raising and lowering the legs will ensure lower abdominal isolation and eliminate cheating movements associated with leg swinging. A more advanced program will also include the use of curl-ups on an incline board, both in the symmetric and diagonal patterns. Additionally, adding manual resistance through a workout partner or holding a weight plate securely across the chest can add to abdominal strength. A progressive resistance program *must* be used. The musculature must be challenged continually if maximal benefit is to be attained. Once patients can do three sets of 10 to 15 repetitions of an abdominal exercise with ease, they should progress to the next phase of the program.

In order to apply the muscle fusion, adequate flexibility and spinal range of motion must be attained. Some interesting work presented by Adams and co-workers on diurnal variations and stresses on the lumbar spine notes changes in lumbar disc and ligament extensibility as the day progresses (65). This is based upon creep of the soft tissue structures, leading to increased range of motion. Adams and colleagues point out that bending and lifting activities early in the morning, when applied to nonextensible ligamentous and anulus fibers, will cause the disc to accumulate fatigue damage more easily than the same activities performed later in the day. This concept can be further applied to the need for flexibility of the structures to eliminate repetitive fatigue stress to the intervertebral joint. We should also think of the muscles that attach to the pelvis as "guy wires" that can effectively change the position and symmetry of the pelvis. Considering that the pelvis is the platform that the lumbar spine rests upon, pelvic positioning is the key to postural control of the lumbar spine. Therefore, adequate flexibility of hamstring, quadriceps, iliopsoas, gastrocsoleus, hip rotator, and iliotibial band is important. A note should also be made for the necessity of flexibile neural elements as well.

Dynamic Muscular Lumbar Stabilization Techniques

Stabilization training routines can be divided into basic level and advanced routines. The basic exercises are described in the appendix to this chapter. The basic program has been classified by some as a neurodevelopmental stage of postural control starting from the most primitive postural positions, namely, lying supine or prone, then advancing to exercises performed while kneeling, standing, and progressing to position transition movements. Because meticulous technique is imperative in these exercises, a skilled and experienced physical therapist or exercise trainer must work with the patient in a painstaking manner. Initially, the exercises are performed with one-on-one instruction after which the patient completes the basic exercises as a member of a class.

Each of the exercises is designed to develop isolated and cocontraction muscle patterns to stabilize the lumbar spine in neutral position. Neutral position must be defined for each individual. Neutral spine does not necessarily mean zero degrees of lordosis, but rather the most comfortable position for the individual based upon the biomechanical principles discussed above. The therapist must monitor the patient carefully for optimal positioning while the patient exercises and progresses through each level of the program. Care must be taken to ensure proper form and slow exercise repetition speed. The neurophysiologic principle of central pathway irradiation secondary to increased amplitude of effort must be continually kept in mind (66). Engram motor programming is the goal of the exercise program; therefore, careful repetition with precision of movement is imperative.

Once the patient has graduated from the basic level and is able to demonstrate proper form and technique, these same principles can be applied to the weight training portion of the program. The patient is taught how to get on and off weight training equipment while continuing to adhere to stabilization principles. Care must be exercised while changing the weight stack resistance pin on the machines as well as when lifting and racking free weights. The patient is then taught how to use resistance equipment including free weights, pulleys, and single-station weight machines using cocontraction of the lower abdominal musculature to maintain optimal anteverted pelvic positioning while flattening the lower back against a back support to maintain a stabilized neutral spine.

A specific strengthening program is tailored to the individual. The patient's physical capacity for occupational and recreational activity is used to structure the program. The weight training program is not geared purely towards the truncal musculature, but taken a step further to a total fitness program. Incorporated in this total fitness program are aerobic and anaerobic training. Teaching the individual to stabilize the spine while riding a stationary bicycle, running on the treadmill, and swimming becomes integral to the training program. Patients progress from treadmill walking to treadmill running and finally to supervised running on a track.

Rehabilitation of the injured athlete with lumbar pain requires a highly specialized and advanced program (67). The training program for football linemen incorporates the same principles already discussed. Additionally, in this particular program the tasks of the athlete are broken down into individual components, including stance positioning, back pedaling while pass blocking as well as pulling and dive positions for run play blocking. Stress is placed upon adequate knee flexion and strong abdominal muscles that cocontract with the gluteus maximus to attain the forward pelvic tilt, thereby eliminating excessive lordosis of the lumbar spine during axial loading. The player is taught how to take a blow and use a contraction of his abdominal muscles to stabilize the spine. The player is also taught how to fall and roll with abdominal contraction. The motivated football player finds this type of positioning comfortable, efficient, and powerful. One-on-one drills are designed to reinforce stabilization principles while the player is being pushed and pulled.

During the sports-specific training programs, the athlete progresses through the basic level of exercises, then the advanced level, finally undertaking the sports-specific training. The sports-specific training begins with hands on one-on-one mat work, advancing from isolated to compound movements. The use of video taped exercise sessions and performances of specific athletic techniques is a valuable coaching aid. The principles of athletic spine training can be extrapolated to virtually all sports. Working carefully with the individual coaches is important before designing any training program. Rehabilitating the athlete with back problems requires a team effort that involves clinicians and others as well as the athlete who is impaired.

Torque to the lumbar spine is intrinsic to the playing of many sports, making it impossible totally to eliminate rotational stresses. The goal is to minimize and control stress where possible. Once again, it must be kept in mind that the majority of athletic lumbar spine injuries actually occur in the weight room secondary to repetitive microtrauma before the athlete ever sets foot on the playing field or gymnasium floor.

Nonoperative treatment must meet reasonable time and cost criteria. Early goal setting is imperative. An understanding of the patient's occupation, recreational desires, and functional level will help guide the goal setting. Once a patient reaches a plateau in functional improvement that is not affected by alterations in the program, the supervised program should be discontinued. Patients should be switched to an independent program as soon as possible. The goal of treatment should be to strive for patient independence rather than to foster a dependent relationship. Any dependency on drugs, on physical therapy, or manipulative treatment should be discouraged. Active exercise programs rather than passive treatment should be encouraged, especially in light of their validation (67). Passive modalities and manual treatment use an extraordinary amount of time and money and do little if anything to rehabilitate the patient's function.

As in surgical planning, realistic goal setting is important for aggressive conservative care programs. A 35-year-old patient with a herniated nucleus pulposus can expect relief of back and leg pain and the ability to return to tennis and skiing. The 35-year-old materials handler with the same injury who has a worker's compensation claim for motivational reasons probably will take much longer to improve and probably will not return to his previous job (14a). A patient with this diagnosis and good motivation will need approximately three months of nonoperative care. If the patient is not improved after an aggressive physical rehabilitation program, surgery should be considered.

Obviously, a patient in severe pain inadequately controlled by the principles set forth in this chapter should undergo the appropriate surgical procedure earlier than the suggested three-month time period. Patients with spinal stenosis and neurogenic claudication can benefit from a nonoperative program, but if pain control is not adequate or progressive neurologic deficit ensues, surgery should be strongly considered. Nonspecific low back pain with or without radicular referral should not be treated with supervised physical therapy for longer than 12 weeks. Institution of a self-monitored gym and/or home program at that point is appropriate. Dependency upon analgesic medication, manual therapy, and modality therapy should be strongly discouraged.

In summary, there are many tools to combat pain, but only patient self-responsibility can be expected to prevent recurrences and affect the natural history of the patient's low back pain.

APPENDIX
Two Treatment Phases for Nonoperative Physical Rehabilitation Program for Patients with Lumbar Herniated Nucleus Pulposus and Radiculopathy

I. Pain Control
 A. Back First Aid
 B. Trial Extension Exercises
 C. Trial of Traction
 D. Basic Stabilization Exercise Training
 E. NSAID
 F. Nonnarcotic Analgesics
 G. Corticosteroids
  1. Oral
  2. Epidural Injection
  3. Selective Nerve Root Injection
  4. Facet Injection
II. Exercise Training
 A. Soft Tissue Flexibility
  1. Hamstring Musculotendinous Unit
  2. Quadriceps Musculotendinous Unit
  3. Iliopsoas Musculotendinous Unit
  4. Gastrocsoleus Musculotendinous Unit
  5. External and Internal Hip Rotators
 B. Joint Mobility
  1. Lumbar Spine Segmental Mobility
  2. Hip Range of Motion
  3. Thoracic Segmental Mobility
 C. Stabilization Program
  1. Finding Neutral Position
  2. Prone Gluteal Squeezes
  3. Supine Pelvic Bracing
  4. Bridging Progression
   a. Basic Position
   b. One Leg Raised
   c. Stepping
   d. Balance on Gym Ball
  5. Quadruped
   a. With Alternating Arm and Leg Movements
  6. Kneeling Stabilization
   a. Double Knee
   b. Single Knee
   c. Lunges
  7. Wall Slide Quadriceps Strengthening
  8. Position Transition with Postural Control
 D. Abdominal Program
  1. Curl-ups
  2. Dying Bugs
  3. Diagonal Curl-ups
  4. Diagonal Curl-ups on Incline Board
  5. Straight Leg Lowering
 E. Gym Program
  1. Latissimus Pull-downs
  2. Angled Leg Press
  3. Lunges
  4. Hyperextension Bench
  5. General Upper Body Weight Exercises
  6. Pulley Exercises to Stress Postural Control
 F. Aerobic Program
  1. Progressive Walking
  2. Swimming
  3. Stationary Bicycling
  4. Cross-country Ski Machine
  5. Running
   a. Initially Supervised on a Treadmill

Treatment Phase I: Pain Control

Decisions for use of pain control methods will depend on patient level of function and ability to comply with the prescribed exercise program. All patients are to be enlisted in a therapeutic exercise regimen as tolerated by their level of pain and neurologic loss. The initial stage, back first aid, involves the application of ice, rest in a position of comfort, and basic instruction in body mechanics to facilitate pain free movement. The use of medications will be kept to a minimum. Transcutaneous nerve stimulation may also be used for pain control. Acupuncture may occasionally be used during this phase. A trial of traction (gravity inversion, pelvic traction, or autotraction) is to be used for patients with refractory radicular pain following extension exercises. Traction will be continued in those patients who have a marked reduction of radicular pain.

Nonnarcotic analgesics (i.e., acetaminophen) and nonsteroidal anti-inflammatory drugs (NSAIDs) may be prescribed. Occasionally, a limited course (up to two weeks) of a class-3 narcotic analgesic such as Tylenol with codeine may be prescribed. No patients will receive a schedule II medication, a sedative hypnotic, or a muscle relaxant.

Prescribed bedrest will not be recommended. Patients will be instructed to pursue a level of activity that does not exacerbate their radicular pain or worsen a neurologic deficit. Persistent radicular pain will be treated with corticosteroid therapy. Epidural injections will be the treatment of choice, although in some patients a tapering course of oral corticosteroids will be used. The caudal route of injection is to be used for disc herniation at the L4–5 and L5–S1 levels, and a translumbar approach will be used for disc herniations L3–4 and above. Localization by instillation of nonionic contrast material under fluoroscopic guidance will be used in all cases. Straight leg raising will be assessed at the peak of local anesthesia (10 ml of 0.5% lidocaine). If no relief occurs during this phase, a selective nerve root injection with corticosteroid will be performed at the root level of greatest involvement (as determined by electromyographic study and CT findings). The results of injection therapy will be assessed at 2 to 3 weeks. If disabling radicular pain persists, epidural corticosteroid injection will be repeated. Patients with persistent back pain consistent with facet syndrome will be asked to undergo facet joint corticosteroid injections. Injection therapy will be used to facilitate the patient's functional progress. Decisions to inject or reinject are to be based upon the patient's ability to progress with the active exercise program.

Treatment Phase II: Exercise Training

The key element in the phase devoted to exercise training is the accomplishment of adequate dynamic control of lumbar spine forces in order to eliminate repetitive injury to the intervertebral discs, facet joints, and related structures. This is called stabilization training.

Stabilization exercise routines can be divided into basic and advanced levels. Exercises to improve soft tissue flexibility and joint range of motion must precede the introduction of strengthening exercises. Flexibility training focuses on the musculotendinous units of the hamstrings, quadriceps, iliopsoas, rectus femoris, external and internal hip rotators, and gastrocsoleus. Strict attention is to be paid to maintenance of neutral spine posture while the stretching exercises are performed. Stretching is first performed passively by the exercise trainer and then is included as part of the patient's home program. Continued active assistive stretching is occasionally necessary to fully overcome soft tissue contracture that results from limited mobility and nerve root irritation. These exercises are to be carried out on a daily basis.

The patient is to be trained in active joint mobilization methods, such as extension exercises in prone and standing positions, as well as alternative midrange flexion and extension while in a four-point stance. Abdominal muscle strengthening will begin with simple curl-ups. From this, the patient is to progress to dynamic abdominal bracing using alternate arm and leg movements while lying supine, contracting the abdominal musculature, and holding the spine in neutral position. More advanced exercises will include diagonal curl-ups performed both on the floor and on an inclined board. Once the patient is able to carry out three sets of 15 repetitions, more challenging exercises are to be undertaken. At the end of this stage of the program, lower abdominal muscle strengthening is to be emphasized using straight leg lowering exercises.

Demonstration of proper form and technique is required for the patient to graduate from the basic level. These same guidelines are then to be applied to the weight training portion of the program. Aerobic and anaerobic training is to be incorporated into the total fitness program. Aerobic conditioning will be initiated early in the program in the form of walking. Shortly thereafter, the patient is asked to ride a stationary bicycle and/or to use a cross-country ski machine. Swimming may be encouraged for those patients interested in it, but should not uniformly be used with all patients. These activities are to be first performed under supervision to ensure maintenance of neutral spine posture. Training levels are to be tailored to the patient's age, medical history, and level of aerobic conditioning according to previously established American College of Sports Medicine guidelines. Decisions for advancement to more challenging exercise during the program will be based upon functional progress rather than pain level. The program end point will be determined by maximal function that will not improve further by exercise training or pain control.

References

1. Saal JA. Electrophysiologic evaluation of lumbar pain: establishing the rationale for therapeutic management. Spine 1987; 1:21-46.

2. Farfan HF. Muscular mechanism of the lumbar spine and the position of power and efficiency. Orthop Clin J North Am 1975; 6:135-144.

3. Farfan HF, Cossette JW, Robertson GH et al. The effects of torsion on the lumbar intervertebral joints: The role of torsion in the production of disc degeneration. J Bone Joint Surg 1970; 52:468-497.

4. Liu YK, Goel VK, Dejong A et al. Torsional fatigue of the lumbar intervertebral joints. Spine 1985; 10:894-900.

5. Adams MA, Hutton WC. The relevance of torsion to the mechanical derangement of the lumbar spine. Spine 1981; 8:241-248.

6. Farfan HF. Effects of torsion on the intervertebral joints. Can J Surg 1969; 12:336-341.

7. Schmorl G, Junghann M. The human spine in health and disease. New York: Grune & Stratton, 1971.

8. McCall IW, Park WM, O'Brien JP et al. Acute traumatic intraosseous disc herniation. Spine 1985; 10:134-137.

9. Vernon-Roberts B, Pirie CJ. Degenerative changes in the intervertebral discs of the lumbar spine and their sequelae. Rheumatol Rehab 1977; 16(1):13-21.

10. Adams MA, Hutton WC. The mechanical function of the lumbar apophyseal joints. Spine 1983; 8:327-330.

11. Kirkaldy-Willis W. The three phases of the spectrum of degenerative disease. In Kirkaldy-Willis, W. ed. Managing low back pain. 2nd. ed. New York: Churchill Livingstone, 1988; 117-131.

12. Panjabi MM, Takata K, Goel VK. Kinematics of lumbar intervertebral foramen. Spine 1983; 8:348-357.

13. Cyron BM, Hutton WC. Articular tropism and stability of the lumbar spine. Spine 1980; 5:168-172.

14. Yong-Hing K, Kirkaldy-Willis WH. The pathophysiology of degenerative disease of the lumbar spine. Orthop Clin J North Am 1983; 14:491-504.

14a. Saal JA, Saal JS. Nonoperative treatment of herniated lumbar intervertebral disc with radiculopathy: An outcome study. Spine 1989; 14(4):431-437.

15. Frymoyer J, Hanley E, Howe J, Kuhlmann D, Matteri R. Disc excision and spine fusion in the management of lumbar disc disease. 1978; Spine 3:1-6.

16. Hurme M, Alaranta H. Factors predicting the result of surgery for lumbar intervertebral disc herniation. Spine 1987; 12:933-938.

17. Mayer DJ, Price DD, Rafii A. Antagonism of acupuncture analgesia in man by the narcotic antagonist naloxone. Brain Res 1977; 121:368-372.

18. Eldred E, Lindsky DF, Buchwald JS. The effect of cooling on mammalian muscle spindles. Exper Neurol 1960; 2:144-157.

19. Deyo RA, Diehl AK, Rosenthal M. How many days of bed rest for acute low back pain? A randomized clinical trial. N Engl J Med 1986; 315:1064-1070.

20. Fox EJ, Melzack R. Transcutaneous electrical stimulation and acupuncture: comparison of treatment for low-back pain. Pain 1976; 2:141-148.

21. Lampe GN, Mannheimer JS, eds. Clinical transcutaneous electrical nerve stimulation. Philadelphia: F Davis, 1984.

22. MacKenzie R. Mechanical disorders and treatment of lumbar spine disorders. Waikanae, New Zealand: Spinal Publications, 1981.

23. Schnebel BF, Chowning J, Davidson R et al. A digitizing technique for the study of movement of intradiscal dye in response to flexion and extension of the lumbar spine. International Society for the Study of the Lumbar Spine, 1987.

24. Lantz SA, Schultz AB. Lumbar spine orthosis wearing. Spine 1986; 11(8):834-842.

25. Steiner ME, Micheli LJ. Treatment of symptomatic spondylolysis and spondylolisthesis with the modified Boston brace. Spine, 1985; 10:937-943.

26. VanHoesen LS. Mobilization and manipulation techniques for the lumbar spine. In Modern manual therapy of the vertebral column. Grieve GP. ed. London: Churchill Livingstone, 1986.

27. Lehman JF, DeLateur BJ. Therapeutic heat. In Therapeutic heat and cold. Lehman JF, ed. Baltimore: Williams & Wilkins, 1982.

28. Maigne R. Low back pain of thoracolumbar origin. Arch Phys Med Rehab 1980; 61:389–395.

29. Nosse LJ. Inverted spinal traction. Orthop Dig 1979; 7:35–37.

30. Oudenhoven RC. Gravitational lumbar traction. Arch Phys Med Rehab 1978; 59:510–512.

31. Gillstrom P, Ericson K, Hindmarsh T. Autotraction in lumbar disc herniation: a myelographic study before and after treatment. Arch Orthop Trauma Surg 1985; 104:207–210.

32. Larsson U, Choler U, Lidstrom A, et al. Autotraction for treatment of lumbago-sciatica: a multicentre controlled investigation. Acta Orthop Scand 1980; 51:791–798.

33. Hinterbuchner C. Traction. In Rogoff JB, ed. Manipulation, traction, and massage. Baltimore: Williams & Wilkins, 1980.

34. Onel D, Tuzlaci M, Sari H, Demir K. Computed tomographic investigation of the effect of traction on lumbar disc herniations. Spine 1989; 14:1–82.

35. Haskvitz EM, Hanten WP. Blood pressure response to inversion traction. Phys Ther 1986; 66:1361–1364.

36. Klatz RM, Goldman RM, Pinchuk BG, et al. The effects of gravity inversion procedures on systemic blood pressure, intraocular pressure and central retinal arterial pressure. J Am Osteopath Asso 1983; 82:853–857.

37. Judovich BD. Lumbar traction therapy and dissipated force factors. Lancet 1954; 74:411.

38. Colachis SC Jr, Strohm BR. Effects of intermittent traction on separation of lumbar vertebrae. Arch Phys Med Rehab 1969; 50:251–258.

39. Judovich BD. Lumbar traction therapy—elimination of physical factors that prevent lumbar stretch. JAMA 1955; 159:549.

40. Saal JA. Diagnostic studies for the industrial low back. In Topics in acute care and trauma rehabilitation. Rockville, Maryland: Aspen, 1988.

41. Derby R. Diagnostic block precedure: use in pain location. Spine: State of the Art Reviews. 1986; 1(1)47–65.

42. White AH. Injection techniques for the diagnosis and treatment of low back pain. Orthop Clin J North Am 1983; 14:553–567.

43. Ghosh P. Influence of drugs, hormones, and other agents on the metabolism of the disc and the sequelae of its degeneration. In The biology of the disc. Ghosh P. ed. Boca Raton, Florida: CRC Press, 1988.

44. Lippitt AB. The facet joint and its role in spine pain: management with facet joint injections. Spine 1984; 9:746–750.

45. Takeshi T, Kouzaburou F, Eisuke K. Selective lumbosacral radiculography and block. Spine 1980; 5:68–78.

46. Travell J, Rinzter S. The myofascial genesis of pain. Postgrad Med 1952; 11:425–434.

47. Lewit K. The needle effect in the relief of myofascial pain. Pain 1979; 6:83–90.

48. Frost FA, Jessen B, Siggaard-Anderson J. A control, double-blind comparison of mepivacaine injection versus saline injection for myofascial pain. Lancet 1980; 8:499–500.

49. Melzack R, Stilwell DM, Fox EJ. Trigger points and acupuncture points for pain: correlations and implications. Pain 1977; 3:3–23.

50. Sjolund BH, Eriksson MBE. Endorphins and analgesia produced by peripheral conditioning stimulation. New York: Raven Press 1979.

51. Takagi H. Critical review of pain relieving procedures including acupuncture: advances in pharmacology and therapeutics. II. CNS pharmacology. Neuropeptides 1982; 1:79–92.

52. Watkins LR, Mayer DJ. Organization of endogenous opiate and nonopiate pain control systems. Science 1982; 216:1185–1192.

53. Reichmanis M, Becker RO. Relief of experimentally-induced pain by stimulation at acupuncture loci: a review. Comp Med East West 1977; 5:281–288.

54. Saal JS, Franson RC, Dobrow R, Saal JA, White AH, Goldthwaite N. High levels of inflammatory phospholipase A2 activity in lumbar disc herniations. Spine (in press).

55. Goodman AG, Gilman LS, Gilman A. The pharmacological basis of therapeutics. New York: Macmillan, 1980.

56. Moffett JA, Chase SM, Porteck BS et al. A controlled prospective study to evaluate the effectiveness of a back school in the relief of chronic low back pain. Spine 1986; 11:120–123.

57. Adams MA, Hutton WC. Gradual disc prolapse. Spine 1985; 10:524–531.

58. Gracovetsky S, Farfan H. The optimum spine. Spine 1986; 11:543–573.

59. Dunlop RB, Adams MA, Hutton WC. Disc space narrowing and the lumbar facet joints. Br J Bone Joint Surg 1987; 66:706–710.

60. Flint MM. Abdominal muscle involvement during the performance of various forms of sit-up exercise. Am J Phys Med 1965; 44:224–234.

61. Floyd WF, Silver P. EMG study of activity of the anterior abdominal muscles in man. J Anat 1965; 84:132–145.

62. Walters CE, Partridge MJ. EMG study of the differential action of the abdominal muscles during exercise. Am J Phys Med 1957; 36:259–268.

63. Ekholm J, Arborelius U, Fahlcrantz A, et al. Activation of the abdominal muscles during some physiotherapeutic exercises. Scand J Rehab Med 1979; 11:75–84.

64. Partridge MJ, Walters CE. Participation of the abdominal muscles in various movements of the

trunk in man: an EMG study. Phys Ther Rev 1959; 39:791–800.

65. Adams MA Dolan P, Hutton WC. Diurnal variations in the stresses on the lumbar spine. Spine 1987; 12:130–137.

66. Harris FA. Facilitation techniques and technological adjunctions in the therapeutic exercise. In Basmajian JV. ed. Therapeutic exercise. Baltimore: Williams & Wilkins, 1984.

67. Mayer TG, Gatchel RJ et al. Objective assessment of spine function following industrial injury: a prospective study with comparison group and one-year follow-up. Spine 1985; 10(6):482–493.

Section II

EDUCATING THE PATIENT

4

BACK SCHOOL BACK THEN: A PERSONAL HISTORY

W. Harry Fahrni

In 1952, I found myself in a tribal region in India with a portable x-ray machine that I had managed to borrow for the occasion. After trekking into a village remote from the nearest urban and industrial centers, I carried out 450 individual examinations as well as an x-ray survey of the population. The findings from that field study were very stimulating. They revealed that at least one isolated cultural group living under preindustrial conditions in a semitropical terrain of hills and forests was characterized by a much straighter posture than is seen in European–American society. Those villagers evinced practically no back pain, and they demonstrated minimal spondylotic changes on x-ray. Their cultural habits, unlike ours, did not appear to adversely affect spinal function or structure (1). Stimulated by this experience, I began to develop in Canada an approach to managing back pain patients that focused on training them to change their postural and movement habits.

When we first organized a treatment program for sore backs in the early 1950's, several assumptions guided the details of our treatment programs:

1. No one was immune after the first 4 or 5 years of age.
2. The degree of postural curve varied greatly, but tended to worsen slowly with age after puberty.
3. Pain could commence with mechanical injury or without apparent cause, i.e., simply from the stresses of daily living.

We assumed that we were treating a condition whose cause was related directly to the physical structure of the spine, which would slowly lose physical stability as the curve increased. The treatment program was designed to handle mechanical causes of pain based upon the following priorities:

1. Correction of postural curves while at rest in bed;
2. Correction of postural curves while sitting and standing;
3. Correction of curves by active exercises; and
4. Control of pain by any symptomatic measures suitable to the case, as required.

In this early effort to develop a back school approach, we provided the following education and training:

1. Instruction in how to assume a corrective position of bedrest (supine with knees well supported in bed) and how to use a similar position for rest in nonsleeping hours (supine with trunk elevated 45° and knees flexed to 90° over a support).
2. Start lumbar flexion exercises (supine) and hip flexion exercises (supine) for lumbar curve straightening.
3. Utilize a flexion jacket to facilitate return to work.
4. Develop further curve-correcting exercises as improvement occurs.
5. Control the patient's activity level sufficiently to stay under the level of activity that would block progress, as indicated by (subjective) pain and (objective) muscle spasm.

This treatment program was followed according to these fairly rigid stipulations, so as to allow assessment of the relationship of cause and effect in the program as we compared one case with another. A noticeable improvement in response was documented, but it was not conclusive, as evidenced by the number of failures to respond satisfactorily.

For this reason, we pursued our treatment program with renewed vigor, concentrating further on the postures of physical effort; teaching the use of the pelvic tilt as essential in bending, lifting, and carrying activities; and detailing postural correction on sitting and standing.

We saw the need for improvement in our teaching methods in order to handle our patients in groups. To facilitate this we built a mock-up of a kitchen, with sink, stove, counter, and drawers. We provided a stool of proper height so that a foot could be elevated to allow the elbow to rest on the elevated knee while working at the counter. Various specific postural instructions were demonstrated relating to lifting, carrying, and moving heavy things from one place to another as patients had to do in their homes. Similar instructions were given to construction workers, warehouse workers, and various laborers in a manner directly applicable to their working conditions, A car seat, door, and dashboard with steering wheel also were set up to demonstrate exactly the proper posture required for taxi drivers, truckers, and others. The set-up made it easy to allow group practice sessions in addition to the strictly instructional periods, and patients were able to learn further by comparing notes with each other.

At that time, we were thinking too much of posture and stance rather than of dynamics as the prime factors in the diagnosis and therapy of any malfunction of body mechanics. We thereafter developed measures for coordinating the three curves of the spine in a functional manner such that dynamic factors far superseded static ones regarding corrective measures for a mechanically deranged spine at any level.

Learning of Tai-chi, we came to recognize how that ancient discipline had developed exercises that corrected all three curves of the spine in a functional manner not possible with any of the exercises of which we hitherto had knowledge. After appropriate discussion and trials, we incorporated this method, which resulted in great improvement in the response to our exercise program and the speed with which it would become effective in producing a three-level straightening of the spine.

We were frustrated, however, on seeing the result in patients who straightened their curves beautifully with exercises, but failed to maintain the correction in the activities of daily living, including manual work of various kinds. After much frustration, we recognized the importance of breathing patterns as these relate to the action of the abdominal muscles in the exercise known as the pelvic tilt. On experimenting, we found it quite easy to teach a person to coordinate abdominal breathing with a pelvic tilt while walking. In a matter of a week or so, a patient could establish a synergy between the abdominal muscle action used in the pelvic tilt and the same muscles used in expiration. Once this becomes established, it is equally easy to apply it to diverse activities done while standing, kneeling, working in a crawl-space, or even sitting at a desk, as long as body movement is occurring.

Over the years, our program has undergone many changes, largely due to an expanding recognition of the spine as a neuro-musculo-skeletal unit controlling all movement of the body. Our teaching methods inevitably changed in accordance with our experience and improved understanding. Through this process of experimentation and testing, a premise first established in the 1950s evolved into back school as it is known today.

Reference

1. Fahrni WH. A comparative radiological study of the spines of a primitive population with North Americans and northern Europeans. Br J Bone Joint Surg 1965; 47(B):552.

5

BASIC BACK SCHOOL CONCEPT

Nancy C. Selby

Talking about back school is a little like discussing ice cream. There are so many manufacturers that it is difficult to compare flavors because the variety of ingredients is so great (1). Is vanilla really vanilla, or does it have some special component? Is back school really patient education, or is it a means for evaluating a person's response to pain? Actually, back school can work in many ways. It can include evaluation, prevention, and treatment goals. But, whatever the goals or mixture of goals may be, the foundation for any back program is patient education. Basic back school serves in an important way, an essential way, as an adjunct to the treatment plan prescribed by the physician.

DIMENSIONS OF BACK SCHOOL

Because the problem of back pain is so great, every kind of person is a candidate for back school. Basic back school offers education to the person who has already sustained an injury. In such cases, the discomfort level is usually high enough for that person to have sought help from a doctor or therapist who, one hopes, recognizes the benefits of back education. Enrollment in a back school, however, should not be limited to those who have been injured or are in pain. A person does not need to have a definitive pathology in order to profit from back education. Physician referral is not a prerequisite for enrollment in a back school program, although most people will not attend unless they have seen a doctor at some time and have been told that their back pain is of the type that will benefit from instruction and training.

What are you trying to accomplish when you offer a back school program? Who are your patients? The goals of a basic back school program should be sufficiently comprehensive to meet the needs of patients of all ages, of both sexes, and with variable spine care needs. Yet, basic back school will function best if it is structured by well-defined goals that have been thought out in terms of clear procedures for attaining them.

It is critical to recognize that a great amount of mythology surrounds the experience of a back problem. One of the first responses to back pain is the despair of a vague but frightening realization, "My back's gone out!" It is terrifying for a person who cannot see his or her back, who is unfamiliar with the anatomy and mechanics of the spine, and who cannot straighten up or bend over. Therefore, the overriding goal of any back school program should be to reduce the mythology that plagues a person with back pain in order to provide an increased knowledge base capable of supporting a therapeutic patient response. That must include instruction in anatomy, biomechanics, and ergonomics, although the depth and breadth of coverage will vary from one school to another. Every patient will also need practical experience in posture modification and improved body mechanics, both on and off the job. Each patient needs to generate the body awareness that is essential to take responsibility for his or her own health care. Physical fitness activities in the form of some kind of exercise program are essential, since experience and research have shown that strength and flexibility are protective measures against back injuries (2–4). These goals will set parameters for a back school program.

Establishing the time frame of a back school

program is also important. Enrolled patients are not necessarily disabled and out of work. For that reason, the amount of time available for attending classes may be limited by the conflicting demands of other responsibilities and commitments. Try to establish a certain amount of time for each major topic so that the entire curriculum will be covered. You must be flexible, however, because some groups are very chatty, while others are very quiet.

A study presented in 1982 compared the outcome of a 12-hour back school curriculum with one that required only 4½ hours (5). It was found that a total of 4½ hours of instruction and training was more cost-effective and that the retention of information was virtually the same. Based upon these findings, we conclude that a successful back school can be presented in two or three sessions. It is our experience that two sessions of 2 hours each work very effectively for most patients when they are scheduled approximately a week apart. The third visit lasting a half hour is scheduled for about 6 weeks after the second session. The purpose of the third visit is to allow the patient to see the physical therapist in an individual session when the therapist will review and evaluate the patient's success in pursuing customary activities with appropriate body mechanics based upon well-understood biomechanics and ergonomic principles. It also offers an opportunity to ensure that the patient is exercising in an appropriate manner.

Back school information can be disseminated in several ways. The ratio of one teacher to one student can be very rewarding for both, but the cost may be excessive. For example, if you charge $100 for back school, it is going to be difficult to justify a salary for a competent teacher at a one-to-one ratio, but if you schedule six to eight people to a class, you can still charge $100, but it will be possible to offer the instructor reasonable compensation.

Not only is a class structure more cost-effective for basic back school, but several added benefits accrue from a training point of view. The exchange of information among attendees can be extremely valuable for each member of the group. However, classes should be kept small and intimate. If there are many more than six or eight students in a class, some may be reluctant to discuss their personal worries and frustrations.

First Session

When the goals, time frame, and structure of the back school have been established, the subject matter should be outlined. A short anatomy course for back patients is essential. Anatomy can be presented in several ways. The combination of demonstrating on a plastic spine model and of discussing appropriate graphic illustrations works well to reinforce anatomic and biomechanical concepts. If there are no more than six or eight patients in a class, it should be possible for everyone to have an opportunity to handle the spine model and ask specific questions. Patients seem to be reassured once they become aware of the strength, flexibility, and function of the spine and the surrounding structures. Terms such as disc, nerve, vertebra, facet joint become meaningful to patients who can see the actual object on a model or picture. In a basic back school, explanation and discussion should be limited to simple anatomy and common problems. The patient who has a complicated condition will probably mention it in group discussions. When that happens, the instructor must decide if it is of use to the class to explain the complications in more detail.

The therapist should keep a written or mental list of the most asked questions and try to incorporate information relevant to those questions into the presentation. Patients should be encouraged to interact within the group and to ask questions. It will save time and improve the flow of teaching, however, if the most common questions are anticipated.

After anatomy has been discussed using the spine model and illustrations, patients should view a slide program. At this time, ask them to lie down on mats with their legs propped up at a 90° angle. Most people find this position very desirable, but if not, other appropriate positions can be recommended. The amount of information retained seems to be directly proportional to the comfort of the student.

The nature of the slides presented will vary. In order to reinforce the anatomy instruction, cartoons, analogies, and pathology slides are used in various combinations. Slides essentially are intended to provide a summary of the information presented at the beginning of the hour.

The information presented should focus on

specifics instead of generalities. The first session normally is expected to cover anatomy, the relationship between disc pressure and posture, and body mechanics relating to daily activities in the home and at work. First aid for back pain is also included in the information package, as is a description of the initial exercises that are to be practiced during the week. Although this may sound fairly simple, it should be remembered that most patients during the first session are still undergoing treatment.

Disc pressure as it relates to posture is the next topic of discussion. Nachemson's disc pressure numbers are projected using both male and female models in a variety of different postural situations (6; Fig. 5.1). Seeing the numbers seems to aid in the retention of basic concepts relating to posture and back pain, especially after the patient has had an opportunity to practice the daily living activities of sitting, standing, bending, lifting, and lying down while keeping the Nachemson numbers in mind.

The concept of body mechanics and the need to modify activities is new to most of the participants, who come from varied educational and work backgrounds. In order to maintain group interest, many different activities are pictured and discussed. The slides have been taken by members of the staff in different home situations and work places. The more slides that are shown, the easier it is for the class to overcome an initial inability to transfer from one correct position to another in different work, recreational, and living situations.

Because many patients are still experiencing episodes of muscle spasm during the initial class, the use of first aid techniques is also presented in the first session. We promote ice massage, stretching, and aspirin or ibuprofen and discourage heating pads. If patients are on medication, they probably will not be taking aspirin as an anti-inflammatory drug, but they need to recognize the benefits of over-the-counter drugs so that they do not feel that they need to rush to the emergency room for an episode of back pain and muscle spasm. First aid is entirely a matter of self-help. Whenever a flare-up occurs,

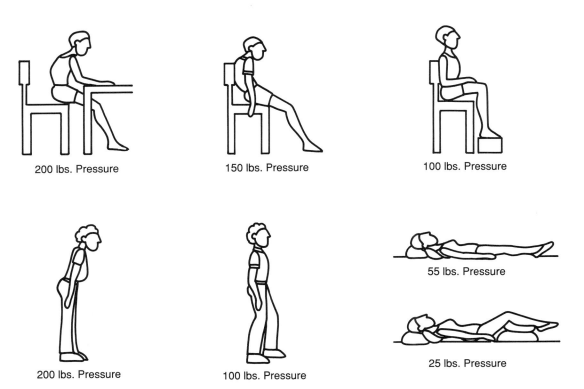

200 lbs. Pressure   150 lbs. Pressure   100 lbs. Pressure

55 lbs. Pressure

200 lbs. Pressure   100 lbs. Pressure

25 lbs. Pressure

Figure 5.1.   Male and female disc pressure in different postures.

flare-up occurs, first aid methods should be tried, at least for several days. It is not necessary to contact a physician unless there is severe leg pain. The symptoms of aspirin overdose and the possible side effects of aspirin usage should also be explained.

Only three or four exercises are presented during the first session. The pelvic tilt, the modified sit-up and the knee-to-chest stretch are recommended for most patients. Occasionally, extension press-ups are recommended if, based on the diagnosis, the therapist feels that they are advisable for a particular patient. Strength and mobility are significant goals of the first basic back school class.

The rather formal classroom situation oriented to the spine model, the slides, and the exercises takes about an hour and 15 minutes, which leaves approximately 45 minutes for instruction in the training laboratory. This is a room with multiple props in which the participants can gain some supervised experience in practical applications and various modifications of daily life activities. The lab should be equipped with mirrors for posture and body mechanics training. During the first two hours, it is wise to target daily home activities, such as ways of brushing teeth, getting in and out of bed, sleeping, sitting, putting groceries away, and standing. They are practiced by everyone in the class. Patients get feedback regarding these activities from the mirrors and from each other. The therapist should request that each patient practice the modifications they have learned during the week between sessions one and two, and they will be asked to report their progress at the next class period. They are also given printed instructions to take with them on the exercises and on first aid techniques.

Second Session

Part two of the basic back school reviews the concepts introduced in part one and presents new information, including positions for sexual intercourse, ways of handling stress, some body mechanics for heavy labor situations, ways of lifting and carrying at home, ways of engaging in recreational activities, and additional exercises for strength and flexibility.

The classroom format remains the same. Again, participants are asked to lie on the mats with their feet up if they can. They are given ample opportunity to share the experiences of the preceding week, and to demonstrate their mastery of the suggested exercises.

Because the information of basic back school must be communicated in only four hours, the concept of good nutrition is merely mentioned. The informational thrust is that if the individual has gained a lot of weight or has decreased activity due to a sedentary life style, it may be a very good idea to shape up. A few specific suggestions are presented. More information is provided in a take-home packet.

Many of the patients are so intimidated by their back pain that they literally are afraid to move. Thus, a sexual relationship can become a worrisome problem. Many are reluctant to share their fears with their physician. Back school can allay those fears. Sexual positions are presented as normal activities that require an awareness of body mechanics and which can be modified just like other kinds of movement. A variety of sexual positions is illustrated for the patient in the information packet (Fig. 5.2). The therapist should encourage all patients to resume normal sexual activities. Patients become more confident of their ability to do this once the subject has been aired.

Individuals with back pain are usually stressed, so relaxation techniques are presented. None is very complex. The instructional emphasis continues to focus on self-help. Progressive relaxation techniques are taught and patients are encouraged to try them as a class activity. Many times they are so effective that patients actually fall asleep. This portion of the program should be given as the last topic before the teaching of additional exercises when the lights will be turned on again and patients will be moving around.

The concepts of body mechanics presented during the second session include those relevant to lifting, carrying, pushing, pulling, and pivoting, as well as others that may be appropriate in terms of individual needs.

Recreational activities are also discussed and encouraged. Patients may need to modify these before they are able to resume them again.

Before the patients leave the classroom setting, they are taught several more exercises by the therapist, who supervises each patient and suggests appropriate programs for each. Exercises may be in flexion or in extension. An ap-

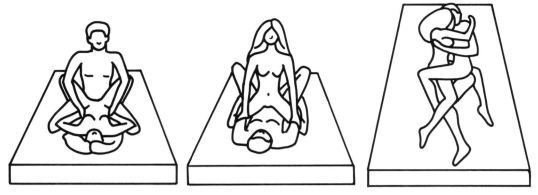

Figure 5.2. Modified positions for sexual activities: *Left,* Woman—may need pillow under hips; keep knees bent. Man—keep knees bent. *Center,* Woman—avoid swayback; avoid bearing too much weight on arms; keep knees forward. Man—keep knees and hips bent. *Right,* Woman—avoid twisting; keep hip of lower leg slightly flexed. Courtesy of Margo Wycoff, Ph.D.

propriate regimen is discussed so that the patients will strengthen muscles and increase mobility and flexibility. Three exercises are usually added and practiced in this session.

The class moves into the training laboratory for a second session of practical experience. As in the first session, props are available. Usually, every class member participates. By this time, the majority of patients have gained a new body awareness with a workable understanding of how body postures and types of movement can reduce instability in the lumbar spine and decrease disc pressure. They need encouragement and feedback from their instructor and from classmates. We find that most patients are willing to change the way they have performed activities in the past, but they need instruction and reinforcement.

When participants have completed the second session, they receive a patient information packet containing virtually all of the information in a comprehensible format. The language is as unsophisticated and nonmedical as possible. Graphics reinforce the concepts of body mechanics, positions, exercises, recreational activities, sexual positions, and first aid techniques. Also included are a written description of relaxation methods, suggestions for weight control, and general do's and don'ts if an episode of pain does occur. In addition, a suggested book list is given in case they want to deepen their understanding of some aspect of the basic back school information.

The third visit takes place approximately 6

weeks after the second and is an individual appointment with the physical therapist. At this time the therapist evaluates the patient's progress, reviews the patient's exercises and physical fitness routines, and reviews techniques of body mechanics relevant to both on and off the job. If the patient is not feeling better, the therapist will probably suggest return to the referring physician for reevaluation.

A report is sent to the referring physician and to any other interested party by the therapist following each back school session. It is of critical importance to keep lines of communication open.

Spouses and family members are encouraged to come to back school with patients because they can reinforce the concepts. Basic back school is short, well defined, has few frills, and is limited to education only. Therefore, it is important that these patients receive all possible encouragement to take responsibility for their own back care.

A study of 1,725 patients from 1979 to 1982 confirmed that the majority gained good insight into their problems and retained enough information to decrease doctor visits and time away from work. Also, most felt they were in control of their backs (7). Similar studies in the Canadian Back School and California Back School have confirmed similar findings (Arthur H. White, personal communication).

Back school should always be thought of as a valuable, conservative resource for both treatment and prevention.

References

1. White AW. Back school and other conservative approaches to low back pain. St. Louis: Mosby, 1983.
2. Keim HA. How to care for your back. Englewood Cliffs, NJ: Prentice-Hall, 1981.
3. Pope MH, Frymoyer JW, Anderson G. eds.: Occupational low back pain. New York: Praeger, 1984.
4. Fardon DF. Free yourself from back pain. Englewood Cliffs: Prentice-Hall, 1984.
5. Hochschuler S, Selby N. Time frames on the back school curriculum. Presented at a meeting of the International Society for the Study of the Lumbar Spine. Cambridge, England, 1982.
6. Nachemson A, Elfstrom G. Intravital dynamic pressure measurements in lumbar discs. Scand J Rehab Med 1970; Suppl 1.
7. Herr LH, Lawlis GF. Back school—a four year follow up study. Presented at the APTA Conference, New Orleans, June 1985.

PATIENT INFORMATION: ANATOMY AND BIOMECHANICS

John Triano
Gregory Cramer

The principal importance of teaching anatomy and biomechanics to patients is to aid them in making the many decisions required daily in the proper care of their painful lower backs. In addition, adequate understanding of the anatomy and biomechanics of the lumbar spine should also help patients prevent future episodes of low back pain by enabling them to better practice their work, recreational, and leisure activities in such a way that the possibility of recurrence is minimized. The purpose of this chapter is to describe those elements of anatomy and biomechanics of the low back region that are most important to give the patient a practical understanding of his or her condition. The spine physician may choose which aspects of the topics discussed best fit each patient.

"PATIENT-FRIENDLY" OVERVIEW OF THE SPINE

The spine and pelvis make up the central column extending from the head to the hip joints. Together, they supply the main support for upright posture and activity. Because the spine is segmented into 24 bones and the pelvis, it is possible to have a great deal of flexibility, as is needed in walking, bending, and sitting exercises. Yet all of these movements potentially can be achieved while an individual carries exceptional loads, as seen, for example, with competitive weight training. In that sport, a person who usually is of hefty bulk may bend forward to pick up as much as several hundred pounds. He or she will then carry that load upward,

straightening out the spine, until the weight is held as shoulder level or higher.

The spine is divided into three functional regions (Fig. 6.1). The cervical region is at the top and is readily recognized as that part that forms the skeleton of the neck. It is the most flexible part of the spine and supports the weight and movements of the head. Beneath it is the thoracic region. The rib cage is suspended from the thoracic spine in such a way that the chest can easily expand for breathing. Human ability to twist in trunk rotation is permitted primarily by this part of the back. The lower back is known as the lumbar region and carries the load of the entire upper body, including the head and arms. While it is most flexible in forward and backward bending, it also allows some side bending and very small amounts of torso rotation.

A number of functional units are strung together to make up the spinal column. In general, they may be categorized as bone, ligament, joint, muscle, and nerves. The bones, called vertebrae, are responsible for the spine's ability to bear relatively large loads or stresses. Ligaments tie the bones together into a loose string and restrict large movements between individual bones, which could prove to be harmful. A special type of ligament, called the intervertebral disc, resides between individual vertebrae and acts as a flexible cushion and spacer. Collectively, two bones and their intervening disc form a joint structure called a motion segment. This joint complex is the smallest functional unit of the spine and is where most problems

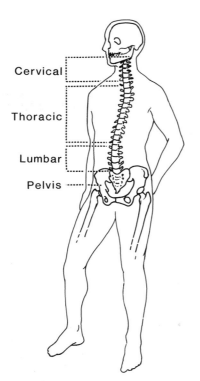

Figure 6.1. Regions of the spine: cervical, thoracic, and lumbar.

are structurally strong and are analogous to the support beams in a building. They bear the loads of body weight and anything that is carried. With proper training and lifting technique, the spine of the weight lifter described earlier can withstand as much as ten times body weight without fracture. It is important to realize that bone is not brittle. In fact, like all bone, the vertebra is somewhat elastic and will compress as a spring or undergo some bending during the course of normal daily activities. As loads are applied and released, the bone can compress as much as 25% of its height without any apparent damage. Without this elastic effect, fractures might occur in young healthy people with as little exertion as running or lifting a laundry basket.

Five lumbar vertebrae are stacked one on top of another with an intervertebral disc between each pair of bones (Fig. 6.2). The bottom vertebra and disc (L5) rest upon the sacrum, a rather large triangular bone that forms the back wall of the pelvis. Each lumbar vertebra consists of two regions, each of which plays a very different role in spine function. The first region is a large block-shaped vertebral body. The second is an arch behind the vertebral body, which surrounds and protects the spinal cord. The ver-

arise. The power driving motion in these joints comes from the back muscles that attach to the vertebrae of the motion segment. Longer trunk muscles that connect the pelvis and rib cage in the front and the back may also contribute to movement. The proper use of these muscles often prevents damage to the spine or allows more normal function to be restored after injury. Finally, nerves pass from openings between the bones and behind the disc to govern the action of the arms and legs and many internal body functions, and to obtain sensory information of the body and its surroundings.

The focus of attention will now be the lumbar region since it is most often the site of spinal problems and complaints. Our primary objective is to understand how the spine works and how to have as normal activity as possible while minimizing risk of injury.

OSTEOLOGY OF THE LUMBAR VERTEBRAE AND SACRUM

Bone is the tissue primarily responsible for the physical strength of the spine. The vertebrae

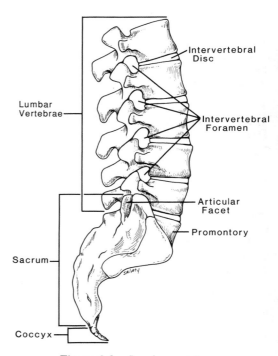

Figure 6.2. Lumbar vertebrae.

tebral body portion acts to carry the compressive weight from the upper torso. The neural arch is irregular in shape and has a number of specialized structures (Fig. 6.3). Many serve as lever arms for muscle attachments to influence bone motion. On both sides of the midline are the articular processes. At the upper end, these overlap with those from the vertebra above. At the lower end, they overlap with the vertebra below. Where they overlap, a special joint is formed, called the facet, which is very moveable and much like a simple knuckle joint of the fingers.

Where the bony processes overlap and form the facets, notice the curved surface and the fact that the upper end faces inward and is cupped, whereas the lower end faces outward and to the side. The lower or inferior articular processes of one vertebra fit very closely together with the superior articular processes of the vertebra below. Where contact is made between them, a smooth cartilage lining secretes lubricating fluid to prevent friction when the joint moves. The close interlocking of the facets causes them to act like rudders, guiding and limiting the motion of each vertebra.

Because of their orientation, the lumbar motion segments operate primarily in forward and backward bending. Some side bending also occurs, but twisting or rotation is very limited. These gliding joints are often thought to be the source of the problem in some people with low back pain. Because the facets are so close together, too much pressure on them can make them irritated and inflamed. Over longer periods, repeated heavy loads may cause them to

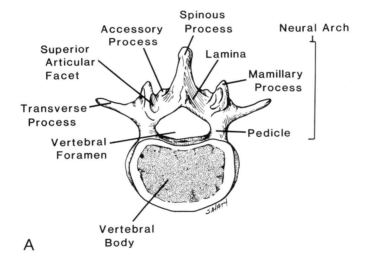

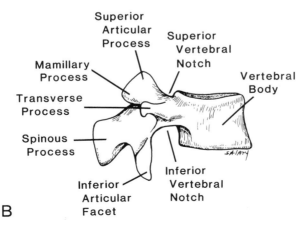

Figure 6.3. Structures of the neural arch.

undergo degenerative changes, which are a form of arthritis.

The arch, acting to protect the spinal cord, can be divided into two different sections. The part closest to the body is known as the pedicle, and there is one on each side. Each pedicle is connected behind to a rather flat plate of bone known as the lamina. The left and right laminae unite behind the spinal cord (Fig. 6.4). From behind, the laminae overlap like roofing shingles to close the spinal canal. The spinal cord travels down the spine in this shelter, and the nerves emit from between the vertebra through the opening formed by the pedicles, articular processes, and intervertebral disc. This opening is called the intervertebral foramen or canal.

Other projections from the neural arch serve as attachment points for ligaments and muscles. The transverse processes protrude from the sides of the vertebra, and the single spinous process points directly backward. The various locations of these attachment sites allow for production of the wide variety of movements seen in the lower back.

The lumbar vertebrae together with the discs stacked one on top of another assume a forward curved shape. Called the lumbar lordosis, the bowed configuration is the normal posture the low back takes during upright stance. The general shape is depicted in Figure 6.2. Lordosis is a unique characteristic of humans, which evolved with the ability to stand erect on two feet. On balance, it seems probable that it is an adaptation of walking upright. During the second year of life, the front block portion of the vertebra begins to take on a wedge shape. That is, it gets taller in the front than in the back. A similar change occurs in the discs between the bones. As a result, the lumbar spine forms an arch and permanently supports the erect posture.

The forward curvature serves as a flexible lever upon which the upper body weight is perched. Like a bent beam, the curved healthy spine may be about ten times stronger when its muscles hold it rigid than it would be if it were straight. While enabling great strength, lordosis also provides for a wide range of movements and postures from bending forward and sitting positions to backward and side bending.

However, some believe that the lordosis may pose a bit of a liability. If it is used improperly, as when postures with too much curve are employed, a set of circumstances can develop in which the facets become easily overloaded. This may be one reason why some women have lower back pain toward the end of a pregnancy. So, a postural balance is desired that serves good strength and flexibility without causing irritation.

The lumbar spine is supported by the sacrum (Fig. 6.5), which is made up of many segments that fuse together during early development and is suspended between the two large hip bones, the ilia. The joint between them is known as the sacroiliac joint. Together, these three bones make up the pelvis. The upper body weight and loads from daily activity that are transmitted down the spine to the pelvis now can be divided equally and transmitted through the iliac bones to the lower extremities. Many muscles from both the trunk and legs attach to the pelvis.

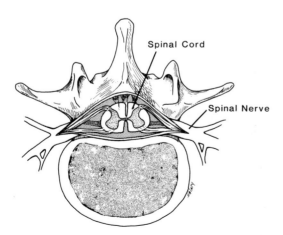

Figure 6.4. Left and right laminae behind spinal cord.

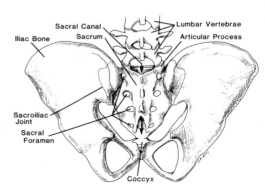

Figure 6.5. Lumbar spine supported by sacrum.

Underneath the sacrum is a rather tiny bone known as the tail bone, or coccyx. Like the sacrum, the coccyx is made up of fused vertebral segments. The coccyx does not support any of the body's weight and moves very little, but some of the muscles of the lower pelvis attach to it.

LIGAMENTS OF THE SPINE

Ligaments are tough fibrous bands that hold all of these bones together. Acting like guiding cables, they are found in almost every conceivable location around the spine where they act to limit movement. Some of them run between the spinous processes of adjacent vertebrae, while others run between adjacent transverse processes. Two of the most important ligaments run along the front and back of the vertebral bodies, respectively. One series runs from the laminae of the vertebra above to the laminae of the next vertebra below (Fig. 6.6). Another completely surrounds and encloses the facet joints so that its lubricating fluid does not leak out. Ligaments can be injured from either sudden stretching or prolonged and repeated loading when they are tight. A torn or over stretched ligament is known as a sprain and usually takes several weeks to heal completely. If it heals in an elongated position, then the joint it protects can become loose or hypermobile.

Probably the best known ligament is the intervertebral disc, located between the vertebral bodies. Each is made up of two parts, an outer fibrous ring called the anulus fibrosus and a gelatinous center called the nucleus pulposus. The anulus is made up of many thin layers, much like an onion cut in half. A herniated or ruptured disc (Fig. 6.6) is a tearing of the outer layers of the anulus. This condition allows the inner nucleus pulposus to push out through the opening. As the nuclear material squeezes out, it can press against the spinal nerves resulting in back pain, leg pain or both. Before the anulus fibers fully tear, there may be a bulging outward toward the nerve that can have the same effects.

Young discs are about 80% water, which accounts in part for their high bending flexibility. As a person gets older, the disc tends to dry out and lose flexibility. Tearing or herniation of a disc in young people probably results more often from repeated wear and tear injury over time. In older persons, because the tissue is less elastic, a single sudden stress might cause it.

Most damage that occurs in the spinal column comes about from either a single injury with high peak loads or prolonged loads using poor posture or mechanical advantage. Depending upon the ligament, it can carry as much as 100 lbs of load and the disc will generally withstand forces beyond those that can fracture the bone. Together, the vertebra and disc can withstand as much as 1440 lbs. Above that, almost everyone becomes injured. One caution is needed. It is important not to take these kinds of numbers too literally, because it does not mean that a person can hold a box that large. As will be explained below, loads this high can be easily generated inside the body by a com-

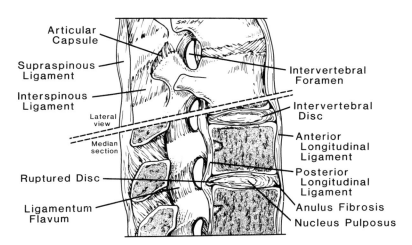

Figure 6.6.   Ligaments.

bination of muscular exertion, posture, and weight lifted.

While the ligaments and disc are extremely strong when used properly, they can be damaged with seemingly innocent tasks that are performed improperly. Underlying their strength is a subtle but very significant weakness. The disc is particularly vulnerable to loads when the spine is twisted or bent. Even persons who have experienced serious spinal injury can return to many normal activities once they understand how the spine works, strengthen themselves accordingly, and begin paying attention to how they use body posture to achieve work or play effort.

SPINAL CANAL AND INTERVERTEBRAL FORAMEN

With the motion segments stacked on top of each other, the arch formed by the pedicles and lamina of the vertebra fashion a canal or tunnel known as the spinal canal. The spinal cord is housed there, protected by the bone and muscles that surround it. The spinal cord is actually much shorter than the spine. It ends at approximately the level of the first lumbar vertebra. The remaining spinal nerves course downward through the canal to the lumbar spine and sacrum. At each level, a nerve branches off the cord and passes through the intervetebral foramen between the vertebra and disc. Blood vessels, lymphatic channels, fatty tissue, and the nerve that returns through the foramen to help supply a portion of the spinal canal itself are also located in this opening (Fig. 6.7). It is at this site that the nerves can occasionally be involved in back problems. This may cause pain to radiate down the back of the leg. Arthritic-like degeneration of the facets or herniation of the disc can trap the nerve in this very small foramen.

Looking at a lumbar vertebra from above, it can be seen that the spinal canal is not circular. In fact, its shape can vary a great deal from one vertebra to another and from one person to another. Sometimes this foramen is much wider than normal from side to side than from front to back, and the spinal nerves in the area can become crowded. When this occurs, there is less tolerance for complications from disc degeneration, arthritis, or excess movement involving the spine. This condition is known as spinal stenosis and may be one of the causes of low

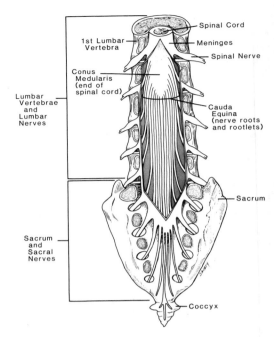

Figure 6.7. Spinal cord and intervertebral foramena.

back and leg pain. Once again, the nerve may be snared, but this time inside the spinal canal before it ever tries to exit.

SPINAL NERVES

The spinal cord and each spinal nerve are covered by a tough set of membranes called meninges. Generally, only one nerve exits through each of the intervertebral foramen. As the nerve leaves the spine, the meninges are replaced by another durable covering that will coat the nerve and all of its branches from the spine to their final destinations. Almost immediately upon exiting the foramen, the nerve divides into two branches. One branch supplies the muscles of the back while the other will travel to either the lower limb, the abdomen or the pelvis. Muscles, intestinal motility, bowel and bladder control, as well as distribution of the blood supply are all influenced by these nerves.

The outer covering of a nerve is needed to help protect it from damage caused by stretching or compressing. As the body moves, the nerve actually slides along the length of the bed in which it rests. Raising the arm from the side to overhead could cause a main nerve in the arm to slide as much as 1.5 inches. Similarly, in the lumbar region, nerves move in and out of the intervertebral foramina. While it would not be very comfortable, the nerve tissue with its outside covering can withstand a suprisingly high-tension load of 13 lbs per square inch. However, the nerves are much more susceptible to pressure. Under abnormal conditions in which the nerve can become trapped, such as with a bulging disc, the sliding action causes the nerve to be dragged over the anulus. That region of the nerve will soon become swollen and inflamed. The covering usually keeps the nerve intact, but inflammation causes pain throughout the course of its distribution. Most often, inflammation of this kind occurs at the bottom of the spine at the level of the L5 disc. Because the nerve that emits from this region goes down into the foot, the disc lesion can be felt as pain in the back of the leg and foot.

The motion segment design is really a compromise between the need for a flexible spine and for protection of the nervous system. When the spine is healthy, this trade-off works well. However, even normal movement can casue problems for the nerve when anything goes wrong. Whether from disc disease, arthritis, or a hypermobile bone, a narrowed intervertebral canal increases the risk of irritation and damage to the nerve. As the spine bends (Fig. 6.8), the foramen changes shape and size. A narrowed foramen simply has less tolerance for a normal range of activities and leads to an increased liability for injury.

MUSCLES INFLUENCING THE LOW BACK

Muscles supply the power for us to move, perform work, and be active in play. They make the spine rigid when heavy loads are carried and orchestrate complicated combinations of activity that are needed to bend, twist, push, pull, or lift. In order to achieve the large number of possible activities, the spine is surrounded by a vast array of muscles (Fig. 6.9). The usage and effects of each muscle depend upon how hard it is contracted, combination with other muscle actions, and posture during use.

Muscle tissue is quite strong. For every square inch of muscle belly in cross-section, approximately 60 lbs of tension are generated. People with good upper body strength tend not to have spinal injury as readily as others. However, muscle fatigues quite easily. An easy experiment can be made by holding a one-pound

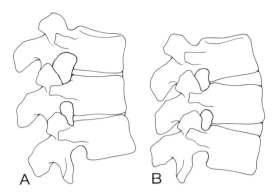

Figure 6.8. Foramen changes shape and size as spine bends.

weight in front of the body at full arm length. After only 5 minutes, the muscles of the shoulder begin to tire and hurt. The same thing occurs in muscles of the spine and is the basis for the frequent shifts in posture that people unconsciously make during the course of the day. In fact, it is really the understanding of muscle strength, posture, and their limitation that serves as the key to reducing the risk of injury.

The muscles of the low back can be divided into three groups that run along the back in various layers. The first of these consists of two large columns of muscle that extend from the back of the sacrum and iliac bones, running on each side of the spinous processes, to the head. These are known collectively as the erector spinae muscles. On each side of the spinous processes, the erector spinae are spread out in three bundles. In general, these longer muscles typically control the activity of the whole lumbar spine region. They help in bending the spine backwards or to the side and, to some extent, contribute to the ability to twist the trunk.

The second group of back muscles are shorter and run from vertebra to vertebra. Bundles of muscle fibers attach between the transverse processes of one vertebra to the spinous processes of the one above. The deeper and closer to the spine that a muscle is, the closer together are the bones that it attaches. A muscle can connect with the next bone above or it may skip from one to six bones before reaching the spinous process to which it will attach. The function of these muscles is similar to that of the erector spinae with two exceptions. They are more influential on twisting the body and they are more directly responsible for governing the

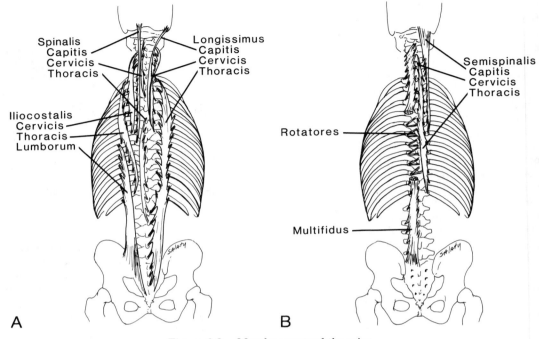

Figure 6.9. Muscles surround the spine.

action of individual motion segments during the coordination of any motion.

The third pair of back muscles is composed of two broad, flat, rectangular muscles, one on each side of the spine, named the quadratus lumborum. Each attaches below to the iliac bones, to the transverse processes of the lumbar vertebrae and also to the lowest rib. While they can help to arch the back in extension, they primarily help to bend the spine from side to side.

Other muscles important to the health and function of the low back are found in the abdomen and legs. Three muscles of the abdomen are probably the most important. They are the rectus abdominis, oblique, and iliopsoas (Fig. 6.10). Once again, the effect of their contraction is to regulate the activity of the lumbar region as a whole rather than influence specific vertebral motion. The rectus muscles on the front of the body next to the midline contribute almost solely to bending the spine forward or helping make it rigid when contracted together with back muscles. Abdominal oblique muscles are positioned to the sides of the body and are the primary rotators of the trunk. They also aid in sideward bending tasks. Together, the rectus and oblique can flatten the lumbar lordosis,

which can be a very helpful maneuver to limit back injury.

The right and left iliopsoas muscles assist in flexing the spine forward and in side bending. Under the right conditions, for example, lying on the floor trying to do a sit-up with legs straight, they initially can contribute to bending the spine backward. These muscles run from the sides of the lumbar vertebrae to the top of the femur.

Two groups of thigh muscles (Fig. 6.11) are also important in protecting the spine. They act as stabilizers for the pelvis and help to keep the base of the spine stable during activity. On the front of the thigh are the quadratus muscles which have one major bundle that attaches to the front of the pelvis at the top of the iliac bone and can cause it to tip forward. This same muscle assists in leg lift exercises if you contract it while lying down. On the back of the thigh are the hamstrings group. They attach at the lower part of the pelvis. Used with the abdominal muscles, they can tilt the pelvis back and flatten the lumbar curve.

Lastly, the gluteal muscles of the pelvis itself cover the broad outer surface of the iliac bones and run to the top of the femur. Their ac-

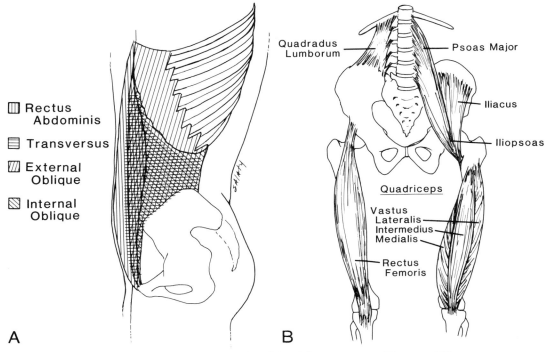

□ Rectus
   Abdominis

▤ Transversus

▨ External
   Oblique

▧ Internal
   Oblique

Figure 6.10. Most important muscles of the abdomen: rectus, oblique, and iliopsoas.

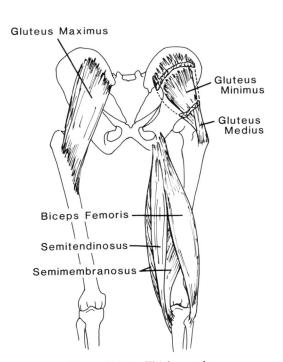

Figure 6.11. Thigh muscles.

tion is principally to help stabilize the pelvis along with the hamstrings.

BIOMECHANICS OF POSTURE AND MOVEMENT

Load Distribution

In order to begin using the back in a safe way and return to normal activities of daily living, it is necessary to understand how these structures work together. The primary objective here is to carry out routine functions and tasks without causing unacceptably high strain to the already damaged tissues of the back. On the surface this can seem tricky because back injuries are often very different from the standpoint of what positions or motions will cause pain. However, there are common principles of mechanics that can guide how we select to use the body. With them, it is possible to find strategies that will improve function for anyone who truly wishes to get better.

Since the objective is to keep back loads at a minimum, it may be useful to first examine how the body weight is shared within the motion

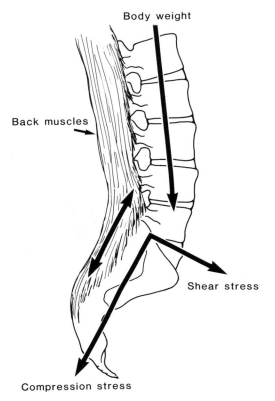

Figure 6.12. Scheme of lower lumbar spine.

Table 6.1.
Back Loads from Lifting with Symmetric Postures (in pounds).

Posture	Compression	Shear	Muscle tension
Bend at knees	628	73	627
Bend at waist	776	112	730
Bend at knees arms extended	892	81	799

Likewise, the amount of forward or backward bending of one bone on another generally influences how the load gets distributed. That is, when the spine is bent forward, the facet joints are disengaged and all of the load, both shear and compression, is transferred to the disc. Conversely, bending backwards presses the facets together and increases the load. See Table 6.1.

Postures and Safe Lifting

The way we choose to perform a given motion or task can tremendously increase the amount of load transmitted to the spine. Posture is a tool and a means of doing work. It is selected according to the job that is to be accomplished. For example, standing up to operate a computer terminal that sits on a desk can be done only with a very stooped posture. Back and neck muscles quickly tire and begin to ache. The option is to use a proper chair that allows a less stressful position.

There are several factors that can be modified voluntarily once they are understood. Figure 6.13 portrays three ways to perform a simple lift of a 20-lb box. The question is, which one is safest. In the first case, the upper body is bent forward without bending the knees deeply while a box is being lifted. Here, the low back muscles must contract very hard to offset the weight of the upper body acting on a long lever arm from the spine. In addition, the 20-lb load is acting on its even longer lever arm. Because of the heavy exertion of the muscles, the lower spine must support a 776-lb force in compression and 112 lbs in shear. To accomplish it, the muscles must exert 730 lbs of tension.

The second case uses a deeper bending of the knees and less bending at the waist. That simple modification of posture saves the equivalent of 150 lbs compression, 39 lbs shear and 103 lbs

segment. Only in a few postures does the vertebra sit in a level position. Figure 6.12 displays a schematic of the lower lumbar spine where most injuries occur. Suppose you are standing and holding a box in front of your abdomen. The weight of the box and the torso would normally cause a fall forward if it were not for the fact that back muscles counteract it. The spine load, then, is increased by the action of the muscles to hold the body in its chosen posture.

The action of these loads is vertically downward on to the motion segment. There it is split into two kinds of components. One is a compressive stress onto the vertebral body and disc. The alternative is a shearing stress parallel to the plane of the disc. This potentially causes stress within the facets. How much of the burden is shared by the vertebral body and the articular processes depends in part upon the slope of the vertebral position. Two things happen. As the vertebra is inclined more, the amount of shear load tends to increase while the disc compression tends to decrease.

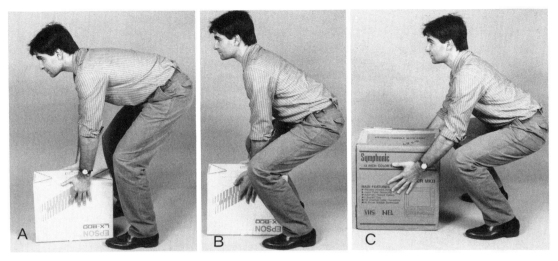

Figure 6.13.   Three ways to lift a 20-lb box.

of muscle tension. All of that reduction in physical stress occurred even though the weight lifted is exactly the same. The aspect that permits such a dramatic difference is that the upper body is more erect and the weight lifted is closer to the spine.

Certainly, the size or bulk of an object can be problematic. To keep the lever arm small, it is often advantageous to bend at the knees, provided that the back can be held upright and the object to be lifted is kept close to the body. On the way up, the object generally travels between the knees. However, with bulky objects, this is not possible and bending at the knees will actually increase the distance between the spine and the object.

Suppose again that a 20-lb box is to be lifted. This time, its dimensions are much larger. Since the box cannot be kept close to the spine, the compressive load jumps to 892 lbs with a muscle tension of 799 lbs. Because the muscle pull in this posture contributes very little to the shear load, it is only slightly increased. Under such conditions, it is actually safer to bend at the waist, because the combined stress from the trunk weight and the load kept close to the body is less than that from the trunk and extended moment arm required to get around the knees when the knee bending posture is used.

Thus far, only symmetric activities have been discussed. Whenever the spine is twisted or bent to the side in asymmetric positions, the effects of weight bearing are severely amplified.

The mechanics become more complex and more muscles are activated in order to realize the desired goal. Moreover, the motion segment is placed in positions that are less able to handle high loads. In practice, the body weight alone can be sufficient to cause damage to the disc if bending and twisting to the side are combined. Table 6.2 shows the comparison of estimated stresses at the midlumbar level between relaxed upright standing, twisted 45°, and twisted plus forward bend of 30°. The midlumbar level is generally horizontal so that no shearing load is present in upright postures.

Fundamentally, any kind of heavy exertion, including bending, should be avoided when the trunk is twisted. Many jobs or activities can be accomplished in such a way that the twist and

Table 6.2.
Back Loads with Combined Twist and Bend* (in pounds).

Posture	Compression	Shear
Stand relaxed	107	0
Stand twisted 45°	108	0
Hold 5 lbs	267	5
Bend 30°	382	41
Bend 30° & hold 5 lbs	515	45

*Adapted from Schultz AB, Andersson GBJ, Haderspeck K et al. Analysis and measurement of lumbar trunk loads in tasks involving bends and twists. Biomechanics 1982; 15(9):672.

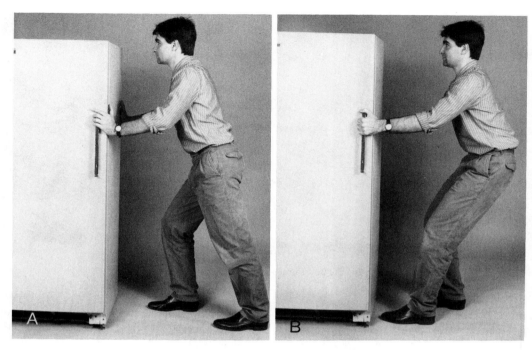

Figure 6.14.   Proper form for pushing and pulling.

bend can be avoided. If that should fail, one should get help. The time saved by attempting the exertion alone is is not worth the risk of loss of work because of an injury.

Push-Pull Tasks

Pushing and pulling jobs are really no different (Fig. 6.14). Now the distance of concern is the vertical distance between the location where the push is applied and the lower back. Optimum hand position is between the level of the elbows and the shoulders. This allows the full effect of the upper body weight. When pulling, a small amount of forward lean of the trunk is helpful. Generally, people are much stronger and safer at pulling than at pushing tasks because they can take better advantage of leg strength and upper body weight.

Prolonged Activity versus Faster Movements

So far, everything explained holds up for short-term static activity or slow-speed movements. However, at both the long-term static end (standing bent over a car engine) and the higher speed dynamic activities (playing tennis), different factors come into play.

For prolonged static postures, changes in both the joint cartilage at the disc and facets as well as in the muscles take place. Consider the fellow bent over his car for 10 or 15 minutes or one who bends over gardening on Sunday afternoon. Everything feels fine until he tries to come back to an upright stance. Then his back feels stiff and sore. As the trunk is bent forward, the muscles may hold the body weight and keep the ligaments and joint from carrying the load. The longer the position is maintained, the more fatigued they become and the burden is gradually shifted from muscle to ligaments and facet joint. The joint fluid is squeezed from between the facet surfaces and they, with the disc, become stiff. If the man has a healthy spine, it loosens up after a few stretches and returns to normal.

The same chain of events occurs when people sit for long periods or assume any constant posture long enough to have muscle fatigue or increased joint pressures. For that reason, it is always wise to take a short flexibility break about every 20 minutes. The joints are loosened and lubricated and the muscles are stretched and relaxed, making for a healthier and more comfortable day.

Finally, a few words should be said about the effect of faster movements. Consider again the description of lifting a 20-lb box. When the lift is made quickly, the load on the spine will be anywhere from 25 to 100% higher. Using the third case in Figure 6.10 as an example, that means the compressive load will range from 1115 to 1784 lbs, depending upon the speed of lift. Since vertebral fracture is more common at loads above 1440 lbs, quick lifting action is clearly not a healthy activity for most to pursue.

SUMMARY

The main features that keep the load on the disc and the loads on the facets smallest are those that keep the weight closest to the spine and are conducted at slow speeds. Sometimes that means that the box or package to be lifted is kept as close to the body as possible. In other cases, where the force acting on the spine comes only from the weight of the body itself, postures should be chosen that keep the center of the body over the pelvis. Twisting activities under load are to be avoided. Strengthening of trunk muscles is an important means of reducing risk of spine disorders. Good body strength and knowledge of proper postural mechanics applied to daily routine help to keep recurring back pain at a minimum.

References

1. Pintar F: The biomechanics of spinal elements. PhD Dissertation. Marquette University, Milwaukee, WI, 1986.
2. Schultz AB, Andersson GBJ, Haderspeck K et al. Analysis and measurement of lumbar trunk loads in tasks involving bends and twists. Biomechanics 1982; 15(9):669-675.

7

VOLUNTEERS IN BACK SCHOOL MANAGEMENT

Elizabeth Kirkaldy-Willis

Medical services in Saskatchewan are free. In reality, this means that we pay for them through taxes. The University Hospital in Saskatoon cannot fund a full-time back school, although it does pay for two therapists and makes a lecture theater available once a week for 2½ hours. Back school is composed of two sessions, a beginners' session and from one to two weeks later, an advanced session. Any physician with admitting privileges at University Hospital can send patients to back school. Consequently, we teach a large number of patients, usually from 10 to 25 in the beginners' sessions and from 25 to 40 in the advanced sessions.

With so many patients, the two therapists cannot give individual time to each. For this reason, we have recruited ten volunteers, all of whom have had back problems and have been through back school. We need six volunteers for each session. In a typical session, one volunteer gives a talk on some aspect of pain. The volunteer has had it and is well qualified to talk about it. Briefly, he or she tells the story of the back problem and how back school helped. The volunteer outlines what he or she has found that makes the pain worse or better. The chief aim of the talk is to get the patients to see that they must become a part of their cure.

One advantage of having volunteers who have had back pain themselves is that patients learn by example. They see volunteers moving, bending, lifting, carrying, and—rarely—sitting during the course of a very busy afternoon. They know that every one had been a patient at one time or another, and they see that it is possible to function normally again.

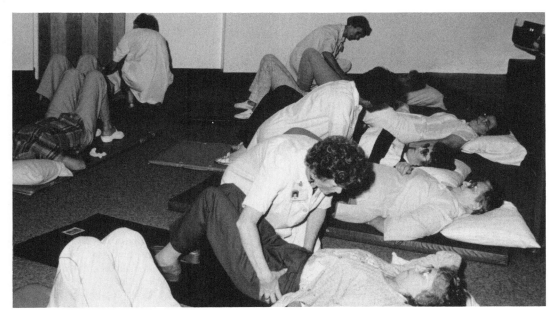

Figure 7.1. Beginners' session.

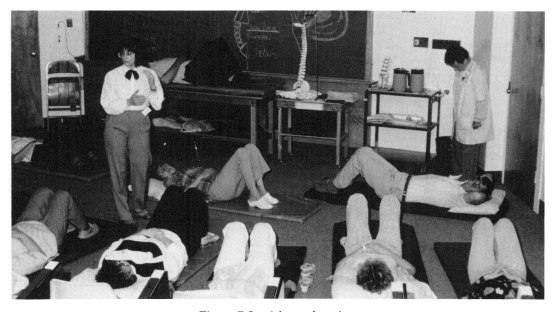

Figure 7.2. Advanced session.

8

BACK SCHOOL FOR CHILDREN

Patricia V. Kunse

In the field of rehabilitation, physical therapists and physicians have established industrial training programs and back schools in response to the increased attention to preventing back injuries. Education is also often used as the key ingredient in managing patients with low back pain (1). It has been demonstrated time and again that education does work to prevent or change the course of certain diseases. Articles in the *New England Journal of Medicine* (2) and the *American Journal of Nursing* (3) report that, merely through education, diabetes, rheumatoid arthritis, and hemophilia (4) can be controlled with a decreased need for emergency room visits and ongoing medical intervention. Scoliosis screening in the schools has decreased the amount of surgery because of early detection of the curves and bracing. Dentists have been so successful with their educational programs in the school system that they are brushing and flossing themselves out of business. Patients can develop an understanding of a disease, take responsibility and, to a large extent, control their pain.

It has also been shown that back schools or body mechanics training programs contribute to a decrease in the amount of time off from work and shorten the episodes of low back pain (5, 6). The success of these training programs makes it reasonable to assume that if education were started prior to the problem, there might be a chance to eliminate some of the problems altogether. The literature suggests that back pain is an uncommon affliction in children (7)—with the exception of athletes (8, 9)—but most children are familiar with the problem of low back pain as it affects the lives of their parents and grandparents. The literature also suggests that while young people can submit their spines to excessive stress and abuse without complaints of pain or disability, there could be an increasing tendency for those over thirty to develop low back pain associated with early postural strain (10).

The need to educate children in preventive back care has been brought up by Boulten-Davies in an article stressing education for the public (11). However, only a few people have attempted to implement preventive back care programs for children, since there are no guidelines as to what should be taught or at what level. Jensen, Spence, and Shepard did a study in 1984 to determine the effect of two teaching methods on children's ability to recall and demonstrate lifting techniques (12) and Donovan in the same year presented a two-day seminar to junior high school students on proper back care (13). With the limited information available from these experiences, Arthur H. White and I set up a prospective study (8) to evaluate a preventive back care program situated in a public school educational system at the high-school level.

Instituting back education in a public school system presented many challenges. Teachers were hard pressed to add new material to an already very full curriculum, no matter how important they thought the subject matter was. In addition, they required considerable education, time, and continued follow-up support to feel confident about delivering what was, after all, specialized material. Schools had little money for supporting such a project, so funding had to be found from outside sources, who in turn wanted guarantees of success before starting. It was gratifying that students were receptive to the information even though most had never experienced low back pain. We found that they did retain the information for a short time even with a limited exposure to the subject matter.

More studies need to be done to test alternative teaching methods and contexts than those of this study. One question under review is the best age at which to begin preventive back care training. In the Acalanes School system, we worked with students in high school. We are currently completing development of a program that will train elementary school children in grades 4 to 6. For either high school or elementary school, we have been reviewing teaching methods that allow an alternative to having the classroom teacher bear the brunt of the training. One of these is team teaching by the physical therapist and the teacher. The physical therapist can present the material, then both the classroom teacher and the physical therapist can guide students through practice and review. We have also found it important to shift the balance from a lecture and verbal testing methodology to one that emphasizes experience with student recognition and performance of the preventive guidelines as its goal.

A long-term goal, one part of which is close to completion, is to develop a teacher's guide and a student manual, as well as a videotape of the training material that will help structure and standardize the information presented. The teacher's guide and the student manual we are developing will be evaluated during a Backs for the Future program (15) we are implementing in the San Mateo County school system. Test instruments are also being developed in conjunction with our teaching materials that quantify both student recognition and performance of the guidelines for preventive back care. We want these instruments to allow us to follow control groups of students and trained students over time, tracking the results of our training program and correlating those results with whatever back pain students may develop as adults.

These shifts in our program, i.e., teaching context, methodology, testing, and materials, will be implemented in the San Mateo County school system soon (15). We believe that through our continued effort to extend and improve our program we can make a significant contribution to the quality of life of our community. We owe it to our children to help them

prevent back pain in later life through instruction in the essentials of spinal anatomy and biomechanics, ergonomic standards, and the maintainence of good health and muscle strength.

References

1. White AH and Zucherman J. The back school approach to low back pain. Musculoskel Med 1984; (11): 13–22.
2. Miller L, Goldstein J. More efficient care of diabetic patients in a county hospital setting. N Engl J Med 1972; 286:1388–1391.
3. Healy KM. Does preoperative instruction really make a difference? Am J Nurs 1968; (January): 62–67.
4. Levine P, Britten A. Supervised patient management of hemophilia. Ann Intern Med 1973; 78:195–201.
5. Moffet JK, Chase S, Portek I, Ennis J. A controlled, prospective study to evaluate the effectiveness of a back school in the relief of chronic low back pain. Spine 1986; 11(2):120–122.
6. Snook S, Campanelli R, Hart J. A study of three preventive approaches to low back injury. J Occup Med 1978; 20: 478–481.
7. Hoffman H. Childhood and adolescent lumbar pain: differential diagnosis and management. In Clinical Neurosurgery (CNS27): Proceedings of the Congress of Neurological Surgeons, Las Vegas, Nevada, 1979. Baltimore: Williams & Wilkins, 1980; 553–576.
8. Clark A. An unusual cause of back pain in a young athlete. Am J Sports Med 1985; 13(1): 51–54.
9. Micheli L. Low back pain in the adolescent; differential diagnosis. Am J Sports Med 1979; 7:362–364.
10. Keegan JJ. Alterations of the lumbar curve related to posture and seating. J Bone Joint Surg 1953; 35:589–609.
11. Boulton-Davies IM. Physiotherapists—teachers of the public. Physiotherapy 1979; 280.
12. Jensen G, Shepard K, Spence S. Comparison of methods of teaching children proper lifting techniques. Phys Ther 1984; 64:1055–1060.
13. Donovan T. Instruction of back care in the school system. American Physical Therapy Association, 1984.
14. Kunse P. Public School Prevention Program. Challenge of the Lumbar Spine. 1986.
15. Kunse P. Backs for the future. Presented to the California Physical Therapy Fund, Inc. 1989.

PATIENT-ACTIVE APPROACHES

9

STRENGTH TRAINING AND FLEXIBILITY

Joel S. Saal
Jeffrey A. Saal

Training programs for the rehabilitation of the lumbar spine progress from floor and manual resistance exercises to the use of resistance equipment. Training for strength and flexibility of the trunk and extremities is integral to the development of adequate postural control and stabilization skills. All patients must demonstrate a baseline level of skill in the floor exercise program before advancing to a gym training program. It is inadequate simply to tell a patient with resolving symptoms of a disc herniation to "go to the gym and work out." A properly structured training program in a gym can minimize the risk of injury through the use of weight training equipment, and maximize the gains from combined and coordinated muscle group activity. That type of training program should conceptually match the program of floor exercises because both are based on the principles of dynamic muscular stabilization of the spine.

It is important to emphasize that every spine patient does not need to commit to an extensive weight training program. The overall rehabilitation program should be designed for an individual patient's needs, with realistic and functional goals. Patients who are avid recreational athletes will usually require additional strength gains attainable only through a weight training program. This is certainly true of professional and high-level competitive athletes. These same considerations exist for patients involved in manual labor or in activities that require performing repetitive tasks with heavy loads.

The training goals of a gym program are similar to those of a floor exercise program. Development of trunk strength is essential for functionally stabilizing the spine (1). Increasing the strength and endurance of extremity musculature will limit the amount of stress placed on the spine and trunk during the performance of daily activities. Patients should be taught to use resistance equipment with spine safe techniques and in spine safe positions.

Extremity strength training techniques are targeted for the muscle groups that stabilize the trunk. These techniques are the ones most commonly used during floor exercises and spine safe lifting and bending. However, the benefits of performing extremity strength exercises are more than the targeting and training of specific sites of extremity strength. In addition, patients are instructed in cocontraction techniques that consist of active use of the trunk musculature to stabilize the spine while an extremity is working against resistance. Specific exercises are targeted for the prime trunk stabilizers, including the abdominal obliques, the latissimus dorsi (including all of its segments), the spine extensors, and the interscapular musculature (middle trapezius, serratus anterior, and rhomboids).

A weight training program must be carried out within the guidelines of the physiology of strength training (2–4). In order to increase muscle strength (power and endurance), a muscle must be exposed to an overload force. Exercising targeted muscle groups to the point of fatigue is essential in order to satisfy the principle of overload (2–4). Fatigue, for the purposes of this chapter, is the point at which an exercise can no longer be performed to a voluntary stimulus. This can be accomplished in weight training exercises by gradually increasing the weight, and using at least three to four *sets* (groups of repetitions of the exercise).

The number of repetitions may be varied depending on whether the patient is to acquire either endurance or power. *Endurance* refers to the length of time that an exercise can be performed with a given weight. *Power* is defined as the amount of work that can be performed (moving a weight through space) in a fixed period of time. Although any resistance exercise trains for both power and endurance, the overall effect depends on the method employed while training. For example, an exercise using a lesser weight performed in four sets of 12 repetitions will primarily train for endurance. The converse is true. An exercise using a heavier weight that generates fatigue in just three or four sets of four repetitions will primarily train for power. Each of these aspects of strength, *endurance* and *power,* is an important component of the training program. Training goals should be assessed for each patient individually to identify the type of training best suited for the targeted muscle groups. Furthermore, the specific targeted muscle groups would be emphasized somewhat differently in a football lineman compared with a recreational athlete who plays tennis and works at a sedentary occupation. The whole of the gym program will therefore have different points of emphasis in different patients.

Training for flexibility is another essential component of a program of spine stabilization. For passive trunk flexion to occur at the hips rather than about the axis of the lumbar spine, adequate flexibility in the hip and leg extensors, hip abductors and external rotators, flexors and knee extensors is important. The hamstrings, gluteus medius, the short hip rotators, quadriceps, iliopsoas, and gastrocnemius-soleus complex are specific sites which should be targeted for training. It is critical that stretching exercises be performed in a spine safe manner. Loaded trunk flexion and torsion are the primary areas of risk. Many of the flexibility techniques taught in school athletic programs and popular exercise video tapes are less than ideal for this reason, and should be avoided. However, flexibility is important, including the flexibility of such structures as the abdominal obliques, the facet joint capsules, and the thoracolumbar fascia. It is important that these stretches be carried out passively in a spine safe manner.

When prescribing flexibility exercises, clinicians need to keep in mind certain facts. Flexibility exercises increase the elasticity of connective tissue, not only that of loose connective tissue, but of the connective tissue of muscle and muscle contractile units (5). Connective tissue behaves viscoelastically (6). This means that it will deform in response to applied force and, if the force is large enough, it will return to a slightly longer length once the force stretching it is removed (7). In addition, a tissue's viscoelasticity will be enhanced in the presence of increased temperature (7, 8). Its increase in length will be greater if force is applied slowly. Thus, one should apply a stretch slowly, for an adequate period of time, after warming the tissue.

Actual lengthening of the muscle contractile units is accomplished by slightly different physiologic principles, but both sets of principles—for tissue elasticity and for muscle contractile unit lengthening—can be applied to good advantage together. The relationship of muscle fibers to each other is governed by neural factors as well as physical principles. Relaxation of incoming neural input is essential for lengthening a contractile unit (9). This relaxation is best accomplished by a stretch that occurs slowly and evenly and is accompanied by gentle contraction of the antagonist muscles. For example, gentle contraction of the ankle dorsiflexors while passively stretching the gastrocnemius-soleus complex facilitates a better stretch (10). Performing stretching exercises both before and after an exercise period has been demonstrated to result in increased flexibility gains (11). The ideal length of time for an individual to hold an isolated stretch is probably 15 to 30 seconds. Continuation of the stretch for a period longer than this will not generate any greater flexibility gains except in the case of pathologic contracture (12, 13).

EXERCISES

Flexibility exercises are divided into techniques that target joint mobility (mobilization exercises) and techniques that are designed to increase the elasticity of the musculotendinous unit (stretching exercises).

Upper Body Exercises

SHOULDER GIRDLE

Lateral Deltoid Raises in Standing Position

While the trunk musculature is actively recruited to maintain neutral position, the lateral deltoids are trained with dumbbell raises (Fig. 9.1). Active cocontraction of the abdominal oblique, transversus, rectus abdominis, and latissimus muscles with combined use of the spine extensors is reinforced. Care must be taken not to allow any forward flexing at the lumbar spine. A head forward posture that might place undue stress on the cervical spine should also be avoided.

Anterior Deltoid Raises in Standing Position

The anterior deltoids are important in daily activities, especially for participating in athletic activity. The principles are the same as those for the lateral raises in standing position.

Posterior Deltoid Raises

The trunk is inclined farther forwards than when performing other deltoid exercises (Fig.

9.2A). Care should be taken to allow no trunk flexion, but to place the trunk by flexion of the hips. Additional recruitment of the glutei stabilizes the trunk in this position. This is a more advanced exercise than the other deltoid raises. It can also be performed using a pulley system (Fig. 9.2 **B, C**). During the pulley exercise, all flexion should occur at the hips, and the weight of the trunk should rest on the nonexercising arm and leg. This will effectively unload the spine. It is very important that there be no flexing at the spine, that flexion occur only at the hips. Keeping the spine in slight extension can reinforce this protective effort.

Dumbbell Extensions

This exercise may be performed while lying prone on a bench, or bent forward at the waist in standing position, supporting the weight of the trunk on the nonexercising arm and leg (Fig. 9.3). The targeted muscle groups are the triceps, medial and long head, and the teres major. These same groups are also stretched during other exercises, but can be trained in relative isolation in this manner to gain additional training for throwing athletes or swimmers, as needed.

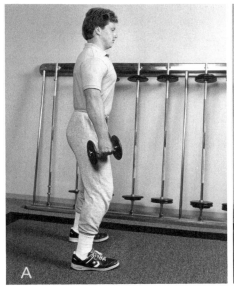
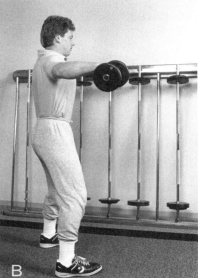

Figure 9.1. Lateral raises.

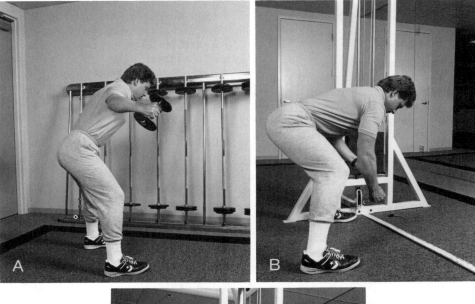

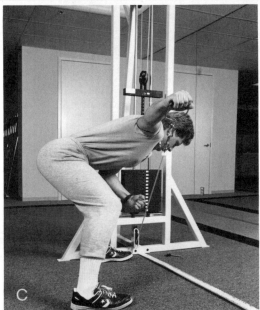

Figure 9.2. Posterior deltoid raises.

Upper Trunk (Interscapular) Training

Seated Rowing

This is an essential and pivotal exercise in the trunk strengthening program (Fig. 9.4). It is also associated with the risk of forced trunk flexion if performed incorrectly or carelessly.

The targeted muscle groups include the shoulder extensors (teres major, posterior deltoid, upper posterior latissimus) and the scapular retractors, including the upper and middle trapezius, rhomboid major and minor, and levator scapulae. This exercise develops the strength to resist the common tendency to thoracic kypho-

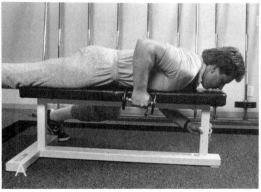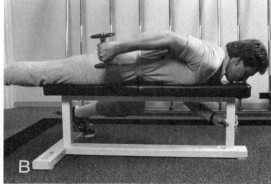

Figure 9.3. Dumbbell extensions.

sis. It must be performed with a stable and nonyielding lumbar posture with no flexion at the lumbar spine. Use of hip flexion is made to attain the starting posture of the exercise, but thereafter all motion occurs at the shoulders and scapulothoracic joint. No forward flexion, either at the hip or spine, is allowed against the resistance to the weight. The weight is pulled toward the waist, with the elbows kept close to the trunk. At the end of the motion, the weight must be returned to starting position with care.

Standing Rowing

This exercise requires the same principles and targeted muscle groups as the seated rowing exercise (Fig. 9.5). In the standing position, more emphasis is placed on the glutei and the lower spine extensors. Again, care must be taken to avoid any undue lumbar spine flexion. Using the extension line from a pulley station can reduce the risk of forced trunk flexion as the weight is lowered.

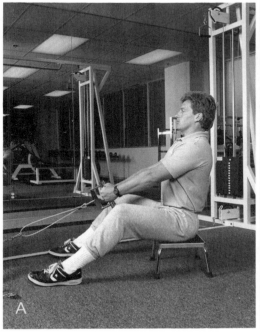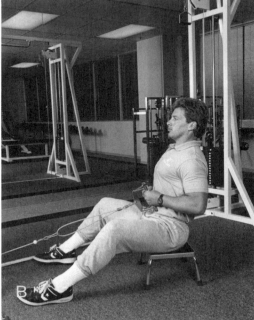

Figure 9.4. Seated rowing.

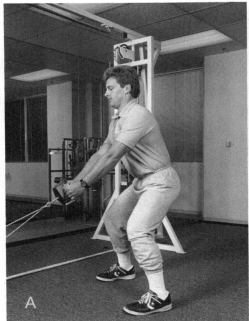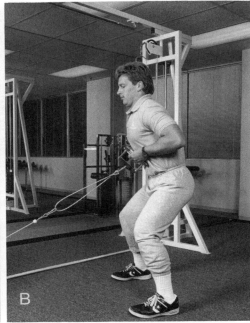

Figure 9.5.   Standing rowing.

Prone Flyes

This exercise trains the posterior deltoid and middle trapezius. Care should be taken not to allow excessive extension of the cervical spine, and the scapulae should be actively retracted (or pinched together) during its performance. To increase the effect on the cephalad scapular stabilizers (upper fibers of the middle trapezius, upper trapezius, levator scapulae, spine extensors), an incline bench with a 30° angle may be used.

Latissimus Pull downs

These exercises are part of an essential core of weight training exercises targeted for most spine patients who have advanced to a weight training program. They are performed in three different ways to target different components of the muscle group. The anterior and lower portions of the muscle along with the serratus anterior must be recruited by using a supinated close-hand grip (Fig. 9.6). Care should be taken to minimize thoracic spine extension and lumbar spine flexion. When the hands are placed in the pronated shoulder width position, the weight can be pulled toward the chest with the

trunk inclined backwards (Fig. 9.7). The trunk should be inclined at the hips, with the lumbar spine maintained in slight extension to avoid any forward flexion of the lumbar spine. The most popular method for performing this exercise consists of pulling the weight toward the back of the neck using a wide grip. Care must be taken to minimize forward head posture and lumbar spine flexion. Once body weight or a weight slightly less than body weight can be lifted, this muscle group can be best trained performing pull-ups to a stationary bar. The pull-ups are the most functional activity for this muscle group, and the exercise can be performed with the same relative positions as with the pulley bar.

Incline Bench Press with Dumbbells

The purpose of this exercise is to train the anterior deltoid and the clavicular and superior aspects of the sternal head of the pectoralis major (Fig. 9.8). It is important functionally because many daily activities require a propulsive motion similar to this action. Additionally, this exercise helps to promote balanced trunk strength in maintaining a shoulders-back profile.

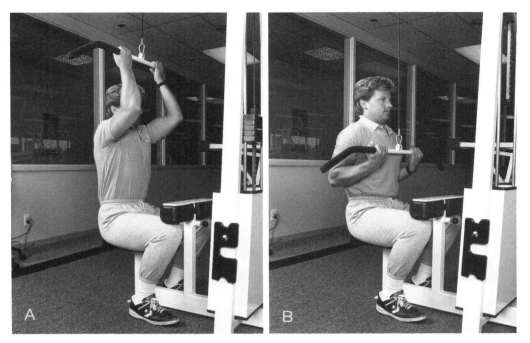

Figure 9.6. Latissimus pull-downs.

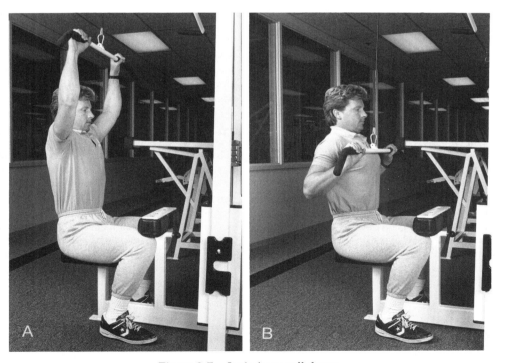

Figure 9.7. Latissimus pull-downs.

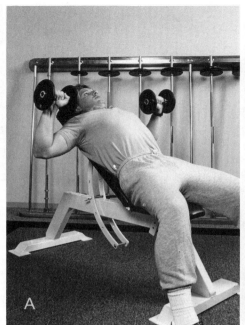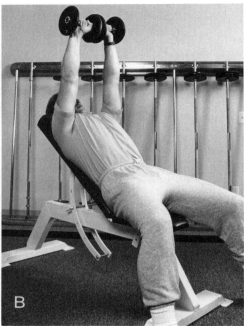

Figure 9.8.   Incline bench press with dumbbells.

Flat Bench Press with Barbell

The bench press is a standard part of any weight training program. Its function is similar to that of the incline dumbbell press, primarily training the sternal head of the pectoralis major and the triceps.

Cable Crossovers

A large variety of exercises can be performed with the use of pulleys (Fig. 9.9). One of the most important uses of pulleys is the standing cable crossover. This exercise trains the sternal portion of the pectoralis major and part of the clavicular head and, to a lesser degree, the long head of the biceps. The key to this exercise is the maintenance of a stable trunk with cocontraction of the lower abdominals, the glutei, and lower spine extensors while weight is moved by the upper extremities. The elbows are kept at approximately 15° of flexion, the hands open, and all of the motion is performed in horizontal adduction. No active elbow or wrist flexion is used. The exercise ends with arms crossed over one another in front of the chest.

Dumbbell Bicep Curls

This exercise is important for developing strength during elbow flexion, an important functional activity (Fig. 9.10). Additionally, it is important to ensure combined contraction of the abdominal muscles, and the glutei and spine extensors for maintenance of stable neutral posture which resists the pull of the weight.

Dip

This is an extraordinarily important exercise because of the cocontraction of several important muscles in a functional pattern (Fig. 9.11). The lower fibers of the pectoralis, the triceps, and the latissimus play a role here. Additionally, the combined contraction of the abdominal musculature to prevent arching or lurching while the body is lowered and raised smoothly trains functional stabilization patterns.

Lunges with Weight

Lunges with weight are part of the progression of lunges that are part of the floor program (Fig. 9.12). They are designed to train cocontraction

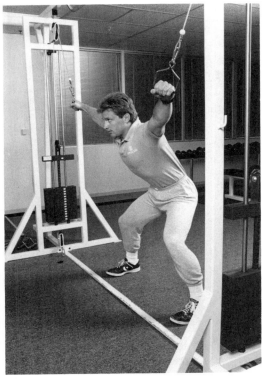

Figure 9.9. Cable crossovers.

of the lower abdominals, the glutei, and quadriceps.

Angled Leg Press

This exercise is an advanced training method (Fig. 9.13). The angle of motion reduces the stress on the patellofemoral joint while obtaining a functional pattern of contraction of the quadriceps, hamstrings, and glutei. It is important to include a slow lowering of the weight, as the eccentric component is the most functional (closest to natural human movement) portion of the exercise.

Hamstring Curls

It is very important that extension of the lumbar spine is minimized during this exercise. Patients with severe facet arthropathy and patients with severe central stenosis may not be able to perform this exercise without increased symptoms.

Seated Knee Extensions

Training of quadriceps strength is an essential component of a weight training program. How-

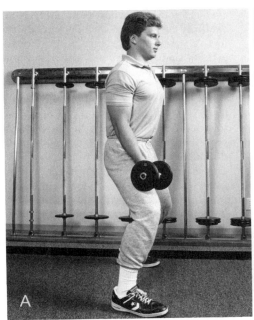
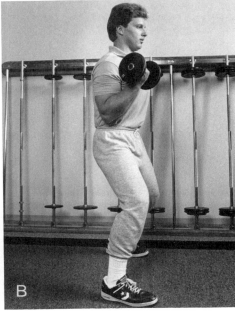

Figure 9.10. Dumbbell bicep curls.

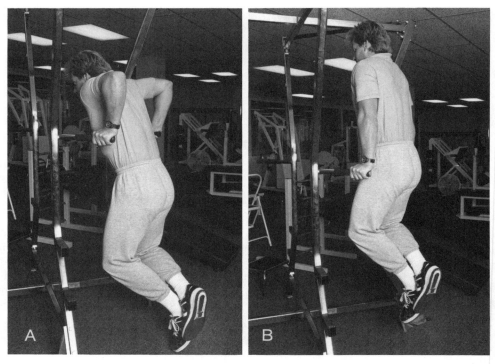

Figure 9.11. Dip.

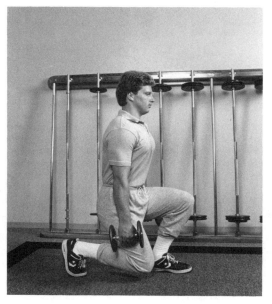

Figure 9.12. Lunges with weight.

ever, the role of this particular exercise must be carefully evaluated in each patient. This will effectively train strength in a range of quadriceps activity that is functional, although not as specifically functional as the angled leg press. It also has the disadvantage of increasing patellofemoral stress when performed with high weights and through the full range. Therefore, in order to avoid injury to the patella (especially inpatients with a history or symptoms of chondromalacia patellae), the weight must be raised and lowered smoothly, ideally form a starting point of 45° of knee flexion. It is equally important to avoid any lurching or arching of the lumbar spine in the terminal phase of the lift. The patient should be instructed to keep the lumbar spine pressed flat into the seat cushion, if necessary, with a lumbar roll placed for comfort.

Calf Raises

Calf raises can be incorporated into the program to add additional training to the gastroc-

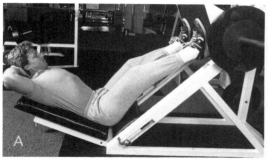
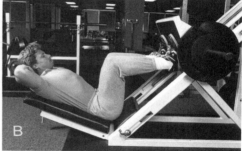

Figure 9.13. Angled leg press.

nemius-soleus complex. Good achilles flexibility is important prior to initiating the exercise.

Incline Board Curl-ups

As trunk strength increases, performing supine abdominal curl-ups will become easier. In order to continue to maintain strength (remember the overload princple), the amount of resistance or the number of repetitions must be increased. At the point where a patient can perform 100 to 120 curl-ups, it is time to move toward the in-

cline bench to increase the resistance. The adjustment of the angle of the bench can place the stress on the lower abdominal and obliques, as well as change the level of difficulty. It is important to keep the buttocks as the close to the leg support as possible. Maintenance of the lumbar spine flat against the bench is also important to protect the spine from injury. The trunk should only be raised so that the shoulder blades clear the bench. This exercise is performed straight ahead for the rectus (Fig. 9.14**A**) and when training the left (Fig. 9.14**B**)

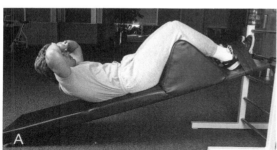
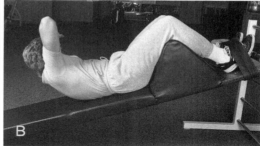
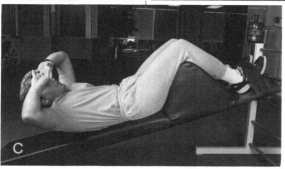

Figure 9.14. Incline board curl-ups.

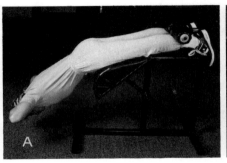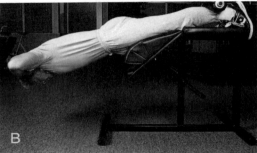

Figure 9.15. Hyperextension bench.

and obliques (Fig. 9.14**C**). These are performed as alternating curl-ups.

Hyperextension Bench

Spine extensor strength is trained by combining its use in the stabilization of the trunk with that of the muscles described in the preceding exercise (Fig. 9.15). However, to isolate the spine extensors with the glutei and train them safely, the hyperextension bench can be used very effectively. It is important to limit the degree of extension to the upper limit of normal lumbar lordosis in standing. This is accomplished by lowering the trunk from supine (0°) position to 60° trunk flexion. The trunk is then raised by a cocontraction of the spine extensors and the glutei to 0° and no higher. This will avoid excessive stress to the facet joints and neural elements of inpatients with stenosis. The spine extensors should not be used alone to lift the trunk; if they are, the patient will rapidly experience muscle fatigue and, possibly, low back pain.

Elevated Chair with Leg Raise and Lowering

An advanced exercise that further trains the lower abdominals is the leg raise from an elevated chair (Fig. 9.16**A**). A passive straight leg raise of 90° is necessary before this can be attempted. This is an essential exercise for the training of trunk strength in athletes. The abdominal muscles are used primarily in resisting the lowering of the legs. Therefore, the legs should be smoothly raised, avoiding any lurching or arching, followed by a slow lowering of the legs in unison. Until adequate strength is available for lowering the legs fully extended, the exercise can be performed productively with the knee flexed (Fig. 9.16**B**).

SUMMARY

Weight training programs are very effective in the rehabilitation of the lumbar spine patient. There are a myriad of exercises that can be used to attain goals for strength. The program must

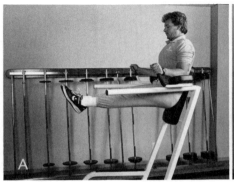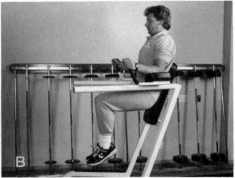

Figure 9.16. Leg raising and lowering from elevated chair.

be individually designed for each patient considering vocational and recreational interests. Adequate flexibility is essential for all lumbar spine patients. This strength and flexibility program must also be tailored for the individual, although there are several stretches that must be performed by all patients. Individual structuring of a program that is based on the physiologic principles of training for strength and flexibility can result in a more successful return to activity for the lumbar spine patient.

References

1. Saal JA, Saal JS. Nonoperative treatment of herniated lumbar intervertebral disc with radiculopathy: an outcome study. Spine 1989; 14(4):431–437.

2. Asterand PO, Rodahl M. Work physiology: physiologic basis of exercise. New York: McGraw Hill, 1986.

3. Brooks and Fahey. Exercise physiology: human bioenergetics and its applications. New York: Wiley, 1984.

4. Brooks and Fahey. Fundamentals of Human Performance. New York: Macmillan, 1987.

5. Saal JS. Aerobic and anaerobic training in the injured athlete. Rehabilitation of Sports Injuries. Saal JS. ed. Philadelphia: Hanley & Belfus, 1987.

6. Haut R, Little R. A constitutive equation for collagen fibers. Biomech 1972; 5:423–430.

7. LaBan M. Collagen tissue: implications of its response to stress in vitro. Arch Phys Med Rehab 1962; 43:461–466.

8. Lehmann J, Masock A et al. Effect of therapeutic temperature on tendon extensibility. Arch Phys Med Rehab 1970; 51–481–487.

9. Sherrington CS. The integrative action of the nervous system. New Haven: Yale UP, 1961.

10. Knott M, Voss DE. Proprioceptive neuromuscular facilitation. New York: Harper & Row, 1956.

11. Moller M, Oberg B, Gilquist J. Stretching exercise and soccer: effect of stretching on range of motion in the lower extremity in connection with soccer training. Intern J Sports Med 1985; 6:50–52.

12. Kottke F, Pauley D, Ptak R. The rationale for prolonged stretching for correction of shortening of connective tissue. Arch Phys Med Rehab 1966; 47:345–352.

13. Saal JS. Flexibility training In Rehabilitation of Sports Injuries. Saal JS. ed. Philadelphia: Hanley & Belfus, 1987.

10

PREGNANCY AND EXERCISE

Sandra Dutro
Lindsay Wheeler

It is well known that during pregnancy a woman is likely to develop back pain. According to a 1983 study by Melpomene, 46% of all pregnant women complain of back pain (1). There are two reasons: The first is the obvious physical strain created by the growing uterus; the second is the hormone relaxin. Relaxin is a peptide hormone thought to increase ligament laxity, soften cartilage, and cause proliferation of the synovium (2, 3). Concentrations are highest in the first trimester, probably preparing the woman's body to accommodate the gravid uterus. Relaxin levels drop approximately 20% after the first trimester but continue to be elevated until just a few days after delivery (4, 5). It is believed that at least the more dramatic changes are reversed within 3 months following delivery (6).

While relaxin is probably crucial for the changes necessary to accommodate the growing fetus and to make delivery possible, the resulting decreased stability of the pelvis and lumbar spine is an obvious liability.

A factor that may play a secondary role is the increased fluid retention in pregnancy. Fluid retention is well known as a contributor to the increased frequency of the various nerve entrapment syndromes associated with pregnancy (7, 8). Given the large number of back pain symptoms associated with local inflammation, it is logical to suspect that the edematous connective tissue will also play a role in increasing the pregnant woman's chances of experiencing back pain.

There are two ways of minimizing development of back pain during pregnancy and the child care that follows. One is careful body mechanics and the other is exercise.

The exercises below are designed especially for the pregnant woman. They are gentle and easy to control and therefore safe for the average perinatal woman. They are also rigorous enough, if done regularly, to maintain the tone and flexibility so valuable not only during the pregnancy and delivery but also, and perhaps more importantly, during the demanding stresses of the child care that follows.

You may note that we mention maintaining muscle tone and do not speak in terms of strengthening. While pregnancy is certainly not a time for muscle stagnation, it is equally not a time to begin major strength development. The key during pregnancy is to maintain good tone with a minimum of strain. The ideal time to begin a strengthening program is before becoming pregnant (9, 10).

Most of what is presented here is derived from yoga because yoga is an ideal source of low impact exercises for strengthening and flexibility. In addition, Yoga is ideally suited to the increased sensitivity and internal focus that many women are aware of during pregnancy and the postpartum period.

Four words of caution: First, while many of the exercises are common and the instructions are straightforward, many others involve complex postural awareness and should be prescribed with some instruction. Second, these exercises are not designed specifically to "cure a bad back." Done correctly by the right person, they are certainly capable of acting therapeutically but they should not be prescribed indiscriminately. Third, done in the order listed in the summary at the end of the exercise descriptions, the routine includes warm-ups and cool-downs. If the exercises are done in a different order, it will be important to include both a warm-up and a cool-down period. Fourth: pregnancy is not a time for a woman to push herself physically. The instructions for these exercises are intended to accommodate a wide range of strength and endurance. A pregnant woman should be encouraged to do only as much as she is comfortably able to do.

CHILD'S POSE

This first exercise is a yoga posture known as the child's pose. The child's pose is a relaxing stretch that can be beneficial for countering the hyperlordosis of pregnancy. Many women are also relieved to discover a position that allows some time prone. Below are three variations, each adapting to progressively more advanced stages of pregnancy.

1. This variation can be done during the first trimester. Kneel with the top of your feet against the floor and your knees and feet far enough apart to make room for your belly. Begin by sitting on the backs of your legs. Bend forward so that your forehead touches the floor and your arms lie relaxed and straight next to your legs. Relax.
2. As the pregnancy progresses, your knees will need to be further apart, your toes will point more directly toward one another. Instead of rounding your back, keep your back straight and stretch your spine forward from your hips. Lower your chest between your knees. Stretch your arms over your head. In the early stages of this trimester, your buttocks will sit as close to your feet as flexibility allows. Later in the pregnancy your belly will force your buttocks higher (Fig. 10.1A).
3. In the last trimester, it will be more comfortable to use pillows on which to rest your upper body. To do so, begin by kneeling on your hands and knees, your toes pointed toward one another, your knees apart, and two or three pillows in front of you. Stretch your spine forward from your hips, lowering your chest down to rest on the pillows. Your forearms should be supported comfortably on the floor in front of you. Your buttocks will be higher than your spine or head (Fig. 10.1B).

Duration: 15 seconds to 1 minute.

PELVIC TILT

The pelvic tilt is a classic exercise for pregnant women. It is a gentle and simple method to help maintain tone and symmetrical range of motion in the lumbar paraspinal musculature, abdomen, and pelvis—areas susceptible to the hormonal and mechanical stresses of pregnancy.

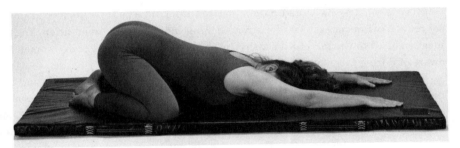

Figure 10.1.   A. Child's pose, 2nd trimester.

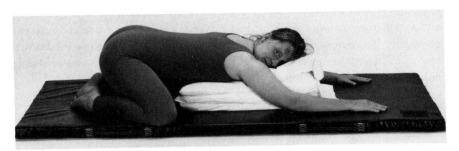

Figure 10.1.   B. Child's pose, 3rd trimester.

Assume a hook lying position (i.e., lie on your back with your knees bent and shoulder distance apart and your feet flat on the floor, approximately 6 inches in front of your knees). Rest your head on a pillow and keep it relaxed. Exhale as you use your abdominal and gluteal muscles to press your lower back towards the floor, As you do your pubic bone will be slightly lifted toward the ceiling. Relax. Repeat.

Done correctly, this movement will cause you to bring your lower ribs and your pelvis closer together. If, when your low back is closer to the floor, you find that you have raised your chest, relax your chest and allow your ribs to come closer to your pelvis.

Duration: 5 to 20 repetitions, holding pelvic tilt for 5 seconds.

Cat Stretch

In cases of women who have difficulty lying supine because of compromised circulation due to pressure of the uterus on the aorta and vena cava (11–13), the pelvic tilt should be performed on all fours or while lying on your side.

Assume a position on all fours with arms and thighs parallel. Exhale as you arch your back upward and lower your head, trying to round your spine to a safe and comfortable position, feeling a mild stretch (Fig. 10.2A). This position is similar to that of an alley cat, but with head down and muscles relaxed. Inhale as you return to the neutral position (Fig. 10.2B). If you are comfortable extending your lower back let your belly lower toward the floor as your face turns upward and you inhale.

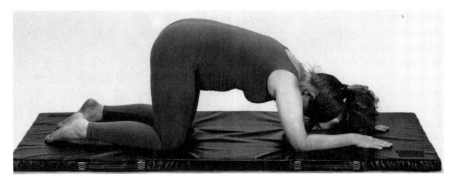

Figure 10.2. **A.** Pelvic tilt; cat stretch.

Duration: 5 to 20 repetitions, holding pelvic tilt for 5 seconds.
You can also try a sidelying pelvic tilt (Fig. 10.2C).

HIP, GROIN, LEG AND BUTTOCKS

Well known for its importance in minimizing the chances of back injury, good flexibility of the hip and groin also has an obvious advantage during childbirth.

Hip Stretch 1

Begin in a hook lying position. Place the outside of your left ankle on your right thigh close to your knee. Place your right hand just below your bent right knee (or on your thigh behind your knee) and your left hand on the inner side of your left knee. Now pull your right knee into your chest as you press your left knee away from you. You should feel a stretch at the back of your left buttock. Hold the position, breathing comfortably, until you feel yourself begin to tire. Relax and repeat on the other side (Fig. 10.3).

Duration: For most, it will be best to begin with 5 to 10 seconds. As you become comfortable with the exercise, duration can be extended to 1 to 2 minutes.

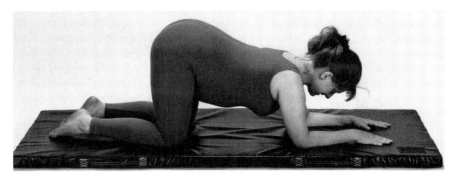

Figure 10.2. **B.** Neutral

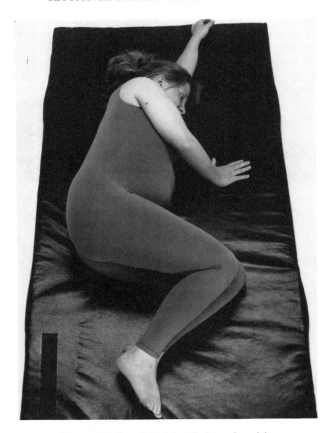

Figure 10.2.   C. Pelvic tilt, lateral position.

Hip Stretch 2

Begin again in a hook lying position. Bring one knee toward your chest. Grasp the inside and bottom of your right foot with your right hand. Pull down on your foot. In this position the bottom of your foot should be facing the ceiling and your knee

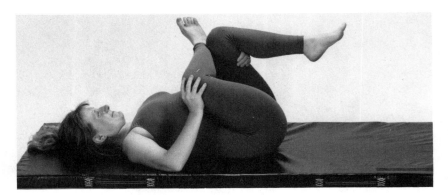

Figure 10.3.   Hip stretch 1.

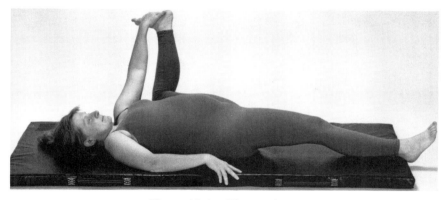

Figure 10.4. Hip stretch 2.

should be forming a right angle. Let your thigh and knee drop toward the floor along the side of your torso. Relax and repeat on the other side (Fig. 10.4).

Duration: For most it will be best to begin with 5 to 10 seconds. As you become comfortable with the exercise, duration can be extended to 1 to 2 minutes.

Note: These two hip stretches are particularly beneficial for women with sacro-iliac dysfunction.

Groin Stretch

Sitting erect, preferably with your back against a wall, place the soles of your feet together in front of you. Grasp your shins and use the leverage of your grasp to help support yourself. This leverage will make it easier for you to sit up straight. Gently bring your feet as close to your pubis as you are comfortably able without sacrificing the position of your back. Let your knees drop toward the floor. Feel the stretch in your inner thighs. You should not bounce your legs or force the stretch but you can use your forearm to increase the stretch gently. Hold, breathing comfortably until you feel yourself begin to tire. Relax and repeat (Fig. 10.5**A**).

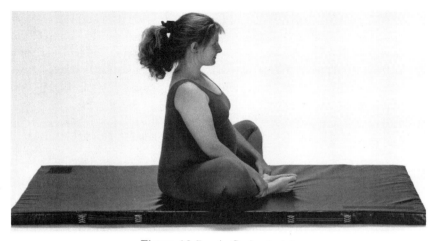

Figure 10.5. **A.** Groin stretch.

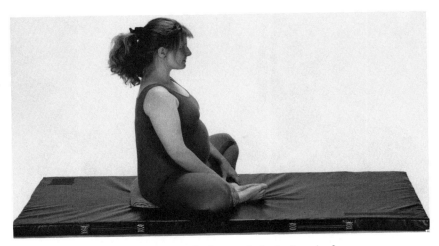

Figure 10.5. **B.** Groin stretch, buttocks raised.

Note: To help you comfortably maintain the normal spinal curves while you are doing this exercise, you may find it useful to place a blanket folded to a thickness of 3 or 4 inches under your buttocks so that your buttocks are higher than your feet (Fig. 10.5**B**).

Duration: For most it will be best to begin with 5 to 10 seconds. As you become comfortable with the exercise, duration can be extended to 1 to 2 minutes.

Hip Flexor Stretch

Beginning on hands and knees, bring your left foot forward to the outside of your left hand: This will cause your left leg to form a right angle. As you do so, be careful that all bending takes place at your hips. (Do not bend at your waist). This will allow your spinal curves to remain in their neutral position. (An alternative way to get into this position is to lower yourself into a half kneeling position first, i.e., your left leg is bent in front of you with your left foot flat on the floor and you are kneeling on your right knee.) Now slide the right knee back until you feel a stretch in the front of your right groin. Breathing slowly hold this position and let the right groin and thigh relax further. You may want to slide your right leg further back to increase the stretch as your muscles relax. Hold, breathing comfortably until you begin to tire. Repeat on the other side.

Duration: For most it will be best to begin with 5 to 10 seconds. As you become comfortable with the exercise, duration can be extended to 1 to 2 minutes.

Squat

Squat as shown below (Fig. 10.6 **A,B**). If hip, leg and back flexibility do not allow you to squat low enough for comfort, try placing a book under your buttocks (Fig.

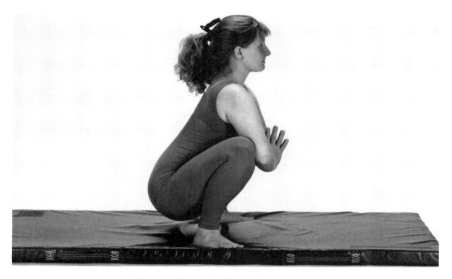

Figure 10.6. **A.** Squat, lateral view.

10.6C). Your feet will be slightly turned out. Be sure that your knees are directly over your feet and that your feet do not roll inward. Hold, breathing comfortably until you feel yourself begin to tire. Relax and repeat.

Duration: For most it will be best to begin with 5 to 10 seconds. As you become comfortable with the exercise, duration can be extended to 1 to 2 minutes.

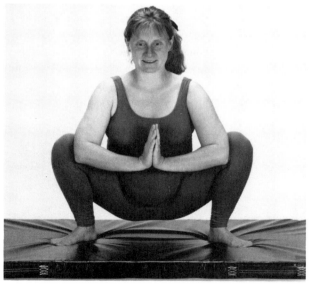

Figure 10.6. **B.** Squat, anterior view.

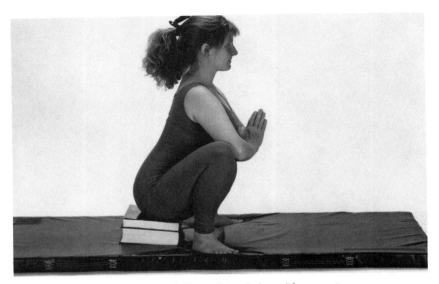

Figure 10.6. C. Squat, lateral view with support.

Bridge

This is one of the most popular and possibly one of the best overall strengthening exercises for pregnant women. It is gentle, it stimulates circulation to the vulnerable pelvic and lumbar region of the body, and it strengthens buttocks, legs, and low back.

Assume a hook lying position. Do a pelvic tilt. Holding the pelvic tilt, inhale as you lift your buttocks off the floor until your pelvis, abdomen and legs form a straight line (do not arch your back). Exhale as you lower. Repeat three times (Fig. 10.7).

Duration: For most it will be best to begin with 5 to 10 seconds. As you become comfortable with the exercise, duration can be extended to 1 to 2 minutes.

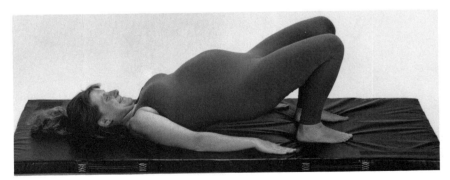

Figure 10.7. Bridge.

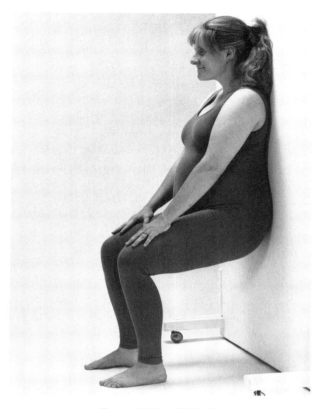

Figure 10.8.   Wall slide.

Wall Slide

Stand with your back flat against the wall. Place feet a distance in front of the wall equal to the length of your thighs. Find the most comfortable position for your back, either a pelvic tilt or maintaining the normal spinal curves. Slide down the wall until your legs form right angles with your thighs. Be careful not to drop so far that your knees are in front of your feet. Hold until you begin to tire. Straighten (Fig. 10.8).

If discomfort, difficulty in maintaining balance, or lack of strength make it difficult for you to hold a 90° angle, begin with your feet closer to the wall and slide down the wall as far as you are comfortably able. The larger angle between the back of your leg and the back of your thigh will give you more control.

Duration: For most it will be best to begin with 5 to 10 seconds. As you become comfortable with the exercise, duration can be extended to 1 to 2 minutes.

ABDOMINAL TONE

When working with pregnant women, it is crucial to address the question of abdominal tone not only because of the role of abdominal muscles in maintaining lumbar stability and protecting the back, but also because pregnant women are concerned with the cosmetic effects of lost abdominal tone. This concern may result in women carrying out an exercise program that will do more harm than good.

Diastasis recti, the stretching and separation of the rectus abdominis muscles, is a common occurrence during pregnancy. According to a 1986 study by Boissonnault, 27% of all second trimester women and 66% of all third trimester women test positive for diastasis (14). The etiology of this stretch injury is still unproven but it is believed to be due to the simultaneous softening of the abdominal connective tissue as the abdominal wall becomes distended (15). Regardless of the cause, a severe diastasis is not only unattractive, it can also compromise one's capabilities in the activities of daily living (16).

Prevention seems to include good muscle tone and avoidance of stressful increases in intraabdominal pressure.

Depending on the extent of the separation, a diastasis recti may or may not result in a bulge of the abdominal wall upon an increase in intraabdominal pressure. The contraction of a curl-up is an especially famous example. For this reason, the pregnant woman must take special care when working the abdominal muscles. The first exercise below takes into consideration and compensates for an existing diastasis while the second allows a somewhat more vigorous workout with minimal risk to the rectus abdominis.

1.   Assume a hook lying position. Take a normal breath and exhale fully, pulling your abdomen and ribs as close to the floor as you are able. You should feel a contraction of both upper and lower abdominal muscles. Release the contraction and let your lungs fill with air again. The key to the protective element of this exercise is the exhalation during the contraction (17). Be sure to pay attention to your timing. Repeat (Fig. 10.9A).

(*Note:* the practitioner should be careful to observe the patient performing this exercise, being especially conscious of contraction of both upper and lower abdominals and of the breathing pattern.)

Duration: Up to 2 minutes.

To tone diagonal muscles, continue to contract abdominal muscles and with your head still resting on the ground raise one knee toward your chest as you si-

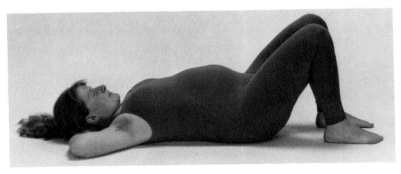

Figure 10.9. **A.** Abdominal contraction.

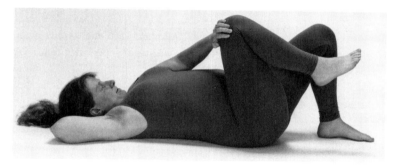

Figure 10.9. **B.** Oblique abdominal contraction.

multaneously bring your opposite arm to meet your knee. Press isometrically, knee against hand (Fig. 10.9**B**).

Duration: Hold each position 5 seconds, two to ten times per side.

2. If your abdominal muscles are strong and accustomed to exercise, you may try lifting head and neck off the floor as you perform exercise one (Fig. 10.9**C**). To avoid strain to the muscles of your neck, concentrate on keeping musculature relaxed. Similarly, do not pull your head forward and lose the normal cervical curve. It is helpful to keep your eyes directed at a spot on the ceiling to prevent you from pulling your head forward. Some find it helpful to cradle their neck in their interlocked fingers. Continue breathing with normal inhalation and full exhalation. If you see or feel a soft bulge protruding from the center of your belly stop and return to variation number one.

Duration: For most it will be best to begin with 5 to 10 seconds. As you become comfortable with the exercise, duration can be extended to 1 to 2 minutes.

Note: Noble has hypothesized that by placing your hands across and on opposite sides of the abdomen and pulling hands towards the midline, you will minimize the tendency of the muscles to separate (18). The success of this approach has never been demonstrated scientifically, but it does have an inherent logic.

Duration: For most it will be best to begin with 5 to 10 seconds. As you become comfortable with the exercise, duration can be extended to 1 to 3 minutes.

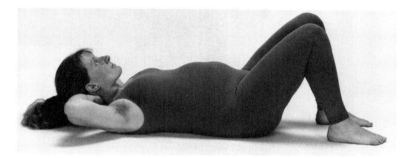

Figure 10.9. **C.** Abdominal contraction, raised head and neck.

UPPER BACK, CHEST, AND NECK

With the mechanical stresses of pregnancy and child care one tends toward hyper-kyphotic postures. These exercises will help counter the postural tendency and to reduce stress.

The first five can be done any time, standing or sitting. They can be done either as an organized set or individually.

Shoulder Roll

Sitting or standing erect, roll your shoulders backwards with a continual circular motion, making your circles as full as you can (Fig. 10.10).

Duration: 10 to 20 times.

Chest Stretch

Sitting or standing erect, place your hands behind your neck, elbows pointing side-ways, away from your body. Press elbows back as far as you can. Relax, repeat (Fig. 10.11).

Duration: Hold 10 seconds, one to three times.

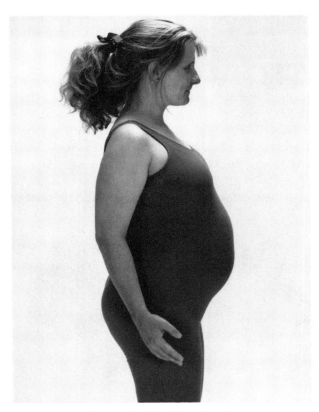

Figure 10.10. Shoulder roll.

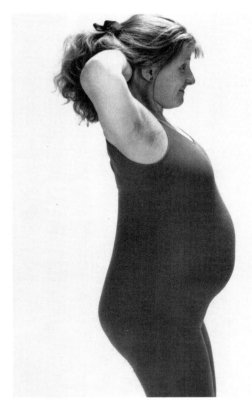

Figure 10.11. Chest stretch.

Rotational Shoulder Stretch

Sitting or standing erect, place your right hand over your right shoulder as if to scratch as far down your spine as possible. The palm of your hand should be flat and facing your back. Place your left hand behind your waist and move it up your spine as far as possible. The palm of your hand should be flat and facing away from your back. If you can reach, clasp your hands together and then pull your hands in opposite directions. Be careful not to exaggerate your lumbar curve while attaining this position, especially if you are standing (Fig. 10.12**A**).

You may not be able to clasp hands. If not, hold a towel in the upper hand and grasp the dangling end of the towel with the other hand. Move your hands as close together as possible without straining. Relax a moment to adapt to the stretch, then gently pull hands in opposite directions. Change sides and repeat (Fig. 10.12**B**).

Duration: For most it will be best to begin with 5 to 10 seconds. As you become comfortable with the exercise, duration can be extended to 1 minute.

Chicken Wings

Stand erect, chin tucked toward your neck and feet shoulder distance apart. Bend your arms at the elbows so that yuor arm and forearm form about a 120° angle.

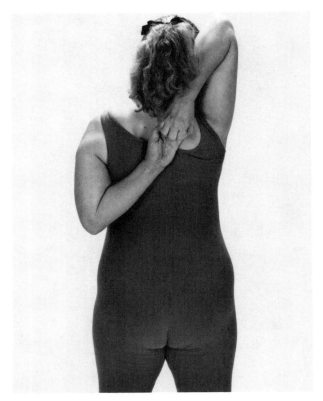

Figure 10.12.   A. Rotational shoulder stretch.

Raise elbows so that they are approximately 3 inches below shoulder height. Squeeze shoulder blades together by pulling elbows behind your back and toward one another. Use abdominal and gluteal muscles to help you avoid arching your back (Fig. 10.13).

Duration: Hold 5 seconds, five to twenty-five times.

Pectoral Stretch

Stand erect facing a corner, approximately arm's distance away from the corner, feet shoulder distance apart and chin tucked. Place hands on each wall at shoulder height and a distance from the corner that is equal to the length of your forearm. Adjust foot position so that feet are the same distance or slightly further from the corner than your hands. Slowly lean toward the wall bringing shoulder blades together and feeling the stretch. Repeat with hands 6 inches above the elbow.

Duration: Hold 5 to 10 seconds, three times in each position.

Shoulder and Upper Back Stretch

You will need to use a chair without arms and with a firm seat for this stretch.

Kneel in front of the seat of the chair and grasp the back of the chair, your elbows

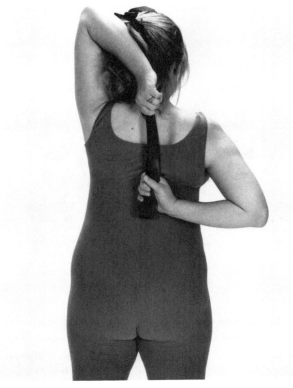

Figure 10.12. **B.** Rotational shoulder stretch with belt.

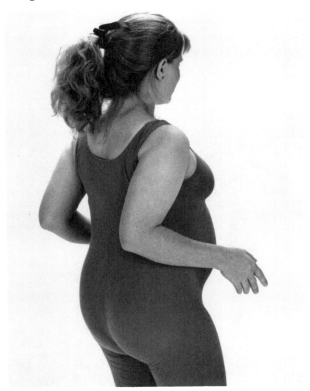

Figure 10.13. Chicken wings.

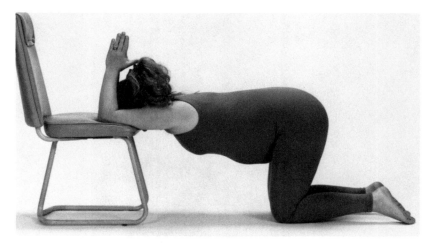

Figure 10.14.   Shoulder and upper back stretch.

in line with your shoulders and the seat. Depending on the length of your arms and the chair, your elbows will be at about the center of the seat. Now walk backwards on your knees so that your upper arms lie on the seat. Your knees should be hip width apart and directly under your hips. Clasp your hands and press down with your elbows and upper arms. Notice your posture and be careful to maintain the normal spinal curves. Breathe evenly and comfortably. You will feel stretching in your shoulders and across your upper back (Fig. 10.14).

Duration: For most it will be best to begin with 5 to 10 seconds. As you become comfortable with the exercise, duration can be extended to 1 minute.

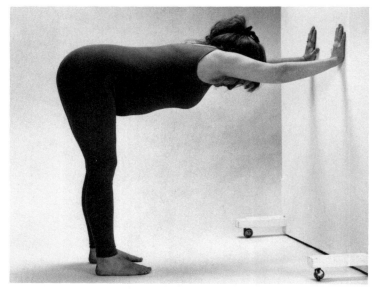

Figure 10.15.   **A.** Straight back stretch, hands even with waist, 90° hip angle.

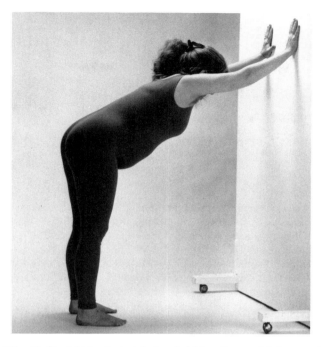

Figure 10.15.   B. Straight back stretch, hands higher than waist, increased hip angle.

Straight Back Stretch

Place your hands shoulder width apart on a wall at about waist height or higher, depending on your flexibility. The more flexible you are the lower your hands will be. Walk backwards so that your arms straighten and your legs are under your hips, hip width apart. Lower your head, bringing your ears between your extended arms. Begin to stretch out your entire spine. To accomplish this push your buttocks up and out behind you, flatten your mid-back (thoracic spine), extend the top of your head toward your hand support and press your hands into your hand support. Rotate your upper arms outward. You may want a mirror or a spotter to guide you in moving your back so that it becomes as flat and straight as possible. Hold, relax and repeat (Fig. 10.15).

Note: Alternatively you may place your hands on a table, desk, or ledge that is waist height or greater.

Duration: For most it will be best to begin with 5 to 10 seconds. As you become comfortable with the exercise, duration can be extended to 30 seconds.

SUMMARY

Exercises are performed in this order:

1. Pelvic tilt
2. Child's pose
3. Squat
4. Hip Stretch 1

5. Hip Stretch 2
6. Groin Stretch
7. Hip Flexor Stretch
8. Bridge

9. Wall Slide	14. Chicken Wings
10. Abdominal Set	15. Pectoral Stretch
11. Shoulder Roll	16. Straight Back Stretch
12. Chest Stretch	17. Pelvic Tilt
13. Rotational Shoulder Stretch	18. Child's Pose

Acknowledgment

We are grateful to Kathleen Coco for modeling.

References

1. Castor L. Pregnancy and fitness: a bibliography. The Melpomene Report 1983; 2:23.
2. Bryant-Greenwood G. Relaxin as a new hormone. Endocrine Reviews 1982; 3(1):62–87.
3. Martin LL. Health care for women. New York: JB Lippincott, 1978; 128.
4. O'Byrne EM, Carriere BT, Sorensen L et al. Plasma immunoreactive relaxin levels in pregnant and nonpregnant women. J Clin Endocrinol Metab 1978; 47:1106.
5. Eddie LW, Lester A, Bennett G, et al. Radioimmunoassay of relaxin in pregnancy with an analogue of human relaxin. Lancet 1986; 1(8494):1344–1346.
6. Romen Y, Artal R. Physiological and endocrine adjustments to pregnancy. In Exercise in pregnancy. Artal R, Wiswell RA, eds. Baltimore; Williams & Wilkins, 1986:59.
7. Friedman MJ: Orthopaedic problems in pregnancy. In Exercise in pregnancy. Artal R, Wiswell RA eds. Baltimore: Williams and Wilkins, 1986:215.
8. Kopell HP, Thompson W. Peripheral entrapment neuropathies. Huntington, WV: Krieger, 1976.
9. Artal R, Wiswell RA eds. Exercise in pregnancy. Baltimore: Williams and Wilkins. 1985.
10. Shangold M, Mirkin G. The complete sports medicine book for women. New York: Simon and Schuster. 1985.
11. Kerr M, Scott D, Samuel D. Studies of inferior vena cava in late pregnancy. Br Med J 1964; 1:532.
12. Kerr M. The mechanical effects of the gravid uterus in late pregnancy. J Obs Gyn Br Comm 1965; 72:513.
13. American College of Obstetricians and Gynecologists. Guidelines for exercise during pregnancy and postpartum. Washington D.C. 1985.
14. Boissonnault J. The incidence of diastasis during the childbearing year. Unpublished manuscript, 1986.
15. Mac Lennan A. The role of relaxin in human reproduction. Clin Reprod Fertil 1983; 2:77.
16. Wilder E. Obstetrics and gynogologic physical therapy. New York: Churchill Livingston, 1986.
17. Noble E. Essential exercises for the childbearing year. Boston: Houghton-Mifflin, 1982.

11

THE McKENZIE METHOD

Ronald G. Donelson

As I began my orthopedic practice in 1978, my enthusiasm for sports medicine paralleled my dislike for treating low back pain. In that first year of private practice however, I was introduced to the then-new "McKenzie approach" to low back pain by a local physical therapist. This "unorthodox" treatment utilized extension rather than the flexion to which I was accustomed. The impressive treatment results I was seeing, however, progressively drew my attention. With time, I was also attracted by the commonality of the mechanical principles underlying this approach and those in other areas of orthopedics.

With greater use and understanding on my part, the McKenzie approach has proven to be of immense assistance in effectively evaluating and treating low back pain patients. It is a very rare patient who now requires hospitalization or surgery. The selection of surgical patients, and therefore surgical outcomes, is much improved because of the invaluable information obtained from the mechanical evaluation process.

Because I now have a productive understanding of the low back pain problem and its solution, my previous dissatisfaction in treating low back pain gradually dissipated; my clinical time is now totally devoted to the care of these fascinating patients. I have likewise ceased performing surgery altogether and function strictly in an office setting evaluating and treating this needy patient population.

It is not within the scope of this brief chapter to cover the extensive work of Robin McKenzie. His text, *The Lumbar Spine, Mechanical Diagnosis and Therapy* (1), is highly recommended as perhaps the most pertinent and practical book written on the low back.

But if this McKenzie approach is so good, where are the studies to prove that it is better than the natural history of the untreated disease?

All treatments for low back pain must ultimately address this question and demonstrate improved rate of recovery over the simple passage of time. Quite simply, as many as 90% of low back patients recover within 3 months, regardless of treatment. If recovery from low back pain were this simple however, this book would likely not have been published.

Another very important statistic is that 60 to 70% of patients with low back pain have recurrent episodes, which usually become progressively more severe. So the challenge is not just the isolated acute episode, most of which resolve without treatment, but the prevention of future episodes. It is to this very issue that the McKenzie approach contributes so much.

To study a problem as complex and subjective as back pain requires rigid criteria in a prospective, randomized, blinded comparison study. One such study (2) was reviewed by DiMaggio and Mooney (3) and compared the McKenzie program with the Cottrell 90/90 Back Trac system and traditional back school in the treatment of all low back patient types, exclusive of those symptomatic for more than 1 year, postsurgicals, and those with neurologic deficits or significant radiographic findings. While overall study conclusions were limited by a larger than expected patient attrition rate, the results are noteworthy.

In the first week of treatment, when just the passage of time (and no other treatment) results in a 40 to 50% recovery rate, 97% of the McKenzie group responded favorably, while only 50% and 38% of the traction and back school groups, respectively, improved.

Clearly something more than just the passage of time contributed to these patients' recoveries. In fact, one would be hard pressed not to conclude that the underlying pathology is in some way being more specifically addressed by the McKenzie program than by the other two treatment programs. The success of the McKenzie method lies in the fact that each patient is mechanically assessed to determine the proper individual treatment.

In two separate comparison studies (4, 5), the McKenzie approach proved to be much more effective than Williams' exercises in the rapid return of range of motion and straight-leg raising, the average time spent in treatment, rapidly diminishing pain, and fewer recurrences.

CENTRALIZATION: THE BASIS FOR THE McKENZIE APPROACH

Centralization is the rapid movement of perceived pain from a peripheral location toward the midline or center of the back or neck. It was first observed in 1956 by McKenzie during a routine clinic appointment with a patient experiencing low back and leg pain for 3 weeks. The patient was inadvertently positioned prone on a table that had its head elevated causing hyperextension of the lumbar spine. In this position, rapid abolition of his leg pain occurred and remained so, even after ceasing that position.

Lumbar end-range extension was explored in subsequent patients, many of whom responded favorably and quickly as described, but the pain in others was made much worse by this position. Subsequent trials with other positions and movements identified other pain behavior categories that were later described by McKenzie.

In a study of patients with low back and radiating leg pain (6), the centralization phenomenon occurred in 87% of the patients during the evaluation period. Ninety-eight per cent of patients with symptoms for 4 weeks or less whose pain centralized during evaluation had excellent or good results. Of those whose pain could not be centralized during initial assessment, only 27% had good or excellent results.

Four patients (5% of the study group), none of whom attained centralization, underwent surgery. Three of these had extruded disc fragments that were predicted during the therapist's attempt at treatment and then confirmed by CT scan.

This progressive elimination of the distal symptoms with repeated end-range movements and positions would seem to indicate that the underlying pathology is being addressed (6–9). Elimination of the distal pain followed by the central pain and return to full function would seem to be the ultimate goal of treatment. Conversely, any treatment that intensifies the pain or causes it to extend further down the leg would seem to be counterproductive and an aggravation of the pathology.

FURTHER PERSPECTIVE

Because it occurs so commonly and is so rapid, centralization of distal pain is likely the most dramatic demonstration of the McKenzie approach to spinal pain. Other patients, however, with no peripheral pain, can eliminate their central pain just as rapidly and it will remain abolished as long as the spine is not bent in the direction opposite to that which centralized the pain.

It is in the sorting out and treatment of simple low back pain, without referred symptoms, that McKenzie's subsequent investigation of pain behavior with end-range positions and movements has proven to be so useful. Subgroups of simple low back pain can also be identified, which then respond to specific treatments (8).

It should not be surprising that proper care of a complex problem like low back pain requires an evaluation and treatment system of some sophistication. The McKenzie program has over 40 treatment exercise combinations. Flexion, extension, and transverse side gliding (Fig. 11.1–11.3), and occasionally a flexion/rotation combination, may need to be done in different sequences and combinations, sometimes standing, sometimes nonweightbearing (recumbent), but always determined by monitoring the patient's pain location and intensity while being tested. Space simply does not allow for great detail in this presentation.

McKENZIE CATEGORIES OF LOW BACK PAIN

McKenzie describes three separate categories of mechanical pain (1), each of which can be iden-

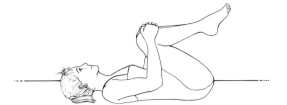

Figure 11.1. Flexion.

tified through the mechanical testing routinely performed with each patient. Patients may fall in one of these categories solely or in some combination of the three.

It must again be emphasized that these categories were not predetermined by McKenzie, but came as the result of his repeated clinical observations of pain behavior responding to repeated end-range movements and positions. The naming of each category is based upon its correlation with pain behavior known elsewhere in the body where the underlying pathology is better understood.

Table 11.1 summarizes these three categories of low back pain in terms of historical and mechanical characteristics on assessment, and lists the specific treatment for each.

A brief description of each category follows, while details of how to differentiate one from the other during testing must be left to McKenzie's text (1) or courses.

Postural Syndrome

It is not true that all patients presenting with low back pain must have underlying pathology; the simplest form of mechanical low back pain has no underlying pathology. It can be the result of the mechanical deformation of free nerve endings within normal periarticular structures.

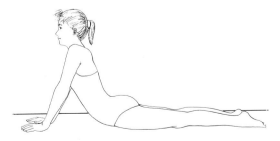

Figure 11.2. Extension.

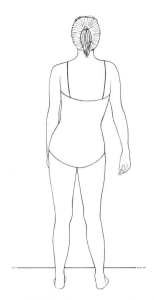

Figure 11.3. Transverse slide gliding.

A shoulder placed into a hammer lock position, or a finger bent backward and held there, can cause severe pain, yet absolutely no pathology exists. Treatment for the pain is the simple cessation of the end-range stretch of the offended normal tissues. The precise identity of the pain-producing tissues under stretch is of no importance in identifying the needed treatment for the pain, removal of the end-range stretch.

Pain similarly occurs in the low back when soft tissue structures are overstretched, most commonly at end-range flexion. Postural lumbar pain typically is central and appears only when normal supporting soft tissues are placed on end-range overstretch. The maintenance of end-range stretch with slouched sitting, hanging on our ligaments, will create this pain, yet no pathology need exist. The pain disappears when the stretch is removed.

As with hammer-lock pain, it is important to note when examining patients with lumbar end-range postural pain that no pain, limitation of movement, or other positive findings can be found. Their pain can only be reproduced with return to the sustained position of end-range overstretch (best tested with prolonged slouched sitting). The pain is then quickly abolished by movement, relieving the end-range stretch.

Treatment simply involves the avoidance of

Table 11.1.
McKenzie's Three Categories of Lumbar Pain and Their Respective Characteristics

	Posture	Dysfunction	Derangement
Age	Usually under 30.	Usually over 30.	Usually 20–45.
Pain	Intermittent;	Intermittent;	Constant or intermittent.
	Central.	Central	Local or referred.
		(Referred only in	
		adherent root).	
History	Gradual onset;	Gradual onset.	Often sudden onset or
	No reason;	Follows chronic poor	following sustained
	Sedentary occupation.	posture; trauma,	position.
		derangement,	History of recurrence.
		degenerative	
		spondylosis.	
		Now chronic.	
Worse	Static load at end-range.	End-range movement.	With certain movements,
		End-range position.	sustaining certain
			positions.
Better	Change position or when	Better with regular	With other movements
	moving.	activity.	and other positions.
Exam	Full, painfree movement,	No deformity, pain at	Poor posture, Deformity
	poor prolonged sitting	end-range only.	common.
	or standing posture	Stops shortly.	Causes pain increase or
	produces pain.	Pain radiates only	decrease. Pain
		with adherent	centralizes/
		nerve root.	peripheralizes and
			remains better/worse
			as result.
Treatment	Correct posture.	Exercise in the	Correct deformity.
	Educate.	restricted direction	Exercise in centralizing
		& produce stretch	direction. Teach self-
		pain.	correction.
		Correct posture.	Essential to correct
		Educate.	posture.
			Educate.

prolonged positions, usually by frequent interruption of them and improvement of posture. Educating the patient to comply with posture correction, therefore, is the essence of treatment.

While it would seem appropriate to think of a stretch on ligaments and joint capsules as the source of this type of pain, we must also consider the vulnerability of the intervertebral disc when end-range stress is applied to this joint. This may in fact represent the very earliest of stages that progress toward disc injury, terminating with the posterior disc protrusion found in imaging studies and at surgery. While some central low back pain then may be simply postural, with no pathology present, it may lead to progressive asymmetrical disc pathology if untreated.

Derangement

A displaced bucket handle meniscus tear is often referred to as an internal derangement of the knee. The term derangement implies displacement and might also be used to describe a displaced long-bone fracture or dislocated shoulder.

The presence of sudden severe pain when such an injury and displacement occurs, as well as the rapid relief when reduction is performed, form the characteristic pain pattern associated with any derangement. The clear treatment protocol predictably begins with mechanical reduction of the derangement. If the injury has the capacity to heal and stabilize, reduction must be maintained and protected to allow adequate healing before recovery of mobility and strength can be undertaken without threatening displacement again.

McKenzie found a large group of low back patients who had similar pain response characteristics:

1. The onset of pain is usually rather sudden. In a matter of an instant, a few minutes, hours, or a day or two, patients change from normal to significantly disabled.
2. Until reduction is attained, pain persists and is usually increased during midrange movement rather than only at end-range, as in the other McKenzie categories.
3. Prior to treatment, pain is usually constant and often no position of comfort can be found. Often described as an "ache" at rest, the pain increases significantly with movement of the injured joint.
4. There often may be gross loss of movement and/or acute deformity (acute lumbar kyphosis or scoliosis).
5. These patients are usually between 20 and 45 years old.
6. Certain end-range movements or positions will significantly increase or peripheralize the pain, while movements and positions in other directions will reduce, centralize or abolish the pain (increasing vs. reducing the displacement).

Those patients whose pain behavior fit this pattern were noted also to have other unique characteristics:

1. The patients invariably have poor sitting posture.
2. The symptoms are most frequently felt not only centrally in the lumbar region, but also adjacent to the spine, and/or radiate distally into the buttock and leg in the form of pain, paresthesiae or numbness.
3. The initial occurrence of symptoms is usually spontaneous, requiring no apparent violence or obvious trauma to the lumbar spine.

It seems far more than coincidental that the majority of patients with referred peripheral pain, when tested mechanically as described by McKenzie, prove to have the characteristics of the derangement syndrome as described here. This is the same group of patients that, by any and all other forms of evaluation, would be thought to have pain of discogenic origin.

To further implicate the disc as the source of pain in derangements, those patients whose pain cannot be centralized have subsequently been found to have either a free extruded fragment or a positive discogram in the face of all other imaging studies being normal. Both of these groups have had good surgical results, the former with discectomy, and the latter with anterior interbody fusion.

The conclusion that seems increasingly valid is that a well-performed McKenzie evaluation monitoring the patient's pain behavior is a most helpful functional assessment of the intervertebral disc and that McKenzie's derangement syndrome could easily be renamed disc syndrome.

REPEATED END-RANGE MOVEMENTS: ESSENTIAL TO THE McKENZIE ASSESSMENT

Many patients who attempt to extend their lumbar spine during an acute episode have an initial increase in pain. This initial pain often leads to incorrect treatment decisions. The uniqueness of the disc mechanism of the spine requires unique methods of evaluation. The shifting of nuclear content is not rapid and requires time to occur. If the nucleus is displaced, the initial attempt at end-range movement may find painful obstruction to movement, while repetition seems to provide the nucleus the opportunity and necessary time to respond, if it is capable. Changes in pain location are observed most readily when the joints are taken to their end-range, which is consistent with the greater response expected when the adjacent endplates are positioned at their greatest angle to one another.

SURGICAL DISCS

There is a small group of low back patients with peripheral pain that does not centralize with repeated movements, and some patients actually intensify their peripheral pain with repeated extension. This group also includes patients with neurologic deficits, constant pain below the knee, and prolonged symptoms. Most importantly, these patients tend to have extruded disc fragments on imaging and at surgery. The hydrostatic disc mechanism is no longer intact, and is therefore unable to respond to the mechanical testing and treatment we have been describing.

Indeed, in the study group of 87 patients with peripheral pain referred to above (6), of the 53 with symptoms for under 4 weeks, only six patients did not centralize their leg pain with repeated end-range extension movements. The other 47 patients all experienced centralization during testing and all but one of these (98%) had a good or excellent outcome with the McKenzie treatment. Of the six who did not centralize, four proved to have irreversible disc pathology (three with extruded discs) and all four had excellent results with surgery. No other patients in this series underwent surgery.

Centralization has proven therefore to be a very reliable and helpful predictor of the state of the disc. Its occurrence predicts excellent outcomes with the McKenzie treatment while its absence most commonly represents irreversible disc pathology. Repeated end-range test movements would appear therefore to be an early functional test of the hydrostatic disc mechanism, information that is clearly unavailable with the standard imaging studies.

The McKenzie methods have proved helpful also as a predictor of the presence of surgical disc pathology, as described by Kopp (8). Of a group of hospitalized patients with disc symptoms, those who did not regain their normal range of lumbar extension in the first 2 days of hospitalization using McKenzie extension exercises had a high incidence of extruded disc fragments or an incompetent anulus. In contrast, those patients who quickly regained their extension range improved without the need for surgery. It would appear that the posteriorly displaced nucleus, if excessive or prolapsed, obstructs extension. If it can be moved forward with the extension exercises, however, the extension range of motion returns, and the patient is successfully treated without surgery.

Postoperatively, patients can benefit from early and regular lumbar end-range extension, initially avoiding lumbar flexion, to prevent recurrent posterior nuclear shifting. The regular performance of straight-leg raising can also prevent nerve root adherence in scar tissue (often lumped with postoperative arachnoiditis). This return to early joint movement, while still respecting the actual pathology (avoiding prolonged flexion), is the same postoperative care we routinely select after any other joint surgery.

DISC DERANGEMENTS WITHOUT PERIPHERAL PAIN?

Without this form of mechanical evaluation, patients with only central low back pain would be nonclassifiable. Many of these nonspecific low back patients are discogenic, representing an early stage in the pathogenesis of asymmetric disc disease. These patients with no peripheral symptoms otherwise respond exactly as they would with a derangement. When these patients are tested with repeated end-range movements (usually extension), their central pain will abolish and remain so as long as they avoid moving in the opposite direction (flexion). The mechanism for this pain likely involves stimulation of the central anulus, bringing about midline pain (10, 11).

"ANTERIOR" DISC DERANGEMENTS

There is yet another very small group of patients with lumbar pain, occasionally radiating to the inguinal region, that improves with *flexion* and worsens with extension. These anterior derangements must be treated with flexion positions and movements. Anterior displacement of disc contents seems likely and the clinical setting is consistent with this, for it tends to occur with pregnancy, rear-end auto accidents, and in prone sleepers, situations involving extension stress to the lumbar spine and an increased and/or fixed lordosis when standing. Those with anterior derangements are usually unmistakable when appropriately tested for they cannot achieve lumbar curve reversal into flexion with initial attempts at forward bending. Treatment response is usually rapid with repeated flexion exercises.

Dysfunction

McKenzie uses the term "dysfunction" to describe the common condition where range of movement is limited because of adaptive shortening of soft tissue structures about a joint. Such would occur as a result of repair after trauma, surgery, or excessive nuclear displacement, or as a result of disuse of a specific range of movement over a prolonged period.

Pain occurs when end-range is prematurely limited by these shortened tissues as they are placed on over-stretch, mechanically stimulating nociceptive pain receptors. Pain is experienced with end-range stretch only, and not during midrange movement, unless the joint surfaces (nuclear displacement) are also disturbed by a derangement. The end-range pain does not worsen with repetition unless excessive force is applied that damages rather than merely stretches the shortened structures.

Only when scarring involves a nerve root will dysfunction pain be experienced peripherally. It is otherwise always central in location.

In the lumbar spine, loss of end-range extension occurs most commonly in patients over 30 years of age who have poor sitting posture and are nonexercisers. Poor posture appears to be the most common cause of lumbar dysfunction in those who also rarely take their lumbar spine into full end-range extension. The loss of extension range typically develops progressively with age.

The second cause of adaptive shortening (dysfunction) is the contracture of fibrous repair of soft tissue trauma. Scar tissue is relatively inelastic in comparison to the surrounding healthy soft tissues, which are capable of further extendibility if not limited by the adjacent scar.

Postlaminectomy pain due to scar tissue contracture can limit both lumbar range of movement and create nerve root tethering with peripheral pain. Postoperative prevention of contracted scar through frequent end-range joint movement and straight leg raising can greatly contribute to the prevention of postsurgical pain.

TREATMENT OF DYSFUNCTION

Treating a dysfunction involves the frequent stretching of the shortened tissues without causing further traumatic injury, just as one would treat a knee or elbow contracture after casting. If treatment is to be effective, end-range stretch discomfort (strain) must be experienced, yet pain that persists after the stretch is released indicates overstretching that causes irritation of the already sensitive shortened structure(s).

It will usually take 4 to 6 weeks to gain sufficient remodeling of the short structures to bring about full range of movement. The presenting pain typically fades as full range of movement is restored, providing there is no other joint pathology.

The most common dysfunction in the spine is limited lumbar extension. This requires passive end-range extension stretching, best accomplished with the frequent performance of press-ups (Fig. 11.2), a passive gravity assisted end-range extension stretch. Strain or mild pain must be experienced for the stretch to be productive.

Using the press-up for this purpose is in direct contrast to the use of this same exercise for treating a disc derangement. End-range movements in treating a derangement are desirable to bring about reduction of displaced disc contents while monitoring centralization or abolition of pain as an indication of the effectiveness of the exercise. In treating pain from a dysfunction however, pain (or strain) is an essential goal of the exercise if it is to be effective whereas, with derangements, we are effective if we are abolishing pain.

Many asymptomatic patients with limited lumbar extension range subsequently develop acute pain from a posterior derangement. The inability of such a patient with extension dysfunction to achieve full extension compromises a critically important means for prevention of posterior migration of disc contents. Extension creates an anteriorly directed force on the nucleus, preventing posterior shifting and keeping the disc out of trouble.

To assist in appreciating the distinctiveness of these three categories of mechanical low back pain, compare their characteristics by again reviewing Table 11.1. Many patients possess a combination of these three categories that can also, with more experience, be accurately sorted using these repeated testing movements.

I have found the vast majority of instances of low back pain to be included in these categories or some combination thereof. Other more commonly used low back pain diagnoses (acute muscle spasm or strain, facet pain, spinal instability, pain from arthritis, spondylolysis, or spondylolistheses) are noticeably almost absent with this assessment system. Most patients with such radiographic findings demonstrate with McKenzie testing methods that their pain is rather typical of one or more of the three categories described. It must be appreciated that a patient with radiographic findings is not immune to back pain from the nonradiographic causes experienced by the majority of the low back pain population.

POSTURE: HOW IMPORTANT IS IT?

Regardless of the mechanical category, the importance of a lordotic lumbar spine in treating most low back pain cannot be overemphasized. Those with postural pain must simply establish and maintain a lordosis while sitting and restore their lordosis more frequently when performing prolonged forward bending activities. The pain will abolish and remain so.

Prolonged loss of the lordosis allows for slow posteriorly directed nuclear shifting resulting in low back pain. If this specific stress is maintained long enough, the pain may progress peripherally. Cadaver discs placed under sustained flexion/compression stress and subsequently studied for nuclear changes have demonstrated this posterior migration of the nuclear gel (10, 12). Maintaining, frequently restoring or, especially, increasing the lordosis counteracts and prevents both the clinically observed pain and the cadaveric posteriorly directed nuclear changes.

Little experience is needed with this approach to conclude with McKenzie that poor sitting posture is the number one predisposing factor to low back pain. Wilder and colleagues demonstrated that one hour of sustained flexion predisposed the disc to more rapid failure when further force was applied than found in those discs not initially exposed to the sustained flexion (13).

In a well-controlled, randomized, prospective study (14), 210 patients with low back and leg pain were assigned either a sitting posture with a lordosis or one with a kyphotic lumbar spine. A significant difference was found in their pain response to these sitting positions over 48 hours, with no other treatment intervention. The lordotic sitting posture resulted in much less back and leg pain and a significant shift of the most peripheral pain towards the low back. In other words, centralization of pain occurred by simply restoring the lumbar lordosis in sitting. There was no such reduction, however, in the intensity of back and leg pain in the kyphotic sitting group, nor was there any reduction in the peripheral location of the pain.

SELF-TREATMENT LEADS TO EFFECTIVE PROPHYLAXIS

The McKenzie assessment identifies the direction of movement the patient must pursue and that which must be avoided in order to successfully self-treat current pain. The responsibility is then placed on the patient. At that time, since pain is such an available and effective teacher, self-treatment teaches which positions, movements, and activities bring on, abolish, or prevent the pain. An appreciation quickly develops that the pain is self-inflicted and preventable. After recovery from the acute episode,

a combination of good posture and timely exercises in the proper direction enables the patient to prevent future episodes and also to know what is effective as first aid at the first sign of low back symptoms (1, 15).

The prevention or early successful self-treatment of a recurrence may well be McKenzie's most significant contribution to the care of low back pain. If recurrences are prevented, the disability and the high cost to our society of caring for this health problem can be greatly reduced.

IS THERE A PLACE FOR MANUAL THERAPY?

Occasionally, the patient-generated force applied to the soft tissue structures with self-treatment is simply of insufficient magnitude to treat the underlying pathology effectively. In the occasional disc derangement, additional force may be needed to initiate or complete the reduction of the nuclear displacement. Additional force is occasionally needed also to stretch a long-standing extension dysfunction (adaptive shortening) effectively.

In each case, the necessary direction of movement has already been determined, based on pain response to test movements, but complete abolition of symptoms has not occurred simply because of the insufficiency of the patient's self-induced forces. Manual procedures may then be required to achieve greater force to move the patient in the predetermined direction. The patient has already demonstrated a sense of responsibility in self-treatment but needs help in applying additional forces.

Manual therapy is thus simply an extension of self-treatment forces. But contrary to the views of osteopaths, chiropractors, and many physical therapists who manipulate almost every patient, it is not only unnecessary but counterproductive to manipulate routinely in order to effectively treat the occasional patient who requires it. As soon as we manually treat patients who are capable of self-treatment, we deprive them of a most valuable educational experience (self-treatment) that will teach techniques and responsibility (vs. dependency) that will serve them well in the essential area of preventing recurrences.

EXPERTISE

After the initial exercise regimen has been determined, often only partial resolution of a patient's symptoms occurs. Retesting will then reveal the need for a change in the movements to complete the abolition of pain. With over 40 treatment combinations, the effective abolition of all symptoms and the restoration of full lumbar function requires a high level of expertise with the McKenzie system on the part of the physician and physical therapist.

As with any other sophisticated diagnosis/treatment system, expertise is achieved through formal training followed by extensive clinical experience in evaluating and treating many patients.

SUMMARY

The complexity of low back pain requires a sophisticated system of evaluation to identify the nature of the underlying problem and to define appropriate treatment. The McKenzie approach uses a wide variety of exercise regimens individually geared to each patient depending on the pain behavior observed during a dynamic repeated end-range test movement protocol. Affecting the location and intensity of pain would indicate that the underlying mechanical disorder is being directly and specifically influenced.

Each patient learns the mechanical nature of the lumbar disorder and then self-treats the acute pain. In doing so, she or he learns the nature of the problem and how to prevent future episodes, which clearly constitutes one of the greatest benefits of the McKenzie approach.

References

1. McKenzie RA. The lumbar spine: mechanical diagnosis and therapy. Waikanae, New Zealand: Spinal Publications. 1981.
2. Vanharanta H, Videman T, Mooney V. McKenzie exercises, back trac and back school in lumbar syndrome. Presented at annual meeting of the International Society for the Study of the Lumbar Spine, Dallas, Texas, June 1986.
3. DiMaggio A, Mooney V. The McKenzie approach: exercise effective against low back pain. J Musculoskel Med (December) 1987; 63–74.
4. Nwuga G, Nwuga V. Relative therapeutic efficacy of the Williams and McKenzie protocols in back pain management. Physiother Prac 1985; 1:99–105.
5. Ponte DJ, et al. A preliminary report on the use of the McKenzie protocol versus Williams protocol in the treatment of low back pain. J Orthop Sports Phys Ther 1984; 6:130–139.
6. Donelson R, Silva G, Murphy K. The centralization phenomenon: its usefulness in evaluating and treating sciatica. Abstracts of The International Society for the Study of the Lumbar Spine, Dallas, Texas, 1986 (Accepted for publication: Spine).
7. DiMaggio A, Mooney V: Conservative care for low back pain: what works? J Musculoskel Med (September) 1987; 27–34.
8. Kopp JR: The use of lumbar extension in the evaluation and treatment of patients with acute herniated nucleus pulposus, a preliminary report. Clin Orthop 1986; 202:211.
9. The Quebec Task Force on Spinal Disorders: treatment of activity-related spinal disorders. Spine 1987; 12:7S, S22–S30.
10. Adams MA, Hutton WC. Gradual disc prolapse. Spine 1985; 10(6):524–531.
11. Cloward RB. Cervical diskography: a contribution to the etiology and mechanism of neck, shoulder and arm pain. Ann Surg 1959; 150:6.
12. Krag M, Seroussi R, Wilder D, Byrne K, Trausch I. Internal displacements from in vitro loading of human spinal motion segments. Abstracts for the International Society for the Study of the Lumbar Spine, Dallas, Texas, 1986.
13. Wilder DG, Pope MH, Frymoyer JW. The biomechanics of lumbar disc herniation and the effect of overload and instability. J Spinal Disorders 1988; 1:1, 16–32.
14. McKenzie RA, Williams M, Hawley J, Van Wijmen P, Reed R, Farry S, Jack M, Laslett M. A comparison of the effects of two sitting postures on back and referred pain. Abstracts of The International Society for the Study of the Lumbar Spine, Miami, Florida, 1988.
15. McKenzie RA. Prophylaxis in recurrent low back pain. N Zealand Med J 1979; 89:22–23.

12

STABILIZATION OF THE LUMBAR SPINE

Arthur H. White

DEFINITION

After working with thousands of patients and many therapists of various backgrounds and training, I would define stabilization training as follows: A patient is trained to move her or his spine in such a way as to find the least painful position. The spine is then held in that "neutral" position while performing ever increasing tasks.

A simpler definition might be that stabilization means bracing, holding, or fusing a diseased and painful spinal segment in a pain-free, balanced or neutral position through the sole use of voluntary musculature.

The simplest form of stablization is abdominal bracing. The voluntary tightening of the abdominal muscles and the additional bracing of the diaphragm to increase intraabdominal pressure has been known for decades to give support to the spine. This is a technique used in preventing spinal fracture in ski jumping and in pulling out of rapid dives in jet planes. We have all used such abdominal bracing when receiving blows during contact sports. With such abdominal bracing, the spine is not necessarily placed in any predetermined position. It is simply supported in whatever position it happens to be in at the time of the muscular diaphragmatic contraction.

Stabilization includes the practice of abdominal bracing, but with accessory muscles presetting the diseases or painful spinal segment in a known position. Sometimes this known or preconceived position is determined strictly on the basis of pathological diagnosis. At other times the position is found and learned through the experience of pain. Since so many painful spinal conditions do not create pain at the time of change of position, it can sometimes take many hours, days and maybe even weeks to determine where the position of neutral balance is for a diseased segment. This may require doing a specific exercise program with the spine held in one position of flexion or extension, and then following the patient for 24 hours clinically to see whether or not that particular exercise program has had any ill effects on the patient. Of course, all other aspects of the patient's life and activity have to be controlled during such evaluation.

TECHNIQUE

There is no one perfect techique for teaching individuals how to stabilize. The technique may depend upon the specific diagnosis, the coordination of the patient, the past experiences of a patient with regard to athletic endeavors, and many other factors. For example, patients who have been highly trained in the martial arts will find that the concepts taught in stabilization come quite easily. Other individuals who have primitive or detrimental movement patterns may never be able to accomplish satisfactory levels of stabilization training. A short period of testing of an individual can determine which level of stabilization training a patient should enter, which could be anywhere from lying down to running.

An average patient with a disc problem but no significant neurological loss would begin stabilization training lying supine. Tightening the abdominal musculature is first practiced with the use of partial sit-up exercises, setting the diaphragm and learning to breathe while doing so. Various forms of pelvic tilt are practiced

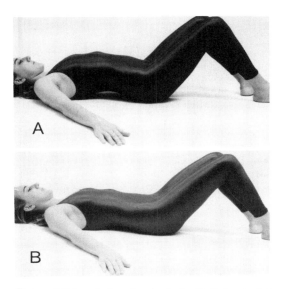

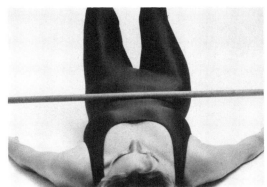

Figure 12.2. Stick balanced across the abdomen.

Figure 12.1. **A.** Lumbar lordosis. **B.** Spine is flat with use of pelvic tilt.

until a comfortable position of spinal pelvic alignment is obtained. A maximum levl of pelvic tilt flattens the lumbar spine firmly against the surface on which the patient is lying (Fig. 12.1). A hand can be placed behind the lumbar lordosis to ensure maximum forceful flattening. Some patients will need maximum lordosis for comfort. Once the optimum position is achieved, the abdominal musculature is contracted and the diaphragm is braced. Motion of the extremities can then begin, first by lifting one extremity at a time slowly as the therapist verifies the patient's ability to maintain the stabilized neutral position while doing so. The extremities are then raised faster and alternately until the patient is doing a bicycling motion with the legs at the same time as a waving motion of the arms from side to side and overhead. This is called a dying bug exercise because it looks like a bug expiring on its back with its legs waving. It is again necessary to stress that there should be no pain, and the patient should show no evidence of spinal motion. This can be accentuated by balancing a stick horizontally across the patient's abdomen or chest (Fig. 12.2), or by placing a hand behind the patient's back with a finger in each interspinous space to feel for any motion that is occurring.

Stabilization training can also be done with the patient lying prone. This is slightly more difficult than lying supine for most patients.

While lying prone the patient is asked to alternately raise one extremity, and then the other, and then two simultaneously. It is easier to observe the patient's spine for motion in this position.

The next logical progression from the prone position is that of kneeling. A patient kneels, finds the neutral balanced pain-free position with a cat-like rounding of the back and then relaxing into lordosis (the humpsag exercises) (Figs. 12.3, 12.4). Once the neutral balanced pain-free position is found in this kneeling position, the patient then practices raising one extremity, then another, and eventually two extremities without having pain or having any motion of the spine (Fig. 12.5). Again, a good test to determine if pelvic stability is being maintained is to have the patient balance a stick horizontally across his or her back while watching in the mirror to see if the stick wavers or falls off.

There are numerous varieties of floor exercises with Swedish balls, large air-filled rubber

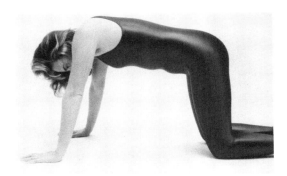

Figure 12.3. Round back.

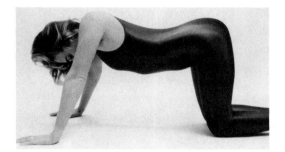

Figure 12.4.   Relaxing into lordosis.

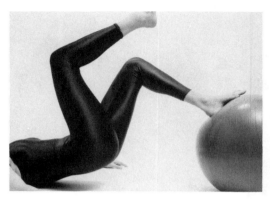

Figure 12.6.   One-legged bridge on Swedish ball.

balls that can be used for balancing the legs upon as the patient lies supine in a hip and knee flexed position (90/90) (Fig. 12.6). The ball creates less stability than the floor and requires greater strength and stabilization control to avoid spinal motion (Fig. 12.7). Stabilization can next be carried into the standing position. In standing stabilization, mirrors are extremely valuable for permitting patients to watch themselves as they find their neutral position. They may use a wall to back up against when they first attempt to find their neutral stabilized position. They then move away from the wall and begin moving one extremity after another, leading eventually to standing on one foot, perhaps even with a weight in one hand (Fig. 12.8).

Increasing degrees of force to attempt to offset the patient's stability are then introduced. This includes such things as jousting between patient partners. Two patients face each other and grasp a stick or baton that is mutually held between them (Fig. 12.9). They then try to force each other off center. This is somewhat akin to Little John fighting Robin Hood on the bridge with his staff. Instead of striking, however, the

opponents simply slowly exert displacing forces under the direction and supervision of a therapist. The therapist assesses each individual's stabilizing capabilities as the patients joust.

As a patient's physical demands increase in activities of heavy labor and contact sports, the stabilization training needs to be increasingly aggressive. Until this point in the training, the stabilization has been relatively impractical. The things that they have been doing are rarely applicable to daily activities. At this point in training, patients need to move about more freely and actively as they do in their daily lives. This can include such activities as walking rapidly with weights in their hands while maintaining stabilization. It can be done on a treadmill at first so that the therapist can easily test and verify good stabilization techniques.

Once verified, patients are allowed to take long walks on their own, remaining pain-free and testing their endurance for up to hours of walking stabilization. Low impact aerobics and dancing programs can be done utilizing stabilization techniques under more enjoyable and

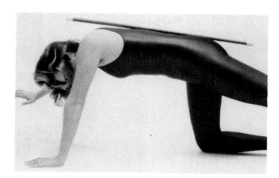

Figure 12.5.   Raising one extremity.

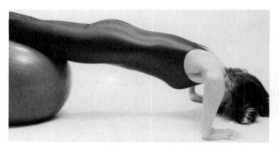

Figure 12.7.   Push-up balanced on Swedish ball with spine in neutral position.

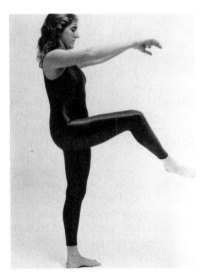

Figure 12.8. Standing balanced on one leg in neutral position.

aerobic circumstances. Jogging can be practiced on a treadmill with stabilization, and then practiced daily by the patient. This is a whole new way to jog. It is difficult to breath while tightening the abdominal musculature. The impact of the foot hitting the ground produces vibration through the leg and pelvis into the spine. This vibration is cushioned by stabilization of the spine, not only with the abdominal musculature, but also with the use of greater

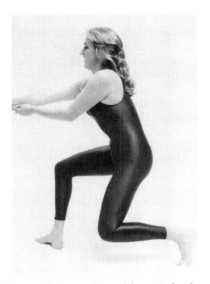

Figure 12.9. Pulling with neutral spine.

amounts of knee flexion and more use of the quadriceps and hamstring muscles to cushion part of the vibration on the spine.

Contact sports require patients to receive blows by other individuals. This frequently entails unexpected trauma or very short warning to allow preparation to receive a blow. Through practice, therefore, the patient must learn to stabilize rapidly and then receive blows of increasing intensity. We have developed training for professional athletes in competitive sports by having them train in martial arts. Martial artists, of course, have dealt with blows, trauma, and human interaction for centuries. Very specific techniques in different schools have been developed and honed to a very fine training program.

There is no activity simulation program better than the required activity itself. If a patient is a baseball player at second base, there is no better place to train than at second base. All of the required positions and motions are analyzed for efficiency, stabilization and energy conservation. The required changes are taught and practiced until they virtually become a natural reflex for the patient. They may require jumping, falling, rolling, throwing, catching, kicking.

It is amazing to me, and probably the crux of all low back pain problems, that many athletes and physically highly accomplished individuals are seemingly untrainable, with habit patterns of movement that lead to injury after injury. Perfect body mechanics are not a requirement for superb athletic performance.

We have known for years that teaching patterns of movement and posture can greatly improve athletic and artistic prowess. Similarly, the martial arts can advance individuals from a brown belt to a black belt, for example, by demonstrating more and more perfect movement, posture and body mechanics. There is no end to the training that we can do in posture, strength, body mechanics and, now, stabilization.

MENTAL STABILIZATION

Simply to use stabilization exercises and expect a patient to become pain-free and normally active is not to take advantage of one of the biggest tools that we have in health care: the human brain. We can program the brain to help us accomplish any task in a more rapid fashion. It has been widely demonstrated that mental imaging and mental programming allow athletes to accomplish much greater feats of strength and coordination.

Some spinal practitioners have stated for years that all the training that is necessary to prevent and control back pain is an awareness of the back. They simply tell their patients, "think back" before they take on any task which may lead even remotely to back pain. This simple type of awareness conceivably puts an individual in a better position of preparedness for doing a physical activity. Even getting out of bed can be traumatic to a degenerative spine. An individual who is aware of the back problem before getting out of bed is more likely to move slightly differently, to tighten the abdominal muscles and "reflexly" protect the spine without conscious attention and without having to take an extensive training program in stabilization.

STABILIZATION EDUCATION

Patients undergoing stabilization training generally have had basic back school. They are in stabilization training in order to accomplish higher levels of activity than they have been able to do previously, given their underlying pathological conditions. They want to be able to move more freely, more rapidly, and in a way that they might consider "normal." Their education, therefore, needs to constitute considerably more than helpful hints and first aid. They should have already been doing abdominal, gluteal, and quadriceps exercises for months. They should have made changes in their environment by altering their seats, workstations, and home environment.

Education for stabilization training, therefore, begins with motivation and theory. Patients already understand at their level of capability the underlying disease process that is creating their pain. It is explained that this underlying diseased spinal segment or other process can endure voluntary efforts in a position of comfort and noninjury. Patients already know that there are times when they can be pain-free and can find positions of comfort. It is easy from there for the patients to understand that if they can maintain the diseased spine in the position of comfort (neutral position) they can increase physical activities if they are strong enough and coordinated enough to maintain that neutral position. When patients see

some of the physical and coordinated feats that human beings are able to accomplish in athletics and acrobatics, it quickly becomes clear to them that it is simply a matter of practice, time, and strengthening to maintain spinal positioning and alignment.

Exaggeration is sometimes helpful in demonstration and motivation. For example, a clinician can demonstrate to a patient in the examining room that she or he can bend laterally to fully 45° and still run around in circles maintaining the neutral position. Similarly, patients can see that if they have a rock in their shoe under the heel that they could, if necessary, walk for miles on their toes without putting pressure on the rock. When these types of examples are extrapolated to spinal postioning and maintenance of stabilization, the patient can at least understand the theory. Additional motivation is accomplished by getting patients to express what they are willing to do to regain normalcy in life activities. Patients frequently make statements such as, "I would do anything to be able to play golf again," or "Surgery is such a frightening thing to me that if there is anything else known to medical science, I will do it." The clinician can quickly capitalize on these statements by countering with "There is something you can do, but it won't be easy," or "How hard are you willing to work?" There is no limit to how strong you can get, how coordinated you can get, and how well you can balance your diseased spine.

If the patient still does not understand the condition, the principles to be used, and the theory of stabilization, demonstrations are in order. It may take a few sessions to get patients to feel that they are accomplishing that which has been described.

Some therapists prefer to simply train patients and let them gain the understanding and feeling for stabilization in the process. The process can go much more quickly with informed and highly motivated patients. Simply doing the stabilization training for an hour a day and spending the other 23 hours in nontraining will take much longer, cost more money, and be much less successful than working with a knowledgeable, well-motivated patient who will attempt to use the basic principles 24 hours per day. Occasional sessions with a therapist to problem-solve and learn new techniques will permit advancement rapidly to higher levels of stabilization.

A quick demonstration by the clinician of one of the stabilization, t'ai chi, or yoga positions, which are somewhat difficult to achieve for the average person, can serve as a good example to the patient of what can be achieved and will challenge some patients to perform. The patient can then be asked to achieve the same position, such as a one-legged, straight back stance (Fig. 12.8). Most patients will not be able to achieve this position. If they can, they have high stabilization potential. After just a few tries, they find they are able to do it better and better, and begin already to understand the principles, theory, and challenge.

SUMMARY

It is always amazing to me how resistant patients can be and how resistant the public generally is to new ideas, new training, physical exercise, and anything called "therapy." A statement we hear frequently is, "Oh, no, not more therapy. I've already done therapy." We no longer use the term therapy, but only the term training. Even then, the patient interprets it as "therapy." Part of the reason is the unfortunate fact that most patients have been given much too much of modalities and not enough exercise and responsibility.

Changing habitual patterns requires considerable mental energy. Spending such mental energy is for some reason distasteful to human beings. Convincing a patient of the need to expend the mental energy required for stabilization is our biggest problem in the stabilization field. The second biggest problem, from a physician's standpoint, is getting the therapist or trainer to convince and motivate the patient. It is much easier for a therapist, and certainly more lucrative, simply to give a class or teach stabilization to those who show up. Convincing patients to show up or come back to suffer these physical and mental energy drains takes time, personality, communication, and psychology. Few of us have an overabundance of any of those items. Thus, many patients miss out on stabilization, have surgery in lieu of stabilization, or are relegated to living with their condition or taking other "therapies" with the impression that "I tried stabilization and it didn't work."

In our changing medical economy, we cannot let our patients, our therapists, our trainers, or ourselves deprive our patients of what we know is best for them because we are lazy, poor salespeople, or not assertive enough. The physician, impelled by socioeconomic realities, can require that a patient achieve a certain level of stabilization before being permitted to take advantage of some of the less strenuous and more pain-relieving avenues of treatment, such as acupuncture or physical therapy modalities. The therapist must fight hard to avoid the all-too-frequent attitude of "pain-relief now, hard work later." The therapist has the tools to give pain relief and has been taught to give pain relief. It is easier, faster, and more lucrative to give pain relief than to give training. Strict guidelines need to be drawn by the physician and the insurance carriers as to how much manipulation, how much of modalities, how much training, and how much surgery is appropriate for any given diagnosis. It is, in short, not only the patient who needs reeducation about old habits.

13

LUMBAR PROTECTIVE MECHANISM

Vicky L. Saliba
Gregory S. Johnson

The primary goal of physical therapists who evaluate and treat patients presenting with lumbar pain is to help the patients to responsibly manage their back dysfunction and prevent future recurrence (1–6). Back pain can be directly correlated to a pathological state, such as nerve impingement, joint degeneration, foraminal stenosis, disc disease or segmental instability; or, the pain can remain undiagnosed despite exhaustive testing (7–10). In either situation, the physical therapist is to identify the biomechanical and neuromuscular dysfunctions related to the exacerbation and perpetuation of the symptoms and the degenerative process. These dysfunctions may include poor posture and body mechanics, poor muscular responsiveness and strength, and limited flexibility of soft tissue and articular structures (1, 2, 6, 10–19). Once these dysfunctions are identified and measured, the treatment program is designed to assist the patient in achieving adequate flexibility, strength, responsiveness, and coordination to learn the postures and movements that will control symptoms and retard the degenerative process (1, 2, 9, 13, 20). Primary components of the treatment program are back education and training (3, 4, 6, 21–27).

Back education and training are founded on the premise that the lumbar spine is less traumatized when the patient utilizes an efficient alignment (4, 28, 29), has an effective base of support, and exhibits an inherent ability to brace or stabilize the lumbar spine during loaded or repetitive activities (3, 13, 20, 30, 31). This inherent mechanism of stabilization, whether reflex or volitional, we call the *lumbar protective mechanism* (LPM) (3, 32). This chapter presents an evaluation and treatment process in which the therapist identifies, assesses, and retrains this protective mechanism.

The initial step in a back education and training program is to identify a mechanical correlation to the patient's subjective complaint (7, 10). This requires a complete history and subjective and functional evaluation (7, 8, 10, 33, 34). The functional evaluation includes an analysis of the patient's range of motion, strength, endurance, habitual postures, presenting body mechanics, and functional capacity during tasks such as lifting (21, 22, 26, 28, 35). Specifically, the therapist identifies the patient's ability to assume a balanced alignment and to maintain this alignment during the tested activities of daily living.

ALIGNMENT

An analysis of the vertical relationship of the structures of the spine provides an initial source of information with regard to the patient's habitual postures and movement patterns (5, 10, 28). Efficient alignment allows for equal weight distribution through the spine, therefore transferring the weight of the upper body and any object carried, pushed, or pulled directly to the base of support. Observation of the patient during functional tasks such as sitting, standing, lifting, carrying objects, pushing and pulling, coming to standing, and returning to sitting reveals the patient's position and use of the cervical, thoracic, and lumbar spines. The therapist assesses as well the segmental relationship of these three spinal segments and any changes that occur during functional activities.

An important objective assessment of the patient's vertical alignment is the vertical compression test (3, 32). This test provides the therapist and patient kinesthetic feedback as to how weight is transferred through the spine to the base of support. The patient is asked to stand in a comfortable, natural stance. The therapist then applies vertical pressure through the shoulders feeling for any give or buckling in the spine (Fig. 13.1). During the procedure, the patient is asked to relate any increase or reproduction of symptoms. In the presence of postural deviations, the therapist usually feels an instability at the level of dysfunction and the patient often reports pressure or pain from the vertical compression in the same area.

The vertical compression test, when used correctly, can help the patient recognize existing postural deviations and their functional and symptomatic effects. Deviations such as an increased lumbar lordosis, posterior angulation of the thoracic spine, anterior shear of the pelvis or regions of instability (36–38), prevent efficient weight transfer through the spine. When the natural segmental relationship of the three spinal curves is interrupted, the spine no longer efficiently transfers the weight to the pelvis, but concentrates the force of the vertical loading at the biomechanically altered segment. This con-

centration of force appears to facilitate a progressive breakdown of the structural and neuromuscular stability at those segments (13, 38). We suggest that the presence of such dysfunctions also inhibits the trunk muscles' natural tendency to stabilize the lumbar spine in a midrange or neutral position during repetitive, loaded, or stressful activities.

LUMBAR PROTECTIVE MECHANISM

Training the patient to maintain the lumbar spine in a balanced alignment during stressful activities is a primary component of the spinal rehabilitation program (3, 13, 20, 30, 31). Before education and training, the therapist must evaluate the reflex or volitional responsiveness, and strength and endurance of the intrinsic and extrinsic trunk muscles necessary to stabilize the lumbar spine in response to external force. The lumbar protective mechanism protects the spine both by holding the individual vertebrae stable in relation to each other and maintaining an efficient alignment and segmental relationship of the thoracic, lumbar, and pelvic regions (31, 32).

An assessment of the patient in various postures and movements identifies the components that need to be addressed during education and training. The following evaluation procedures are primarily influenced by the principle of *proprioceptive neuromuscular facilitation* (PNF) (39, 40). Specifically, manual contact, resistance, approximation, and diagonal patterns provide a framework for consistent testing.

Primary assessment of the LPM is performed with the patient standing. The therapist applies appropriate manual resistance to the patient's shoulders or other regions of the body in anterior, posterior, rotational and diagonal directions (Figs. 13.2 and 13.3). Initially, no instructions are given, so that the patient's natural responsiveness can be assessed. If there is a delayed or diminished response, the patient is instructed to maintain a stable position against the therapist's resistance. Once a response is elicited, the strength and endurance of the LPM is assessed by increasing and maintaining resistance (3).

The functional effect of the patient's available responsiveness, strength, and endurance is clarified by further testing. The patient is asked

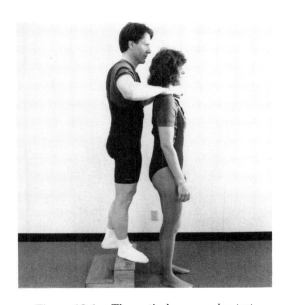

Figure 13.1.   The vertical compression test.

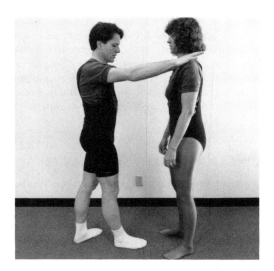

Figure 13.2. Testing the lumbar protective mechanism in standing with straight anterior-posterior resistance.

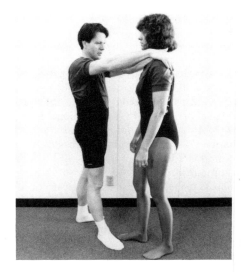

Figure 13.3. Testing the lumbar protective mechanism in standing with diagonal resistance. Note: the patient can be in either a bilateral stance or a straddled stance.

to perform several movements while sitting and standing as well as lifting and push-pull activities (Figs. 13.4, 13.5, 13.6). In each movement, the patient is observed to determine if the spine is positioned and stabilized in a balanced alignment, allowing the work to take place in the hips, legs, ankles, and upper extremities (3, 30, 41).

EDUCATION AND TRAINING OF ALIGNMENT AND STABILIZATION

To educate a patient is to influence the patient's thought process by altering knowledge base and kinesthetic awareness so as to expand the options for decision making. Education of the spinal patient also involves the identification of existing patterns and instruction directed at helping the patient to replace these patterns with more efficient ones. This process can be considered successful only if the information imparted is learned by the patient. The patient should be able to exhibit a balanced alignment, stabilization, and efficient body mechanics in any given activity of daily living. This learning process requires repetition and positive feedback (40, 42).

The techniques used to educate and train a patient can vary widely. However, if the goal is to influence the patient's kinesthetic awareness, the principles of PNF provide a clinically proven framework for enhancing neuromuscular facilitation and reeducation (39, 40). Manual contact, appropriate resistance, visual cues, verbal feedback, traction, and approximation all facilitate a specific response from the patient. This specific response is important in training posture and movement, as well as in

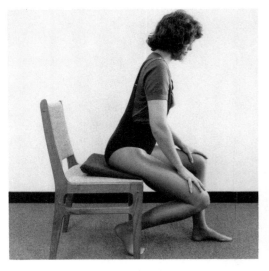

Figure 13.4. Testing the lumbar protective mechanism in active sitting. The patient is observed to determine if the spine is positioned and maintained in a balanced alignment.

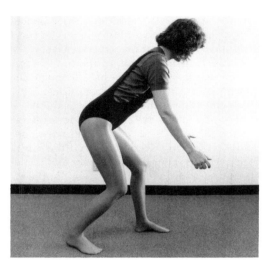

Figure 13.5. Testing the lumbar protective mechanism in active standing or bending. The patient is observed to determine if the spine is positioned and maintained in a balanced alignment.

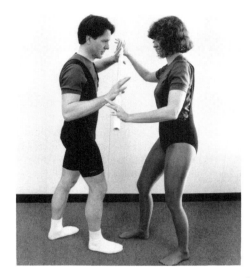

Figure 13.6. Testing the lumbar protective mechanism during resisted activities. The patient is observed and monitored through kinesthetic feedback to determine if the spine is positioned and maintained in a balanced alignment as well as to determine the patient's muscular responsiveness and recruitment.

teaching exercise. Each time a new exercise is given, the patient is manually guided through the exercise using the PNF principles. This ensures the appropriate recruitment of muscles and prevents substitution and compensation. This response is then learned through repetitive exercises and activities that require the patient to maintain the newly learned posture or movement (3, 39, 40).

The circumstances that influence the presence and effectiveness of the lumbar protective mechanism are a naturally balanced alignment, utilization of appropriate principles of body mechanics, and well-conditioned musculature (3).

Alignment and Body Mechanics

Factors that inhibit the assumption of a naturally balanced alignment include existing posture patterns and structural limitations such as decreased soft tissue and articular mobility (11, 32, 43, 44). The therapist, utilizing visual, verbal, and manual techniques of PNF facilitates the patient to correct any nonstructural postural deviations identified in the evaluation and assume a more balanced alignment. This process of retraining through awareness highlights for the therapist the structural deviations that must be addressed with soft tissue (5, 32, 45, 46) and joint mobilization (7, 33, 34, 47, 48) and

PNF stretching techniques (39, 40, 46). These restrictions can include soft tissue restrictions in the scalenes, iliopsoas, pectorals, and hamstrings, and limited spine and rib mobility that prevent the assumption of a completely balanced alignment.

Once a more balanced alignment is achieved, the vertical compression test is repeated, noting any improvements in weight transference and pain. If there is any noted improvement, the therapist then retests the LPM to reassess the patient's responsiveness, strength, or endurance. Clinically, most patients demonstrate an improved LPM when there is an improvement in alignment (3, 32). For this reason, we suggest that the initial step of the actual education and training process be directed at any identified postural deviations. This is coupled with the training of the following four basic body mechanic principles (3):

1. Base of support;
2. Utilization of proper axis of motion;
3. Weight shift or momentum;
4. Weight acceptance or balance.

These basic principles, when applied to body mechanics and exercise, enhance the maintenance of an efficient alignment and facilitate the action of the lumbar protective mechanism. These principles also provide a foundation from which the patient can begin to solve problems and take on an active role of self-responsibility (9, 13, 23, 24, 49).

Exercise

The development of well-conditioned musculature involves a program that consists of relaxation, flexibility (3, 11, 13, 43, 44, 50–53), stabilization (3, 13, 30), and strengthening exercise (3, 11, 13, 14, 20, 30, 44, 54, 55). This program is designed specifically to improve dysfunctions identified in the initial objective and functional evaluation and enhance the structural changes facilitated with manual techniques. Initially, the patient's strength and flexibility are rated and measured (1, 17, 20, 43). These data assist the therapist in establishing parameters for developing the exercise program and allow for accurate assessment of any gains or improvements. Equally important, any deviations in strength and flexibility that can be mechanically correlated to the patient's pain further emphasize the patient's role in rehabilitation.

The relaxation and flexibility exercises address those limitations that restrict the patient from assuming a more balanced alignment, using the proper axes of motion, and recruiting maximal strength response from key muscle groups (Fig. 13.7) (11, 12, 20, 31, 56–59). These exercises are initially performed three or four times a day to gain a rapid improvement and then tapered to four or five times a week.

While efficient function of the lumbar protective mechanism depends on alignment and proper body mechanics, the most critical factor influencing this mechanism is the available responsiveness and strength of the lower trunk muscles (3, 11, 12, 31, 54, 57). The patient's ability to brace or selectively recruit the intrinsic and extrinsic muscles necessary to stabilize the lumbar spine is initially assessed in the supine hook lying position. The therapist gently applies pressure to the anterior and lateral walls of the trunk and asks the patient to tense muscles or press out against the pressure. If a diminished or inefficient response is observed and palpated, the patient is immediately trained in bracing exercises (3, 32, 49). To perform these exercises, the patient locates the specific area of diminished response, presses his fingers deep into the soft tissue, and attempts to push the fingers out using the trunk muscles. This process is enhanced with the added facilitation of resisted hip flexion as illustrated in Figure 13.8. The patient is also instructed to maintain the response to develop endurance within these muscle groups.

Once the patient demonstrates the ability to produce and maintain an efficient bracing contraction, the program then incorporates progressive stabilization exercises (3, 13, 30). This progression is designed to improve the strength and endurance of the abdominal and lower trunk muscles during both open kinetic and closed kinetic activities (Figs. 13.9 and 13.10).

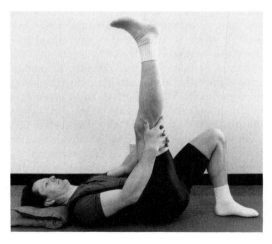

Figure 13.7. The hamstrings muscle group can be stretched in supine position with resistance applied to the hip extensors during an active contraction of the quadriceps at the patient's end range of motion.

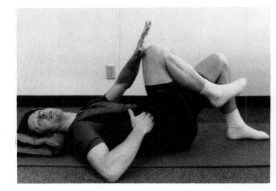

Figure 13.8. Finger-tip pressure and resisted hip flexion enhance the responsiveness and strength of the trunk muscles' ability to brace.

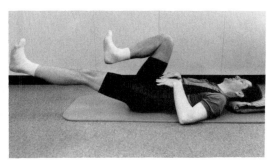

Figure 13.9. Superimposed extremity movement during bracing further enhances the strength and endurance of the muscles that stabilize the lumbar spine. The fingers can remain in the area of greatest weakness to facilitate the maintenance of the bracing contraction.

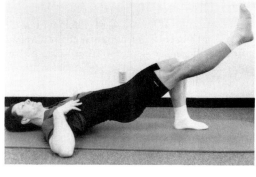

Figure 13.10. Bridging with leg extension while bracing places a greater demand on the trunk stabilizers.

This exercise program progresses to include the addition of weights to the extremities as well as graded external force to the trunk during weight shift and movement over fixed distal extremities. This resistance is facilitated with the use of pulleys or a sports cord. This resistance, applied to functional activities, ensures the carryover of the improved strength and stabilization to activities of daily living. It is this phase of training that becomes specific to the patient's work, home, or recreational activities.

The responsiveness of the LPM is retrained to its maximum potential as the patient's stabilization strength and endurance improves. This quick adjustment (39) or balancing component is challenged with such activities as medicine ball tosses, two-person resisted push-pull exercises, selective Swedish ball exercises, and the use of equipment which varies the base of support such as the profitter or circular balance board.

In conjunction with the stabilization exercises, the patient is placed on a general strengthening program to address any weakness identified in the key muscle groups of the trunk and extremities (3, 6, 11, 13, 14, 20, 30, 43, 44, 54). These exercises are prescribed to achieve two primary goals. First, the patient exercises the trunk and extremities while maintaining a balanced, pain-free position of the trunk, promoting the use of the LPM during loaded and repetitive activities. Examples include repeated squats incorporating forward bending at the hips and resisted lifting patterns with the upper extremities. Second, the patient facilitates general strength and coordination of the trunk muscles through controlled concentric and eccentric movement of the spine, as with progressive controlled rotation of the lower trunk (50, 3, 60).

Throughout the rehabilitation program, exercises are continuously modified to meet the patient's progressive needs. At all times, the exercise program should be directed at improvement in specific functional tasks. In addition, the length and intensity of the exercise program should correlate with the patient's lifestyle and work, home, and recreational demands (Fig. 13.11).

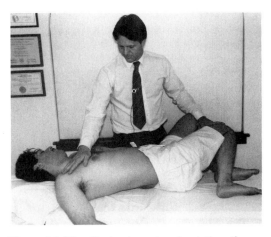

Figure 13.11. During lower trunk rotation, the patient is manually assisted performing movement with proper sequencing and coordination.

SUMMARY

The fundamental premise of back education and training is the maintenance of a balanced, pain-free alignment of the lumbar spine during repetitive, loaded, or resisted activities while allowing the movement and work to take place in the hips, legs, ankles, and upper extremities. This is accomplished through dynamic stabilization of the intrinsic and extrinsic trunk muscles (LPM) and utilization of other key muscle groups. The goal is to retrain dynamic movement that allows a fluid transfer of weight and force throughout the movement, not allowing the weight or force to become fixed in the lumbar spine. This requires the education and training of posture and movement as well as the facilitation of a responsive and strong lumbar protective mechanism and overall flexibility, strength, endurance, and coordination through exercise.

Acknowledgment

We thank Cheryl Wardlaw, PT and Jeffrey Ellis, PT for invaluable assistance in the preparation of this chapter.

References

1. Mayer T, Gatchel R, Kishino N, et al. Objective assessment of spine function following industrial injury. Spine 1985; 10:482–493.
2. Mayer T, Gatchel R, Mayer H, et al. A prospective two-year study of functional restoration in industrial low back injury. JAMA 1987; 258:1763–1767.
3. Saliba VL, Johnson, GS. Back education and training. course outline. San Anselmo, CA: The Institute of Physical Art. 1988.
4. Hultman G, Nordin M, Ortengren R. The influence of a preventive educational programme on trunk flexion in janitors. Applied Erg 1984; 15:127–133.
5. Johnson G, Saliba V. Soft tissue mobilization. In White AH, Anderson R. Conservative care of low back pain. Baltimore: Williams & Wilkins, 1991.
6. Waddell G. A new clinical model for the treatment of low-back pain. Spine 1987; 12:632–644.
7. Grieve GP. Common vertebral joint problems. London: Churchill Livingstone, 1981.
8. Kirkaldy-Willis, WH. Managing low back pain. 2nd ed. New York: Churchill Livingstone, 1988.
9. White AH, Rothman RH, Ray CD. Lumbar spine surgery: Techniques and complications. St. Louis: CV Mosby, 1987.
10. Jull GA. Examination of the lumbar spine. In: Grieve G, ed. Modern manual therapy of the vertebral column. London: Churchill Livingstone, 1986; 547–558.
11. Janda V. Muscle weakness and inhibition (pseudoparesis) in back pain syndromes. In: Grieve G, ed. Modern manual therapy of the vertebral column. London: Churchill Livingstone, 1986.
12. Lewit K. The contribution of clinical observation to neurological mechanisms in manipulative therapy. In Korr I, ed. The neurobiologic mechanisms in manipulative therapy. London: Plenum Press, 1978; 3–25.
13. Saal JA. Rehabilitation of sports-related lumbar spine injuries. Phys Med Rehab: State of the Art Reviews 1987; (4):613–638.
14. Biering-Sorensen F. Physical measurements as risk indicators for low-back trouble over a one-year period. Spine 1984; 9:106–119.
15. Cady L, Bischoff D, O'Connel E, et al. Strength and fitness and subsequent back injuries in firefighters. J Occup Med 1979; 21:269–272.
16. Liemohn W, Snodgrass L, Sharpe G. Unresolved controversies in back management—a review. J Orthop Sports Phys Ther 1988; 1:239–244.
17. Mayer T et al. Objective assessment of spine function following industrial injury. Spine 1985; 10:482–493.
18. Smidt G, Herring T, Amundsen L, et al. Assessment of abdominal and back extensor function—a quantitative approach and results for chronic low-back pain patients. Spine 1983; 8:211–219.
19. Thorstensson A, Nilsson J. Trunk muscle strength during constant and velocity movements. Scand J Rehab Med 1982; 14:61–68.
20. Smidt G. Trunk muscle strength and endurance in the context of low back pain. In Grieve G, ed. Modern manual therapy of the vertebral column. London: Churchill Livingstone. 1986.
21. Bergquist-Ullman M, Larsson U. Acute low back pain in industry. Acta Orthop Scand (Suppl) 1977; 170:1–117.
22. Kvien TK, Nilsen H, Vik P. Education and self-care of patients with low back pain. Scand J Rheumatol 1981; 19:318–320.
23. Linton S, Kamwendo K. Low back schools—a critical review. Phys Ther 1987; 67:1375–1383.
24. Matmiller AW. The California back school. Physiotherapy 1980; 66(4):118.
25. Moffett J, Chase S, Portek I, Ennis J. A controlled, prospective study to evaluate the effectiveness of a back school in the relief of chronic low back pain. Spine 1986; 11:120–123.
26. Simmons J, Dennis M, Rath D. The back school: a total back management program. Orthopedics 1984; 7:1453–1456.
27. Zachrisson-Forsell M. The Swedish back school. Physiotherapy 1980; 66(4):112.

28. Nordin M, Ortengren R, Andersson G. Measurements of trunk movements during work. Spine 1984; 9:465.

29. Steindler A. Mechanics of normal and pathological locomotion in man. Springfield, IL: Charles C Thomas, 1935.

30. Morgan D. Concepts in functional training and postural stabilization for the low-back-injured. Top Acute Care Trauma Rehabil 1988; 2(4):8–17.

31. Morris J, Lucas D, Bresler B. Role of the trunk in the stability of the spine. Bone Joint Surg 1961; 43A:327–351.

32. Johnson GS, Saliba VI. Functional Orthopedics I, course outline. San Anselmo, CA: Institute of Physical Art, 1984.

33. Maitland GD. Vertebral manipulation. 5th ed. London: Butterworth, 1986.

34. Paris S. S-1 course notes. Atlanta: Institute for Graduate Health Sciences, 1977; 3.

35. Andersson GBJ. Epidemiologic aspects of low-back pain in industry. Spine 1981; 6:53–60.

36. Farfan H, Gracovetsky S. The nature of instability. Spine 1984; 9:714–719.

37. Howes RG, Isdale IC. The loose back: an unrecognized syndrome. Rheumatol Phys Med 1971; 11:72–77.

38. Paris S. Physical signs of instability. Spine 1985; 10:122–124.

39. Johnson GS, Saliba VL. PNFI: the functional approach to movement reeducation. San Anselmo, CA: Institute of Physical Art, 1981.

40. Knott M, Voss DE. Proprioceptive neuromuscular facilitation. 2nd ed. London: Ballière, Daintily & Cogs, 1968.

41. Aston J. Aston patterning. Mill Valley, CA. Aston Training Center, personal communication.

42. Johnson G, Saliba V, White A. Back school: principles in action. Video teleconference syllabus. April 18, 1989.

43. Kendall HO, Kendall FP, Boynton DA. Posture and pain. Huntington, NY: Krieger, 1977.

44. Sahrmann SA. Diagnosis and treatment of muscle imbalances associated with musculoskeletal pain. Dec. 6, 7, 1988.

45. Cyriax J. Textbook of orthopedic medicine: diagnosis of soft tissue lesions. London: Ballière-Tindall, 1984.

46. Evjenth O, Hamberg J. Muscle stretching in manual therapy: a clinical manual. Alfta, Sweden: Alfta Rehab Farlag, 1985.

47. Bourdillon JF. Spinal manipulation. 3rd ed. London: Heinemann, 1982.

48. Mennell JM. Joint pain. Boston: Little, Brown, 1964; 6.

49. Heston WM. Responsible self-management: a pragmatic approach to the treatment of low back pain. Cont Orth 1985; 11:55–57.

50. Feldenkrais M. Awareness through movement. New York: Harper & Row, 1977.

51. Kottke F, Pauley D, Ptak R. The rationale for prolonged stretching for correction of shortening of connective tissue. Arch Phys Med Rehab 1966; 47:345–352.

52. Saal JS. Flexibility training. Phys Med Rehab 1987; (4):537–554.

53. Tollison CD: Stretching exercises. Orthop Rev 1988; 17:35.

54. Gracovetsky S, Farfan HF, Helleur C. The abdominal mechanism. Spine 1985; 10:317.

55. Komi PV. Training of muscle strength and power: interaction of neuromotoric, hypertrophic and mechanical factors. Int J Sports Med 1986; 7:10–15.

56. Cailliet R. Low back pain syndrome. 3rd ed. Philadelphia: FA Davis, 1981.

57. Klausen K. The form and function of the loaded human spine. Acta Physiol Scand 1965; 65:176–190.

58. Micheli L. Low back pain in the adolescent—differential diagnosis. Am J Sports Med 1979; 7:362–364.

59. Stokes I, Abery J. Influence of the hamstring muscles on lumbar spine curvature in sitting. Spine 1980; 5:525–528.

60. Saudek C, Palmer K. Back pain revisited. J Orthop Sports Phys Ther 1987; 8:556–566.

14

ALTERNATIVE SOMATIC THERAPIES

Brian Miller

Since the turn of the century and especially with the advent of the human potential movement in the 1960s and '70s, a category of human wellness has evolved which has come to be known as somatics (1). Somatics involves the study of the human being and the most fundamental expression of human life, i.e., movement, with an emphasis upon the first-person, internal, subjective experience rather than the ofttimes exclusionary third-person, external, objective perspective more common to traditional scientific investigation. These studies can be approached from various viewpoints, as will be demonstrated here, each of which can be found to have a symbiotic relationship with the traditional sciences, each enriching the other and adding to the fullness and sense of completion of the others' understanding.

Within the health care professions, the best known and most fully developed of these disciplines have been referred to as alternative approaches (2). These approaches have been receiving increased attention from traditional health care practitioners who deal with disorders of the locomotor system including that broad area encompassed by low back pain. The physical therapy profession, in particular, has begun to embrace these therapies and integrate their various philosophies, concepts, and techniques into its mainstream, orthopaedic manual therapy, in particular.

Although there are numerous somatic approaches, this chapter will focus upon several that have received the widest acclaim and acceptance and have had the greatest impact upon physical therapists. These are the Alexander Technique, the Feldenkrais Method, Rolfing (Structural Integration), the Trager Approach, and Aston Patterning. Although space

limitations preclude an indepth exposition of each of these therapies, this chapter will provide an overview to direct the inquiring clinician to further exploration of this topic.

ALEXANDER TECHNIQUE

The Alexander Technique (AT) is the grandfather of the somatic therapies. It was developed around the turn of the century by an Australian named F.M. Alexander. Although he had no formal training as a scientist or a medical practitioner, his discovery of this technique through a disciplined, systematic, and logical process of self-study is surely an outstanding example of the scientific method in action (3).

This technique is a method of psychophysical education that teaches people better use of themselves such that posture and movement become more poised, fluid, and graceful. Its goal is education rather than therapy. Use of this technique nevertheless often yields therapeutic results since improved and more efficient posture and movement will very frequently result in improvement or resolution of symptoms.

The essence of the Alexander Technique involves what is known as "use." Use is a difficult concept to define succinctly since it embraces the entire realm of human action including posture, movement, breathing, and speech. It refers to the quality of that action and the way the total pattern of action responds to stimuli. The AT recognizes that thought processes cannot be divested from the action of the body, and encourages action that is preceded and accompanied by conscious attention rather than action that is an unconscious, possibly harmful, reaction to a given stimulus.

Bad use is most frequently evident in the form of a subtle activation of the startle reflex preparatory to initiating any kind of activity. The startle reflex has been described by Jones and others (4, 5). Its extreme state is represented by the brief somatic retraction and muscular cocontraction that occurs as an instinctive protective reaction in response to a strong, sudden stimuli such as an unexpected loud, frightening noise. While this dramatic reaction is short-term and subsides as quickly as it appears, the startle reflex can also persist indefinitely in a much more subtle form. It becomes a habitual remnant that is unreasoned and serves no worthwhile function. This somatic reaction is very common with long-term exposure to chronic stressful factors including emotional states like anxiety. In fact, the muscular pattern present with this low-level startle reflex is inextricably intertwined with anxiety as its somatic representation.

The somatic configuration most characteristic of the startle pattern is a forward and downward translation of the head relative to the trunk. The focus of the AT is to teach the individual to inhibit this unconscious reaction. Inhibition or deactivation of this habitual stereotypical response (or of any other pattern of muscle activation that is excessive, improperly distributed, or in some way effortful, uncoordinated, or inappropriate) is desirable and constitutes good use. While bad use is inefficient and frequently detrimental, good use is characterized by inhibition of unnecessary effort and clarity of (intended) direction yielding a kinesthetic perception of freedom and ease. The resultant posture and movement looks and feels better. Mastering this process gives the individual a clear choice of conscious action over unconscious reaction.

An upward direction of the body manifests itself when this inhibitory process is utilized, suggesting the activation of some sort of reflex postural mechanism. This sense of *up* is governed by the direction of the top of the head and is accompanied by feelings of lengthening and elongating through the spine. The upward direction is initiated by the teacher giving the student verbal orders and using manual contact to convey the same orders kinesthetically.

The verbal orders consist of directing the neck to be free, the head to go forward and up, and the torso (back) to lengthen and widen. (*Note:* The statement of "head forward and up"

is not the same as the standard orthopaedic conception of a forward head; rather, the occiput goes forward in a flexion direction relative to the axis while the entire cranium displaces vertically upward and somewhat posteriorly.) Because language is linear, the directions are sequential, yet their occurrence is virtually simultaneous or, as Alexander stated, "All together, one after the other" (6). An analogous situation would be a locomotive pulling a train. The locomotive initiates the movement yet the entire train moves simultaneously.

Concurrently with the verbal orders, the teacher's hands are used to invoke a dynamic relationship of the head on the neck whereby a sense of effortless poise and balance is achieved, a sense that extends to the rest of the body and the relationship of the head and neck to the trunk, the shoulder girdles to the trunk. This kinesthetic message is ultimately of far greater significance than the verbal orders although the verbal directions do serve as a starting point. Alexander called this particular head-neck-torso relationship the primary control. Although it is compared to the righting reflexes discovered by Magnus, the exact nature of this phenomenon has yet to be elucidated.

Simply telling students that their actions have gone astray and must be corrected is not enough. Faulty use of the self necessarily involves somewhat faulty and distorted sensory appreciation. Therefore, when students think they are doing one thing, they are often doing something else very different. This faulty sensory appreciation requires the presence of a teacher to provide an accurate kinesthetic image of the desirable head-neck-trunk relationship and to provide feedback and guidance of a kinesthetic, tactile, and verbal nature throughout the learning process. Having this external frame of reference available allows students to become aware of their habitual use and enables them to institute positive changes.

A typical Alexander lesson lasts 30 to 45 minutes. The student is fully clothed and often the work begins with the student sitting in a chair. Less frequently, a table may be used when the Alexander work is performed with the student in a recumbent position (known as tablework). The teacher's hands are used to induce a relationship among head, neck, shoulders, and back that instills a feeling of kinesthetic lightness. Once this impression of lightness is experienced in a stationary position, the progression is made to creating this experience during motion. As long as this optimal relationship is maintained, the student can easily carry out normal activities without the accustomed sense of effort and strain (4). In the early stages of learning this relationship, much input is needed from the teacher. As the student becomes more familiar with the AT, less input is required and the student acquires the ability readily to assume the proper relationship with little or no input. Consequently, a transition occurs from being teacher-dependent to being teacher-independent (capable of self-education or treatment). The number of lessons required to make this transition is, of course, highly variable but ranges anywhere from one (rarely!) to twenty or thirty on the average. The perception of kinesthetic lightness from a single demonstration persists, at least for a short time, but the memory of it can linger for life (4). Further lessons serve to reinforce and amplify this feeling and refine the applications of the technique.

By using light pressure, which by its very quality and nature suggests an upward direction (rather than simply pulling or pushing upward), the teacher establishes the balance or poise of the pupil's head in such a way that the muscles of the neck (mainly the posterior musculature and particularly the suboccipital muscles) are encouraged to release and thereby lengthen. The occiput tends to roll or glide forward out of occipito-atlantal extension into a more neutral position with this procedure, the tone of the posterior musculature is reduced to the minimal level necessary to maintain an erect position, and the entire neck lengthens vertically. Applying too much pressure or applying it too quickly or otherwise being overly hurried or urgent with the directing hand pressure can prevent the desired effect from resulting. When the Alexander Technique is properly carried out, the head will feel well balanced and rest easily on the neck, like a golf ball on a tee. The head will seem almost weightless, to teacher and student alike, and respond in a friction-free, fluid manner to any manual input. Having achieved this sense of equipoise, the teacher proceeds by extending this sensation of release through the entire length of the spine and eventually, the rest of the body. The teacher does this in the same manner, by using a light, persuasive, directional style of touch

coupled with verbal suggestions to gently guide the student towards a more ideal configuration.

The teacher and student then progress to maintaining this improved head-neck relationship during the performance of everyday movements such as coming to standing from sitting, walking, raising an arm, and talking. In the process, the student's body can be felt to lengthen and become more vertical, and will seem lighter in its responsiveness to movement. Movements will be easier and smoother, the student will feel taller and more relaxed (although most teachers are loath to use the word "relax," students will often use the word as a descriptor), and the student's overall bearing will be one of grace and composure.

To understand the AT more fully, it is important to be aware of its various concepts such as use, inhibition, direction, primary control, and faulty sensory appreciation. An additional concept is the attention the AT places upon the "means whereby" rather than "end-gaining," which describes the process-orientation of the AT. When the focus is upon the end or goal of action, the action is performed habitually, the concern being not on performance but rather on achievement of the goal. When attention is kinesthetically directed towards the process involved in attaining a goal, awareness is enhanced such that the quality of the action can improve substantially and the goal is more economically and less stressfully attained. This is what occurs when one pays attention to inhibition or direction while performing a movement rather than just doing the movement with no regard to "how."

The AT is not directed toward alleviating or treating symptoms. Rather, it is directed toward improving use and thereby, indirectly, addressing symptoms by eliminating factors that would tend to produce symptoms such as dysponesis (7) (bracing, holding, efforting) and inefficient movement patterns. It deals with the use of the entire organism, even with specific problems such as low back pain. Wilfred Barlow, M.D., an Alexander teacher, underscores this concept: "It is wrong to treat a painful back as a local condition. Back pain is always accompanied and preceded by general misuse" (8).

The universality of the AT allows it to be applied in almost any context, from doing therapeutic exercise to performing activities of daily living, from receiving manual therapy to going through back school. Although applying its concepts assiduously can be helpful with acute pain, it is not uncommon for the pain to obscure awareness and make it difficult to focus on anything other than the pain. Like many of the other somatic therapies, the AT is most effectively utilized in instances of chronic and subacute pain and dysfunction rather than highly acute pain.

FELDENKRAIS METHOD

The Feldenkrais Method (FM) is an elegant, gentle, nonintrusive method of reprogramming the central nervous system by utilizing nonthreatening, nonhabitual passive and active movement to explore the interdependency of thinking, feeling, sensing, and moving. This process develops kinesthetic awareness and achieves a sensory-motor integration that allows improved motor learning ability and expanded potential for learning. It was developed by Moshe Feldenkrais, a renowned Israeli physicist. There are two interrelated formats for the method. The first is an intensive hands-on, one-to-one teaching known as Functional Integration (FI). FI utilizes the practitioner's touch and handling skills to communicate change in the student's neuromuscular organization and to translate those changes into efficient, economical, easy movement. The second consists of verbally directed group lessons in movement exploration known as Awareness Through Movement (ATM). ATM uses the attentive repetition of nonstrenuous, active movements, performed in a planned sequence, to change the patterns in the brain that organize and control movement (9).

Functional Integration

The hands-on technique is so named because the functions of the teacher and the student are neurally integrated in a cybernetic mode so that the more sensitive and discriminating nervous system of the teacher detects small differences essential to the learning process and communicates those differences to the student by means of skillful touch and handling. The nature of this two-way communicative feedback system between the teacher and student is such that a Functional Integration lesson takes on a dance-like style. The action of the teacher

serves to propose certain conditions and the teacher notes the student's responses to these tactile and kinesthetic proposals. The teacher then guides the student according to the nature of these responses and the interaction of these responses with the teacher's plans for the theme and direction of the lesson. Feldenkrais, in fact, compared the interplay in FI to dancing and the way a skilled dance partner can, through guidance, allow a poorer dancer to perform well.

Bringing the student's awareness to small distinctions and building upon those distinctions, leading the student to learn new, more efficient options for movement is the fundamental goal of the lesson. This goal is achieved by the quality and sensitivity of the teacher's touch and by a variety of unique and interesting movements. A core principle underlying this quality of touch is the teacher's intent. Precision and specificity of intention allow the tactile and kinesthetic message being communicated to the student to be the clearest possible. The clarity of the message increases the likelihood of its absorption and retention. In addition, the sensitivity with which students are touched allows them to feel understood and to be understood at a very deep level, creating an ambience of safety and security that is essential to learning. Effective learning also requires motivation. By introducing nonhabitual positions and movements that are interesting and pleasurable and arouse curiosity yet are meaningful and relevant, the teacher can evoke and sustain the desired motivational state.

The teacher produces these movements in the student by projecting touch (in the form of pushing or pulling, for example) through the bones of the student's skeleton so as to create a trajectory of movement. This trajectory is ultimately dictated by the structural constraints of the skeleton and its articulations. In other words, the ideal path of action is that which the skeleton would follow if there were no interference by muscles. Any deviation from this movement pathway indicates superfluous or parasitic muscle activity that hampers fluid, efficient movement.

Because the FM is a learning-based approach, the sessions are referred to as lessons, the practitioner as a teacher, and the patient as a student. The lesson is designed to teach the student, by means of functional integration, about a particular movement (or movement sequence) relevant to the problem or need. To more clearly explain what is involved in the process of FI, Rywerant has proposed the concept of a *manipulon,* a unit of communicative manipulation (10). He uses this concept to discuss the methodology involved in an FI session. Although the manipulon is a somewhat artificial construct and belies the flowing, integrative nature of a session, it is a useful way of categorizing aspects of a lesson for didactic purposes. The various classifications of manipulons include exploratory, conforming, leading, and integrative manipulons, each of which will be explained in turn.

To offer the possibility of change in a movement pattern, the teacher first needs to be aware of what the student habitually does. The teacher first looks carefully to note various structural and functional features such as bony and articular position and alignment, muscle tonus (its level and distribution), and patterns of muscle activity. Then the teacher begins a tactile and kinesthetic "inquiry" into the pupil's structure and neuromuscular functioning. Using skills of palpation (touch) and moving various body parts (handling) in an exploratory type manner and correlating this information with what is seen, both with regard to the student's resting state and responses to these manual "investigations," the teacher gathers information that will determine the content and direct the course of the lesson. This process is known as an exploratory manipulon.

During the lesson, the teacher monitors not only the ongoing movement but also other related movement functions, such as breathing. By observing the student's breathing, the teacher will be aware of the degree of relaxation, the response to various inputs, and the processing of the newly presented information.

The teacher then needs to convey this information to the student. By joining the student's system and accurately matching the responses without attempting to correct them, the teacher allows the student to become more fully aware of the prevailing way of functioning. For example, if the student performs a movement in an inefficient trajectory, the teacher shows the exact path of that very trajectory, with particular emphasis on the deviation from the ideal path. Or if the student overactivates a muscle, the teacher shows precisely how that was done and how to do the movement well. This process

of showing the student what he or she is doing by congruently matching it is known as a conforming manipulon (10).

Once the student understands what she or he is doing, the teacher can begin to show alternative paths of action and lead toward other possibilities. The manner in which the student is led is important. The leading should at first be light (with little effort), small, and slow so that attention can be directed to every point in the trajectory. The movements should be pleasurable, interesting, or unusual so that the student's curiosity and desire to perform the movement are aroused, and yet safe and nonthreatening so that conscious or unconscious protective responses are not provoked. As the lesson proceeds, the teacher may choose to develop the movements into faster and more expansive ones. This progression is known as a leading manipulon (10).

The leading manipulon can assume many forms. One particular form, a juxtaposing manipulon, compares and contrasts one situation with another. It may be comparing a condition or structure on the one side of the body with the other side, it may be comparing one position or movement with another. One ubiquitous form used in the FM is that of relative conjugate movements (10). This technique contrasts movement performed with the proximal part fixed and the distal part mobile, with movement performed with the distal part fixed and the proximal part mobile (in the instance of muscles, looking at movement with a reversal of origin and insertion).

Another leading manipulon is the confining manipulon (10), which is characterized by encouraging movement in one directiion, particularly the direction of greatest ease, and preventing movement or work in another direction. A particular example of this manipulon is the use of effort substitution (10). Here the teacher's effort is substituted for that habitually performed by the student's muscles, allowing the student's nervous system to recognize that effort is no longer necessary and can be reduced.

A third form of the leading manipulon is a positioning manipulon (10). This manipulon involves either supporting the student comfortably in a resting position or transferring him or her from one position to another as easily and effectively as possible. The FM always emphasizes the importance of options—in position, in movement, in life in general. A particular form of this manipulon may involve teaching the student three possible rest positions for a low back problem. Another would be to show an efficient, less stressful way of changing position, for example, from a recumbent to a sitting position. Transfers or transitional movements such as these are always defined by the structural limitations of the joints and the most efficient skeletal path of action.

The integrating manipulon (10) is the form of leading manipulon most vital to helping the student successfully incorporate a useful concept into regular movement patterns. It may involve further completion of the student's image of a concept that was clarified in preceding manipulons or it may present that concept in a new context. Completing the image can be accomplished by correlating movement from one area of the body with movement in another area of the body, demonstrating the whole body connectedness that is manifested with any movement. The greater the number of connections established between various areas of the body in performing an action, the greater the likelihood of the new movement pattern becoming well established in daily activities. Presenting that concept in a new context may involve performing the movement in a new position. Feldenkrais stated that he regularly used about 30 positions (10a). The more positions that a movement can be learned in, the better the assimilation of that movement and its integration into normal motor patterns. Overall, the lesson consists of an interactive weave of evolving manipulons. The integrating manipulon is the thread that binds this fabric together to create a meaningful whole.

In summary, the lesson consists of a methodical presentation of various options for component positions and movements. These components are progressively assembled in a systematic and meaningful fashion into increasingly larger aggregates of movement (again with the emphasis placed upon relevant movement combinations and the possible options they present). Eventually, the student progresses performing a whole, complete movement sequence that is more clear and well defined, easier and more efficient, and less likely to result in pain or damage than previously used motor patterns. Thus, the progression is from habitual, nondifferentiated movements to nonhabitual, differentiated movements to a more clear and efficient integrated movement

sequence that will teach the student new beneficial movement possibilities. The result is improved differentiation of the various parts of the body and of the relation between them with a subsequent lessening of tonus, an increase in conscious (cortical) control, and a concomitant shift away from limbic system influence.

Awareness Through Movement™

The second format in the Feldenkrais Method is Awareness Through Movement (ATM) lessons. These are group experiential lessons in movement exploration and awareness in which the participants are verbally guided through a structured sequence of movements. The style of these lessons simulates the exploratory learning natural to infants. The lessons are very similar to FI in their purpose and intent, in the sensitive way in which they are conducted (with slow, small, easy, questing movements with frequent interruptions for rest and processing), and in the results obtained. The differences are the absence of any manual contact from the teacher and the fact that ATM is less appropriate for serious problems where one-on-one help (as provided by FI) is indicated. ATM lessons can be used apart from FI with problems of a minor nature or they may be used as an adjunct to FI. In this adjunctive role, they may serve as a home exercise program designed to further develop movement awareness, or the basic movement sequence can be adapted into a stretching or strengthening exercise, done with a new sense of awareness and improved efficiency. (*Note:* This latter application is not a traditional aspect of the FM.)

The lessons are usually done lying on the floor (to minimize the influence of antigravity muscular responses). The participants are encouraged to attune their awareness to subtle internal sensations and feelings and to cultivate the quality and scope of this attentiveness. Attention is directed to how and where movements are initiated, how the movement is transmitted through the body, what prevents the movement from going farther, and what adjustments would allow it to proceed farther. Awareness is also brought to breathing, participation of the *entire* body, and quality, quantity, and location of contact with the supporting surface.

The lesson progression follows a pattern similar to an FI lesson, starting with the various possible options of small component movements, summing and expanding these movements into progressively larger, meaningful movement combinations that eventually evolve into a new or more fully clarified, complete movement sequence. ATM lessons take about 45 minutes on the average, about as long as an FI lesson.

A classic example of an ATM lesson is the pelvic clock (11), which teaches how to differentiate a multitude of possible movements of the pelvis and then examines the relationship of these movements to the spine, head and lower extremities. By cultivating sensitivity and releasing unnecessary muscle tension, participants acquire a sense of freedom and ease in posture, movement, and breathing. Reduction or elimination of chronic discomfort, and a positive feeling of physical and emotional well-being are frequent by-products of learning these new movement options. In summation, the ATM lessons allow an individual to explore the tremendous capacity the nervous system has for self-correction and self-improvement without requiring a teacher other than oneself.

The Feldenkrais Method is oriented toward improving function, not treating symptoms. A lesson is directed toward what an individual needs to do better and is designed to reprogram the neuromotor system into more efficient patterns of action that will allow the improvement to occur. Almost always, however, the improved function can't help but result in the decrease or elimination of symptoms.

While the method does not specifically deal with the standard medical diagnoses, it does address neuromotor inefficiencies or deficiencies that can result in or exist concomitantly with conditions normally associated with low back pain. Typical examples of neuromotor dysfunction that could result in back pain include a nonextending trunk where there is overactivity of the flexors; habitual overactivity of the extensors; a fixated, nonrotating trunk; excessive lateralization of function; inefficiency of timing; and general hypertonicity (1, 10, 12). Ultimately, however, the goal of the Feldenkrais Method is to teach the individual to learn how to learn movement.

ROLFING (STRUCTURAL INTEGRATION)

Rolfing, or Structural Integration, is a somatic therapy developed by Ida Rolf, a biochemist and physiologist. It is a structurally oriented approach based on improving the vertical alignment of human structure in the gravitational field and achieving that end by deep manipulation of the fascia (connective tissue) of the body. Since most human beings are significantly out of ideal alignment with gravity and function better (on many levels) when this alignment is optimized, it is desirable to make use of the plasticity of human structure to improve our structural organization.

The fascia is always amenable to change and can respond to the proper application of force by undergoing a plastic deformation. This deformation allows the normal length, alignment, orientation, and mobility of the fascia to be regained, thereby facilitating improvement in the skeletal alignment as well. Rolf looked upon fascia as "the organ of structure" and recognized that an orderly restoration of fascial freedom around a vertical "core" axis in the body would enable gravity to support and maintain the integrity of the body rather than act as a disorganizing and harmful stressor.

The conceptual model of Buckminster Fuller's "tensegrity" structure is often used by Rolfers to explain how fascia is involved in the support of the body (13, 14). A tensegrity structure is one that maintains its integrity through tensile forces. Such a model can be made of wires. Applying an external compressive force results in increased tension being created and distributed through the wires. The mechanism by which the various fascial envelopes and planes of the body provide for support and movement is postulated to be similar.

Rolfing is generally performed as a series of 10 sessions, each about an hour to an hour and a half long, spaced about a week apart. Every part of the body is worked on, but especially those areas where the body is most misaligned vertically. Each session involves working on particular areas of the body specific to that session and then ensuring optimal relationships of that area with other regions of the body by balancing the changes obtained in that particular region with the remainder of the body. In dealing with a problem such as back pain, symptoms per se are not addressed directly. Treatment focuses upon a structural reorganization of the connective tissues and, as such, structure and the movement of that structure, rather than pain, are used as treatment guidelines. Often, however, once structural dysfunctions are resolved, symptoms decrease or are eliminated. Care is taken, nonetheless, to avoid creating new symptoms or exacerbating existing ones.

Furthermore, the symptomatic areas are not the only ones addressed. Structural Integration recognizes that treatment of these regions only can often be successful in the short-term alleviation of symptoms but results in the recurrence of symptoms in the long term since the underlying causes have not been corrected. Consequently, it is vital to include in treatment those areas of the body that are nonsymptomatic but are contributing to and perpetuating the problem. Very often, the different regions of the body are considered as distinct, separate entities unto themselves because of traditional anatomical didactic methodology that looks at "parts." In truth, they are continuous and the distinction is only an artificial one, meant for the sake of teaching purposes but often carried through and considered as reality. The interactive and integrative nature of the various regions of the human body requires that the organism always be considered in its entirety and treated as a whole, not simply as a collection of parts.

Before starting treatment, full length photographs are taken of the patient. These pretreatment pictures are then compared to pictures taken at the completion of the 10th session to give the client a posttreatment comparison. In this way, the patient not only has an internal kinesthetic frame of reference for noticing changes, but an external visual frame of reference as well. The Rolfer assesses need for intervention in several ways. Visual inspection reveals how the various regions of the body (head, neck, thorax) line up vertically and determines if sufficient spatial dimension has been achieved in the fascial tissues. Watching the patient's movements enables the Rolfer to see where restrictions persist in the system. Rolfers look at the body with more of an artistic and esthetic eye rather than in the conventional orthopaedic manner that a traditional health care practitioner would use.

A low treatment table is utilized so that the Rolfer may make maximum use of gravity in applying the techniques. The actual hands-on aspect of Rolfing uses deep pressure applied through the fingers, knuckles, or elbows to mechanically deform the connective tissue. By applying a force and maintaining loading, the therapist guides the fascia through a slow, plastic deformation into a more elongated, resilient configuration. At the same time, the Rolfer instructs the patient to move the specified area while the Rolfer maintains and directs pressure. Thus, the patient's active movement synergistically complements the Rolfer's pressure and allows the force to be functionally directed so that the fascia is accurately reoriented and the movement is freed in the desired direction.

Rolfing has a reputation for being painful that, in its present form, is largely exaggerated. The sensitive application of force, the trajectory of that force application, and most importantly, the cooperation and nonresistance of the patient will generally result in mild to minimal discomfort. The Rolfer must apply strong enough pressure to affect change but must be sensitive to the patient's pain threshold. The realization that any pain is almost always transient in nature, and abates as soon as the Rolfer's pressure is removed, is reassuring to the patient. The Rolfer needs to make the patient aware of how tightening or bracing muscles against the therapeutic pressure very often has the reverse effect from that desired; that is, rather than protecting against pain, this protective action will often magnify or create pain. Judith Aston influenced teaching Rolfers the trajectory of force application (15). She discovered that a curvilinear application of force matches the contours of a person's tissues and is less invasive (and therefore, less painful) than a linear force application. By encouraging patients to take an active role in the process of change and focusing their awareness, cueing their breathing, using appropriate imagery, and directing them toward relaxation, Rolfers can greatly facilitate the releases and the ease with which they occur.

Rolfers make several points about the experience of pain. One is that now Rolfers tend to work *with* their patient rather than *on* their patient. This increased cooperation and active participation of the patient makes pain less likely. In addition, sensitivity allows the Rolfer to work deeply enough to effect change but lightly enough to respect the individual's pain threshold. An interesting but perhaps somewhat euphemistic comment made by some Rolfers is that the pain felt with Rolfing is pain that the person is releasing rather than pain that is being inflicted.

Objective effects of treatment are noted with observation, movement testing, and palpation.

Visually, the body will appear to have more volume, be less contracted inward. Movements will be improved in quality, if not quantity. They will be smoother, more fluid, and even more coordinated. Palpation of tissue will reveal that previously dry, stringy tissue will have a plumper "juicier" (more hydrated) feeling. Likewise, bulgy, overdeveloped muscles will be less knotted, smoother, and softer.

Subjectively, the body will feel more open, more relaxed, and better aligned. Joints will feel freer, as if well lubricated. The patient will have a sense of optimal vertical orientation and, because of this improved relationship with the gravitational field, will feel solidly supported by the ground. The dramatic nature of this improved condition often subsides somewhat, but the patient will retain a certain measure of freer movement and, more importantly, will retain a vivid mental image of freer movement. The patient will realize that this improved condition is possible, can be retained with appropriate attention, and added to with further treatment, increased awareness, and properly applied movement work. An interesting phenomenon noted both subjectively and objectively is that the treatment frequently imparts a certain measure of therapeutic momentum. That is, the patient will often show further improvements at a later date that were not evident immediately after treatment. (*Note:* This phenomenon has been noted with other somatic disciplines as well.) As in every other human experience, however, these long-term changes are not universally experienced or acknowledged. However, their occurrence underscores the primacy of the self-correcting and self-regulating mechanisms of the human body in obtaining positive improvements in the somatic state.

The theme and progression of the sessions are standardized. The sequence was developed by Ida Rolf who felt that it was the most logical and beneficial for creating orderly and lasting change in the body. However, since each body is highly individual, the work in each session will vary according to the nature of the restrictions present.

The first session deals with breathing and thus much of the focus is upon the thorax and its relationship to adjoining structures. This session is concerned with freeing the shoulder girdle from the thorax and establishing the proper relationship and space between the pelvis and the thorax. The second session addresses the foundation or supporting structures of the body, the feet, and legs. The third session deals with the lateral lines of the body. It is designed to establish sides that match the front and back of the body giving the patient a sense of depth and internal volume. The lateral muscles, such as the quadratus lumborum, and the upper extremities are treated in this session. These first three sessions involve the superficial, extrinsic myofascial structures.

The fourth session deals with the pelvis and includes the pelvic floor and various muscles that attach to the pelvis, such as the adductors. The fifth session addresses the psoas muscles and their functional balance with the abdominal muscles as well as their connection with other structures such as the diaphragm. The involvement of the psoas with gait as opposed to frequent overutilization of the quadriceps is also addressed. The sixth session has to do with the spine, especially its foundation, the sacrum. The seventh session deals with the head, face, and neck region and its relationship to the rest of the body. Sessions four through seven tend to deal with the deeper intrinsic myofascial elements of the body.

Sessions eight through ten are integrative in nature. The eighth and ninth deal with the shoulder girdle and the pelvic girdle (the one requiring the most work being first in the sequence). The tenth session acts to tie the body together, top half to bottom half and inner core structures to outer sleeve structures. Once the hands-on work is complete, the client is given instructions for retaining this improved state through appropriate movement and direction of awareness. A separate area of Rolfing known as Rolfing Movement Integration addresses movement reeducation in greater detail.

Rolfing is, by the admission of many of its devotees, not designed to treat an acute problem. Rather, its focus is upon optimizing the structure of the person. As such, it is best applied to the chronic conditions where the fascia has become bound down, shortened, and dehydrated. It can be wonderfully effective in certain situations but the fixed pattern of progression is not suitable for some patients who do better with a more succinct, directed, individualized approach.

TRAGER APPROACH

Trager Psychophysical Integration or the Trager Approach (TA) is a somatic approach developed by Milton Trager, a physician. Its origins were highly intuitive and thus, in many ways, it is the least structured of the major somatic disciplines addressed in this chapter. The goal of the TA is to eliminate psychophysical blocks in the unconscious mind. Trager believes that these thought patterns manifest themselves in patterns of limitation in the body. While this description may sound like that of a psychotherapeutic approach, it should be remembered that many everyday human movements such as walking or driving a car have, to a large degree, been relegated to the unconscious mind. The intent of the Trager work is to communicate a sensorimotor message of positive feelings (lightness, softness, ease, security) from the unconscious mind of the practitioner to the unconscious mind of the patient by way of the practitioner's hands moving the patient's body in a particular way. The movements are rhythmic and wave-like in nature and impart a soothing, undulatory motion to the patient's body. They are designed to convey a sense of openness and expansiveness and allow the patient the safety and freedom to release any unnecessary holding.

Fundamental to the TA is the concept of hook-up, Trager's name for the relaxed state of meditative consciousness that the practitioner assumes for the purpose of being maximally sensitive, perceptive, and in harmony with self and patient. Just as the Alexander Technique requires that the practitioner's use of self be optimal, and the Feldenkrais Method emphasizes the importance of the cybernetic relationship between the teacher and the student and the need for one's own integration and sensitivity, so too the TA recognizes, in its own unique fashion, the need for self-development. This is in the form of hook-up.

The touch employed by a Trager practitioner is a soft, open, sliding, shifting, dynamic touch that communicates a sensory message of an easy and relaxed state of being. The movements utilized have been variously described as rocking, rolling, shaking, shimmering, spreading, and tractioning. Their overall effect is to produce a peaceful, tranquil feeling in the patient, as if being rocked like a baby.

A session is normally one to one and a half hours long. All regions of the body are worked on in a sequence that usually proceeds from head and neck, to anterior legs, to abdomen, to chest, to posterior legs, to shoulders, to low back and buttocks, and finishing with the neck again. Although the routine is somewhat chor-

eographed, each session is unique to that patient at that particular time. Rather than treating the different regions of the body in a separate and isolated fashion, the person is treated in a serial yet integrative fashion. Thus no two treatments are identical and the moves tend to flow into one another creating the image of a rhythmic, fluid "dance."

In addition to the tablework, the patient is shown "mentastics" (mental gymnastics). These are active movements designed to allow the patient to recall and reinstate the sensory impressions gathered from the passive movements performed by the practitioner in the tablework. While the feeling of lightness and openness obtained from the session can fade over time, the patient can recall those feelings and thereby facilitate reproducing them both mentally and physically by performing mentastics. In this way the patient can not only reestablish the beneficial results gained in a session, but further continue the process of development by regularly doing mentastics.

The interchangeability between the tablework and mentastics is emphasized. The tablework consists simply of the practitioner passively performing mentastic movements on the patient in a resting state, while mentastics are simply an active replication or continuation of these movements by the patient.

A common mistake made by those attempting to duplicate Trager movements without appropriate training is to use them in a massage-like manner or to stretch out areas. There is a profound difference between doing the Trager movements and actual Trager work that resides in the feeling state of the practitioner and the resultant intention. Trager never works *on* tissue; the key is working *with* the tissue to communicate positive feeling sensations to the unconscious mind. Restrictions are never directly confronted. Rather patients are shown the possibility of light, easy, free movement within their limitations. In this way, the confines of the restrictions gently fall back, openness and expansiveness begin to prevail, and the unconscious mind is shown the possibility of an improved way of being. The entire process is very gentle and noninvasive, one of coaxing and persuasion rather than force and coercion.

Because of the nature of the Trager Approach, it can be highly effective in achieving deep relaxation and in eliminating or reducing functional holding patterns, neuromuscular hypertonus, or other problems involving inappropriate muscle guarding or bracing. Since these conditions frequently play a significant role in the genesis and/or proliferation of low back-pain, it can be seen that the TA can play a significant role in this area. While it cannot correct a true structural holding pattern, it is surprising how, with the right sensitivity, holding patterns that were often thought to be structural resolve, and thereby show themselves to have been functional restrictions only. Because of the constant movement involved, one must be cautious in applying this technique when there is high joint irritability or latent pain (16), where inflammation is present (as in a nerve root impingement), and when the patient is prone to motion sickness.

While the language used by Trager practitioners often has more to do with transcendental meditation than with medicine, the reasons for Trager's success are based in neurophysiology and the behavioral sciences. The astute health care professional must be careful to put aside prejudice of a method simply because a standard medical frame of reference and terminology are not utilized. Many patients have been helped by this approach who would otherwise have obtained incomplete or unsatisfactory treatment through the standard medical systems.

ASTON PATTERNING

Aston Patterning (AP) is an integrated system of movement education, three-dimensional soft tissue body work, environmental modification, and fitness training developed by Judith Aston, an educator and innovator in the somatic field as well as an ergonomic product designer. It is unique among the somatic disciplines in its completeness. AP includes a comprehensive formal evaluative system, manual techniques that are applicable to a wide range of dysfunctions in the neuromusculoskeletal system, movement education procedures, a number of exercise programs—each designed to develop a particular aspect of fitness, and an array of fundamental concepts that allow the work to have an extraordinary scope of application (15, 17).

The evaluation procedures include both a subjective and an objective component. A detailed history is taken first. Then pretreatment testing is performed that includes viewing the body structurally while at rest and then observing the person performing either a simple functional movement task or a movement specific to AP, such as arcing (which will be explained later in this discussion). Features noted during observation include alignment and dimensions and proportions. Alignment deals with the placement of the body and its parts. The relationship of parts in space and the distribution of weight bearing through those parts are two aspects of alignment. Dimension and proportion concern the internal volume of the body or a body part and how that volume is distributed with regard to its component dimensions of length, depth, and width. Regions of decreased dimension are areas that will require attention. This decrease may be determined by comparison with the contralateral side, with adjacent parts, or with the body as a whole.

The observed movement can be a simple functional one, such as coming to standing from sitting, walking, or a movement associated with the person's normal activities of daily living, occupation, or recreation. It may also include an activity unique to AP, such as arcing. Arcing is an apparently simple flexion-extension movement of the whole body that can be enacted and studied in an increasingly detailed fashion. It is a complex movement-awareness activity that serves a number of purposes including teaching such movement concepts as balanced weight transfer, use of momentum, breathing for release, eye tracking, acknowledging asymmetry, and finding neutral.

Palpation is performed using Aston's three-dimensional touch, a particular way of using touch in congruency with the practitioner's body so that maximum sensitivity is obtained. Salient findings are placed on a body chart and correlated with those obtained through observation. These findings will direct the treatment. The manual techniques utilized in AP fall into three categories. One such technique, functional massage, is designed especially to reduce and normalize tone. The hands are used in a three-dimensional fashion in alternately opposite directions with broad contact over large surfaces, giving patients a sense of feeling their own shape and allowing them to release functional holding patterns.

The most commonly used manual technique is called myokinetics. It utilizes highly localized three-dimensional spiralling strokes. As in functional massage, the spiralling nature of the strokes is designed to match the contours of the body, whether these are surface contours or contours of the tissues. To preserve the integrity of the tissue while performing this work, the practitioner avoids compressing tissues by using gentle and very specific strokes that alternately stretch and release the tissues. The practitioner also avoids any needless trauma that may result from working through more superficial tissues by creating slack in these tissues. This slack allows the tissues to be moved aside while the work is directed to the appropriate layer of tissue. Myokinetics is directed toward the myofascia and is used to remove restrictions and rehydrate this tissue.

The deepest work is called arthrokinetics. It addresses restrictions at the joint level. Rather than using linear movements traditionally associated with joint mobilization, the practitioner "spirals down" to the articular level and thus can achieve a deep effect without violating the more superficial tissues. This broad range of manual techniques utilized in AP allows restrictions to be treated on both the functional (neurological and behavioral) and the structural (myofascial and articular) levels.

At the core of AP is movement education known as neurokinetics. In fact, the purpose of the manual technique is to allow or sustain changes that are produced with movement education. Movements are broken up into "units of work" such as sitting-to-standing or an arm unit for tasks involving upper extremity activity. The goal here is not so much to teach how to move but to teach how to learn and integrate principles of movement into the particular unit of work and, eventually, all other movements. As in other aspects of AP, an individual, problem-solving approach is employed. A key factor in the success of the movement education is the adroit application of verbal and nonverbal (tactile and kinesthetic) communication skills.

An additional aspect of AP is Aston Fitness. This is exercise training tailored to the individual to improve proportion, muscle tone, joint resiliency, cardiovascular conditioning, and lightness in movement. There are five sequences of exercise and movement:

1. horizontal loosening (lying on the floor) using weight in motion,
2. vertical loosening (standing) using weight transfer,
3. stretching,
4. toning (using weights and a device called a toning platform to facilitate alignment, and
5. cardiovascular conditioning.

The key to AP is the Aston Paradigm, a set of principles underlying all aspects of this body work system. The first concept is that of the wisdom of the body. That is, the body has a reason for being in the condition it is in, and to implement effective and lasting change, one needs to understand and deal with the underlying causes. Respecting the integrity of the body is another principle. This principle has many ramifications but one aspect of it involves the understanding that the body compensates in various ways to maintain balance. This compensation can be in space (by displacement) or spatial dimension, in force or effort (with tension), in movement (hypermobility counterbalancing hypomobility), and in time (timing or sequence of movement). A third principle is that of alignment of body parts including the alignment of part to part, part to whole, the whole to gravity (for weight bearing), and the whole to environmental constructs (such as shoes, chairs). The latter consideration (the attention to environmental factors and appropriate modification of those factors) can range from modifying shoe lacing patterns to utilizing a system of wedges and supports developed by Aston for optimizing sitting alignment.

Other concepts include: all movement following an asymmetrical three-dimensional spiral, arrangement and utilization of base of support, awareness of cooperative movement, the principle of matching, the implications of holding patterns, and the use of weight in motion. These concepts further underscore the uniqueness of many aspects of the Aston Paradigm in recognizing and finding practical application for certain principles of physics within the scope of human movement.

The level of integration between body work, movement education, and environmental modification, the recognition of and respect for asymmetry in structure and movement, and the individualized problem-solving approach to each patient are aspects of AP that are unique both in other somatic disciplines and in the more traditional manual therapies. Because of the meticulous attention to proper positioning prior to initiating manual techniques and the unusual adaptability of its range of techniques, AP is suitable not only for the chronic low back patient but also for the acute patient. Its various positioning and movement principles can be utilized as a sophisticated foundation for any back school or back conditioning program.

Both standing on its own and as an adjunct to standard physical therapy, AP can be of great value for a very wide range of low back complaints. It would behoove all health care professionals involved with treating low back pain to investigate this discipline further.

HELLERWORK

Another somatic discipline that developed as an offshoot of both Rolfing and Aston Patterning is Hellerwork. Developed by Joseph Heller, a past president of the Rolf Institute, it is remarkably similar to Rolfing in its format with the difference that an eleventh session is added and each session includes relevant movement education and deliberate, purposeful verbal dialogue. The eleventh session does not, however, involve body work. Rather, its expressed purpose is "completion, self-expression, and empowerment" (18). The movement-education aspect is influenced by the work of Judith Aston, with whom Heller trained. The verbal dialogue component examines the relationship between a patient's emotions and attitudes and somatic configuration. Thus, Hellerwork integrates deep connective tissue body work, movement education, and verbal dialogue. Because of its similarities, its applicability to the problem of low back pain is the same as that discussed in the section on Rolfing (19).

Each of these somatic therapy approaches possesses its own distinctive philosophies, concepts, and techniques and yet, in many ways, they resemble one another. First of all, they all have a holistic orientation. Webster (20) defines holism as "the view that an organic or integrated whole has a reality independent of and greater than the sum of its parts." Although the word has been greatly overused, if we examine the way each of these approaches looks at back pain, the word is quite appropriate. This definition and these approaches are in agreement with the growing recognition that the body operates according to systems theory. No structure or function exists in isolation. There is an interrelation on many levels, including the mechanical and neural. Thus, these approaches generally deal with the soma as a whole, even if the problem appears to be a local one. Such things as head and shoulder position, organization of the cervical musculature, thoracic cage mobility, ventral soft tissue status, hip joint mobility, and the foot's shock absorbing function, are but a few of the multitude of factors that can affect the degree of stress placed upon the lumbar spine. Therefore, treatment of back pain is never limited to addressing only the suspected local anatomical origin of the pain but includes the entire organism, both from a structural and from a functional and behavioral perspective.

This holistic perspective suggests that a medical diagnosis such as a bulging anulus may explain the present source of pain but fails to address adequately those influences that preceded and, eventually, precipitated the present problem and are perhaps still present and operating in such a manner as to interfere with the healing process. Such influences may arise from dysponetic states (7), inefficient or aberrant movement patterns, fascial restrictions, or other atypical (from a medical perspective) yet ubiquitous dysfunctions that may involve not only the low back but other areas of the body as well, particularly the remainder of the weight-bearing skeleton.

This holism also acknowledges that the mind and body are inseparably interactive, and a dualistic separatist approach not only belies reality but also may prolong or misdirect the therapeutic process. These approaches go beyond the oft mentioned but mainly theoretical recognition of body-mind unity and provide practical strategies based upon applications of this concept. Employing these somatic approaches elucidates how thoughts, feelings, and emotions are intimately associated and interwoven with the somatic state of the human organism. For example, most of these approaches recognize how certain negative emotional states (such as chronic anxiety) can result in a predictable somatic configuration (cocontractive retraction with flexion predominance, along with certain idiosyncratic variations) that, if allowed to exist over the long term, may be a contributory factor in the genesis of low back pain.

Training for each of these approaches carries a strong emphasis upon refining manual therapy and teaching skills. Central to this refinement is the theme that self-improvement and self-development are essential in enabling the practitioner to achieve the highest skill levels. Whether this is viewed in terms of the "use" of an Alexander teacher, the "hook-up" of the Trager practitioner, or the neuromotor reprogramming and expansion of the self-image that the Feldenkrais practitioner undergoes, the net result is that developing sensitivity and awareness of oneself allows one to be maximally sensitive and aware of others and enhances evaluative skills and therapeutic effectiveness, not to mention one's own sense of well-being.

Further similarities exist among these methods. In terms of clinical application, they each integrate hands-on manual therapy with movement reeducation procedures and acknowledge how these therapeutic formats go hand in hand. In terms of therapeutic intent, they seek to optimize function and/or structure rather than focus upon symptoms. Although this approach is indirect, it is often very effective in reducing or eliminating symptoms in chronic pain disorders where the reliability of pain as an index for directing treatment is uncertain.

The somatic approaches differ from traditional manual therapeutic approaches in placing much emphasis upon using attention to propioceptive sensations as a way of changing neuromuscular function (1). Some of these approaches also view the myofascial system as a possible direct or indirect source of symptoms. The sophistication of the theoretical justification for each of these somatic methods is highly variable. As with many other manual therapies, however, there is limited research available at present (4, 21–24). The exception is a series of surprisingly thorough investigations that were conducted on the Alexander Technique (4). Nevertheless, the degree of clinical insight and expertise inherent in these approaches is impressive and has, in fact, contributed significantly to improving physical therapy skills in this area.

It is hoped that health care practitioners will investigate these somatic approaches further (with prejudices put aside and with open-minded yet discerning interest), learn and adopt what is useful from them, and utilize both these approaches and their practitioners to expand the range and effectiveness of care available to our patients, broaden our therapeutic perspectives, and increase our therapeutic options.

References

1. Hanna T. The body of life. New York: Knopf, 1980.
2. Johnson G, Saliba V. Functional orthopaedics I course notes. Fairfax, CA: Institute for Physical Art, 1985.
3. Alexander FM. The use of the self. Downey, CA: Centerline Press, 1984.
4. Jones FP. Body awareness in action: A study of the Alexander technique. New York: Schocken Books, 1970.
5. Tengwall R. Systems in conflict: Postural reflexes & postural dysponesis. Somatics 1983–84; IV(3):57–61.
6. Maisel E. ed. The resurrection of the body, the essential writings of F. Matthias Alexander. New York: Delta Books, 1980.
7. Whatmore GB, Kohli DR. The physiopathology and treatment of functional disorders. New York: Grune & Stratton, 1974.
8. Rickover R. Fitness without stress: A guide to the Alexander technique. Metamorphous Press, 1988.
9. Wildman F. The Feldenkrais method professional training program. 1989.
10. Rywerant Y. The Feldenkrais method. San Francisco: Harper and Row, 1983.
10a. Feldenkrais M. Awareness through movement. The 1975 annual handbook for group facilitators.
11. Feldenkrais M. Awareness through movement. New York: Harper and Row, 1977.
12. Hanna T. Somatics. Reading, MA: Addison-Wesley, 1980.
13. Kirkby R. The probable reality behind structural integration. Bull Struct Integ 1975; 5(1):5.
14. Robbie D. Tensional forces in the human body. Orthopaed Rev 1977; VI(11):45–48.
15. Aston J. Course notes from overview, seeing, PT-1A, PT-1C, etc. Mill Valley, CA: The Aston Training Center. 1986, 1987.
16. Maitland GD. Vertebral manipulation. 5th ed. Boston: Butterworth, 1986.
17. Low J. The modern body therapies. part four: Aston patterning. Massage Magazine 1988; 16:Oct./Nov.
18. Heller J, Hanson J. The client's handbook. Hellerwork Practitioners Association, 1985.
19. Heller J, Henkin WA. Bodywise. New York: St. Martin's Press, 1986.
20. Webster's new twentieth century unabridged dictionary. New York: Simon & Schuster, 1983.
21. Garlick D. ed. Propioception, posture and emotion. Kensington, Australia: The University of New South Wales, 1982.
22. Hunt VV, Massey WW, Weinberg R, Bruyere R, Hahn PM. A study of structural integration from neuromuscular, energy field, and emotional approaches. Rolfing research conducted at UCLA. Unpublished.
23. Weinberg RS, Hunt VV. Effects of structural integration on state-trait anxiety. J Clin Psychol 1979; 35(2):319–322.
24. Witt PL, MacKinnon J. Trager psychophysical integration: A method to improve chest mobility of patients with chronic lung disease. Phys Ther 1986; 66:214–217.

Section IV

INJECTION PROCEDURES

15

THERAPEUTIC BLOCKING PROCEDURES

Garrett Kine
Richard Derby

Regional blocking procedures have been utilized for a multitude of painful conditions. These procedures, when combined as diagnostic and therapeutic tools, are particularly efficacious in the management and treatment of spinal disorders. Current rational utilization of therapeutic blocks necessitates an appreciation of their strengths and limitations and the forenotion that these be considered an adjunctive therapy and not an exclusive treatment modality in and of themselves. The plethora of pathologic and emotional overlays in the patient population with lower back pain must be carefully considered so as to most appropriately apply these interventional therapeutic modalities in those individuals who would most benefit by their adjunctive role. The applications of steroids near sites of pathology will often open a treatment window where physical therapy and other interventional maneuvers may be directed with increased effectiveness. In this chapter we will outline the basic anatomical rationale for the proper placement of regional blocks so that clinicians of various backgrounds and experience can most appropriately seek those professionals skilled in these maneuvers.

Typically, blocking procedures utilize a combination of a local anesthetic with a steroid. The use of a local anesthetic provides comfort to the patient, diagnostic information as to the proximity of the needle to the pain generator and, occasionally, the breaking of a neuronal self-propagating pain generator. This self-propagating neuronal cycle is perhaps best typified by the hyperactive reentry cycle seen in the sympathetic dystrophies. Here the selective application of a local anesthetic may break the vicious cycle and, in a sense, reset it as evidenced by ablation of symptomatology for a duration longer than that expected by the local anesthetic. In other block procedures, the aim is to use the local anesthetic as a vehicle to deliver anti-inflammatory medications as close as possible to the site of pathology. This is perhaps best seen in the current use of epidural steroid injections in lower back pain of discogenic origin. Additionally, some practitioners believe the volume of local anesthetic delivered between tissue layers may in fact in some way deter the early formation of adhesions following tissue injury and thereby abate the process of scarring, whose formation may lead to distress in the patient (1).

RATIONALE

The use of epidural steroids has appeared in the literature since the 1950s. The presumptive rationale for its use is based on the theory that there may be a mechanical, chemical, or autoimmune response in lower back pain that will lead to an inflammatory process. Currently, corticosteroids are the most potent anti-inflammatory medicines at our disposal. The procedure for epidural steroids is to apply the medication as close as physically possible to the site of the actual inflammatory process. This enables the clinician to achieve a maximal benefit to risk ratio. Possibly a similar level of anti-inflammatory properties could be delivered to the site of pathology through oral medication, but the inherent risks associated with such high doses of steroids renders this treatment unfeasible.

The efficacy of epidurally applied steroids remains controversial (2–4). Most studies in the literature are open-ended trials with few controls. Interpretation of results is complicated by secondary gain issues and other psychosocial complexities (5). At best, it would be safe to say that properly delivered steroids near the site of pathology will in all likelihood produce a window of relief for a difficult-to-predict period of time. The general consensus is that the highest hopes of benefit reside in those patients whose duration of symptoms is of an acute rather than chronic nature, whose segmental pathology involves a single rather than multiple levels, whose pain originates from disc protrusions rather than stenotic bony structures, and who have not undergone previous lumbar surgical interventions (1–3). This last prerequisite may be due to the difficulty involved in accurately delivering steroid mixtures to postsurgical patients where the epidural space is rendered noncontinuous.

PROCEDURAL CHOICE

Rational decision-making toward appropriate choice for selection of a particular block over another mandates anatomical knowledge of the structures involved coupled with a clinical acumen to best determine the pain generator in a particular patient. For example, in a patient whose posterior elements are the major contributor to distress, a facet joint injection would certainly have a higher potential for benefit over that of an epidural steroid injection. Anatomical derangements observed on imaging studies do not absolutely correlate with the true pain mechanisms. This is particularly evident in studies comparing the radiographic findings of hypertrophic zygoapophyseal joints with the relief obtained through injections into these facet joints. Suffice it to say that clinical judgment and observational skills coupled with diagnostic and imaging studies plus a history and physical examination will lead to the most potentially beneficial procedural choice.

Within the realm of epidurally applied steroids, certain anatomical considerations should be considered. The spinal structures must be visualized in a three-dimensional perspective. If one considers disc protrusions as an entity, it must be appreciated that the actual pathologic mechanical compressions occur on the ventral aspect of the spinal cord and its related struc-

tures. Epidurals applied from a translumbar approach are placed on the dorsal surface of the epidural space and must therefore track ventrally to maximize proximity to the lesion. Disc protrusions may cause compressive phenomena on exiting nerve roots. This being the case, centrally applied epidural steroids might not reach nerve roots through the exiting foraminal openings where the nerves are being compressed. Here it might be appropriate to administer a selective nerve root block at the exit zone of the foraminal opening where the steroids may be able to track medially and contact the site of disc protrusion in the lateral recess. This might also be true with the entity of foraminal stenosis, where it may be appropriate to administer steroids both proximally and distally to the lesion, such as in combining an epidural steroid injection with a selective nerve root block at the appropriate level (Fig. 15.1).

In the postsurgical patient, other complexities are involved, although the rational approach to these patients remains the same. In a patient who has had previous surgery at a particular level and continues to have irritative mechanisms at this same level, it would be inadvisable to attempt to apply a translumbar epidural at this exact surgical level as there is undoubtedly surgical scarring and probable obliteration of the epidural space. Not only would the risks of dural puncture be significantly increased, but the steroids themselves would most likely not be delivered to the appropriate site. It would be more appropriate in this case to deliver the steroids either above or below the postsurgical spinal segment, or to place the steroids to the side at the foraminal

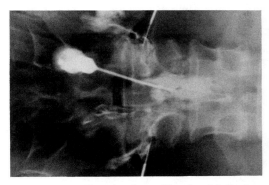

Figure 15.1. Translumbar epidural at L5–S1 from paramedial approach combined with bilateral selective nerve root blocks at L5. Courtesy of Ron Wiley.

openings and hope that they will track towards the site of pathology. The more common and practical of these procedures will be discussed in turn.

RISKS OF INJECTION

The risks of injection may be classified as either immediate or long-term potential complications. The immediate complications include reactions to the medications in the block as well as the risks of the technical performance of the procedure itself.

Generally, there are two classes of medicines used in the performance of a block—local anesthetic and steroid—as well as any analgesic or anxiolytic agent that may be delivered for the patient's comfort. The toxicity of local anesthetics is well recognized. It may manifest itself as a true allergic reaction or, more commonly, as a cardio- or neurotoxic phenomenon. The potential for these complications is of an acute nature. Under proper surroundings where resuscitative equipment is immediately available, and with skilled personnel to watch for these potential complications, the risks of adverse effects are minimized. Rising blood levels of local anesthetics can lead to a decrease in the seizure threshold as well as eventual frank seizures and ultimately a cardiovascular collapse. Techniques that limit the total dose of local anesthetic delivered, those insuring placement of the local anesthetic into nonvascular structures, and the careful observational skills of the practitioner directed to signs of increasing blood concentration (tinnitus, perioral numbness) will protect against these preventable mishaps.

Local anesthetics inhibit neuronal conduction. When they are used in a generalized block such as an epidural application, both sensory and motor blockade will occur. Although certain local anesthetics, such as bupivacaine, have been touted as producing a somewhat more selective sensory than motor block, the inevitability of motor blockade must be appreciated when certain anesthetic concentrations are delivered to perineuronal tissues. The patient's safety can be ensured by judiciously observing the patient in the reclined position until the full motor blockade is ensured. Motor strength can then be assessed prior to trials at ambulation. Because fine motor coordination may be altered, should any signs of instability be rec-

ognized, the patient must remain recumbent until the anesthetic actions have dissipated.

Concurrent with the motor and sensory blockade is the inevitable sympathetic blockade. This can lead to vasopooling in the lower extremities, which might precipitate orthostatic changes on attempts at ambulation. It is generally recommended that all patients should be initially evaluated in the sitting position for any light-headedness or reflex tachycardia secondary to the partial sympathectomy in the lower extremities. It should be appreciated that the sympathectomy might outlast the motor and sensory block.

Of concern during the performance of any epidural procedures is avoidance of an inadvertent dural puncture. Although in initial trials the subarachnoid application of steroids was considered to be equal in efficacy, the consequence of deliberate dural puncturing is apparent. It is thought that subarachnoid steroid application has an increased incidence of meningitis, arachnoiditis, and infection when compared to epidurally applied steroids (6–8). The immediate complications of dural puncture are twofold. Relatively small volumes of local anesthetics applied subarachnoidly can produce a profound motor, sensory, and sympathetic block. Cerebral spinal fluid is freely mobile and rostral spread of local anesthetic may induce a total spinal blockade. If the dose is high enough, the patient will require ventilatory and hemodynamic assistance. Intrusion into the subarachnoid space may leave a hole leading to a postdural-puncture headache. This headache might become extremely severe at times and, should visual or auditory changes occur, emergency medical treatment is necessitated. Generally, the headaches will acquiesce and the dural leak will close with strict bed rest and oral hydration. Occasionally, an epidural blood patch may be performed with the patient's own blood to hasten healing of the dural puncture leak.

Sympathectomies induce vasopooling and its accompanying hemodynamic consequences. This afterload reduction is generally well tolerated in the healthy individual. For those individuals with compromised hemodynamic stability, short-term supportive care may be indicated.

The safety of the judicial use of steroids is well established. Transient increases in water retention and blood glucose levels may be noticed in certain individuals. The long-term sequelae of large doses of glucocorticosteroids are well recognized. The maximum number of allowable steroid injections has not been well defined. Logic dictates the use of a minimal quantity of steroid to achieve maximal beneficial results. Steroids must be viewed as a temporizing mechanism except in those cases where all other therapeutic interventional maneuvers have been exhausted and who still are experiencing disabling pain or neurologic compromise. Naturally with high-dose steroids, cushingoid syptoms and arthritic degeneration are potentialities, although even relatively small doses of steroids have been reported to induce transient hypercorticism (9).

REGIONAL BLOCKING PROCEDURES

Optimally, blocking procedures are performed under fluoroscopic guidance (2, 10, 11). Although a majority of blocking procedures in the community are accomplished without fluoroscopic aid, fluoroscopic visualization helps ensure proper needle placement and minimizes the potential for adverse sequelae. Utilization of a water-soluble contrast demonstrates the potential flow of the anesthetic and steroid mixture. Difficult blocks may be performed with greater accuracy and confidence that the steroid will reside in the contiguous proximity of the pathologic lesion. The epidural space and the surrounding tissues possess a rich venous supply which one must be careful to avoid. An accidental intervascular injection can be easily recognized by the distinctive flow of contrast material, which should be looked for prior to introducing a potentially threatening large dose of local anesthetic. Naturally, radiologic safety measures must be ensured for both the patient and the medical personnel.

Epidural Block

The epidural space is a potentially continuous space from the occiput to the sacral hiatus. It surrounds the dural sac and its contents and forms sleeves for the exiting spinal nerves through their foraminal openings. An epidural block may be considered a very generalized block. The extent of the block is related to the volume of injectate used and the physical characteristics of the individual patient. As mentioned above, the translumbar approach to epidural steroids places the solution at the dorsal aspect of the epidural tube. Pathology that is lateralized or more ventral necessitates flow of injectate to this location. It is generally recommended to attempt to place the steroid at the same segmental level as the pathology. The exception to this, of course, would be if the patient has had previous surgery at this level.

A caudal epidural may be viewed as an alternative approach to the epidural space. Generally, a single shot injection is administered with a 22-gauge needle through the sacral hiatus. The cephalad segmental spread is dictated by volume or injectate and impediments (scarring, stenotic compression) to rostral flow. The perceived advantage of a caudal epidural approach lies in its lessened risk of dural puncture and in those situations where a translumbar approach might be inappropriate. In persons who have degenerative spine disease with closure of the interlaminar space or in those who have had previous surgery at a lower segmental level, the caudal approach to the epidural space might be the only feasible option in administration of steroids at the lower levels. In general, it is recognized that the caudal approach is most useful for the lower two segmental levels, especially in view of the fact that there would be considerable nontherapeutic steroid dilution with steroid dead space should this approach be attempted for lesions above the L4 level.

When working without fluoroscopic guidance, the skilled practitioner typically administers an epidural steroid injection with the patient in the lateral fetal position with the side of dominant pathology toward the table. Gravity will influence anesthetic spread to some degree (12; Fig. 15.2). In persons whose bony landmarks might not be easily palpated, sometimes

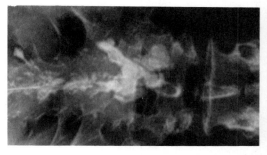

Figure 15.2. Caudal epidural showing primarily unilateral flow. Courtesy of Ron Wiley.

the sitting position is preferred with utilization of a midline approach. Under fluoroscopic guidance, a prone position is typically preferred with final needle position lateralizing from the midline toward the site of dominant pathology.

Pain relief might be expected to be twofold. Initial relief as a result of the local anesthetic supplies reassuring evidence that the delivered injectate has reached the level of pathology. This relief will wane in concordance with the duration of local anesthetic effect. The second period of relief generally takes several days to a week to exert its maximal therapeutic effect. A prolongation of the alleviation of pain greater than the period of local anesthetic suggests an ongoing chemical and/or mechanical injury.

Pain has a protective role in the physiologic makeup of the individual. Nociceptive impulses warn against repeated mechanically disruptive patterns. The patient must be cautioned that the steroids do not strengthen the supporting structures, nor do they shrink a potentially herniated disc. The patients must maintain appropriate protective behavior patterns both during the local anesthetic and the steroid phase of pain relief.

Selective Nerve Root Block

Sensitized spinal nerve roots are a well-recognized cause of radicular-type pains. Selective spinal nerve root blocks, often termed paravertebral nerve root blocks, are means by which to localize irritative foci as well as administer anti-inflammatory medications in close proximity to the mechanical irritant. Selective lumbosacral radiculography has both diagnostic and therapeutic potential (13).

The technique for a selective nerve root block requires the placement of the needle as close to the foraminal exit zone as is possible. Optimally, this is done under fluoroscopic guidance with the appropriate level identified. The needle is generally introduced between 4 and 8 cm from the midline and directed to contact the transverse process. This allows judgment of approximate depth so as to attempt to avoid a paresthesia of the nerve root, which can be quite distressing to the patient. After the needle depth is noted, the needle is then directed caudally to pass off the inferior edge of the transverse process and is advanced approximately 0.5 to 1 cm. Injection of radiopaque contrast agent should then outline the nerve root. A more lateral approach to the foraminal opening allows closer proximity to the exiting nerve and more medial flow of steroid agent into the foraminal opening. Selective nerve root blocks may be performed under a lateral fusion, although this is a somewhat more technically difficult procedure. The sacral nerve roots may be blocked via the posterior sacral foramen. Localization of the posterior foramen is best accomplished by anatomical knowledge of the fluoroscopically visible anterior foramen in relation to the posterior foramen and their proximity to surrounding bony landmarks. An approximate 15°-tilt may line up the two foramina and permit better visualization (14). Generally, much smaller doses of local anesthetic are administered when performing a selective nerve root block than with the lumbar epidural, as large volumes exert a large pressure phenomenon that can be quite distressing to the patient.

Facet Joint Injections

The lumbar zygoapophyseal joints are now well recognized as a potential source of lower back discomfort that may additionally radiate to the gluteal region and thighs (15). Short of true diagnostic facet blocks, there is no definitive radiologic criterion, physical examination finding, or segmental pain distribution that will consistently correlate with the proper diagnosis of facet syndrome (16, 17). Aggravation of symptoms with posterior element loading, extension rotation maneuvers, or paravertebral tenderness will only lead to a clinical suspicion of facet joint syndrome. Performed as a diagnostic and/or therapeutic maneuver, the injection of the zygoapophyseal joints may lend credence to this diagnosis.

Interarticular or capsular inflammation may be due to increased subluxation stress from anterior element breakdown, spondylolisthesis, or posttraumatic injury. Again, as in the case of epidural steroid injections, the empirical placement of steroid mixtures within the interarticular capsule is based on the presumption that there are potential benefits from their anti-inflammatory properties or simply from some neurolytic effect on the capsular nerve endings.

The efficacy of facet joint injections is difficult to assess. The multitude of open trials have varied considerably in techniques and solutions applied. It is recognized that if the block be performed for diagnostic purposes, then small vol-

umes of injectate (1 to 1.5 ml) should be utilized. Greater volumes with increased pressure
will cause the steroid solution to extravassate
beyond the capsular limits, which potentially
permits flow into the adipose tissue and the superior recess of the facet joint and thereby into
the epidural space surrounding the spinal nerve
(18). Another means that has been devised to
evaluate the facet joint pathology is to block the
innervation of the facet capsule. This is performed through blocking of the medial branch
of the dorsal primary ramus in its course over
the superior end at the base of the transverse
process at levels above and below the targeted
facet capsule. This block is often utilized as a
prognostic factor toward the consideration of
denervation rhizotomy.

With fluoroscopic guidance, the technique
for facet joint injection is quite simple (Fig.
15.3). The patient is placed in a lateral oblique
position at an angle that will best visualize the
articular surface of the joint itself. A 22-gauge
spinal needle may then be passed from a spot
overlying the facet joint with the needle progressing in a manner parallel to the radiographic rays. It is generally possible for the needle tip to enter the capsule and the joint itself.
A normal joint should have a tight capsule and
allow only 1 to 2 ml of solution to be injected.
In general, a degenerated level may have a
stretched or ruptured capsule and large volumes of injectate will be allowed.

Facet joint injections are not a cureall (19).
At best, they may temporize the symptomatology during periods of flaring and allow more rigorous physical therapy and other strengthening
maneuvers. Attempts at denervating facet capsules have been fraught with controversy.
Chemical, thermal, and surgical rhizotomies

have high failure rates and, in general, the
nerves will regenerate over time. At best, one
might expect 1 to 2 years of maximal relief.

SUMMARY

The management of lower back pain will often
require a multidisciplinary objective outlook. If
conservative interventional treatment modalities prove ineffective, more invasive interventional maneuvers should be considered. Therapeutic blocking procedures may be just the
impetus needed to allow the further progression
of conservative treatment. Epidurally applied
steroids appear to be most effective for lower
back pain associated with radicular symptoms.
The weight of statistical data and clinical impression is that this is indeed a relatively safe
and potentially effective method of care. Except
in those cases where there is an ongoing progressive neurologic deficit, or where there is an
absolute contraindication to the procedure, a
patient deserves a fair trial of therapeutic
blocking procedures.

References

1. Morelle P, Hoogmartens M. Epidural injections
   in the treatment of chronic sciatica. Acta Orthopaed Belgic 1987; 53 (2):170.
2. White A, Derby R, Wynne G. Epidural injections
   for the diagnosis and treatment of low-back pain.
   Spine 1980; 5(1):78.
3. Liebergall M, Fast A, Olshwang D, Magora F,
   Floman Y. The role of epidural steroid injection
   in the management of lumbar radiculopathy due
   to disc disease or spinal stenosis. Pain Clinic
   1986; 1(1):35.
4. Benzon H. Epidural steroid injections for low-
   back pain and lumbosacral radiculopathy. Pain
   1986; 24:277.
5. Arnhoff F, Triplett HB, Pokorney B. Follow-up
   status of patients treated with nerve blocks for
   low-back pain. Anesthesiology 1977; 46:170.
6. Dougherty JH Jr, Fraser RAR. Complications following intraspinal injections of steroids. Report
   of two cases. J Neurosurg 1978; 48:1023.
7. Nelson DA. Dangers from methylprednisolone
   acetate therapy by intraspinal injection. Arch
   Neurol 1988; 45:804.
8. Delaney TJ, Rowlingson JC, Carron H et al. Epidural steroid effects on nerves and meninges.
   Anesth Anal 1980; 59(8):610.
9. Stambough JL, Booth RE, Rothman RH. Transient hypercorticism after epidural steroid injection. J Bone Joint Surg 1984; 66-A(7):1115.

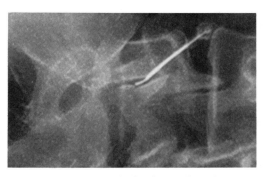

Figure 15.3. Intraarticular facet joint injection at
L5-S1. Courtesy of Ron Wiley.

10. El-Khoury GY, Ehara S, Weinstein JN, Montgomery WJ, Kathol MH. Epidural steroid injection: A procedure ideally performed with fluoroscopic control. Radiology 1988; 168(2):554.
11. Stewart HD, Quinnell RC, Dann N. Epidurography in the management of sciatica. Br J Rheumatol 1987; 26:424.
12. Krempen JF, Silver RA, Hadley J. An analysis of differential epidural spinal anesthesia and pentothal pain study in differential diagnosis of back pain. Spine 1979; 4(5):452.
13. Tajima, T, Furukawa K, Kuramochi E. Selective lumbosacral radiculopathy and block. Spine 1980; 5(1):68.
14. Dooley JF, McBroan RJ, Taguchi T, Macnab I. Nerve root infiltration in the diagnosis of radicular pain. Spine 1988; 13(1):79.
15. Fairbanks JCT, Park WM, McCall IW, O'Brien JP. Apophyseal injection of local anesthetic as a diagnostic aid in primary low-back pain syndrome. Spine 1981; 6(6):598.
16. Carrera GF, Lumbar facet joint injection in low-back pain and sciatica. Radiology 1980; 137:661.
17. Helbig T, Lee CK. The lumbar facet syndrome. Spine 1988; 13(1):61.
18. Moran R, O'Connell D, Wash WG. The diagnostic value of facet joint injections. Spine 1988; 13(12):1407.
19. Murtagh FR. Computed tomography and fluoroscopy guided anesthesia and steroid injection in facet syndrome. Spine 1988; 13(6):686.

16

PROLOTHERAPY IN THE TREATMENT OF LOW BACK PAIN

Thomas A. Dorman

Prolotherapy has its roots in the art of sclerotherapy used by herniologists before the era of aseptic surgery. Scarring of connective tissue was induced by various irritants to provoke contracture of fascial layers and control hernias. In antiquity the scarring was provoked by searing and from the first third of the last century by injection with irritants or sclerosants. It was Geroge Hackett, an industrial surgeon active in the United States in the mid-1950s, who recognized that the injection of mild irritants into ligaments in the back and other parts of the body where strains had occurred can strengthen these structures and correct a number of painful conditions. Are scarring and contracture the only mechanism of action of these irritants, or does a genuine refurbishing take place? The hypothesis that, with certain agents and appropriate injection techniques, a genuine hypertrophy of ligaments can be induced and that this hypertrophy would contain tissue that was akin to the natural ligament, rather than scar, was the brain child of this worker. He coined the term *prolotherapy* (from Latin *proles*—offspring) to make this point. The testing of this hypothesis needs to be based on histologic and biomechanical studies. Hackett's book contains reports of a number of uncontrolled histologic studies that point in this direction (1). A number of irritant solutions were used and, in his day, hospitalization for the injections, which were putatively painful, was not uncommon.

It was at about that time that the Dalmas Company in the United Kingdom introduced an agent for the sclerosis for varicose veins and touted it also as a proliferant for ligaments. M.J. Ongley, an orthopaedic physician from New Zealand, was instrumental in popularizing this agent, referred to by the company as P25G and, since a misprint in one of the early editions of Cyriax's *Textbook of Orthopedic Medicine,* also known as P2G. It consists of phenol, 2.5%; glucose, 25.0%; glycerine, 25.0%; and pyrogen-free water to 100.0%. This solution is mixed with an equal volume of 0.5% lidocaine for injection. It is estimated that over 100,000 injections of this substance have been given in the last 30 years without untoward effect. This contrasts with dangerous complications reported with the use of psyllium seed oil extract or zinc sulfate when injected inadvertently into the lumbar theca, which have been responsible for two known deaths and three cases of paraplegia (2-4). Sodium morrhuate, a fish oil extract, is also in frequent clinical use, sometimes in combination with Ongley's solution. Many experienced users prefer to use morrhuate only in areas away from the midline to avoid any possibility of inadvertent introduction into the subarachnoid space.

Safety

Both phenol and glycerine have been injected intentionally into the subdural space, at 5% and 100% respectively, for pain relief in cancer patients (5-7). When the subjects subsequently died of their cancers, autopsies revealed only minor changes in the C fibers. It is, therefore, likely that the occasional inadvertent intrathecal injection of small amounts of Ongley's solution is harmless. Animal experiments to confirm this are needed. It is, however, normal practice to avoid intradural injections.

Effectiveness

A double-blind animal experiment at Iowa State University, where the medial collateral ligament of rabbit knees was injected, showed the effect of sodium morrhuate as a proliferant. The tensile strength, actual size of the ligaments, and amount and size of collagen fibers as judged by light and electron microscopy increased (8). This began the contemporary trend confirming Hackett's uncontrolled work, the data of which remained dormant for the last 30 years, probably because of the complications of the intrathecal injections already mentioned. The effectiveness on the mechanics of injured

ligaments in human knees has been the subject of a recent report based on a computer-assisted device for measurement of the dynamic function of knee ligaments in the live human subject using Ongley's solution (9). Another recent study of patients presenting with low back pain attributed clinically to ligament incompetence has demonstrated an increased facility of movement. Three patients were subjected to biopsies before and after treatment by a protocol that included prolotherapy with Ongley's solution to the relevant low back ligaments. These cases showed hyperplasia of fibroblasts and a significant increase in collagen as judged by light microscopy and an increase in the size of the collagen fibers as judged by transmission electron microscopy (10). The light microscopy changes are illustrated in Figure 16.1. The electron microscopy changes are shown in Figure 16.2.

Figure 16.1. A, Light microscopy before prolotherapy; H & E stain; ×250. **B,** Light microscopy after prolotherapy; H & E stain; ×250. Note increase in wavy lines representing collagen and increase of fibroblast nuclei

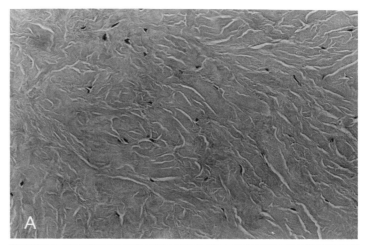
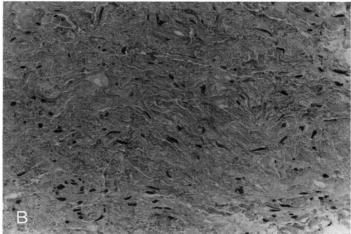

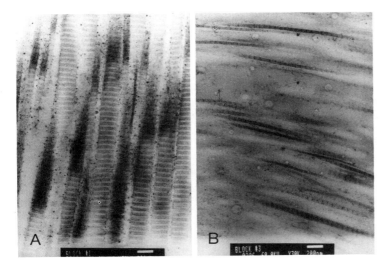

Figure 16.2. **A,** EM micrograph of collagen fibers before prolotherapy. **B,** EM micrograph of collagen fibers after prolotherapy. Note increase in number and size.

Clinical Trial

A complete treatment protocol, which included prolotherapy as its main component, has been the subject of a double-blind controlled study in which 81 patients were divided into placebo and active treatment groups. The important variables were those of re-position of the sacrum into the midline after anaesthesia and the use of Ongley's proliferant injections six times at weekly intervals. The placebo group had a sham manipulation and injections of saline. Both groups took part in an exercise program consisting of repeated back flexion (11). The findings of the study are summarized in Figures 16.3 and 16.4. A recent retrospective survey claims long-term benefit from this form of treatment (12).

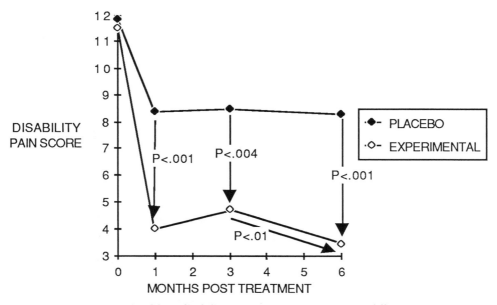

Figure 16.3. Mean disability pain scores at posttreatment follow-up.

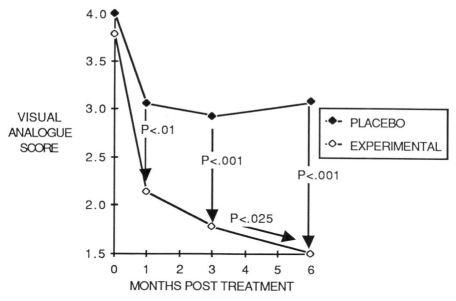

Figure 16.4. Mean visual analogue pain scores at posttreatment follow-up.

PATHOLOGY

Position of the Sacrum

Viewed in the quadruped position, the sacrum is suspended by the short, strong posterior sacroiliac ligaments. It is the biped human position that alters the mechanics of these members. When there is ligamentous insufficiency, it allows the sacrum to become trapped in a somewhat asymmetrical position between the ilia. It is thought that this is the cause for recurrent episodes of back pain that, in individuals who are subject to this problem, occur typically when rising from a bent posture with twisting, not necessarily involving much weight. As these minor displacements are hard to demonstrate radiologically and do not amount to a true subluxation, the term *asymlocation* has been coined to describe this phenomenon. (See Figure 16.5.)

Ligament Injuries

Chronic ligamentous insufficiency in the low back can result from injuries. It is thought ligaments in the back are more susceptible to injuries that include a rotational as well as a fore and aft component. It seems likely that man, in the modern era of a relatively sedentary life punctuated by unguarded acceleration-deceler-

ation moments, is more prone to these problems. The degenerative process between the vertebrae of the spine involves the three-joint complex of the zygoapophyseal joints and the intervertebral discs (13), and weakening of the abdominal musculature diminishes the contribution to posture from the abdominal mechanism (14). The common denominator for the degenerative process, therefore, is in the structures that bind the vertebrae together, i.e., the ligaments.

PAIN FROM DISC DEGENERATION

Degeneration of the intervertebral discs is an integral part of the pathological process. It is well known that individual episodes of acute leg pain, as well as low back pain, arise from dural pressure or impingement on dural sleeves of nerve roots from displaced or sequestered fragments of ruptured anulus fibrosus and at times from extruded nuclear pulp. Many of these patients have pain from the acute disc problem in combination with pain from the ligament relaxation. The ligamentous component of the problem is best treated with prolotherapy, sometimes after surgery. Nonoperative management of some cases of acute disc disease can be attempted with the orthopedic medical methods discussed here and with manipulation.

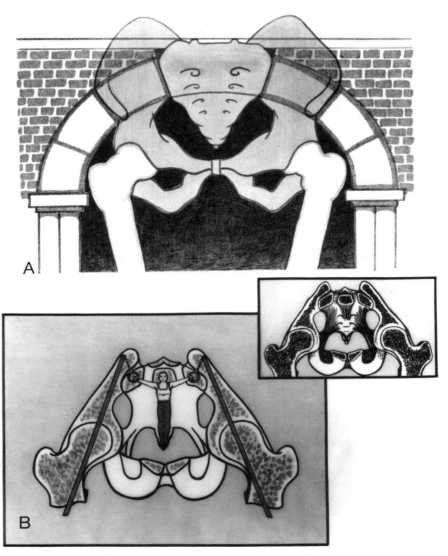

Figure 16.5. **A**, Sacrum can be visualized as a keystone in an arch. **B**, Sacrum in coronal section, as in a quadruped standing *(inset)* and as suspended from the ilia.

DIAGNOSIS

History

It is to Kellgren that we owe the original identification of patterns of referred pain from deep structures including ligaments (15, 16). Recognition of the pattern of pain in any individual is based on matching one's knowledge of characteristic patterns with what the patient describes or draws on his pain diagram.

Diagnosis begins with a meticulous clinical history which should include:

1. An account of the onset of the pain. A gradual onset suggests a chronic strain.
2. Was there an injury? Did the pain begin at the time of the injury or after an interval? The latter suggests a possibility of a sacral or vertebral displacement followed by a ligament strain.
3. Does the pain radiate? A pain diagram is helpful. The experienced clinician will recognize characteristic patterns of referral from deep structures.
4. Is the pain aggravated by movement? Osteoarthritis is an example.

5. Is it worsened by prolonged sitting? Most ligament strains are manifested by the characteristic *ligament symptom* of aching with maintenance of any one position for a long time. How long can you sit before the pain troubles you? is a useful sample question.

6. Is the pain brought on by a particular position? Standing with lumbar spine extended and with the provocation of sensation of numbness down the back of the legs is characteristic of lumbar spinal stenosis with the extension syndrome.

7. Associated symptoms must be elicited. When the patient complains of numbness, the clinician should establish if there is true anesthesia or a numb-like sensation, which in itself is a characteristic manifestation of referred ligament strain.

8. A cough-aggravated pain helps to assess the severity, but unfortunately does not give a clue to etiology.

It goes without saying that evaluation of the patient's general health and problems in other parts of the body should be taken into account.

Examination

Examination follows the cues obtained from the history and pain pattern. It is best to start by evaluating the patient from behind and standing. Extension, side bending, rotation, and forward flexion are inspected. Leg length discrepancy and hip problems must be recognized. Meticulous care in neurological examination of the lumbar plexus is the best guide to nerve root impingement. Each muscle group should be tested correctly against resistance. It is important for the examiner to use muscle strength in a mechanically advantageous position rather than body weight. Slight weakness referable to a myotome is an important sign. The reflexes are tested, including those from L4. A *numb-like* sensation is characteristic of a referred ligamentous sensory phenomenon, in contrast to true anesthesia.

With the patient in the prone position, trigger point examination and the elasticity of each lumbar segment are evaluated. Palpation of the subcutaneous tissues and skin rolling are helpful in some instances and various maneuvers that are useful in evaluating the sacroiliac joints and lumbosacral junction are complementary (17–19).

When imaging and laboratory studies are complete, a diagnosis of chronic ligamentous insufficiency, usually with sacral asymlocation, can be reached.

INDICATIONS FOR TREATMENT

The indication for prolotherapy is simply that of a symptomatic strained ligament. Recognition of the number of syndromes among the many that are responsible for back pain and are likely to respond to this form of treatment grows with experience. It has, however, been found that in very many individuals recurrent episodic low back pain with a chronic background ache is associated with sacral asymlocation and ligamentous insufficiency involving the main stabilizers of the sacrum. It is for this most common problem that M.J. Ongley devised the protocol that now bears his name (11). The treatment routine outlined is that used in the study and can serve as a template. In practice, modifications are made depending on individual circumstances and the clinician's experience.

Treatment Protocol for Asymlocation with Low Back Ligament Relaxation

The patient receives a light intravenous anesthesia, with suitable monitoring. Local anesthesia is used next. The object of the local anesthesia is 1. to break the pain reflex arc; 2. to break up microadhesions by an hydrostatic effect; and 3. to place a fluid in and around the sacroiliac joints to facilitate the manipulation. A 3 inch, 19-gauge needle is inserted just above the L5 spinous process in the midline. The operator needs to have excellent familiarity with the local anatomy and should have practical experience in the technique. The needle serves as probe of the bony landmarks, as well as for injecting. Local anesthetic is infiltrated into the ligaments near, but not into the periosteum. The ligaments which should be infiltrated include the interspinous and supraspinous ligaments between L4 and L5. The base of the lamina is sought by needle feel to inject at the ligamentum flavum. Without being withdrawn from the skin, the needle is reangled subcutaneously and aimed at the two attachments of the lumbosacral ligament, the deep innominate ligaments, the insertion of the ileolumbar ligament at the ileum. Occasionally it is necessary to inject the spinal origin of the ileolumbar ligament. Importantly, the superior and deep sacroiliac ligaments are injected on each side. The posterior aspect of the sacrotuberous ligament and the sacrospinous ligament at their medial edge can sometimes be reached from this midline insertion, but may require a separate skin puncture. The extensor aponeurosis over the sacral multifidus muscle is infiltrated and finally, if there are particularly tender areas, other relevant ligaments are identified and infiltrated separately. It is common to find in cases where the sacrum is rotated anteriorly on the right (as seen from behind) that the right gluteus medius muscle is strained. In some of these cases, the insertion of the muscle along the superior gluteal line can be infiltrated with 10 ml of 0.5% lidocaine followed by a small dose of triamcinolone.

The patient is now ready for manipulation. The purpose of the manipulation is to apply an abduction and shearing force across the sacroiliac joints, gaping them momentarily, allowing the sacrum to spring back into the midline position. To the extent possible, the spine is locked down to the lumbosacral level and one of the thighs is used as a lever for the movement. The technique used is a modification of an osteopathic one. When there is an associated intervertebral disc displacement, there is an advantage in placing the painful side uppermost, but in most cases, the manipulation can be performed in either direction. More force is used than usual in routine osteopathic office work.

The first stabilizing injection is given the next day. A total of 20 ml is injected at each of the six weekly follow-up visits for the stabilization. The injection technique is the same as the one described for the local anesthesia. The same needle insertion point is used and contact with the same structures made, except that no attempt is made to enter the sacroiliac joints with the proliferant. Droplet injections of about 0.2 ml to each site are infiltrated. It usually requires 10 ml to inject the portion of the area between L4 and S1 and both innominates. The second 10 ml are used for the ileolumbar and other ligaments described. After the stabilizing injection flexion exercises are initiated. The patient can expect stiffness and pain from the injection in the first one to two days and this is best treated by frequent flexion exercises. Usually, by the time of the next injection—in a week—the discomfort has abated and the underlying pain not yet returned. It is usual to find some residual pain and tenderness at some ligamentous site or other, which needs to be infiltrated. By the fourth proliferant injection, most patients begin to experience some relief.

EXERCISES

During the rehabilitation period, patients are encouraged to stay at their regular occupation, though severe exertion and lifting are not advised. This admonition is particularly true for those who have not been active before. Unaccustomed exercise should be taken up gradually while the back muscles are regaining strength. It has been shown that exercises, in their own right, strengthen the attachment of tendons and ligament to bone (20). Though some experienced prolotherapists do not advocate exercise (21), it is the distinct impression of this author and the group of prolotherapists active in coastal California, that healing in the presence of movement has a great benefit, presumably by disrupting any adhesions that might tend to form between moving layers of fascia and ligament. Therefore, rehabilitation with exercise is advised.

The hamstring muscles are often tight in patients with chronic low back pain and asymlocation. Rehabilitation will depend in part on stretching them out. The supervision of a trained physiotherapist is an advantage, though many patients manage adequately with the help of some office guidance and written handouts. The exercises consist of repeated full flexion and extension of the low back. Repetition within the range of tolerance is recommended, say 50 bends thrice a day. Additional exercises are often adapted to individual cases.

FOLLOW-UP

Follow-up visits are planned at about monthly intervals, usually decreasing as the back is stabilized and the pain controlled. The gluteus medius phenomenon sometimes recurs during the rehabilitation period and should alert the physician to possible recurrent asymlocation of the sacrum. There are many structures in the low back and after a prolonged period of disability it is usual for one or other to be a source of symptoms in the recovery period. Persistent attention to detail by the physician and persistence with the flexion exercises by the patient is found to be very rewarding in the majority of cases.

Facet Syndrome

The term facet syndrome was coined by Ghormley in 1933 (22) and the pattern of pain that arises from the zygoapophyseal joints, as they should properly be called, demonstrated by Mooney in 1975 (23). The L4–5 and L5–S1 joints refer pain into the posterior part of the buttock and down the back of the leg and the L3–4 joint a little more laterally. The pain is aggravated by straight leg raising. Diagnostic facet injections have become quite useful in modern practice. It is thought, however, that zygoapophyseal joint dysfunction is a component of the whole constellation of chronic ligamentous insufficiency in the low back. The zygoapophyseal joints are treated with Ongley's proliferant injection as part of the routine he devised for the low back. The frequency with which the facet syndrome occurs in isolation remains unknown.

Lumbar Spinal Stenosis

The size of the lumbar spinal canal varies among individuals and there is a general tendency for it to become narrower with aging, in part because of the tricomponent degenerative process of the apophyseal joint and the discs (24). Back pain associated with disc disease has been shown to have a positive correlation with the narrow spinal canal (25). The mechanics of degeneration have been described by Kirkaldy-Willis (26). The presence of spondylolisthesis can aggravate the problem, as can rotational displacement in the lumbar spine (27). The gradual narrowing can be associated with two groups of symptoms.

FLEXION SYNDROME

The patient complains of pain, numbness or discomfort in the lower limbs, usually affecting both the calves and the thighs, in that order of importance when walking. Typically, this is most troublesome when the patient walks uphill and it tends to be relieved when walking downhill. The symptoms are usually different from the pain of vascular claudication in several respects:

1. Symptoms are usually symmetrical.
2. In vascular insufficiency, almost always, one limb or group of muscles is more affected than the other.
3. When the pain is provoked by walking, it does not usually compel the patient to stop and rest, as is the case with vascular insufficiency.
4. If the patient rests after the pain is provoked, the length of time necessary to relieve the symptoms is longer in spinal stenosis than in vascular insufficiency of the muscles.
5. In vascular insufficiency, relief is not dependent on altering posture and is provoked by a constant level of work. At a lower level of work, the patient may be able to continue walking for a long period.
6. Backache is common, but not invariable, in spinal claudication.
7. In spinal claudication, one of the symptoms is a numb, cramp-like, burning paraesthesia (28). Spinal claudication is thought to be due to an inadequate blood supply to the lumbar spinal cord and corda equina, usually in association with a narrow canal.

An individual will usually slightly flex the lumbar spine with walking uphill and the slight reduction in the volume of the canal accounts for the symptom being worse in the slightly flexed position, in contradistinction to walking downhill, when the natural lordosis is slightly increased.

EXTENSION SYNDROME

The extension syndrome consists of a group of symptoms and signs that arise from a narrowing of the posterior recesses of the trefoil-shaped canal and the intervertebral foramina. They are brought on when the spine is extended, i.e., when the patient stands straight, or enhances the lordosis with leaning back or walking downhill. Patients will typically recount that they have a numb-like sensation and pain, usually in the posterior aspect of the legs and thighs, in that order, often spreading to the heel and sole of the foot and sometimes to the lateral aspect of the foot. With slight flexion of the lumbar spine, as on walking uphill or leaning over a sink, the symptoms are relieved or abolished. These patients always report that sitting is comfortable (29). These symptoms are usually bilateral. The explanation for this is that in extension of the lumbar spine, the posterior recesses—in these spines the canal has a trefoil cross-section—the foramina are narrowed and, being initially only marginal, the slight further narrowing from this posture passes a critical point, provoking the symptoms. When the spine is slightly flexed, however, there is slight gapping or opening of the posterior recess and the foramina, hence the improvement in the symptoms. The known history of this entity is related in an elegant account by Ehni (30).

TREATMENT

Traditionally, this condition has been treated surgically. This author has found that in some instances stabilization of the low back and particularly the ligaments between L4 and S1, as well as the sacroiliac joint by proliferant therapy may control most of the symptoms, which were seemingly due to intermittent spinal claudication. The mechanism for this is not entirely clear, but it may well be that an associated sacral subluxation, as well as rotational displacements between the low lumbar vertebrae, contribute to the narrowing, so that when this is corrected, enough improvement in space occurs to allow the disordered physiology to improve to below the threshold that provokes symptoms. The extension syndrome is sometimes controlled by sinuvertebral blocks at the affected levels. The mechanism for the effectiveness of these injections may be the reduction of surrounding inflammation and desensitization of the nerve sheaths at the impingement sites in the foramina. In any case, it is wise to analyze these symptoms as precisely as possible in each case before planning therapy.

As the results of surgery in spinal stenosis are not guaranteed, it seems possible, at least in cases with not very severe incapacity, to try a conservative approach first. Patients who are able to walk only a short distance are usually elderly and often have a combination of vascular insufficiency with spinal stenosis, so that surgical intervention is not always helpful (27). It may be that the provocation of pain can occur synergistically from both disease processes. This should be kept in mind when individual cases are analyzed. Treatment of one problem might seemingly by serendipity alleviate symptoms previously ascribed to the other (31).

Central Low Back Pain, or "Lumbago"

Central low back pain, when of sudden onset after an injury, can be due to a posterior displacement of a central fragment or bulge of an anulus fibrosus. The differential diagnosis is a tear, with bruise and hematoma, in the interspinous ligament. Protective spasm may occur in the ileopsoas so the patient is bent forward. Anesthetizing the posterior ligaments in the midline by injection will confirm the diagnosis. The usual history is that after lifting, with the trunk in a straight position, there was a sudden tearing or pain in the back that was not very severe and some hours later the pain gradually worsened and the stiffness set in. The patient may have a feeling of a swelling in the back.

Coplans regards most cases of lumbago as due to partial tears in the interspinous ligaments. This was supported by a radiologic study showing vacuolation in this ligament in such cases (32).

Chronic low back ache in the midline, spreading symmetrically to both sides at the level of the iliac crests, and aggravated by prolonged sitting, is often due to a strain of the lumbosacral ligament. Rotations are normal and flexion hurts in full range. There is trigger point tenderness over the ligament. Treatment consists of disinflammation in the first instance, particularly in the acute state, and subsequent strengthening of this area with two or three injections of proliferant. If symptoms persist, one should keep in mind the suprasacral ligament, which is the inferior extension of the same structure.

The lumbosacral distribution of pain is band-like across the back at the level of the lumbosacral joint. Pain, arising from the ligamentous attachments of the middle portion of the sacrum approximately at the level of S3, is distributed across the middle of the buttock in an inverted horseshoe shape. It lends itself to treatment in the midline of the sacrum. The sacrococcygeal ligament leads to pain down the backs of both thighs in the distribution of S1 and 2.

Sacrotuberous Ligament

Pain from this ligament is the most common form of false sciatica. When a person who is standing leans back extending the lumbar spine, the sacrum tends to pivot, so its inferior aspect rises while its superior and anterior aspects move forward slightly, so the sacrotuberous and sacrospinous ligaments are put on the stretch. A patient who complains of pain in the upper outer buttock with radiation down the side or back of the thigh in a broad band, possibly as far as the bottom of the heel, often associated with a numb-like sensation, should be suspected of having a strain at the sacral attachment of the sacrotuberous ligament. It is best to palpate and inject the sacrotuberous ligament with the patient in the side lying position with the knees flexed. This condition responds well to injection treatments, but when the back is very tender, it is best to reduce the inflammation with a local anaesthetic and triamcinolone first and consider prolotherapy a week later.

Sacrospinous Ligament

From the pattern of pain in the buttock and its distribution down the leg, it is possible to judge whether the sacrotuberous or sacrospinous ligament is involved. Sacrospinous pain is characterized by a thin line of referred pain through the center of the buttock and in the natal fold. The sacrospinous ligament is attached under the sacrotuberous ligament. When injecting the sacrospinous ligament, the therapist should aim not only at its origin on the sacrum, but also at its insertion into the spine of the ileum.

Piriformis Syndrome

An early description of this entity can be found in James Mennell's book (33). In diagnosis a modification of the straight leg raising test can be tried. When the leg on the affected side is raised with the knee straight and pain shoots down the leg as a result, the leg is replaced on the couch until the acute episode of pain subsides. Next, the hip is rotated externally to the full extent and the leg raised again slowly, with the knee straight. The moment discomfort returns, the angle is noted and the limb is lowered slightly until the pain is just relieved. At this point, the hip is rotated internally to the full extent. Reprovocation of the pain is considered a positive sign for the piriformis syndrome. It is not uncommon for the sciatic nerve to emerge into the gluteal region in two parts, one behind and one partly through the piriformis muscle.

Occasionally as a result of an injury or an inflammatory process, the element of the nerve that pierces the muscle is irritated in this tunnel. When the leg is raised in external rotation, the muscle is relaxed, but it is stretched with internal rotation and it is this tightening that reproduces the pain down the leg at a degree of elevation that is otherwise just below pain threshold. On rectal examination, the muscle is found to be tender, particularly when stretched by passive internal rotation of the thigh. It has also been pointed out (35) that the piriformis muscle is closely associated with the gluteus medius and is an abductor of the thigh in the sitting position. Resisted abduction inducing pain in this position is an additional sign implicating the muscle. In these cases the bow string sign is positive at straight leg raising of about 80°, and there is tenderness in the sciatic notch.

Simple stretching of the nerve used to be tried to relieve the pain, but is not currently advocated. A steroid injection, suitably diluted in 0.5% lidocaine, just below the greater sciatic notch is often curative. Failing this, the muscle fibers should be divided superficially to the element that pierces the muscle. This will afford adequate decompression. An excellent early description of this entity was written by Haggart (35).

Gluteus Medius Syndrome

The gluteus medius is the major abductor of the hip. It is an L4 structure predominantly, with contributions from L5 and S1. A strain in this muscle is a common cause of pain in the buttock. In standing it is active in maintaining balance, stopping the person from tipping forward.

Helweg recognized the importance of pain arising from the posture, which maintains isometric action of this muscle in relation to altered use and in association with underlying pathological entities, such as osteoarthritis of the hip. He regularly identified abnormalities in the buttock muscles by palpation and described relative atrophy from dysfunction (36). He described the distribution of pain down the leg, identifying the muscles as a source of referred pain and local tenderness, refuting the then prevalent theory of inflammation in the sciatic nerve in all cases of sciatica.

The gluteus medius syndrome can arise from sacroiliac ligamentous insufficiency occurring with right sacral subluxation in right-handed individuals. This phenomenon is not always symptomatic. When the pelvic ring is asymmetric, with one ileum forward (in osteopathic terminology), the gluteus medius on one side is more active than the other. In right-handed individuals, this is typically on the right side. Macnab pointed out that, because the muscle is an abductor of the thigh, it can be used to test the sacroiliac joint indirectly (37). In cases of pelvic ligament relaxation, it is advisable to stress the pelvic ring before testing for an involved gluteus medius. This can be done by asking for several sit-ups. The knees and hips may be partly flexed. The rectus abdominis pulling on the pubis will twist an unstable pelvic ring. Dysfunction of the gluteus medius muscle will then be detectable by weakness if it is examined at a mechanical disadvantage. The patient lies on the good side, the low back extended, the upper leg elevated in abduction and extended to about 20°. The patient then rolls 10° forward to keep balance. Weakness or pain on abduction in this position is usually referred to as the gluteus medius syndrome. The apparent weakness or giving way of the muscle in this situation can, on occasion, be tempered by correcting the sacroiliac subluxation, either by manipulation or, when there is easy mobility, by the leg lengthening maneuver, i.e., abduction, external rotation, flexion, adduction, and replacement on the couch (38).

A partial tear or inflammation at the origin of the muscle from the ileum may develop in a chronically strained gluteus medius. Gluteus medius pain is important in the differential diagnosis of sacroiliac pain and other L4 dermatome pains. The pain may come on while walking uphill and needs to be separated from hip pain proper. The inferior fasciculus of the muscle may give pain in the distribution of S1 and needs to be separated from pain arising in the sacrotuberous ligament and piriformis muscle. On prone examination trigger point tenderness is sought at the origin of the gluteus medius under the superior gluteal line with firm pressure. A more subtle feature of a strain in this muscle can be discerned in the standing patient with forward flexion. If the two buttocks are compared, the affected side with the contracting muscle is a little firmer, more prominent, and less round. With forward flexion of the trunk, both muscles eventually relax at 10 to 14° flexion, but the asynchrony is noted.

The gluteus medius syndrome can be provoked by the flexion exercises that are recommended after low back manipulation prolotherapy, particularly when the patient leans forward rather than folds the body down with the neck flexed. The treatment is the same. Testing the muscle may bring out subtle weakness of a nerve root, commonly an L5. This is an interesting contrast to the pattern of referred pain from the gluteus medius, which is usually in an L4 distribution.

Ileolumbar Ligaments

The origin of the ileolumbar ligament is in part from the L1-2 scleratome and in part from L3-4. Pain can be referrred to the groin and upper medial aspect of the thigh from the former origin, or into the buttock and lateral aspect of the thigh and down the medial aspect of the leg on the other. The ligaments join the iliac crests and the tips of L5 and L4. They infrequently require treatment on their own as a problem here is usually associated with sacral subluxation. One should remember that the origin of the ileolumbar ligament is from the inner rim of the iliac crest. When coming to the injection with a proliferant from the midline, a 3-inch needle is just long enough to reach the origin of the ileolumbar ligament on each side. If the ileal insertion alone is to be treated, it is helpful to have the patient lie with the painful side up over a pillow, to give some lateral flexion.

Suprasacral Ligament

Pain from the inferior part of the suprasacral ligament can radiate in the distribution of S2 down the back of the thigh, often bilaterally, but may be felt mostly as a band across the low back. It can be precipitated by prolonged sitting, standing, or lying. In treatment of the suprasacral ligament, a band across the back of the sacrum is infiltrated so the proliferant is injected, not merely in the midline, but down to the little bumps or spines along the back of the sacrum, these being just medial to the sacral posterior foramina.

Spondylolisthesis

Spondylolisthesis, either between L4 and L5, or between L5 and S1, is reported in 6% of the population and may be congenital. Acquired spondylolisthesis from ligamentous insufficiency is the common variety seen by orthopedic physicians. The results of prolotherapy are rewarding. However, it has been found that at least eight follow-up stabilizing injections are needed, with particular attention to the spondylolisthetic level. It should be kept in mind that the presence of this form of slippage is often without symptoms and the demonstration of spondylolisthesis on x-ray is not in itself sufficient to make a diagnosis (37).

Postlaminectomy Pain

The use of prolotherapy injections is not contraindicated in cases of postlaminectomy pain. As mentioned earlier, the injurious pathological process that causes the phenomenon of disc degeneration is responsible also for chronic ligamentous insufficiency. It is, therefore, not surprising that many cases correctly treated with laminectomy have an additional problem with ligaments, and these patients quite often respond to a suitably modified prolotherapy program.

References

1. Hackett GS. Ligament and tendon relaxation treated by prolotherapy. 3rd ed. Springfield Il: Charles C Thomas, 1958.
2. Hunt WE, Baird WC. Complications following injections of sclerosing agent to precipitate fibro-osseous proliferation. J Neurosurg 1961; 18:461–465.
3. Keplinger JE, Bucy PC. Paraplegia from treatment with sclerosing agents—Report of a case. JAMA 1960; 73:1333–1336.
4. Schneider RC, Williams JI, Liss L. Fatality after injection of sclerosing agent to precipitate fibro-osseous proliferation. JAMA 1959; 170:1768–1772.
5. Maher RM. Further experiences with intrathecal and subdural phenol. Lancet April 23, 1960; 1:895.
6. Nathan PW. Intrathecal phenol to relieve spasticity in paraplegia. Lancet Dec 19 1959; 2:1099.
7. Churchill-Davidson HC. ed. A practice of anaesthesia. 5th ed. Chicago: Year Book, 1984:919–926.
8. King Liu Y, Tipton C, Matthews RD, Bedford TG, Maynard JA, Walmer HC. An in situ study of the influence of a sclerosing solution in rabbit medial collateral ligaments and its junction strength. Conn Tiss Res 1983; 2:95–102.
9. Ongley MJ, Dorman TA, Eek BC, Klein R, Lundgren D. Ligament instability of knees: a new approach to treatment. Man Med 1988; 3:152–154.
10. Klein R, Dorman T, Johnson, C. Proliferant injections for low back pain: histologic changes of injected ligaments and objective measurements of lumbar spine mobility before and after treatment. J Neurol Orthop Med Surg 1989; 10:123–126.
11. Ongley MJ, Klein RG, Dorman TA, Eek BC, Hubert LJ. A new approach to the treatment of chronic back pain. Lancet July 18, 1987; 143–146.
12. Bourdeau Y. Five-year follow-up of sclerotherapy/prolotherapy for low back pain. Man Med 1988; 3:155–157.
13. Kirkaldy-Willis WH. Managing low back pain. 2nd ed. New York: Churchill Livingstone, 1988.
14. Gracovetsky S, Farfan H, Helleur C. The abdominal mechanism. Spine 1985; 10(4):317–324.
15. Kellgren JH. Observations on referred pain arising from muscle. Clin Sci 1938; 3:175.
16. Kellgren JH. On the distribution of pain arising from deep somatic structures with charts of segmental pain areas. Clin Sci 1939; 4:35.
17. James P. Backache. Philadelphia: Blackiston's, 1931.
18. Mennell JM. Back pain: Diagnosis and treatment using manipulative techniques. Boston: Little Brown, 1960.
19. Stoddard A. Conditions of the sacro-iliac joint and their treatment. Physiotherapy 1958; 44:97–101.
20. Bunting CH, Eades CC. The effect of mechanical tension upon the polarity of growing fibroblasts. J Exp Med 1926; 44:147–49.
21. Barbor R. Sclerosant therapy: The theory of treatment of ligamentous disturbance by a dextrose sclerosant. Reunion Sobre Patologia de la Columna Vertebral. Murcia, Spain. March 30, 1977.
22. Ghormley RK. Low back pain with special reference to the articular facets with presentation of an operative procedure. JAMA. 1933; CI:1773.
23. Mooney V, Robertson J. The facet syndrome. Clin Orthop No. 115. March-April 1976.
24. Kirkaldy-Willis WH. Managing low back pain. New York: Churchill Livingstone, 1983.
25. Porter PW, Hibbert CS, Wicks M. The spinal canal in symptomatic disc disease, J Bone Joint Surg 1978; 60B:485–87.
26. Kirkaldy-Willis WH, Wedge JH, Yong-Hing K, Reilly J. Pathology and pathogenesis of spondylosis and stenosis. Spine 1978; 3:319–28.
27. Faran HF. A reorientation in the surgical approach to degenerative lumbar intervertebral joint disease. Orthop Clin North Am 8:9–21.
28. De Villiers. Combined neurogenic and vascular claudication. SA Med J 1980; 19:650–54.
29. Simkin PA. Simian stance: A sign of spinal stenosis. Lancet Sept. 18 1982; 52–53.
30. Ehne G. Effects of certain degenerative disease of the spine, especially spondylosis and disk protrusion, on the neural contents, particularly in the lumbar region: Historical account. Mayo Clinic Proc 1975; 50:327–337.

31. Johansson JE, Barrington TW, Ameli M. Combined vascular and neurogenic claudication. Spine 7(7): 150–158.
32. Kohler R. Contrast examination of lumbar interspinous ligaments. Acta Radiol 1959; 52:21.
33. Mennell J. The science and art of joint manipulation. London: Churchill, 1952.
34. Klein R. Personal communication.
35. Haggart GE. Sciatic pain of unknown origin. J Bone Joint Surg 1938; 20(4).
36. Helweg J. Sciatica or myopathia of the posterior region of the leg. Copenhagen: Arnold Busch, 1925.
37. Macnab I. Backache. Baltimore: Williams & Wilkins, 1977.
38. DonTigny R. Function and pathomechanics of the sacroiliac joint. J Am Physical Ther Assoc 1985; 65(1):35–43.

Section V

MOBILIZATION AND MANIPULATION

17

STANDARDS OF CARE: MANIPULATIVE PROCEDURES

John Triano

APPROPRIATENESS

Scientific interest has only recently focused upon the questions of appropriate treatment for spine disorders. Combined costs of therapy and payments for disability may be higher in these conditions than for any other entity. Policy makers alerted the society's consciousness for work-related musculoskeletal injury in 1984 by proposing a national strategy (1) to seek solutions to high costs and loss of productivity. With the collaboration of engineering scientists and health professionals in the study of how spines work, an extraordinary accumulation of new knowledge has developed in the past two decades. Yet, in the sense of strict scientific rigor, few of the existing treatment methods used by health care providers have been subjected to high-quality randomized trials. Evidence gained from retrospective, cohort, and nonrandomized studies indicates that the physician is faced with making choices among clinically based options. Against this backdrop, government agencies, the insurance industry, and professional associations struggle with controversy concerning the appropriateness of the treatments that are chosen.

The professional uncertainty hypothesis described by Wennberg and his associates (2) lends some perspective to this current sociomedical climate. Indications from diverse clinically based data (3) lead to robust treatment variations in common practice. The persistence of widely differing viewpoints about appropriate methods of care results from an absence of tested theory.

Given this situation, there is little justification for omitting the practice of spinal manipulation as an early intervention for spinal disorders (4). More controlled trials of manipulation have been performed to test the theory of its clinical utility than for any other treatment. Table 17.1 lists outcomes from nine studies. Scientific methodologists (5) continue to debate over the proper interpretation of the less impressive findings reported in two of them. Even taking these outcomes in the most pessimistic light, seven of the nine investigations demonstrate therapeutic benefit from manual

Table 17.1.
Outcomes of Nine Studies

Study	Outcome
Evans et al. 1978 (6)	Tx. > codeine phosphate
Rasmussen 1979 (7)	Tx. > shortwave diathermy
Hoehler et al. 1981 (8)	Tx. > placebo
Godfrey et al. 1984 (9)	Tx. = massage & electrostimulation
Gibson et al. 1985 (10)	Tx. = shortwave & electrostimulation
Waagen et al. 1986 (11)	Tx. > placebo
Meade et al. 1986 (12)	Tx. > hospital Tx.
Ongley et al. 1987* (13)	Tx. > placebo
Hadler et al. 1987 (14)	Tx. > mobilization

*Manipulation coupled with injection.

procedures over alternative, more traditional treatments. Clearly, indecision about the potential value and appropriateness of these manual procedures is reduced substantially by such research findings.

Relief from pain and the correction of altered intervertebral and regional mechanics and their sequelae are important objectives. However, persistence of pain is insufficient grounds for continuing with a course of treatment indefinitely. The current clinical challenge is to determine how best to optimize therapeutic benefits while a more fundamental study of causation continues. The most pressing issue may be to identify the frequency and duration of application that will yield maximum effects in the shortest time.

The current social intent is to press forward with programs designed to limit the fiscal consequences of health care for third-party payers. Cost-containment strategy emphasizes the question of appropriateness of treatment, but it does not offer a solution for setting reasonable criteria for selection. The ultimate judgment on the acceptability of a treatment plan still resides with each patient who is suffering. Informed participation in the therapeutic decision making role remains the only ethical option. In this way, tolerance of uncertainty of the value of specific procedures can be taken into account. The attending clinician may then proceed with applying his or her view of what appears to constitute the best available treatment.

The suitability of care is often decided in retrospect by examining the frequency of patient visits and the duration over which a treatment plan was carried out. The relevance of these variables may vary widely according to the circumstances of each case. Factors of lifestyle, somatization, and occupational biomechanics become important modifiers of early treatment outcomes. Monitoring treatment must ultimately depend upon knowledge of the expected course to recovery and documentation of mitigating factors. The physician must quickly grasp the implications of patient response and react to the effects of modifiers. As an elegant model of clinical decision making for common back impairment, monitoring criteria have been seriously lacking. Opinions of prognosis are often based upon biases inbred in the clinician's discipline. Each provider moderates methods of treatment empirically as experience

with back disorders accumulates. Regional disparity in the rate and kind of treatment is a natural result (15), in part, because no standard of care has evolved that is systematically linked to patient outcomes.

As a consequence of the existence of so much variability, a serious mismatch exists between common practices in prescribing treatment and strategies used to assess results. A simple example is conveyed by observing the many clinical terms used to describe back pain. The nomenclature often implies assumptions about the location or severity of an underlying lesion. Experience has shown the terminology to be presumptuous. In contrast, DRG listings lump 165 primary diagnoses together under code number 243 for medical back problems. Only a few entities are satisfactorily predictable as pain producers (Table 17.2). Pathoanatomic diagnoses can be achieved only in about 10 to 20% of patients (16), and some of these will remain clinically silent during much of the course of the illness.

OUTCOME PROSPECTS

A greater understanding of the nature of back-related disorders from continued fundamental studies of spine function and pathology is likely to emerge in the future. In the interim, however, we must rely upon available sources of information to formulate standards of acceptable practice. It may be possible to reduce ambiguity in assessing treatment outcomes by means of patient categorization and attention to the natural history of back-related disorders. Two systems of patient categorization are emerging that offer more realistic representations of problems of this sort. Both are based in part upon descriptive groupings defined in terms of the characteristics of clinical presentation. On the one hand, a simple classification of pain distribution and behavior has been proposed (17) that

Table 17.2.
Painful Spine Lesions

Herniated nucleus pulposus
Central canal stenosis
Lateral recess entrapment
Ankylosing spondylitis
Spinal cord tumor
Osseous spinal tumor
Spinal infection

is tied directly to clinical outcomes. For example, a person categorized with leg pain extending below the knee will respond more slowly and less completely than a person presenting with back pain alone or with back pain and associated leg pain. On the other hand, the Quebec listings (Table 17.3) are descriptive of the patient's status at any given time. Classification is not fixed, but is revised depending upon clinical progress and can reflect clinical management changes along the way.

Historically, descriptive analyses such as these are consistent with earlier schools of thought in chiropractic, which placed less emphasis on diagnosis and more on response to trial therapy. Moreover, when clinical diagnoses are lumped into descriptive groups, as is done in the DRG or Quebec schemes of classification, patterns in the course of the treated and untreated conditions emerge (15, 16, 18–20). These observations describe a natural history that can serve as a reference criterion for setting treatment expectations. The most important outcome measures available are the rate of return to work, continued use of health care services, and recurrence of back-related injuries (21).

Separately, a presumptive model of spinal motion segment pathology has been developed and linked with clinical observations, including the tendency for conditions to evolve over time. From systematic observations of spine pathology and functional morphology, a plausible pathoanatomical explanation for the long-term behavior of back disorders has been advanced (22). The hypothesis that the natural history of spine disorders can be described in terms of three degenerative stages is now well known. Most patients fall into Stage I. Stage I, the dysfunctional phase, may occur as a primary problem or in conjunction with other pathology. Dysfunctions of this kind may be responsible for up to 90% of chronic low back pain complaints (23).

Diagnostic entities based upon functional descriptions have been proposed (Table 17.4). While remaining to be validated, these entities are clinically serviceable. Studies of the cervical spine have shown that some diagnostic elements of the pain syndrome can be functionally identified (24, 25). Case management can be adjusted according to the rate of response and the perception of tissues involved. Table 17.4 lists these descriptions, including treatment alternatives and the presumed role that manipulable lesions may play.

Regardless of how the patient's impairment is classified diagnostically, clinical decision making for the majority of back pain sufferers can be rationally organized. The natural history of back pain gives a defensible basis from which a measurable plan of action can be made.

Standards in patient management require close attention to three elements of the treatment plan. They are

1. criteria for selecting treatment procedures.
2. close monitoring of response in comparison with the expected outcome of natural history, and
3. flexibility of the protocol when less favorable responses are encountered.

Table 17.3.
Quebec Task Force on Spinal Disorders Functional Categories

Pain without radiation
Pain with radiation
  a. proximal
  b. distal
  c. neurologic signs
Plain radiographic evidence of nerve compression
  a. spinal instability
  b. fracture
Confirmed nerve root compression
Spinal stenosis
Postsurgical rehabilitation status
Persistent or recurrent postsurgical pain
  a. symptomatic or occasional mild pain
  b. spinal or radicular debilitating pain
Chronic pain syndrome
Other diagnoses

TREATMENT DYNAMICS

Over 40 different manipulative and/or adjustive procedures are currently available for treatment of the lumbopelvic spine alone. This technical diversity is often masked by the apparent ease of performance that a skillful manipulator demonstrates. Currently, literature references to manipulation often are made as if all clinical circumstances are expected to respond identically. As with any other form of therapy, it is likely that manual procedures follow dynamic principles much like those that govern pharmacokinetics. That is, treatment response will depend upon threshold effect, dosage, duration of administration, and additive effects from

Table 17.4.
Therapeutic options commonly used in conjunction with manipulation for treatment of back related disorders.

Presumptive Diagnosis by Presentation Characteristics	Manipulable Lesion*	Adjunctive Therapy								% Total Cases
		Exercise/ Stretch	Rehabilitation Exercise	Electrotherapy Modalities	Muscle Technique	Spray & Stretch	Biofeedback	Acupuncture	TNS	
Disc-HNP	2	+	+	+	−	−	+	+	+	14
Stenosis										
lateral	2	+	+	+	−	−	+	+	+	13
central	2	+	+	+	−	−	+	+	+	5
Spondylolisthesis	2	+	+	+	+	−	+	+	−	8
Instability	2	+	+	−	+	−	−	−	−	4
Sacroiliac syndrome	1	+	+	+	−	−	−	+	−	23
Posterior Jt syndrome	1	+	+	+	+	−	+	+	−	22
Myofascial syndrome	1/2/0	+	−	−	+	+	+	+	−	6

*1. The primary problem is a manipulable lesion.
2. A manipulable lesion is present as a secondary problem.
3. A manipulable lesion is not involved.

combination with other agents (Table 17.5). Scientific studies of the relative efficacy and mechanism for different procedures have only recently begun (13). For example, the mechanical response of a motion segment may be influenced by a number of modifiers. Local muscle tone and the patterning of recruitment during voluntary movement affect the distribution of stresses that are transmitted through the spinal tissues. The passive mechanical properties of disc, ligaments, and muscle may be altered by inflammatory or degenerative processes. Pathologic barriers imposed by intraarticular adhesions or meniscoid entrapments may be present and are thought by some to constitute potential mechanisms for disrupting normal mechanics. Finally, the occupational hazards of prolonged static postures or high-peak spinal loads can inhibit responses. The body's healing processes must proceed and inflammation subside, for example, before the effects of prolonged antalgic loading of the spine can be mitigated. Application of a single manipulation, as often reported in research protocols, is not a realistic clinical approach. Occasional anecdotes recall speedy response from single treatments, but experience shows that such cases are the exception rather than the rule.

No controlled studies are available that systematically evaluate the relative effects of frequency and duration of treatment. However, descriptive information about treatment response is available.

The treatment plan is divided into four phases (Table 17.6), each having distinct objectives that allow for both passive and active benefits. When the patient exhibits acute distress, efforts to reduce soft tissue and joint stresses are applied to diminish inflammation and

Table 17.6.
Stages of Treatment Goals & Objectives

1. Acute intervention
    a. To promote anatomical rest
    b. To diminish muscular spasm
    c. To reduce inflammation
    d. To alleviate pain
2. Remobilization
    a. To increase the pain-free motion
    b. To minimize deconditioning
3. Rehabilitation
    a. To restore strength and endurance
    b. To increase physical work capacity
4. Lifestyle adaptations
    a. To modify social and recreational activity
    b. To diminish work environment risk factors
    c. To adapt psychological factors affecting or altered by the spinal disorder

swelling. A short term of reduced mobility to limit the joint loading effects of gravity may be warranted. Passive forms of treatment, including the manual and palliative procedures listed in Table 17.4, may be used with deference to the type of mechanical lesion present. Once pain and discomfort have abated, the area is remobilized with low-speed and minimal-load exercises directed to improve flexibility without incurring mechanical stress. As the range of pain-free motion is improved, a gradual increase in exertion can be introduced. Finally, when a maximal range of motion is achieved, rehabilitation for strength and endurance can begin. It is beneficial to proceed to the rehabilitation phase as rapidly as possible and to minimize dependence upon passive forms of treatment. Studies have shown a clear relationship between prolonged limited activity and risk of failure in returning to preinjury status. Often a complete resolution of pain is not possible until the patient begins to focus on increasing the number and kind of activities in which to participate. Even then, some residual pain can be expected, although it will be offset by the benefits of increased productive functioning.

Clearly, the duration and intensity of in-office treatment for the uncomplicated case should not extend beyond the duration observed in reports of the natural untreated course. As a minimal standard, the patient's progress in comparison with the natural history helps to set an upper limit on the time during which a case should be followed without modification of the treatment plan. Figure 17.1 de-

Table 17.5.
Factors of Treatment Dynamics

Threshold	minimum rate and magnitude of joint load needed to effect change
Dosage	frequency of treatment necessary and sufficient to maintain effects while healing occurs
Duration	minimum of treatment interval to obtain stability in response
Combination	potentiation of response by simultaneous treatment applications

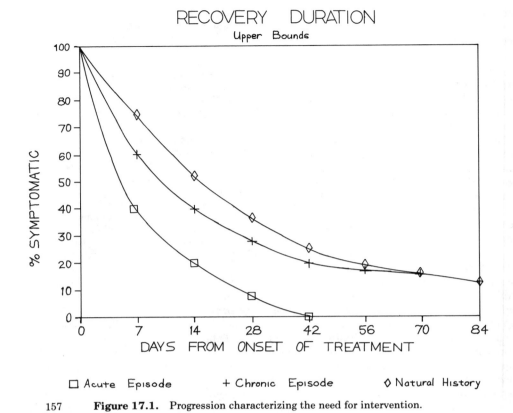

Figure 17.1. Progression characterizing the need for intervention.

fines the progress believed to characterize the majority of low back pain patients who require intervention. Each episode of back disorder can be perceived in the context of its own time course and can be described in stages of acute, subacute, chronic, or recurrent. Some controversy exists about definitions for each category. They appear to be loosely based upon the duration of absence from work or upon an assessment of relative clinical improvement. Table 17.7 lists three sets of definition, representing aggressive, intermediate, and conservative time limits for each stage. Recurrent episodes of back pain are not listed separately, since they

are treated in the same manner as acute cases. Differences in the decision cutoffs chosen in the separate studies reflect the relative values each group placed upon intervention to avert chronicity. Upon one fact there is agreement. Of those whose symptoms persist for more than 3 to 4 months, more than half will still be disabled at the end of a year.

Descriptive studies of the frequency and duration of care for spine disorders managed with manipulative procedures have been presented by Phillips (26) and Wickes (27). Patients seen by physicians trained in manipulation are characteristically indistinguishable from those

Table 17.7.
Time Course of Back Pain Stages

	Quebec Study (1987)	Frymoyer (1988)	Mayer & Gatchel (1988)
Acute	0 to 7 days	0 to 6 weeks	0 to 8 weeks
Subacute	7 days to 7 weeks	6 to 12 weeks	8 to 16 weeks
Chronic	more than 7 weeks	> 12 weeks	> 16 weeks

whose seek nonmanipulative care. Severity of injury being similar, the natural history and course of the condition will also be the same. Reporting on 3,943 cases under treatment, Phillips and Butler (28) found a mean number of 12.5 treatments required with a standard deviation of 13.1. Separately, Phillips (29) reported a mean of 9.02 treatments in 871 people with spine-related complaints. Patients fit all categories—acute, subacute, and chronic. Symptoms had been present for fewer than 30 days in 57%, for 60 to 180 days in 11%, and for longer than 180 days in 22%. The mean length of case management was 11.4 days. Twenty-four per cent were attended for a week or less while 56% received care for up to 30 days. One hundred and three cases (30) of lumbosacral pain were treated with up to four sessions of manipulation. They were followed for 1 to 3 years. Recurrence of symptoms appeared in only 11.7% during that time.

These statistics describing clinical experience with manipulation fit well within guidelines based upon natural history outcomes. An intriguing observation was made by Wolk based upon an investigation of differences in treatment patterns that distinguish chiropractic and traditional medical providers in workman's compensation cases. In a study of 17,198 claims for DRG code 243, the total cost and duration of management were accumulated considering all prescribed and physician performed procedures, but excluding hospitalization. Overall, a significantly higher frequency of treatment was noted for the chiropractic providers using manipulative procedures, but the total cost was less (31). Manipulative services on work-related back disorders averaged 29 office-based procedures per patient. Medical services were given 13 times per case. Additional costs from hospitalization were four times more frequent for medical treatment than for chiropractic. The average total disability period under traditional medical management was 58 days, contrasted with 39 days for chiropractic. Cost-benefit comparisons were favorable to manipulative management as well, with a 55.3% lower total cost of care for the latter (32). Conclusions from the study suggest that a more aggressive in-office intervention early in the course of treatment may ultimately result in reducing the amount of disabling injury and the necessity of engaging in more extensive inpatient procedures. These conclusions closely resemble determinations derived from functional rehabilitation and from the recommendations of the Ontario study for an earlier aggressive treatment approach.

Whether the patient's episode of pain is a first acute occurrence, a recurring pattern, or a flare from a chronic back, a substantial reduction in symptom severity should be expected within 10 to 14 days. An accompanying expansion in activities of daily living is a normal event. Rehabilitation and return to preepisode status should be achievable within 6 to 8 weeks for the majority of cases. Importantly, these kinds of recovery patterns are expected in every diagnostic category. Based upon return-to-work data, the Quebec study strongly urges that a 7-week episode duration be used as a critical cutoff point for any given treatment plan. Cases persisting without substantial improvement beyond then should be subjected to an intensive diagnostic reevaluation.

The presence of pathologic or anomalous structures may retard progress (33). Reinjury and exacerbation from unexpected events will also alter expectations. Circumstances such as these call into effect the artful practice of patient management. The ability of the attending clinician to identify the primary problem is a major factor in minimizing the time of patient suffering (15). Figure 17.2 displays a decision algorithm used to sort out these cases. Its value lies in helping to clarify and distinguish physician and patient responsibilities in working toward case resolution. The overriding concern is a focus upon the patient's rate of improvement in comparison with that predicted by the natural history.

The patient who experiences sufficient severity or duration of back discomfort will seek consultation. From that time forward, treatment is divided into the four stages of intent described above. Case management includes decisions about timing in the implementation of each stage. Some minimal variation can be expected from case to case as this derives from circumstances in the patient's habits, lifestyle, or occupation. These elements should be sought actively whenever the progress of treatment approaches or intersects the estimated time line of Figure 17.1. A systematic interview with the patient, including members of the family, will often reveal influences competing with treatment objectives. Trial therapy should be implemented again, incorporating a treatment plan for correcting these factors.

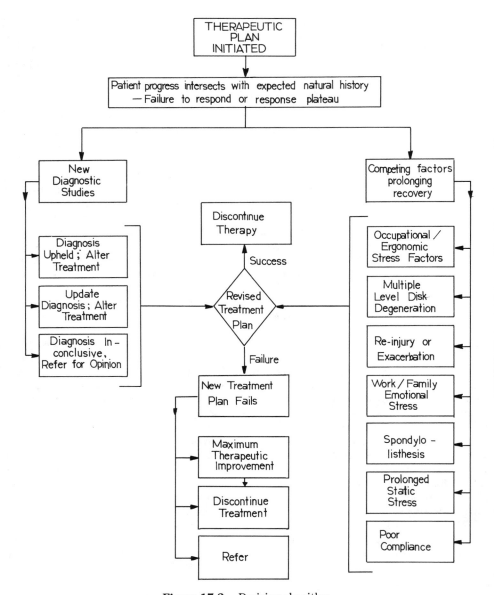

Figure 17.2. Decision algorithm.

If extenuating circumstances are not evident, or if a renewal of trial therapy fails to bring about an adequate rate of improvement, it is wise to reconsider the initial diagnosis. Special testing may be warranted, depending upon the level of suspicion and the reaction to renewed treatment. Whether or not the diagnostic impression is upheld, by this time a change in the therapeutic plan needs to be instituted. Failure to achieve a satisfactory response after working through the scenario laid out in the algorithm should result in an assessment for maximum therapeutic improvement or a referral and a second opinion. Patients who would tend to progress into a state of chronicity often can be aggressively rehabilitated at an earlier stage of their disorder.

SUMMARY

A large number of unknown factors continue to plague our understanding of the nature of most spinal disorders. Manipulative and adjustive procedures constitute an important option in the initial management of back-related pain episodes. While efforts continue to further understand pathoanatomical and functional features, a systematic method for adopting outcome expectations has been proposed. Even very complex cases can be managed within a time frame that avoids or reduces the risk of chronicity or the development of physician dependence. Treatment based upon documented therapeutic need can be more rationally based when factors of natural history and modifying factors from the patient's lifestyle and environment are considered.

References

1. Proposed national strategy for prevention of leading work-related diseases and injuries. Assn of Schools of Public Health, 1986.

2. Wennberg J, Barnes B, Zubkoff M. Professional uncertainty and the problem of supplier-induced demand. Soc Sci Med 1982; 16:811-812.

3. Mulley A, Eagle K. What is inappropriate care? JAMA 1988; 260(4):540-541.

4. Haldeman S. Presentation to American Back Society, Orlando, FL, Spring 1988.

5. Hoehler F, Tobis J. Appropriate statistical methods for clinical trials of spinal manipulation. Spine 1987; 12:409-411.

6. Evans D, Burke M, Lloyd K, Roberts E, Roberts G. Lumbar spinal manipulation on trial: Part 1—Clinical assessment. Rheum & Rehab 1978; 17:46-53.

7. Rasmussen T. Manipulation in treatment of low back pain (a randomized clinical trial). Man Med 1978; 1:8-10.

8. Hoehler F, Tobis J, Burger A. Spinal manipulation for low back pain. JAMA 1981; 224:1835-1838.

9. Godfrey C, Morgan P, Schatzker J. A randomized trial of manipulation for low-back pain in a medical setting. Spine 1984; 9:301-304.

10. Gibson T, Grahame R, Harkness J, Woo P, Balgrave P, Hills R. Controlled comparison of shortwave diathermy treatment with osteopathic treatment in non-specific low back pain. Lancet 1985; 2:1258-1260.

11. Waagen G, Haldeman S, Cook G, Lopez D, KeBoer K. Short term of chiropractic adjustments for the relief of chronic low back pain. Man Med 1986; 2:63-67.

12. Meade T et al. Comparison of chiropractic and hospital outpatient management of low back pain: a feasibility study. J Epidem Com Health 1986; 40:12-17.

13. Ongley M, Klein R, Dorman T, Eek B, Hubert L. A new approach to the treatment of chronic low back pain. Lancet, July 18, 1987; 143-146.

14. Hadler N, Curtis P, Gillings B, Stinnett S. A benefit of spinal manipulation as adjunctive therapy for acute low-back pain: A stratified controlled trial. Spine 1987; 12:703-706.

15. Mayer T, Gatchel R. Functional restoration for spinal disorders. Philadelphia: Lea & Febiger, 1988:7.

16. Frymoyer J. Back pain and sciatica. JAMA 1988; 318:291-300.

17. Leblanc F. ed. Scientific approach to the assessment and management of activity-related spinal disorders. Spine 1987; 12:16-21.

18. Roland M, Morris R. A study of the natural history of back pain, Part I. Development of a reliable and sensitive measure of disability in low back pain. Spine 1983; 8:141-144.

19. Roland M, Morris R. A study of the natural history of low back pain, part II. Development of guidelines for trials of treatment in primary care. Spine 1983; 8:145-150.

20. Valfors B. Acute, subacute and chronic low back pain: clinical symptoms, absenteeism and working environment. Scand J Rehab Med 1985; 11(Suppl):1-90.

21. Mayer T, Gatchel R, Mayer H, Kishino N, Keeley J, Mooney V. A prospective randomized two year study of functional restoration in industrial low back injury utilizing objective assessment. JAMA 1987; 258:1763-1769.

22. Kirkaldy-Willis W. Managing low back pain. New York: Churchill Livingstone, 1983:75-128.

23. Kirkaldy-Willis W. Presentation to The American Back Society, Orlando, FL, Spring 1988.

24. Jull G, Bogduk N, Marsland A. The accuracy of manual diagnosis for cervical zygapophysial joint pain syndromes. Med J Aust 1988; 148:233-237.

25. Bogduk N. Neck pain: An update. Aust Fam Physician 1988; 17:75-80.

26. Phillips R. Physician selection in low back pain patients. PhD Dissertation, U. of Utah Dept. of Sociology, 1987.

27. Wickes D. Demographic characteristics and presenting complaints of initial visit patients at Lombard Chiropractic Clinic. Unpublished internal data, 1980.

28. Phillips R, Butler R.: Survey of chiropractic in Dade County, Florida. JMPT 1982; 5:83-89.

29. Phillips R. A survey of Utah chiropractic patients. ACA J Chiroprac 1981: 15:113-128.

30. Guifu C, Zongmin L, Zhenzhong Y, Jinaghuz W. Lateral rotary manipulative maneuver in the treatment of subluxation and synovial entrapment of lumbar facet joints. J Trad Chin Med 1984; 4:211-212.

31. Wolk S. An analysis of Florida workers' compensation medical claims for back-related injuries.

American Public Health Association Meeting, Boston November 1988.

32. Wolk S. Chiropractic versus Medical care: a cost analysis of disability and treatment for back-related workers' compensation cases. American Public Health Association Meeting, Boston November 1988.

33. Herrin G, Chaffin G, Mach R. Criteria for research on the hazards of manual materials handling. NTIS PB83-151902, 1974.

18

SOFT TISSUE MOBILIZATION

Gregory S. Johnson
Vicky L. Saliba

Over the past several decades our capacity to diagnose and understand the mechanisms that lead to lumbar pathology has expanded, largely due to scientific and clinical advances made within the medical, physical therapy and affiliated professions (1–5). Significant progress has also been made in the area of conservative care of lumbar dysfunctions (6–9), including the use of a biomechanical and systematic approach to soft tissue mobilization (10). This approach is organized both to treat myofascial pain and to improve the patient's biomechanical ability to achieve and maintain a balanced posture and learn and perform efficient body mechanics. The approach is always coupled with a specific conditioning and flexibility program.

Soft tissue moblization (STM) is intended to be utilized as a component of a complete manual therapy program that includes evaluation and treatment of articular and neuromuscular dysfunctions. The approach encompasses the evaluation of the soft tissue system and application of specifically directed manual therapy techniques to facilitate normalization of soft tissue dysfunctions (10, 11).

Our purpose is to define soft tissue mobilization and describe its contribution to the conservative care of the lumbar spine. This chapter will 1) define the relevant soft tissue structures; 2) outline a specific system of subjective, objective and palpatory evaluations; 3) present basic treatment techniques; and 4) conclude with clinical correlations to develop an anatomical and biomechanical rationale for the use of soft tissue mobilization in the treatment of lumbar pain and dysfunction.

SOFT TISSUE COMPONENTS

The four primary soft tissues of the body are epithelial, muscular, nervous, and connective tissue (12, 13). All soft tissue structures have individual and unique functions while integrating together into a dynamic biomechanical unit (3, 14). Grieve emphasized this by stating that "the nerve, connective tissue, muscle and articular complex produce multiple and varied arthrokinetic systems which are functionally interdependent upon each other" (3).

Many authorities have stated that dysfunctions of the soft tissue system play a primary role in the onset and perpetuation of lumbar symptoms (3, 4, 15–18). Trauma is the most common precipitant of soft tissue pain and functional impairment (19). Trauma in its broadest sense includes external macrotraumas and internal or external microtraumas (Fig. 18.1). The resulting soft tissue dysfunctions may be the primary source of symptoms, or changes in posture and biomechanical capacity may alter the dynamic balance and distribution of weight, precipitating or perpetuating related symptomatology and pathology (3, 4, 16, 20, 21).

Most soft tissue dysfunctions in the lumbar spine can be specifically identified through an organized and precise subjective and objective evaluation. The therapist should have a working knowledge of the body's normal functional anatomy, biomechanics, and neuromuscular patterns to conduct and interpret this evaluation and to provide effective treatment. An understanding of soft tissue pathokinetics is essential to correlate the objective findings to pos-

External Macrotraumas	Internal or external Microtraumas
Blows Falls Improper heavy lifting Surgery Whiplash	Faulty posture Improper neuromuscular mechanisms Poor body mechanics Muscular imbalance Improper foot wear Repetitive stressful activities Poorly organized work surfaces Nonsupportive sitting and sleeping surfaces Chronic anxiety or depression Overweight

Figure 18.1. Macrotraumas and microtraumas.

sible soft tissue dysfunction. Soft tissue mobilization primarily addresses the evaluation and treatment of three soft tissue structures: irregular and regular connective tissues, skin, and skeletal muscle (12, 22).

Connective Tissue Structures

Connective tissue structures are of mesodermal origin and vary widely in density and function, ranging from bone to adipose tissue to blood. The primary structures evaluated and treated by soft tissue mobilization are the regular (dense) connective tissues such as tendons and ligaments, and the irregular (dense and loose) connective tissues such as fasciae, intrinsic elements of muscle, capsules, and aponeuroses. The physical properties and fiber orientation of these different connective tissue structures are complex and varied (23; Fig. 18.2).

Irregular connective tissues, primarily the fascial system (Fig. 18.3),

- ensheathe and permeate all tissues and structures (13, 22, 24),
- supply the mechanical supportive framework that holds and integrates the body together and gives it form (13, 24),
- supply pathways for nerves, blood vessels, and lymphatic vessels (19), and
- provide for space and lubrication between all bodily structures (12, 19, 24).

The fascial system is composed of laminated connective tissue sheaths of varying thickness and density which extend from the periosteum of bone to the basement membrane of the dermis. They are continuous throughout the body and are interconnected with the connective tissue structures of muscle (intrinsic elements,

tendons and aponeuroses), the articular structures (ligaments and capsules), and the intrinsic elements of peripheral nerves (endoneurium, perineurium, and epineurium; 12–14, 22). Because of this ensheathing organization, fasciae allows structures to have independent three dimensional mobility and function, while connecting the system together into an integrated functional unit (12, 19).

Hollingshead states, "If it were possible to dissolve out all the tissues of the body so as to leave only the fibrous (irregular) connective tissues, the essential organization of the body would still be represented and recognizable" (14).

Fascia is composed primarily of collagen fibers, which have high tensile strength and minimal extensibility (25, 26) because of three factors represented by the stress strain curve: elasticity (crimped nature), viscoelastic properties, and plasticity (27, 28; Figs. 18.4, 18.5).

Fascia, however, has a high degree of extensibility due to the weave, wavy helical configuration, and multiplanar orientation of the collagen fibers (Fig. 18.2 **A**; 29). Therefore, fascia is capable of adapting, providing support, and withstanding compressive, tensile, and sheer forces from all directions (12, 13, 30).

FUNCTIONAL JOINT CONCEPT

Gratz defined the normal spaces that are maintained between all structures by fascia as "functional joints," that is, a space built for motion (31). Each functional joint allows the adjoining structures, from individual muscle fibers to the large muscle bellies, to move in mul-

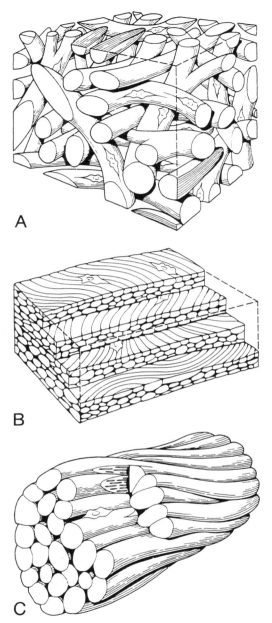

A

B

C

Figure 18.2. Three types of arrangement of collagen fibers. *A*, dense irregular connective tissue; *B*, a ligament; *C*, a tendon. (Reproduced with permission from Warwick R, Williams PL. Gray's Anatomy. 35th Br ed. Philadelphia: WB Saunders, 1979:40.)

tidimensional directions in relation to each other (18, 19).

We have expanded the functional joint concept to include the space that is maintained be-

tween each collagen fiber by the amorphous ground substance (23), a viscous gel containing a high proportion of water (60–70%) and long chains of carbohydrate molecules called mucopolysaccharides, principally glycosaminoglycans (GAGs; 13, 22, 32). The primary glycosaminoglycans are hyaluronic acid, chondroitin-4 and -6 sulfate, and dematin sulfate (22). Hyaluronic acid absorbs water and provides lubrication, while the chondroitin-sulfates maintain proper cohesiveness and viscosity (12, 13, 22, 33).

In a healthy state, the three-dimensional mobility that exists at these functional joints is termed *normal play* (10, 34). The degree of normal play varies according to the functional needs of the individual structures. Within the lumbar region there are thousands of functional joints separating soft tissue structures from each other and from the adjacent bony structures.

These functional joints between soft tissues, like the articulations of the spine, may become restricted and limit normal extensibility, accessory mobility, and biomechanical function of the tissues. This state of dysfunction is defined as *restricted or decreased play*. Tissues that are in a state of decreased play are clinically identifiable through skilled palpation, range of motion testing, and observable alteration in function (10, 34).

Mennell noted that "it is very remarkable how widespread may be the symptoms caused by unduly taut fascial planes. Though it is true that the fascial bands play a principal part in the mobility of the human body, they are often conducive to binding between two joint surfaces" (35).

An exact scientific explanation for restricted play and decreased extensibility of tissues has not yet been provided, and further research is needed to provide more in-depth physiological understanding. There are, however, some possible physiological explanations which include the following.

Scar Tissue Adhesions. Following an injury, laceration, or surgery, fibroblastic activity forms new connective tissue fibers to reunite the wound as part of the postinflammatory fibroblastic phase (Fig. 18.6) (36, 37). These fibers are formed through random fibroblastic activity. If the appropriate remodeling stimuli are not applied during the healing process the scar will be inextensible and nondynamic (15, 25, 38,

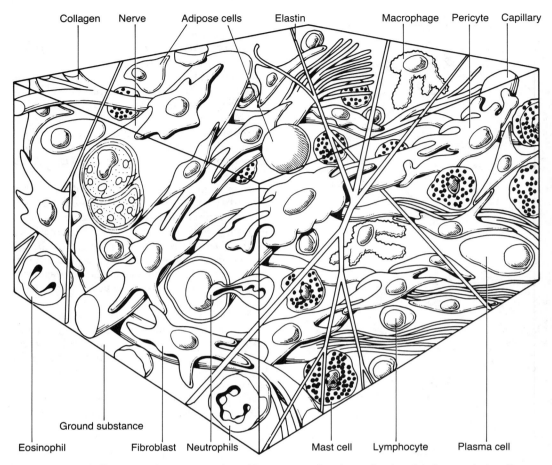

Figure 18.3. A diagrammatic reconstruction of loose connective tissue showing the characteristic cell types, fibers, and intercellular spaces. (Reproduced with permission from Warwick R, Williams PL. Gray's Anatomy. 35th Br. ed. Philadelphia: WB Saunders, 1979:32.)

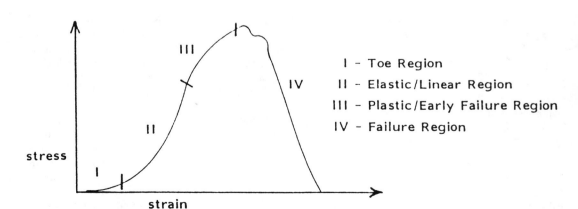

Figure 18.4. Stress strain curve.

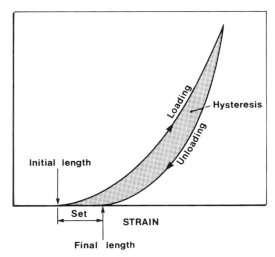

Figure 18.5. Hysteresis. When unloaded, a structure regains shape at a rate different from that at which it deformed. Any difference between the initial and final shape is the "set." (Reproduced with permission from Bogduk N, Twomey LT. Clinical anatomy of the lumbar spine. Edinburgh: Churchill Livingstone, 1987:56.)

39). Most scar tissue produces localized adhesions (15) that create a restrictive matrix with spider-web-like tentacles that can alter and limit normal mobility of structures and articulations in the surrounding region (1, 40).

Hollingshead states that scar tissue "may be a major factor in altering the biomechanics of the whole kinematic chain, placing strain on all related structures" (14). The abnormal strain caused by adherent and inextensible scar tissue may contribute to a chronic inflammatory process and further perpetuate symptoms (1, 15, 41). The scar tissue matrix may also compromise neurovascular and lymphatic structures affecting the fluid balance, the exchange of metabolites, and the removal of waste products from the region.

Lymphatic Stasis and Interstitial Swelling. An increase in interstitial fluids alters the mechanical behavior of the structures and restricts normal mobility of the functional joints. This fluid imbalance may possibly be related to immobility, poor lymphatic drainage, scar tissue blockage, or inflammation (42, 43).

Ground Substance Dehydration. Research conducted to determine the effects of forced immobilization on the periarticular tissues of various mammalian populations has revealed that such immobilization contributes to soft tissue changes and the development of an identifiable limitation of joint mobility (44–47). Biochemical and biomechanical compensations have been found to correlate with this restricted mobility within the ligaments, tendons, capsule, and fascia (32, 45).

One of the biochemical changes is a decrease in the level of GAGs within the ground substance. This includes a reduction in the level of hyaluronic acid (40%) and a decrease of chondroitin-4 and chondroitin-6 sulfate (30%; 48). As a result, there is a marked reduction in the water content (4.4%) within the soft tissue matrix (44, 45) and the interfascial planes (32). Ground substance dehydration creates a deterioration in the viscoelastic properties, a reduction in the critical fiber distance, an alteration in the lubrication between the fibrous elements, and a decrease in the spacing of the functional joints of fascial planes (23, 44, 49, 50). A result of dehydration is that the ground substance becomes more viscous (thixotropy) leading to increased tissue rigidity and stiffness, and thus requiring more force to elongate the tissues (44, 46).

Intermolecular Cross-linking. When the ground substance becomes dehydrated and the critical fiber distance is diminished, there is a higher potential for, and a significant increase in, formation of additional intermolecular cross links fibers (Fig. 18.7; 29, 44, 49–51). These intermolecular cross-links restrict interfiber mobility and extensibility and may be partially responsible for restricted soft tissue mobility and play. Furthermore, it has been shown that this reduced mobility affects the synthesis and orientation of new collagen fibrils, which further contributes to the pathogenesis of restricted fascial mobility (44).

Response to Treatment

It is reasonable to postulate a correlation between these research findings and the clinically identifiable decreased mobility and play found in dysfunctional soft tissues. Clinically, through the application of STM, the mobility of these dysfunctional soft tissues can be improved. These improvements may be a result of one or more of the following factors:

1. an alteration of the scar tissue matrix (1, 52),
2. a redistribution of interstitial fluids,

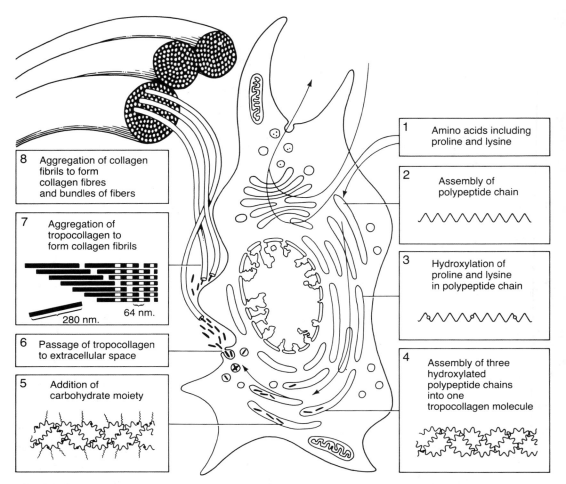

Figure 18.6. Genetic types of collagen and their distribution in connective tissues. (Reproduced with permission from Warwick R, Williams PL. Gray's Anatomy. 35th Br. ed. Philadelphia: WB Saunders, 1979:38.)

MODEL OF COLLAGEN CROSSLINK AT THE MOLECULAR LEVEL

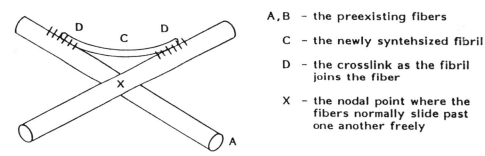

A,B – the preexisting fibers

C – the newly syntehsized fibril

D – the crosslink as the fibril joins the fiber

X – the nodal point where the fibers normally slide past one another freely

Figure 18.7. Idealized model of collagen crosslink at the molecular level. (Reproduced with permission from Akeson WH, Amiel D, Woo SL-Y. Immobility effect on synovial joint: The pathomechanics of joint contracture. Biorheology 1980; 17:95–110. © Pergamon Press Ltd.)

3. the stimulation of GAG synthesis restoring normal or improved lubrication and hydration,
4. the breaking of restrictive intermolecular cross-links (44,46),
5. the mechanical and viscoelastic elongation of existing collagenous tissues through the phenomena of creep and hysteresis as demonstrated by the stress strain curve (Fig. 18.4; 27, 30), and
6. a neuroreflexive response that may alter vascular, muscular, and biochemical factors related to immobility (53–58).

Skin

The skin is composed of two layers, an outer epidermis, which is of ectodermal origin and the deeper dermis, which is of mesodermal origin (59). The skin is continuous with the deep fascia and underlying structures because the superficial fascia is attached to the basement membrane of the dermis (13).

Because of the orientation and weave of the collagen and elastin fibers, the skin demonstrates considerable mechanical strength and a high degree of intrinsic flexibility and mobility. This *intrinsic mobility* allows considerable extensibility and the skin's elastin content provides the ability to recoil to its original configuration (27, 39). Because of the pliability of the superficial fascia, the skin also has extensive *extrinsic mobility* in all directions in relation to deeper structures (14, 22). In regions superficial to joints, the skin's mobility allows it to fold and stretch in response to the underlying articular and soft tissue movements (15, 39).

Response to Treatment

Dysfunctions of intrinsic and extrinsic mobility of the skin can be improved through the application of specific soft tissue techniques. These structural improvements are often clinically associated with dramatic reduction in pain and improved musculoskeletal function. These improvements may be related to the following possibilities:

1. more efficient biomechanical function,
2. local and general changes in the vascular and lymphatic circulation (42, 56), and
3. a neuroreflexive inhibition of muscle tone and pain, which may be a response to existing pathology in deeper structures (54, 56), including that of underlying spinal dysfunctions (3, 60, 61).

Skeletal Muscle

The muscles of the lumbar spine produce and control dynamic motion, as well as stabilize and protect the vulnerable spinal structures through reflex and volitional muscular bracing (10, 13, 22, 62). The two basic components of skeletal muscle are the muscle fibers (the contractile components; and the surrounding connective tissue sheaths (the noncontractile components).

The connective tissue components are the endomysium, perimysium, and epimysium (Fig. 18.8). They envelop each muscle fiber, fascicle, and muscle belly respectively and invest at the muscle's terminus to form the tendon, fascia, or aponeurosis (13, 22). These connective tissues provide for:

1. the mechanical and elastic characteristics of muscle for broadening during contraction and lengthening during passive elongation (functional excursion; 1, 63). They may be the major component affected by passive muscle stretching (40);
2. the elastic property of muscle, possibly due to the parallel arrangement of these sheaths with the contractile components (64);
3. the tension regulation of the muscle which influences contractile strength (40), ability to withstand high impact loads, and adaptive and recoil capability (65);
4. the support, cohesion, and protective restraint of the muscle (66);
5. the space and lubrication for normal extensibility and play of
   a. the intrinsic contractile elements, and

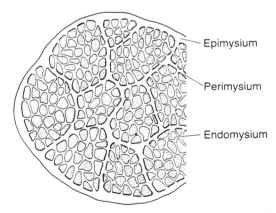

Figure 18.8. Connective tissue components of muscle. (Reproduced with permission from Ham A, Cormack D. Histology. Philadelphia: JB Lippincott, 1979.)

b. the muscle belly (through the epimysium) in relationship to surrounding structures (14, 15);

6. A soft tissue continuum (the myofascial unit) as they interconnect with each other, as well as the loose connective tissue and fascia surrounding the muscle through the superficial epimysium (18); and

7. A conduit for blood vessels and nerve fibers (13, 22, 67).

DYSFUNCTIONS OF THE MYOFASCIAL UNIT

For the proper protection of articular and soft tissue structures, the movement control of the neuromuscular system must be precise and allow for few deviations (19, 68, 69). Several authors believe that the myofascial unit is often the primary precipitator of pathology and symptoms (4, 17, 70). Many report that dysfunctions of this unit are often preceded by faulty posture, poor neuromuscular control, and altered recruitment patterns (19, 68, 71–73). These conditions often lead to length-associated muscle imbalances (between antagonistic muscle groups) and affect the balanced force production, coordination, fine motor control, and distribution of forces necessary to protect the spinal segment during dynamic and static postures (3, 19, 68).

Kirkaldy-Willis has proposed a model, "the myofascial cycle," that schematizes a degenerative cascade of lumbar pathology (Fig. 18.9; 4). This cycle begins with a minor trauma or emotional disturbance that causes a chronic neuromuscular response. This response facilitates chronic muscular changes such as fibrosis, weakness, limited extensibility, and altered recruitment patterns. Specifically in cases where the multifidi become dysfunctional, significant alteration of the arthrokinematics of the spinal segment may occur leading to possible facet and disc deterioration (74).

Efficient neuromusculoskeletal function requires normal joint and soft tissue mechanics in conjunction with well-coordinated neuromuscular control. Normal voluntary and involuntary neuromuscular control is developed primarily through learned activities. Various factors may precipitate a state of altered recruitment patterns (19, 68). Janda has observed that when altered recruitment patterns exist, muscles that are composed primarily of tonic (slow twitch) fibers become chronically facili-

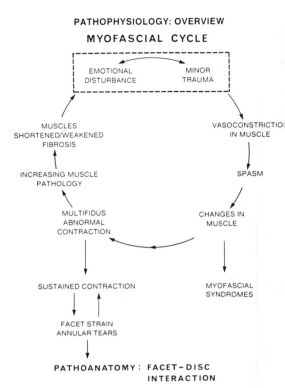

Figure 18.9. Myofascial cycle. (Reproduced with permission from Kirkaldy-Willis WH, Hill RJ. A more precise diagnosis for low back pain. Spine 1979; 4:102.)

tated and respond to stressful situations and pain by increased tone and tightness, while muscles that are primarily composed of phasic (fast twitch) fibers are inhibited, becoming weak, atrophied and overstretched, thus creating length-associated muscle imbalances (Figs. 18.10 and 18.11; 62, 68).

An example of altered recruitment patterning is seen in the inappropriate activation and tightness of trunk extensors (during attempted trunk flexion), which further inhibits weak and lengthened lower abdominals. This imbalance alters the normal neuromuscular, postural, and mechanical dynamics of the lumbar spine. Appropriate treatment for this condition would include soft tissue mobilization and stretching of the shortened extensors (10, 16, 62, 68), strengthening of the weakened flexors (16, 75, 76), neuromuscular reeducation to restore proper movement and recruitment patterns (19, 71, 72, 77), and body mechanics training to change stressful ADL patterns (76).

Muscle Hypotrophy   Muscle Hypertrophy

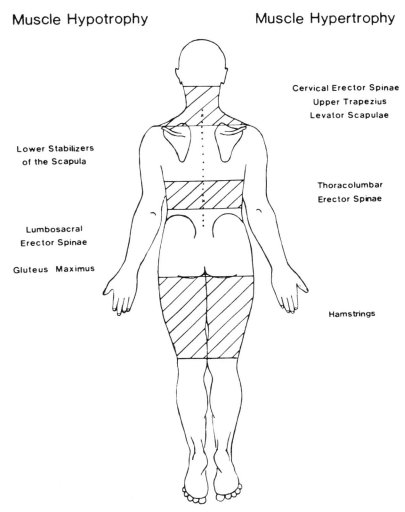

Cervical Erector Spinae
Upper Trapezius
Levator Scapulae

Lower Stabilizers
of the Scapula

Thoracolumbar
Erector Spinae

Lumbosacral
Erector Spinae

Gluteus Maximus

Hamstrings

Figure 18.10. Depiction of the layer syndrome. (Reproduced with permission from Jull GA, Janda V. Muscles and motor control in low back pain. In Twomey LT, Taylor JR, eds. Physical therapy of the low back. New York: Churchill Livingstone, 1987:253–278.)

Patients with lumbar dysfunction who manifest poor posture due to soft tissue dysfunctions often have difficulty performing dynamic, coordinated, and balanced motions while simultaneously maintaining trunk stability and controlled mobility. Soft tissue mobilization directed toward improving posture often elicits an almost immediate improvement in neuromuscular control, recruitment patterns, and stabilization abilities (10, 76).

The primary structural dysfunctions of the myofascial unit include:

• restrictive scar tissue,

• restricted muscle play,
• weakness or increased tone through impaired peripheral and central innervation,
• restricted extensibility and play of the connective tissue elements (fibrosis),
• adaptive muscle shortening possibly through the loss of sacromeres (15, 18, 43, 75, 78),
• injury of the musculotendenous structures (40), and
• generalized hypertonus (1) and localized myofascial trigger points (17).

Grieve states that "tone in striated muscle is due to three sets of influences:

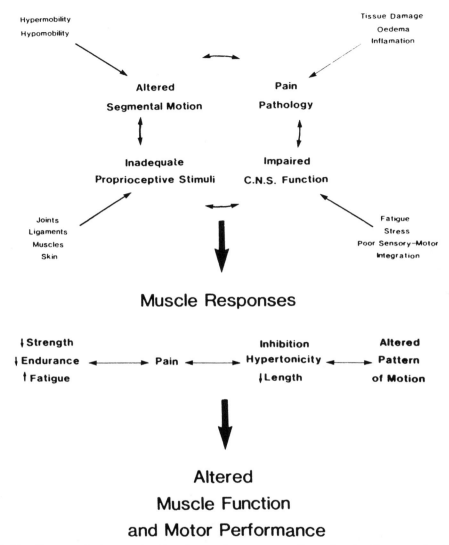

Figure 18.11. Sources of adverse stimuli and muscular responses. (Reproduced with permission from Jull GA, Janda V. Muscles and motor control in low back pain. In Twomey LT, Taylor JR, eds. Physical therapy of the low back. New York: Churchill Livingstone, 1987:253–278.)

- the elastic tension of the connective tissue elements,
- the degree or extent of interdigitation overlap of the actin and myosin elements, and
- the number of motor units which are active." (3)

The number of active motor units can be related to multiple factors, such as trauma (3, 18), scarring from disease or injury (18), supraspinal influences (3), protective spasm, chronic reaction to situation stress, and repetitive habitual holding and movement patterns (10, 79).

Myofascial trigger points are defined by Travell and Simons as "a hyperirritable spot, usually within a taut band of skeletal muscle or in the muscle's fascia that is painful on compression and that can give rise to characteristic referred pain, tenderness, and autonomic phenomena" (17). Simons reports that the palpable hardness identified with myofascial trigger points may be caused by increased fibrous connective tissue, edema, altered viscosity of muscle, ground substance infiltrate, contracture of muscle fibers, vascular engorgement, and fatty infiltration (17). Within the system of STM myofascial trigger points are included in the category of specific or general muscle hypertonus.

Muscle hypertonus and myofascial trigger points can be identified in most cases of lumbar pain and dysfunction. These conditions may be the primary source of symptoms (17), or a secondary source through a reflex response to underlying or related pathology. In addition to local and referred pain, increased muscle tonus and myofascial trigger points may also precipitate altered movement patterns (62) and restricted range of motion (1, 2, 4, 17). Because of the individual variability of response to pain and the possibility that referred pain or protective spasm may be caused by the hypertonic state, the location of muscle tone or tenderness is often not a reliable indicator of the location of the source of pathology (3).

Both muscular hypertonus and myofascial trigger points have been shown to normalize quickly in response to a treatment program of soft tissue mobilization. However, if the hypertonus or trigger points are in response to a secondary source, the objective signs often partially or completely return within a short time (10).

EVALUATION

A specific and organized evaluation system is an integral aspect of a rehabilitation and manual therapy program. The following components of evaluation are avenues that can assist the therapist in identifying musculoskeletal dysfunction: 1) client's subjective report, 2) structural analysis, 3) motion analysis, and 4) palpation. Specific aspects must be integrated into these evaluations to assist in identifying the condition of the soft tissue system.

Subjective Evaluation

Many of the factors that cause or precipitate soft tissue dysfunctions can be identified through a careful subjective evaluation. Cyriax states that most soft tissue dysfunctions have a "distinctive history" (80). Within the framework of a normal subjective evaluation there are certain questions that are important in determining soft tissue involvement.

Precipitating Trauma or Activity. It is important to identify carefully the direction of trauma and the movement pattern that occurred. This information helps in understanding the presenting symptoms, in analyzing the structural deviations, and in identifying which soft tissues should be evaluated. It is often important to know the patient's emotional state at the time of injury (19).

Previous Traumas. One should look for earlier traumas that may have precipitated soft tissue changes, alteration in the biomechanics of the kinematic chain, or performance of normal motor function. These alterations may contribute to the presenting symptoms.

Previous Surgeries. Question especially for abdominal surgeries or spinal surgeries, since the scar tissue may affect normal lower quadrant function.

Duration of Symptoms. Inquire primarily about those symptoms related to the chronic protective spasm and inactivity that could precipitate fibrotic changes within muscles and a remodeling of soft tissues.

Stressful Employment and Leisure and Recreational Activities. Identify repeated patterns of postural dysfunction and aberrant movement patterns that may create dysfunctional soft tissue and muscular changes.

Postural and Sleeping Habits. Identify prolonged and habitual positions that may cause adaptive shortening of soft tissues.

Objective Evaluation

Careful objective evaluation provides a means to assess the physical and functional status of the whole patient. Objective evaluation will assist in identifying abnormal postural and functional components both in the symptomatic region and in related asymptomatic regions.

Examples of asymptomatic postural dysfunctions are a forward head due to tight anterior lower cervical soft tissues, or unilateral or bilateral pronated ankles due to intrinsic or extrinsic soft tissue or articular abnormalities.

Data gathered through the objective evaluation will assist in 1) the development of a treatment plan, 2) setting of realistic goals, and 3) objectifying the effectiveness of treatment (62). Objective evaluation includes three components:

- structural analysis
- movement analysis
- palpation.

STRUCTURAL ANALYSIS

Through careful observation, the postural and soft tissue components are analyzed for patterns of dysfunction that are directly or indirectly related to the lumbar symptomatology. They are observed through the analysis of vertical alignment and positional relationship of segments, and soft tissue contours and proportions.

Evaluation of the Vertical Alignment and Positional Relationships of Movement Segments

Efficient posture can be defined as the arrangement of skeletal and soft tissue structures in a balanced relationship allowing for efficient weight distribution, shock absorption, and optimal coordinated intersegmental function (neutral posture).

Poor posture is often a major factor in the pathogenesis and perpetuation of lumbar symptoms (19, 81). Careful assessment of vertical alignment and the relationship of individual movement segments (thighs, pelvis, lumbar spine, thoracic spine) to each other can assist in identifying many of the postural and mechanical dysfunctions which are related to the presenting symptoms (81). Improper alignment places abnormal stress upon sensitive spinal structures and affects normal weight distribution, shock absorption, segmental biomechanics, and energy expenditure. These alterations can precipitate pathology and symptoms in the articular and soft tissue structures.

Poor skeletal alignment is most clinically significant in patients who sustain faulty posture for extended periods of time, especially where additional stress is imposed on the spine by frequently carrying loads. Poor alignment is usually a result of two distinctly interrelated factors: 1) structural and mechanical limitations (e.g., articular immobility and soft tissue adaptive shortening and contracture), or 2) habitual patterns of functional holding and posturing (e.g., poor kinesthetic awareness and emotional or attitudinal posturing) (68, 79, 82).

Observational evaluation begins with a global view of the patient, which guides the therapist to regions in need of specific assessment. One should note overall body type, contour, integrity, and balance of the patient's posture. This global assessment often reveals general patterns of imbalance and poor alignment, which may place stress on lumbar structures.

An organized regional assessment should begin with an analysis of the base of support, then progress superiorly to an evaluation of each movement segment's position and relationship to the segment below and above (Fig. 18.12). Special attention is given to evaluate the symptomatic region or regions with a focus on capacity to assume a neutral posture (10, 62, 81).

The *vertical compression* test is utilized to evaluate the vertical integrity of the lumbar spine. The test is performed in a standing or sitting position, by manually applying a vertical force through the patient's shoulders, while noting the quality of weight distribution and transmission of force through the spine (Fig. 18.13). When vertical compression is applied to an efficient neutral alignment, the structure

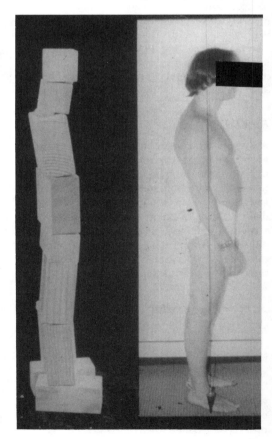

Figure 18.12. Positional relationships of movement segments.

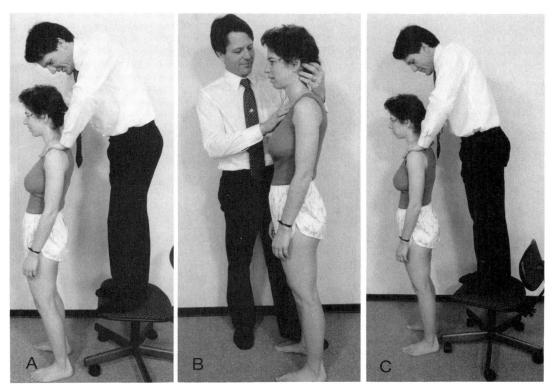

Figure 18.13. Vertical compression test (*A*); correction (*B*); retest (*C*).

feels solid under the therapist's hands without any noticeable buckling of the thoracic or lumbar spine. However, when it is applied to an individual with poor alignment, there is observable and palpable buckling at the segments of inefficient weight distribution. This usually occurs in transitional zones where the direction of the spine changes. These *transitional zones* are often symptomatic and also inappropriately utilized as the primary axis of motion during functional activities. This excessive over-utilization of individual segments often precipitates degeneration, low-grade inflammatory response, hypermobility, and associated soft tissue adaptations (83).

Once the segments of poor skeletal alignment are identified, the therapist attempts to attain a more balanced neutral position through manual and verbal cues. Vertical compression is again applied both to reevaluate the vertical integrity and to provide the patient with further kinesthetic feedback of the more stable and balanced alignment. Those segments that can not be repositioned because of

structural limitations are identified for more in-depth soft tissue evaluation and treatment. The most important and frequently identified alignment problem is improper positioning of the pelvis and rib cage in relationship to the lumbar spine (10, 76).

Except in cases where a forced posture controls pain (such as maintaining a pelvic tilt to open the intervertebral foramina in cases of advanced foraminal stenosis), increased muscular effort should not be utilized to assume an improved posture against underlying soft tissue tension. The effort of forcing a fixed posture often causes secondary compensations, biomechanical stresses, and structural shortening (10, 71). Therefore, restrictive soft tissues should be normalized through soft tissue mobilization and stretching so that an improved alignment can be assumed with greater ease. This decreased effort enhances patient compliance and comfort. With improved postural alignment, increased emphasis should be placed on body mechanics training and a conditioning exercise program to strengthen weak muscles, stretch shortened structures, reeducate proper movement patterns, and improve kinesthetic awareness and balancing reactions.

Soft Tissue Observation

Soft tissues are evaluated for:

- the condition of the surface (texture and color changes, scars, dryness and moisture),
- the proportions of soft tissue bulk (between the front and back, right and left, inferior and superior),
- the contours, by assessing the body's outline for circumferential and segmental bands, regions of bulges or protrusions, and flattened or tightened areas,
- three dimensional structural proportions, checking for obvious imbalances of length, width or depth. (79)

Observation of the soft tissue often reveals abnormal patterns of tissue tension. These patterns often occur in spiral zig-zag configurations affecting available movement (Fig. 18.14). These compensatory restrictive patterns may perpetuate symptoms and require treatment to assist with the rehabilitation of the regions of pathology and symptomatology. Any noted proportional imbalances of soft tissue development require further evaluation and the initiation of an appropriate muscular conditioning program.

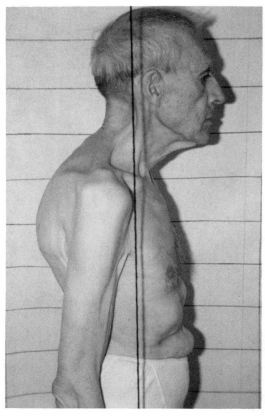

Figure 18.14. Evaluation of patterns of spiral and zig-zag soft tissue compensations.

Movement Analysis

Once postural abnormalities and soft tissue changes are identified, it is important to evaluate the mobility of the involved regions while the patient performs physiological and functional movements. Restricted tissues can often be identified during movement analysis through their inability to conform and slide in relationship to surrounding structures and through the altered and restricted mobility of underlying joints. Through careful observation of the patient's ability to perform

- physiological movement patterns,
- normal functional activities, and
- functional movement patterns,

the therapist can identify soft tissue dysfunctions and grade the effects of those dysfunctions on movement performance.

Evaluation of Physiological Motions

Through a conventional active range-of-motion evaluation, important data related to the condition of soft tissues can be gained. This evaluation can be performed in weight bearing postures such as standing, sitting, and quadruped. The evaluator should look for:

- quality and sequencing of motion,
- range of movement (delineating structural and symptomatic limitation),
- effect of movement on intensity, location and type of pain,
- mobility of individual segments,
- ability of soft tissues to elongate and fold, and
- proper utilization of base of support.

Careful assessment and recording of specific limitations of physiological motions provides the therapist with parameters for reevaluation and thus the ability to correlate the effects of soft tissue treatment.

Evaluation of Functional Activities

Observation of an individual performing normal activities of daily living often reveals soft tissue dysfunctions that impede the use of proper body mechanics and contribute to the exacerbation of symptoms. A functional evaluation should include all functional activities frequently performed by the patient, including those listed in Figure 18.15 (76, 79). Functional limitations such as a tight calf compartment, limitations in hip range of motion, and restriction in shoulder girdle mobility are frequently identified through careful analysis. Success of treatment can be gauged through documented improvements in functional abilities (76).

Evaluation of Functional Movement Patterns

Functional movement patterns (11) are specific segmental and whole body active motions that assist in the assessment of motor control and soft tissue and articular mobility. These specific movement patterns were primarily adapted from the Proprioceptive Neuromuscular Facilitation diagonal movement patterns (72, 77) and awareness through movement lessons developed by Moshe Feldenkrais (71). These functional movement patterns offer additional tools for evaluationg specific limitations in dynamic range and sequencing of motion. Patterns such as the pelvic clock, lower trunk rotation, unilateral hip rotation, and pelvic diagonals can provide valuable information about the three-dimensional active mobility and compliance of the soft tissues and articulations of the lower

Functional Activities
_____

Coming to sitting
Sitting
Rising to standing
Walking
Bending
Reaching
Pushing
Pulling
Lifting

Figure 18.15. Evaluation of functional activities.

quadrant. Functional movement patterns such as side-lying arm circles reveal the mobility and compliance of the rib cage and upper extremities.

Palpatory Evaluation

Palpation evaluation is guided by the data gained through the subjective, postural, and movement assessments, and includes the specific assessment of the condition and the three-dimensional mobility of the individual layers of tissues. This assessment begins superficially, while the deeper layers are defined by the individual muscle layers. Soft tissue dysfunctions can exist within a specific layer of tissue or extend through several distinct layers. These restrictions generally have an epicenter and often exist in spiral patterns of adherences. Restrictions that alter normal functional movements are most effectively evaluated during the performance of passive, active, or resisted motion (11).

Tissues tender to normal palpation are considered to be in a state of dysfunction, whether they are a primary or secondary source of symptoms or dysfuncton (10). Through proper palpation, dysfunctional tissues can be identified and any patterns of referred pain can be elicited and evaluated (54, 80).

During a palpatory evaluation, it must be remembered that proper palpation is a critical means of communication that relays to the patient the therapist's clinical competency and caring attitude. A knowledgeable touch is one of the quickest means of developing a patient's confidence and achieving improvements in soft tissue dysfunction (84, 85). Soft tissue dysfunctions are identified through palpable changes in tissue extensibility, recoil, end feel and independent play (10).

EXTENSIBILITY AND RECOIL

Soft tissue extensibility is evaluated through direct pressure to the tissues being evaluated or through elongation of those tissues by joint motion. As soft tissues are deformed through their range of motion, points of increased resistance may be felt. These restrictions or changes in density may exist through only a portion, or through the complete excursion of the tissues. Identification of the tissues' specific restrictive points is important, as the treatment is applied to the adherent tissues at the point of greatest tension (epicenter). Recoil is evaluated as the tissues return to their resting length.

END-FEEL EVALUATION

Tissue end-feel (1) is the quality of tension felt when a tissue is manually deformed through direct pressure to the limit of its physiological or accessory range. In a healthy state, tissues have a springy end-feel that can be compared to the quality of elasticity and recoil felt when a new rubber band is taken to end range. The excursion (range of deformation) of soft tissues varies throughout the body, but the end-feel is consistently springy.

Tissues in a state of dysfunction have a hard end-feel. Clinically it can be demonstrated that soft tissue dysfunctions have specific three-dimensional limitation with an epicenter of precise depth, direction, and degree of maximal restriction. When the specific direction and depth of the restriction is known, treatment can be more specific, more effective, and less invasive (10).

STRUCTURES AND TOOLS OF EVALUATION

Skin and Superficial Fascia Assessment

The skin is first evaluated for changes in texture, temperature and moisture which can guide the therapist to underlying acute or chronic conditions. Next, the skin is evaluated for its intrinsic mobility of extensibility, end-feel, and recoil and its extrinsic mobility of independent play in relationship to underlying structures. There are three primary ways to evaluate the mobility of the skin and superficial fascia; skin sliding, finger sliding, and skin rolling.

Skin Sliding. Utilizing general contacts such as the palm of the hand or specific contacts such as the finger tips to evaluate the ability of the skin to slide in relationship to underlying structures. This procedure reveals patterns and directions of restrictions and assists in identifying the location of those restrictions.

Finger Sliding. Evaluation of the ease in which the finger tips can slide through the skin (Fig. 18.16). In normal tissue, the finger slides with ease creating a wave of skin in front. In restricted regions, there is diminished ease of sliding. Restrictions are identified by specific locations and direction of maximal restriction.

Skin Rolling. Lifting of the skin between the thumb and the index and middle fingers to evaluate the skin's ability to lift from underlying structures. Skin rolling is accomplished by keeping a wave of skin in front of the thumb while the finger pulls ahead and feeds tissue towards the thumb. This evaluation tool is especially effective over bony prominences.

Bony Contours Assessment

Scott-Charlton and Roebuck state that "a great deal of spinal pain may well be pain felt where muscle, tendon, ligament and capsule are attached to sensitive periosteum of the spine" (86). Due to the extensive attachment and proximity of soft tissues to bony contours, such as the iliac crest and each individual vertebra, evaluation of each individual layer provides valuable information related to the overall condition of the soft tissues of the lumbar spine and surrounding regions. This evaluation is performed by sliding the fingers parallel (longitudinally) along the edges of the bone noting any points of adherence and restricted mobility in various layers or depths (Fig. 18.17). Corrective treatment often facilitates functional and symptomatic improvements, perhaps because the normal dynamic soft tissue tension and mobility is restored.

Muscle Assessment

Evaluation of muscles should include assessment of the four conditions of muscle tone, muscle play, muscle functional excursion, and neuromuscular control.

Muscle Tone. Muscles in a state of increased tone will appear harder, more dense, and often quite tender to normal palpation (hypertonus and myofascial trigger points; 3, 10, 87). Specific points of maximal density can be identified in cases where the entire muscle belly is involved as well as in situations where distinct localized points are present. With careful palpation, the specific location, depth, and direction of the increased tone should be located and appropriately treated.

Muscle Play. Play is evaluated through perpendicular (transverse) deformation and

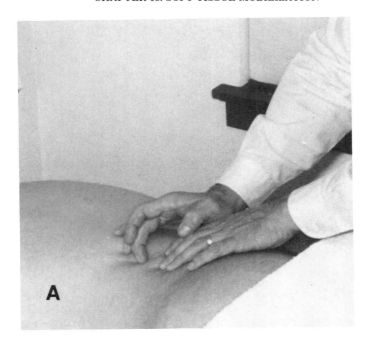

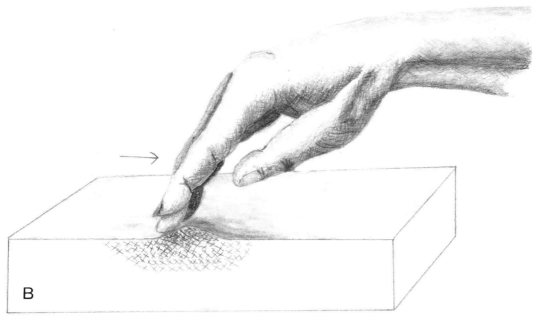

Figure 18.16. A, B. Skin and superficial fascia assessment—finger sliding.

parallel (longitudinal) separation of the muscle belly from surrounding structures. Each restriction is identified for its specific depth and direction.

Muscle Functional Excursion. Muscle length and flexibility are evaluated by stretch-ing the origin of the muscle from its insertion, identifying the specific direction of maximal re-striction and treating with soft tissue mobili-zation including contract or hold relax tech-niques (Fig. 18.18; 72, 88). This state of decreased muscle length may be due to either a

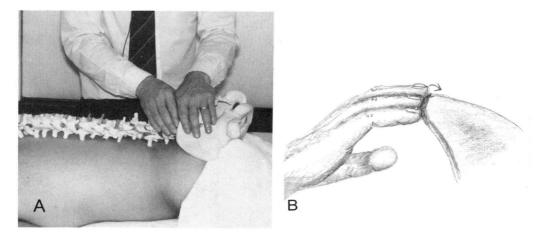

Figure 18.17.   A, B. Assessment of bony contours.

state of chronic muscular "contraction" or a structural "contracture." Evaluation of the ability of a muscle to shorten and broaden is done passively, through transverse fiber palpation to assess the play of the intrinsic components; and dynamically, through palpation of the tissue as they shorten.

Neuromuscular Control. This is effectively evaluated and treated by utilizing the principles and techniques of Proprioceptive Neuromuscular Facilitation (Fig. 18.19; 72, 77). Poor recruitment and sequencing patterns of movement often lead to strain upon the soft tissues, precipitating soft tissue dysfunction. Improvement in neuromuscular control decreases the stress on articular structures and assures long-term maintenance of improvement in posture, available movement, and symptoms (72, 77).

General Three-dimensional Evaluation

Three-dimensional palpation is a means of evaluating the general ease or difficulty with which soft tissues surrounding a segment of the body move. For example, in the evaluation of the mobility of the circumferential soft tissues of the upper thigh, one hand is placed over the region of the quadriceps while the other hand is placed over the hamstrings (Fig. 18.20). The therapist can evaluate the mobility of each layer circumferentially around the leg by moving the tissues in congruent motions of superior or inferior, internal or external circumferential

rotation, or in a motion combining diagonal and spiral directions. Through this evaluation, the therapist can identify those patterns in which the tissues are restricted and those in which they move freely. This distinction will help identify movement patterns that are frequently utilized, producing tissue mobility, and those that are not utilized, creating tissue immobility (11, 55, 79).

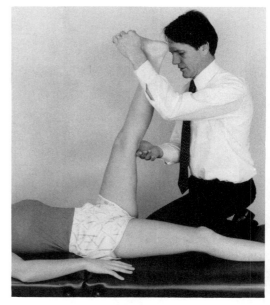

Figure 18.18.   Muscle functional excursion.

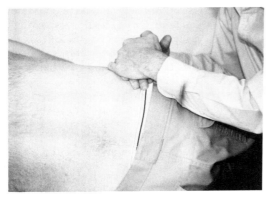

Figure 18.19. Performance of PNF pelvic patterns.

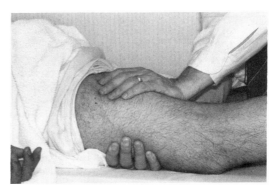

Figure 18.20. Three-dimensional evaluation.

Proprioceptive Neuromuscular Facilitation Pattern

Through PNF one can identify inherent patterns limiting tissue tension. Because of the dynamic spiral nature of PNF patterns, many of the soft tissue restrictions that limit function can be identified (Fig. 18.21). When those patterns of restriction are corrected, the PNF patterns that were previously restrictive should be performed to reeducate movement within the new available range (72, 77).

Associated Oscillations

Associated oscillations are rhythmical oscillatory motions that are manually applied at a rate that will set up a wave action in the soft tissues of the body part being evaluated. The therapist evaluates the ease of motion, the patient's ability to relax, and the independent mobility and play of the soft tissues (10, 11).

TREATMENT

Evaluation and treatment must be interrelated for application of soft tissue mobilization to be effective. Treatment is based upon objective measures such as signs, symptoms, and the mechanical behavior of the spine (8, 89). The success of treatment is also dependent upon the active involvement of the patient with the process through conscious relaxation and appropriate feedback.

Approaches to Soft Tissue Mobilization

There are two general approaches to soft tissue mobilization from which one can evaluate and treat a lumbar patient: localized and biomechanical (11). The *localized approach* focuses primarily upon the painful region, treating the symptomatic structures and dysfunctions within the same local area. The *biomechanical approach* focuses upon improving postural alignment and mobility of related regions of the kinematic chain to reduce the stress upon the symptomatic lumbar region. Observational evaluation and the utilization of functional movement patterns and functional activity

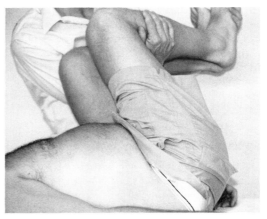

Figure 18.21. PNF lower trunk extension pattern.

evaluations will assist in identifying these related soft tissue dysfunctions. A condition in which the biomechanical approach to a load-sensitive lumbar problem (90) would be useful is tightness and restricted play of a pectoralis minor. This dysfunction usually causes a protraction of the shoulder girdle, limiting its ability to be seated (like a yoke) and centered upon the convexity of the rib cage. This posture affects the normal arthrokinematics of the shoulder girdle and may possibly precipitate an impingement syndrome. There are two potential biomechanical compensations that can result from this dysfunction.

1. The shoulder girdle and arm are positioned anterior to the lateral midline, thus shifting the center of gravity of the upper body asymmetrically anterior of the vertical axis. Most people compensate for this structural limitation by backward bending of the thoracic cage from the thoracolumbar junction or the lumbar spine. This backward bending alters the vertical alignment, accentuating the lumbar lordosis and increasing the strain upon the posterior elements.

2. During activities that load the upper extremities, the weight is normally distributed through the rib cage into the pelvis and lower extremities. However, with scapular protraction, a greater proportion of the weight must be borne by the cervical and scapular musculature, creating an increased strain both on the cervical and lumbar spine.

These related biomechanical compensatory patterns and restrictions may not be symptomatic, but may affect the function of the lumbar spine leading to faulty posture, poor shock absorption, uneven weight distribution, altered movement patterns, and decreased pliability and mobility of the affected soft tissues. These changes often slow down healing of a related injured tissue as the system is unable to conform or respond to the functional demands, hence increasing the likelihood of exacerbation or reinjury.

Principles of Technique Application

The basic approach of this method of treatment is first to evaluate and treat superficial restrictions and then proceed to those of deeper layers. After assessing and localizing a soft tissue dysfunction, the therapist selects a specific soft tissue mobilization technique and applies the appropriate amount of force specifically in the direction of maximal density and/or restriction. The goal in applying soft tissue techniques is to use the least amount of force to achieve the desired results. It is important to be patient and give the tissues time to respond and to allow both the mechanical and viscoelastic effects to occur. Increased force is only utilized as the last resort when all other options for release have been attempted, or when less mobile tissues such as scar adhesions and contractures are present. These tissues may require more force, the exact amount of force being dependent upon the extent of restriction, the degree of discomfort provoked, and the irritability of the patient's condition.

This work will focus on direct techniques, i.e., those applied directly into the barrier or tissue restriction. However, there are instances where an indirect technique (one that treats in the direction of greatest tissue ease or mobility) is valuable, such as treatment of highly irritable tissues.

During application of a soft tissue technique, improvement in the dysfunction is noted through a palpable normalization in tissue mobility or density. If there is a palpable improvement in the restriction, the objective signs should be reevaluated. However, if the status of the restriction does not improve, another technique is chosen. If there is no change after the application of two techniques, the authors find that, as a general rule, it is necessary to reevaluate the region for an underlying or more remote dysfunction.

Treatment Techniques

Techniques are applied by utilizing one hand to apply pressure upon the restriction, while the other hand assists to facilitate a release. The *treatment hand* can apply pressure through specific (fingers or thumb) or general (heel of hand, elbow, forearm) contacts. The pressure is applied in the direction of the restriction and, as it releases the slack is taken up to keep a consistent pressure upon the resolving restriction. One should note that the direction of the restriction often changes as the release occurs, and appropriate adjustments in direction of force are needed to stay with the pattern of release. An inherent aspect of effective application of soft tissue mobilization techniques is the therapist's utilization of proper body posi-

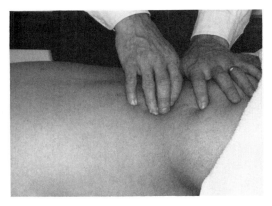

Figure 18.22.   Sustained pressure.

tion and mechanics. The techniques applied by the treatment hand are:

1. Sustained pressure—utilizing a pushing or pulling pressure upon the restriction to improve contractile and noncontractile tissue mobility (Fig. 18.22);
2. Unlocking spiral—sustained pressure with a small amplitude of lateral or rotary motions seeking for the path of least resistance (Fig. 18.23);
3. Direct oscillations—rhythmical repeated end range deformation of a restriction;
4. Perpendicular mobilization—transverse pressure to a muscle belly to improve muscle and soft tissue play (Fig. 18.24);

5. Parallel mobilization—longitudinal pressure to the edge of the muscle belly along the seam between two muscles or along bony contours to improve muscle play and soft tissue mobility (Fig. 18.25);
6. Perpendicular (transverse) strumming—repeated rhythmical deformation of a muscle belly, as one would strum the string of a guitar, to improve muscle play and reduce tone (Fig. 18.26); and
7. Friction massage—repeated cross grain manipulation of soft tissue lesions (1, 41, 80).

The assisting hand facilitates improvement by:

1. Placing tissues on slack—adjusting the surrounding tissues in a shortened range to ease the tension on the restriction (Fig. 18.27);
2. Placing tissues on tension—adjusting the surrounding tissues in a lengthened range to place tension on the restriction (Fig. 18.28);
3. Passive associated oscillations—rhythmic passive oscillations of the body to facilitate relaxation (possibly through the mechanoreceptors; 91); and
4. Manual resistance—to facilitate appropriate contractions and relaxation of the muscles and normalization of the soft tissues being treated.

There are instances where both hands are used together and no distinction is made between the treatment and assisting hands. For example, when performing a three-dimensional technique (which evolves from the three-dimensional evaluation covered under the palpatory

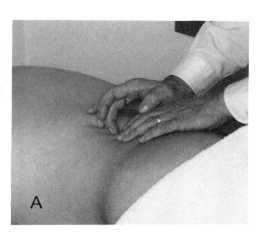

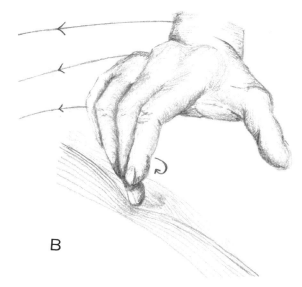

Figure 18.23.   A, B. Unlocking spiral.

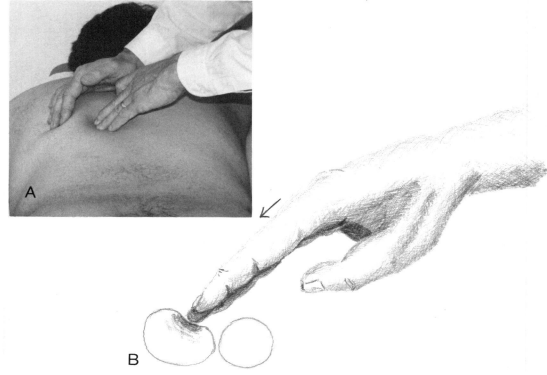

Figure 18.24.   A, B. Perpendicular mobilization.

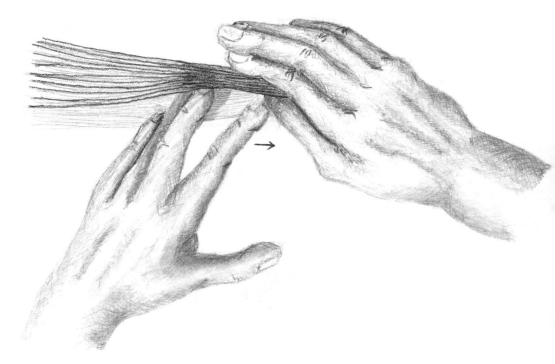

Figure 18.25.   Parallel mobilization.

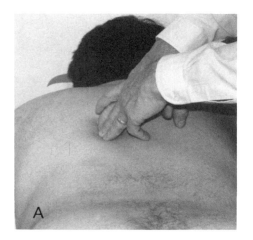

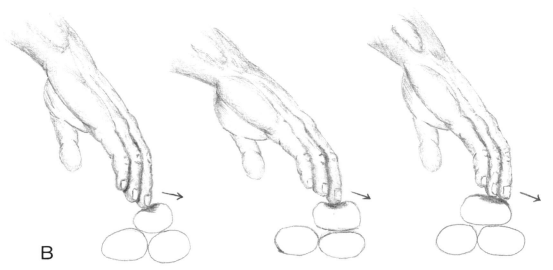

Figure 18.26. **A, B.** Perpendicular (transverse) strumming.

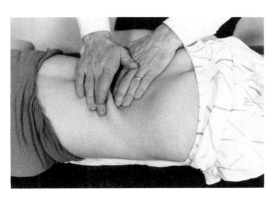

Figure 18.27. Placing tissues on slack with assisting hand.

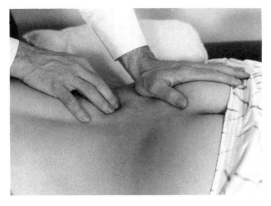

Figure 18.28. Placing tissues on tension with assisting hand.

evaluation section), the two hands function together to improve the mobility of the tissues as an extension of the evaluation process (11, 55, 79).

Treatment appears most effective when the patient is first placed in a comfortable position that allows for the greatest accessibility of the affected tissues, while at the same time promoting the neutral position of the transitional junctions of the vertebral column. Treatment techniques can be performed while the patient attempts to soften or relax the region being treated, or performs small active oscillations, active physiological and/or active functional movement patterns.

In our clinical experience, we have noted that dysfunctions related to scar tissue, decreased muscle play, or fascial tightness generally maintain the improvements following treatment (Fig. 18.29). However, dysfunctions related to hypertonus and swelling and those of a neuroreflexive nature may return with time. A primary factor in the long-term effectiveness of treatment will be training the patient to minimize stressful postures and movements.

As noncontractile and contractile soft tissues regain their normal state of free and independent mobility, decreased tone, and normal physiological lengths, the individual can assume a more efficient alignment and move with greater ease and coordination. New postures and ranges of motion should be reinforced through application of resisted neuromuscular reeducation techniques (72, 77) and emphasis should be placed upon a specific training and rehabilitation program (8, 76).

CLINICAL CORRELATIONS

This overview of clinical correlations is intended to assist the reader in understanding the relevance of soft tissue mobilization to the overall management of a patient, and to illuminate the possible interaction of specific soft tissue restrictions with spinal dysfunction. Most of the functional changes reported are correlations made from observations following normalization of soft tissue dysfunctions.

Lumbar Skin and Superficial Fascia

Improvements achieved through correction of skin restrictions are often dramatic in comparison with the subtlety of the restriction. The

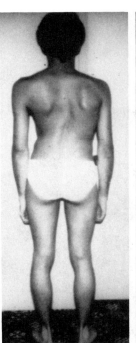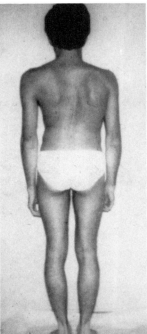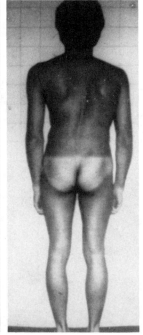

Figure 18.29.   Postural changes following treatment. Initial; after 10 treatments; 1 year after discharge.

most frequently noted functional improvements (increased range of physiological and functional motion, improvement in alignment, segmental spinal mobility, and reduced symptoms) are often noted following the treatment of cutaneous adherences (10, 54).

Lumbar Muscles and Thoracolumbar Fascia

The lumbar muscles (Fig. 18.30) can be divided into three groups and layers (30):

- the short intersegmental muscles—the interspinales and the intertransversarii,
- the polysegmental muscles—the multifidus, rotories, and the lumbar components of longissimus, spinalis, and iliocostalis, and
- the long polysegmental muscles—represented by the thoracic components of longissimus and iliocostalis lumborum that span the lumbar region from thoracic levels to the ilium and sacrum.

The deeper intersegmental and polysegmental muscles, particularly the multifidi, are primarily stabilizers controlling posture and assisting in fine adjustments and segmental movement (4, 14, 22, 92). The multifidus is also believed to protect the facet capsule from being impinged during joint movements because of its attachments to the joint capsule (30). Kirkaldy-Willis reports that uncontrolled contraction of the multifidus may be a primary factor in the production of torsional injury to the facet joints and disc (4). The erector spinae, with the longissimus, spinalis, and iliocostalis, produce the grosser motions of thoracic and pelvic backward bending, sidebending, and rotation that increase the lumbar lordosis (4, 22, 92). Some authors have reported that the erector spinae is active in maintaining upright posture (92).

The extensive thoracolumbar fascia attaches to the transverse processes of the lumbar vertebrae, the iliac crest and iliolumbar ligament, the twelfth rib, the quadratus lumborum, the lateral portion of the psoas major, and the aponeurotic origin of the transversus abdominis (22, 93). Each individual layer of lumbar musculature is separated and compartmentalized by the thoracolumbar fascia and, in an efficient state, can be palpated to have independent mobility from surrounding structures by sliding over them during normal trunk movements. The lumbar musculature is most effectively assessed in the side-lying and prone positions. Its extensibility is most effectively appraised through evaluation of end ranges of PNF trunk patterns.

Restricted play of the erector spinae can limit range of motion of the lumbar spine because of the inability of the muscles to slide normally upon each other. This is especially noted with the motions of side gliding (lateral shear), forward bending, and rotation. When muscles are in a state of increased tone or restricted play, they may have difficulty folding on each other and will restrict motions such as side bending to the same side and backward bending.

Increased tone of the deeper musculature can be the primary source of symptoms and can limit mobility of individual segments. With unilateral soft tissue dysfunction there will often be a deviation to the affected side during forward bending. In conjunction with the improvement of alignment, range of motion, and pain, a patient's ability to better control active movement is often observed following treatment.

When the more lateral intertransversarii lateralis and quadratus lumborum have limited extensibility, the region will often appear shortened and will be restricted in motions such as sidebending and pelvic lateral shear (sidegliding). The quadratus lumborum will often have restricted normal play relative to the erector spinae and psoas, affecting most spinal motions.

Abdominal Scar

Scar tissue in the abdominal region often has far-reaching effects on the function of the lumbar spine, from the restricted mobility of the skin to the deeper layers of scar tissue. Through careful palpation, spider web-like strands of restricted tissue can be traced extending away from the central scar, possibly extending throughout the abdominal cavity and to the posterior wall. If the palpation is performed with superimposed movement (such as a functional movement pattern or PNF pattern), the effects of these limitations and the altered biomechanics can be noted. This restricted matrix can affect proper alignment and functional movements such as forward bending (possibly due to the abdominal tissues' inability to fold upon themselves) and backward bending sec-

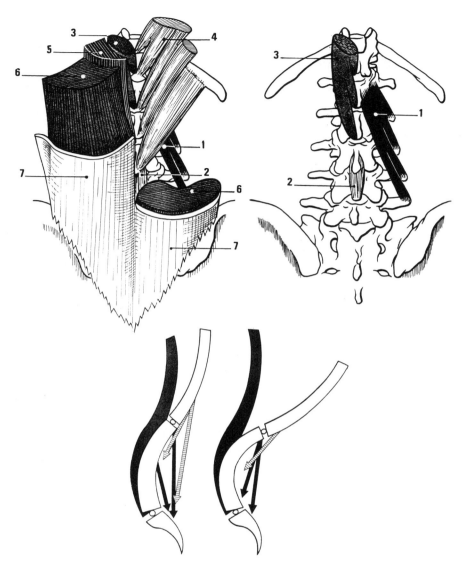

Figure 18.30. Lumbar musculature. *1.* The transversospinalis, *2.* the interspinalis muscles, *3.* the spinalis muscle, *4.* serratus posterior inferior, *5.* the longissimus, *6.* the iliocostalis, *7.* aponeurosis of the latissimus dorsi. (Reproduced with permission from Kapandji AI. The physiology of the joints, Vol. 3. Edinburgh: Churchill Livingstone, 1974.)

ondary to decreased extensibility of the anterior section.

In patients with hypermobilities or spondylolisthesis, dramatic improvement in functional abilities with reduced symptoms has been observed through normalization of abdominal scar. Improvement is often noted in static postures and in the performance of functional movement patterns such as the pelvic clock and lower trunk rotation. Through appropriate soft tissue mobilization, the scar tissue may become more pliable, but the primary effect appears to be improved mobility of the surrounding structures and of the restricted spider web-like matrix. This probably facilitates a more neutral position of the lumbar spine and allows movement to be distributed through the spine into the pelvis more efficiently.

Rectus Abdominis

The rectus abdominis originates primarily from the costal cartilage of the fifth, sixth, and seventh ribs and inserts on the crest of the pubis. It is enclosed between the aponeuroses of the obliqui and transversus forming the rectus sheath that separates it from the other abdominals (22). If the rectus adheres to the underlying structures, motions such as rotation and pelvic lateral shearing are restricted because of the inability of the rectus abdominis to slide over the underlying abdominals. The umbilicus should also be evaluated for free three-dimensional mobility, as restrictions will also affect the mobility of the rectus abdominis.

The rectus abdominis will often be found to be in a shortened state that holds the rib cage down, increasing a forward head posture and thoracic kyphosis. There is often a compensatory backward bending of the thoracic cage, increasing thoracolumbar or mid-lumbar lordosis. We often find shortened rectus abdominis muscles in individuals who do many sit-ups in a flexed position.

Psoas and Iliacus Muscles

The psoas arises from the anterior surfaces and lower borders of the transverse processes of the twelfth thoracic and all of the lumbar vertebrae, creating a muscle with multiple distinct layers (Fig. 18.31). At each segmental level it is attached to the margin of each vertebral body, the adjacent disc and the fibrous arch that connects the upper and lower aspect of the lumbar vertebral body (22, 30). The iliacus originates primarily from the superior two-thirds of the concavity of the iliac fossa and the upper surface of the lateral part of the sacrum, and most of the fibers converge into the lateral side of the psoas tendon (22). The psoas and iliacus are covered with the iliac fascia, which attaches to the intervertebral discs, the margins of the vertebral bodies, and the upper part of the sacrum, and are continuous with the inguinal ligament and the transversalis fascia. The iliopsoas flexes the femur upon the pelvis, or flexes the trunk and pelvis upon the lower extremities. Some authors attribute a distinct postural component to the deeper spinal fibers of the psoas (92).

The iliopsoas muscles are often found to have limited extensibility and play or increased tone at the level of spinal pathology (3, 35, 68,

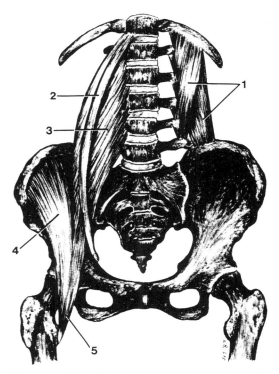

Figure 18.31. Muscles of the anterior spinal column. The intrinsic flexors of the lumbar spine: *1.* two layers of quadratus lumborum, *2.* psoas minor, *3.* psoas major, *4.* iliacus, *5.* conjoined attachment of psoas and iliacus of and around the lesser femoral trochanter. (Reproduced with permission from Dupuis PR, Kirkaldy-Willis WH. The spine: integrated function and pathophysiology. In Cruess RL, Rennie WRJ, eds. Adult orthopaedics. New York: Churchill Livingstone, 1984.)

94). Because of its centralized biomechanical position, minor dysfunction of the psoas can have a dramatic effect upon posture and the length of the lumbar region, and can place excessive stress upon the intervertebral discs and the performance of functional motions (94, 95). Restricted extensibility limits the posterior tilt of the pelvis, which increases lumbar lordosis. Such restrictions can decrease movement in all directions, especially limiting backward and forward bending. The function of the psoas is often altered by dysfunctions in the lower extremities, especially if the dysfunction is unilateral, thus altering the dynamics and the capacity for the two psoas muscles to act symmetrically during spinal function.

Through clinical experience it has been observed that with improved length, play and normalized tone of the psoas, there often results an increase in forward bending of the lumbar spine. This improved mobility is possibly due to the ability of the psoas to fold upon itself and the ability of the transverse processes, which are posterior to the central axis of motion, to separate from each other to allow the spine to bow convexly posteriorly. It has also been noticed that restricted play of a psoas at a specific level can limit mobility of that segment, specifically affecting rotation and sidebending to the opposite side. Often pressure applied to the localized foci of tone will cause referred pain which duplicates the reported symptoms (Fig. 18.32). In many cases normalization of psoas mobility and improved neuromuscular control have facilitated dramatic changes in symptoms and function.

Lower Extremities and Hip

Limited mobility of the myofascial structures of the lower extremities is a primary contributing factor that forces an individual to use the lumbar spine instead of the lower extremities as a primary axis of motion. Several authors have suggested a correlation between poor flexibility of the lower extremities and lumbar symptoms (94, 95). Also, myofascial tightness of the lower extremities may cause a decrease in blood and lymph flow that contributes to restricted mobility, fluid stasis, and greater muscular fatigability.

Of primary importance are dysfunctions that affect extensibility and normal play of the hip rotators, hamstrings, rectus femoris, iliotibial band, adductors, and gastroc-soleus (triceps surae).

Hip Rotators. Restricted play and decreased extensibility of these closely interrelated muscles limits hip mobility and affects pelvic motion and coordination for performance of forward oriented tasks. The ability to rotate the body through the hips over a fixed base of support while maintaining a stable lumbar spine is affected when there is limited extensibility and play of the hip rotators.

Hamstrings. Shortened hamstrings limit pelvic anterior tilt and, therefore, restrict a patient's ability to maintain a neutral spine while bending forward in standing and sitting. Restricted play between the three bellies can cause abnormal torsion on the ilium and affect the eccentric control of lower extremity and pelvic motions.

Rectus Femoris. Decreased flexibility of the rectus femoris restricts the ability of the pelvis to tilt posteriorly upon the head of the femur, often limiting the individual's ability to assume a neutral lumbar position in standing. Restricted mobility of the rectus femoris in relation to sartorius, tensor fascia lata, and the underlying quadriceps affects performance of each muscle's independent actions. Soft tissue restrictions within and around the rectus femoris can also limit hip extension during gait and result in compensatory backward bending in the lumbar spine.

Iliotibial Band. The iliotibial band is an important lateral stabilizer and helps maintain posture during gait (93). Limited mobility of the iliotibial band is probably a major contributor to lumbar immobility and pain (35). Tightness often affects a person's ability to shift weight over the base of support (because of lateral tightness) and to perform any lateral motions. In cases of sacroiliac hypermobility, limited extensibility of the iliotibial band is often seen on the side of hypermobility.

Adductors. As with the iliotibial band, adductor tightness and limited play affect pelvic position, mobility, and the dynamics of lateral movements.

Gastroc-Soleus. When the soleus is shortened, the heel will lift off the ground, decreasing the base of support and impairing balance during bending and lifting activities. This may further contribute to rear-foot deformities such as calcaneal valgus that may cause aberrant lower quadrant function. Ankle coordination can be

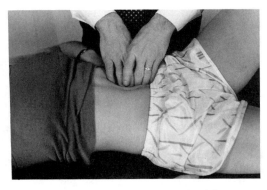

Figure 18.32. Palpation of the body of the psoas.

affected by restricted play between the bellies of the gastroc and soleus and also between the soleus and the deeper toe flexors and posterior tibialis.

SUMMARY

The soft tissues of the body can often be found to be in an inefficient state of mobility and tone, which causes, precipitates, and perpetuates many symptoms of the lumbar spine. Soft tissue mobilization can play a valuable role in the treatment of these soft tissue dysfunctions. Soft tissue mobilization will achieve the optimal results desired when used in conjunction with patient education, body mechanics training, a musculoskeletal conditioning program, and other manual therapy approaches (joint mobilization and neuromuscular education). A well-rounded and comprehensive conservative care program is required in the effort to return a patient to optimal potential while avoiding such nonconservative methods of management as surgical intervention.

Acknowledgments

The authors wish to sincerely thank many of their professional associates for their assistance and guidance in completing this chapter. These include Scott Hubert, MS, PT; Jeffrey Ellis, PT; Larry Elson, PhD; Brian Miller, PT; Brian Hauswirth, PT; Jeni Hartmann, OTR; Linda Little, PT; Sandra Eastburn; and John Palmer, PT; and Bob Steinfield for his creative artistic interpretations. In addition, great appreciation and gratitude is given to Erica Liebman for her complete dedication and invaluable assistance throughout the duration of this project. Without Erica, this chapter most likely could not have been completed.

References

1. Cyriax J. Textbook of orthopaedic medicine: Diagnosis of soft tissue lesions, ed. 8. Baltimore: Williams & Wilkins, 1984.
2. Dvorak J, Dvorak V. Manual medicine: Diagnostics. Stuttgart: Thieme-Stratton, 1984.
3. Grieve GP. Common vertebral joint problems. London: Churchill Livingstone, 1981.
4. Kirkaldy-Willis WH. Managing low back pain. 2nd ed. New York: Churchill Livingstone, 1988.
5. White AH, Ruthman RH, Ray CD, eds. Lumbar spine surgery: Techniques and complications. St. Louis: CV Mosby, 1987.
6. Fisk JR, Dimonte P, Courington SMcK. Back schools, past, present and future. Clin Orthop 1983; 179.
7. Mooney V, Cairnes D. Management in the patient with chronic low back pain. Orthop Clin North Am 1978; 9:543.
8. Morgan D. Concepts in functional training and postural stabilization for the low-back-injured. Top Acute Care Trauma Rehabil 1988; 2(4):8–17.
9. Saal JA. Rehabilitation of sports-related lumbar spine injuries. Phys Med Rehab, State of the Art Reviews 1987; a(4):613–638.
10. Johnson GS, Saliba VL. Functional orthopedics I, course outline. The Institute of Physical Art, San Anselmo, CA, 1989.
11. Johnson GS, Saliba VL. Functional Orthopedics II, course outline. The Institute of Physical Art, San Anselmo, CA, 1990.
12. Gray H. Anatomy of the human body. Philadelphia: Lea and Febiger, 1966.
13. Ham A, Cormack D. Histology. Philadelphia: JB Lippincott, 1979.
14. Hollinshead WH. Functional anatomy of the limbs and back. (A text for students of the locomotor apparatus). Philadelphia: WB Saunders, 1976.
15. Cummings GS, Crutchfield CA, Barnes MR. Orthopedic physical therapy series: Vol. 1. Soft tissue changes in contractures. Atlanta: Strokesville, 1983.
16. Kendall HO, Kendall FP, Boynton DA. Posture and pain. Huntington, NY: Robert E. Krieger, 1977.
17. Travell JG, Simons DG. Myofascial pain and dysfunction: The trigger point manual. Baltimore: Williams & Wilkins, 1983.
18. Woo SL-Y, Buckwalter JA. Injury and repair of the musculoskeletal soft tissues. Park Ridge, IL: American Academy of Orthopedic Surgeons, 1988.
19. Cailliet R. Soft tissue pain and disability. Philadelphia: FA Davis, 1977.
20. Farfan HF. Mechanical factors in the genesis of low back pain. In Bonica JJ, et al. eds. Advances in pain research and therapy, Vol 3. New York: Raven Press, 1979.
21. Wadsworth CT. Manual examination and treatment of the spine and extremities. Baltimore: Williams & Wilkins, 1988.
22. Warwick R, Williams PL. eds. Gray's anatomy. 35th Br ed. Philadelphia: WB Saunders Co, 1973.
23. Akeson W. Wolff's law of connective tissue—The effects of stress deprivation on synovial joints. Unpublished.
24. Krause WJ, Cutts HJ. Concise text of histology. Baltimore: Williams & Wilkins, 1986.
25. Nikolaou PK, MacDonald BL, Glisson RR et al. Biomechanical and histological evaluation of muscle after controlled strain injury. Am J Sports Med 1987; 15:9–14.

26. Bunting CH, Eades C. Effects of mechanical tension on the plarity of growing fibroblasts. J Exp Med 1926; 44:147.

27. Frankle VH, Nordin M. Basic biomechanics of the skeletal system. Philadelphia: Lea & Febiger, 1980.

28. Tipton CM, Matthes RD, Maynard JA et al. The influence of physical activity on ligaments and tendons. Med Sci Sports 1975; 7:165.

29. Nimni ME. Collagen: Structure, function, and metabolism in normal and fibrotic tissue. Semin Arthritis Rheum 1983; 13:1–86.

30. Bogduk N, Twomey LT. Clinical anatomy of the lumbar spine. New York: Churchill Livingstone, 1987.

31. Gratz CM. Air injection of the fascial spaces. Am J Roentgenol 1936; 35:750–751.

32. Donatelli R, Owens-Burkart H. Effects of immobilization on the extensibility of periarticular connective tissue. J Orthop Sports Phys Ther 1981; 3(2):67.

33. Swann DA, Radin EL, Nazimiec M. Role of hyaluronic acid in joint lubrication. Ann Rheum Dis 1974; 33:318.

34. Mennell JM. Joint pain. Boston: Little, Brown & Company, 1964; 6.

35. Mennell JB. The science and art of joint manipulation. Vol. 2. London: Churchill, 1952.

36. Forrest L. Current concepts in soft tissue connective tissue wound healing. Br J Surg 1983; 70:133–140.

37. Woo S, Matthews JV, Akeson WH, Amiel D, Convery R. Connective tissue response to immobility: Correlative study of biomechanical and biochemical measurements of normal and immobilized rabbit knees. Arthr Rheum 1975; 18:257–264.

38. Arem JA, Madden JW. Effects of stress on healing wounds: I. Intermittent noncyclical tension. J Surg Reas 1976; 20:93.

39. Peacock E, VanWinkle W. Wound repair. 2nd ed. Philadelphia: WB Saunders, 1976.

40. Malone TR. Muscle injury and rehabilitation. Baltimore: Williams & Wilkins, 1988.

41. Palastanga N. The use of transverse frictions for soft tissue lesions. In Grieve G, ed. Modern manual therapy of the vertebral column. London: Churchill Livingstone, 1986; 819–825.

42. Ganong A. Textbook of medical physiology. 3rd ed. Philadelphia: WB Saunders, 1968; 833.

43. Lowenthal M, Tobis JS. Contracture in chronic neurological disease. Arch Phys Med 1957; 38:640.

44. Akeson WH, Amiel D, Woo SL-Y. Immobility effects on synovial joint: The pathomechanics of joint contracture. Biorheology 1980; 17:95–110.

45. Amiel D et al. Effects of nine weeks' immobilization of the types of collagen synthesized in periarticular connective tissue from rabbit knees. Trans Orth Res Soc 1980; 5:162–165.

46. Noyes F. Functional properties of knee ligaments and alteration induced by immobilization: A correlative biomechanical and histological study in primates. Clin Orthop 1977; 123:210–42.

47. Peacock E. Comparison of collagenous tissue surrounding normal and immobilized joints. Surg Forum 1963; 14:440.

48. Akeson W. Value of 17-B-oestradiol in prevention of contracture formation. Ann Them Dis 1976; 35:429.

49. Amiel D, Frey C, Woo SL-Y, Horwook F, Akeson WH. Value of hyaluronic acid in the prevention of contracture formation. Clin Orthop 1985; 196:306–311.

50. Woo SL-Y, Gomez MA, Woo YK, Akeson WH. Mechanical properties of tendons and ligaments: The relationships of immobilization and exercise on tissue remodeling. Biorheology 1982; 19:397–408.

51. Meyer K. Nature and function of mucopolysaccharides in connective tissue. Mol Biol 1960; 69–75.

52. Enneking W, Horowitz M. The intra-articular effects of immobilization on the human knee. J Bone Joint Surg 1972; 54A:973–985.

53. Cottingham JT, Porges SW, Richmond K. Shifts in pelvic inclination angle and parasympathetic tone produced by Rolfing soft tissue manipulation. Phys Ther 1988; 68(9):1364–1370.

54. Dicke E, Shliack H, Wolff A. A manual of reflexive therapy of the connective tissue (connective tissue massage) "Bindegewebsmassage." Scarsdale, NY: Sidney S. Simone, 1978.

55. Fabian P. Myofascial Strategies I. Course outline. San Anselmo, CA: The Institute of Physical Art 1988; 8.

56. Korr IM. The collected papers. Colorado Springs, CO: American Academy of Osteopathy, 1979.

57. Levine P. Stress. In Coles MGH et al. eds. Psychophysiology: Systems, processes, and applications. New York: Guilford Press, 1986; 331–353.

58. Ward RC. The myofascial release concept. Course manual—Tutorial on level 1 myofascial release technique. Michigan State University, College of Osteopathic Medicine Sept. 18–29, 1987.

59. Basmajian JV. Grant's method of anatomy. 9th ed. Baltimore: Williams & Wilkins, 1975.

60. Korr IM. The neurobiologic mechanisms in manipulative therapy. New York: Plenum Press, 1978.

61. Stoddard A. Manual of osteopathic practice. London: Hutchinson & Co., 1959.

62. Jull GA. Examination of the lumbar spine. In Grieve G, ed. Modern manual therapy of the vertebral column. London: Churchill Livingstone, 1986; 547–558.

63. Sapega A, Quedenfeld T, Moyer R, Butler R. Biophysical factors in range-of-motion exercise. Physician Sportmed 1981; 9:57–65.

64. Hill A. The mechanics of active muscle. Proc Roy Soc Lond 1953; 141(B):104–117.

65. Komi PV. Training of muscle strength and power: Interaction of neuromotoric, hypertrophic and mechanical factors. Int J Sports Med 1986; 7:10–15.

66. Locker LH, League NG. Histology of highly-stretched beef muscle: The fine structure of grossly stretched single fibers. J Ultrastruct 1975; 52:64–75.

67. Engles M. Tissue response. In Donatelli R, Wooden M, eds. Orthopaedic physical therapy. New York: Churchill Livingstone, 1989.

68. Janda V. Muscle weakness and inhibition (pseudoparesis) in back pain syndromes. In Grieve G, ed. Modern manual therapy of the vertebral column. London: Churchill Livingstone, 1986.

69. Kirkaldy-Willis WH, Hill RJ. A more precise diagnosis for low back pain. Spine 1979; 4:102.

70. Sahrmann SA. Course notes—Diagnosis and treatment of muscle imbalances associated with musculoskeletal pain. Dec. 6, 7, 1988, Bay Shore, NY.

71. Feldenkrais M. Awareness through movement. New York: Harper & Row, 1977.

72. Knott M, Voss DE. Proprioceptive neuromuscular facilitation. 2nd ed. New York: Harper and Row, 1968.

73. Lewit K. The contribution of clinical observation to neurological mechanisms in manipulative therapy. In Korr I, ed. The neurobiologic mechanisms in manipulative therapy. London: Plenum Press, 1978; 3–25.

74. Jowett RL, Fidler MW. Histochemical changes in the multifidus in the mechanical derangements of the spine. Orthop Clin North Am 1975; 6:145.

75. Gossmand MR, Sahrmann SA, Rose, SJ. Review of length-associated changes in muscle. Phys Ther 1982; 62(12):1799–1808.

76. Johnson GS, Saliba VL. Back education and training, course outline. The Institute of Physical Art, San Anselmo, CA, 1988.

77. Johnson GS, Saliba VL. PNFI: The functional approach to movement reeducation. Course outline. The Institute of Physical Art, San Anselmo, CA, 1987.

78. Tardieu C, Tarbary J, Tardieu G, et al. Adaptation of sarcomere numbers to the length imposed on muscle. In Gubba F, Marecahl G, Takacs O, eds. Mechanism of muscle adaptation to functional requirements. Elmsford, NY: Pergamon Press, 1981.

79. Aston J. Aston patterning, The Aston Training Center, Mill Valley, CA.

80. Cyriax J, Cyriax P. Illustrated manual of orthopaedic medicine. Bourough Green, England: Butterworths, 1983.

81. Jull G, Janda V. Muscles and motor control in low back pain: Assessment and management. In Twomey LT, Taylor JR. Physical therapy of the low back. New York: Churchill Livingstone, 1987.

82. Todd ME. The thinking body: A study of the balancing forces of dynamic man. Brooklyn, NY: Dance Horizons, 1937.

83. Paris S. S-1 Course notes. Institute for Graduate Health Sciences, Atlanta, GA, 1977; 3.

84. Miller B. Learning the touch. Phys Ther Forum Western ed., Wed. September 16, 1987.

85. Montagu A. Touching: The human significance of skin. 2nd ed. New York: Harper & Row, 1978.

86. Scott-Charlton W, Roebuck DJ. The significance of posterior primary divisions of spinal nerves in pain syndromes. Med J Aust 1972; 2:945.

87. O'Brien J. Anterior spinal tenderness in low back pain syndromes. Spine 1979; 4:85.

88. Evjenth O, Hamberg J. Muscle stretching in manual therapy: A clinical manual. Alfta, Sweden: Alfta Rehab Forlag, 1985.

89. Maitland GD. Vertebral manipulation. 5th ed. London: Butterworths, 1986.

90. Vollowitz E. Furniture prescription for the conservative management of low-back pain. Top Acute Care Trauma Rehabil 1988; 2(4):18–37.

91. Wyke B. The neurology of joints. Ann Roy Coll Surg 1967; 41:25–50.

92. Basmajian JV. Muscles alive: Their functions revealed by electromyography. Baltimore: Williams & Wilkins, 1978.

93. Donatelli R, Walker R. Lower quarter evaluation: Structural relationships and interdependence. In Donatelli R, Wooden M, eds. Orthopaedic physical therapy. New York: Churchill Livingstone, 1989.

94. Saal JS. Flexibility training. Phys Med Rehab 1987; 1(4):537–554.

95. Farfan H, Gracovetsky S. The optimum spine. Spine 1986; 11(6):543–573.

19

OSTEOPATHIC MANIPULATION OF THE LUMBAR SPINE AND PELVIS

Philip E. Greenman

Manipulation has been a component of the practice of osteopathic medicine since the founding of the profession in 1892. Manipulation is used within the context of comprehensive patient care and is based upon the application of osteopathic philosophy and principles that 1) the body is a unit; 2) the body possesses self-regulating mechanisms; 3) structure and function are reciprocally interrelated; and 4) rational therapy is based upon an understanding of body unity, self-regulating mechanisms, and the interrelationship of structure and function. As a total school of medicine, osteopathic physicians include medical and surgical procedures in addition to manipulation as appropriate for the patient's condition.

LOW BACK PAIN

In patients with complaints of low back pain, with or without radiation to the lower extremities, 60 to 80% are classified as idiopathic and challenge the practitioner to evaluate the pateint adequately and determine a rational treatment plan. The diagnostic process includes a comprehensive history and physical examination. In addition to the standard orthopedic and neurological tests for patients with low back and leg pain, the osteopathic practitioner includes structural diagnosis to identify the presence of somatic dysfunction and its significance in the patient's presentation. It is important to look for the presence of inflammatory, infectious, metabolic, and primary or secondary ma-

lignant disease of the musculoskeletal system. Pathology that requires surgical intervention, such as progressive neurological deficit and the cauda equina syndrome, must be identified if present. Appropriate diagnostic assessment including adequate radiographic imaging, electrodiagnosis, and laboratory testing, is made to identify the anatomical and physiological capacity present. For the structural diagnostic process to be effective, the examiner needs to know how the anatomy is altered by development, previous trauma, and surgical interventions.

Structural Diagnosis

The osteopathic physician uses structural diagnosis to identify somatic dysfunction, which is defined as impaired or altered function of the related components of the somatic (bony framework) system: skeletal, arthrodial, and myofascial structures, and related vascular, lymphatic and neural elements. Somatic dysfunction is the codable diagnosis for the manipulable lesion. The diagnostic triad for somatic dysfunction is:

A, asymmetry of form and function,
R, range of motion alteration, primarily hypomobility,
T, tissue texture abnormality.

The diagnostic process comprises three stages: a screening examination, a scanning examination, and finally, the segmental definition. The screening examination identifies the presence of functional alteration of the musculoskeletal system that may be significant in the patient's presentation. The scanning examination then proceeds to identify the area deemed to be significant. This is followed by segmental definition, which defines the specific manipulable lesion that needs intervention.

The screening examination begins by observation of the gait with particular interest in the function of the lumbar spine and pelvis during the walking cycle. Evaluation of the static posture is made to identify the level of the iliac crest (Fig. 19.1**A**) and greater trochanter (Fig. 19.1**B**) that may indicate anatomical shortening of the lower extremity or a pelvic tilt syndrome due to asymmetrical development of the pelvis. Motion is introduced by instructing the patient to sidebend the trunk to the left (Fig. 19.2**A**) and to the right (Fig. 19.2**B**) and is measured by the excursion of the fingertip down the lateral side of the leg. Observation is made of the participation of the lumbar spine in sidebending to one side and rotation to the opposite. Absence of symmetrical sidebending lumbar mechanics is evidence of significant somatic dysfunction. The standing and seated flexion tests are used to identify the presence or absence of significant restriction of the sacroiliac joints, and to observe the related function of the lumbar spine. The flexion tests are performed by placing the thumbs on the inferior aspect of

the posterior and superior iliac spines (PSIS; Fig. 19.3**A**) and following their movement through a forward bending movement by the patient (Fig. 19.3**B**). The PSIS that moves more cephalicly and ventrally is deemed positive and identifies restriction of pelvic motion on that side. Observation is made of the behavior of the lumbar spine during forward bending (Fig. 19.4), particularly looking for the introduction of lateral curvatures, lumbar dysrhythmia, and the behavior of the lumbar lordosis. Possible restriction of motion within the sacroiliac region, and abnormality of function of the lumbar spine, need to be further evaluated by detailed examination.

Diagnosis of Sacroiliac Dysfunction

The significance of movement restriction of the sacroiliac joints continues to be controversial. Research in humans and animals, both in vivo and cadaveric, has identified the presence of a small amount of movement within the sacroiliac joints. Clinical experience has shown that restriction of sacroiliac motion appears to be highly significant in patients with low back and lower extremity pain. The standing and flexion tests are highly sensitive for restriction within the osseous pelvis and need to be confirmed by other motion tests including the one-legged stork test of Gillet, spring tests, four-point respiratory testing, and gapping testing. Tissue

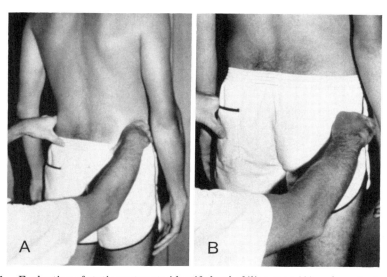

Figure 19.1.   Evaluation of static posture to identify level of iliac crest (**A**) and greater trochanter (**B**).

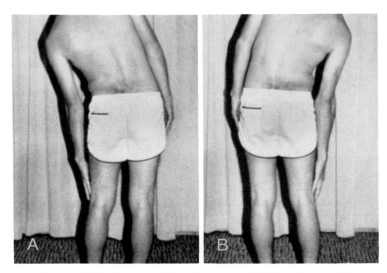

Figure 19.2.   Patient sidebends trunk to left (**A**) and right (**B**).

texture abnormality is evaluated by palpation of the iliolumbar ligament and the posterior sacroiliac ligaments over the upper and lower poles. The sacrotuberous ligaments are palpated at their superior attachment at the inferior lateral angle of the sacrum and the inferior attachment at the ischial tuberosity. Palpation of the lumbar, gluteal, and hip muscles is made to identify the presence of hypertonicity and trigger points, which are commonly related to significant sacroiliac motion restriction.

Palpation is made of paired anatomical structures, looking for the presence of symmetry or asymmetry:

Pubic tubercles and inguinal ligaments,
Medial malleoli,
Ischial tuberosities,
Sacrotuberous ligaments,
Inferior lateral angle of the sacrum,
Posterior superior iliac spine,
Sacral base (sacral sulcus),
Anterior superior iliac spine.

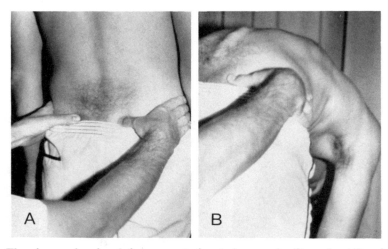

Figure 19.3.   Thumbs are placed on inferior aspect of posterior-superior iliac spine (**A**) and follow through a forward bending movement (**B**).

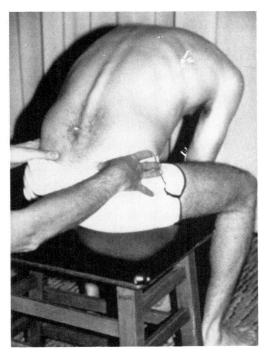

Figure 19.4. Observation of lumbar spine during forward bending.

Combinations of motion restriction, tissue texture abnormality, and asymmetry of the paired landmarks identify one or more of 14 possible somatic dysfunctions within the pelvis.

The criteria for dysfunctions of the symphysis pubis are found in Table 19.1; for dysfunctions of the sacrum between the two innominates (sacroiliac dysfunction) in Table 19.2; and for dysfunctions of one ilium on one side of the sacrum (iliosacral dysfunction) in Table 19.3.

Diagnosis of Lumbar Dysfunction

The lumbar spine is evaluated in the three positions of neutral (Fig. 19.5A), full forward bending (Fig. 19.5B), and full backward bending (Fig. 19.5C). Palpation through the skin, subcutaneous fascia, and musculature looks for tissue texture abnormality overlying the five lumbar segments. The examiner palpates the right and left transverse process of each of the lumbar segments in the three positions. Interpretation of the relative position of the right to left transverse processes allows the examiner to interpret three different motion restrictions within the lumbar spine amenable to manipulation therapy. Two dysfunctions involving a single vertebral motion segment, termed nonneutral (Type II) dysfunctions, have the following characteristics:

1. A single vertebral motion segment involved (two vertebrae and the intervening structures).
2. A flexion or extension restriction present.
3. Restriction of sidebending and rotation to the same side.

Dysfunctions of three or more lumbar vertebrae are termed group dysfunctions. They are also identified as neutral (Type I) dysfunctions and their characteristics are:

1. Three or more lumbar vertebrae involved.
2. Minimal flexion or extension restriction.
3. Restriction of sidebending and rotation to opposite sides.

With freedom of motion of a superior lumbar vertebra on the inferior, the right and left transverse processes appear to remain symmetrical through forward bending, neutral, and backward bending. The interspinous space should open during forward bending and close during backward bending. If something interferes with the capacity of one facet joint to open (flex), the

Table 19.1.
Pubic Symphysis Dysfunction

		Standing flexion test positive	Pubic tubercle height	Tension and tenderness of inguinal ligament
Superior	Right	Right	Right superior	Right
	Left	Left	Left superior	Left
Inferior	Right	Right	Right inferior	Right
	Left	Left	Left inferior	Left

Table 19.2.
Sacroilial Dysfunctions

Dysfunction	Seated flexion test positive	Base of sacrum	Inferior lateral angle position	Inferior lateral angle motion	Lumbar scoliosis	Lumbar lordosis	Medial malleolus prone
Unilateral Inferior Shear (Flexed) (Flexion)	Left	Anterior left	Inferior left	—	Convex left	Normal to increased	Long left
	Right	Anterior right	Inferior right	—	Convex right	Normal to increased	Long right
Unilateral Superior Shear (Extended) (Extension)	Left	Posterior left	Superior left	—	Convex right	Decreased	Short left
	Right	Posterior right	Superior right	—	Convex left	Decreased	Short right
Anterior Torsion	Right (Left on left)	Anterior right	Posterior Left	Left increased on forward bending	Convex right	Increased	Short left
	Left (Right on right)	Anterior left	Posterior Right	Right increased on forward bending	Convex left	Increased	Short right
Backward Torsion	Right (Right on left)	Posterior right	Posterior right	Right increased on backward bending	Convex left	Reduced	Short right
	Left (Left on right)	Posterior left	Posterior Left	Left increased on backward bending	Convex right	Reduced	Short left
Bilateral Flx	Bilateral	Anterior	Posterior	—	—	Increased	Even
Bilateral Extended	Bilateral	Posterior	Anterior	—	—	Reduced	Even

Table 19.3.
Iliosacral Dysfunctions

		Standing flexion test positive	Anterior superior iliac spine supine	Medial malleolus supine	Posterior superior iliac spine prone	Sacral sulcus prone	Ischial tuberosity prone	Sacrotuberous ligament prone
Anterior Rotated	Right	Right	Inferior right	Long right	Superior right	Shallow right	—	—
	Left	Left	Inferior left	Long left	Superior left	Shallow left	—	—
Posterior Rotated	Right	Right	Superior right	Short right	Inferior right	Deep right	—	—
	Left	Left	Superior left	Short left	Inferior left	Deep left	—	—
Outflare	Right	Right	Lateral right	—	Medial right	Narrow right	—	—
	Left	Left	Lateral left	—	Medial left	Narrow left	—	—
Inflare	Right	Right	Medial right	—	Lateral right	Wide right	—	—
	Left	Left	Medial left	—	Lateral left	Wide left	—	—
Superior Shear (Upslip)	Right	Right	Superior right	Short right	Superior right	—	Superior right	Lax right
	Left	Left	Superior left	Short left	Superior left	—	Superior left	Lax left
Inferior Shear (Downslip)	Right	Right	Inferior right	Long right	Inferior right	—	Inferior right	Tight right
	Left	Left	Inferior left	Long left	Inferior left	—	Inferior left	Tight left

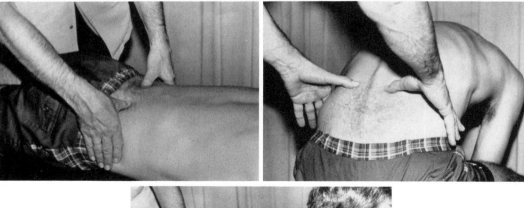

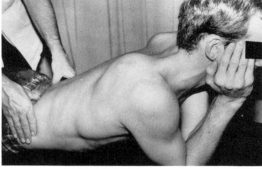

Figure 19.5. Evaluation of lumbar spine in neutral position (**A**), full forward bending (**B**), and full backward bending (**C**).

transverse process on that side appears to become more prominent during full forward bending, and both transverse processes become symmetrical in full backward bending. The motion restriction of the superior vertebra on the inferior is forward bending, sidebending, and rotation to the opposite side of the posterior transverse process. If something interferes with the capacity of one facet to close (extend), the transverse process on the opposite side of the restricted facet appears to become more prominent during backward bending and both transverse processes become symmetrical during forward bending. The motion restriction of the superior on the inferior vertebra is backward bending, sidebending, and rotation to the side opposite the most posterior transverse process.

If the transverse processes of three or more lumbar vertebrae are prominent in all three positions, restriction of this group of segments is of sidebending toward the most posterior transverse processes and rotation to the opposite side. The procedure described is but one means of motion testing of the lumbar spine and is recommended for its simplicity, timesaving, and

reliability across time and multiple examiners. Traditional multiplaner intersegmental motion testing is also useful, but includes elements of an articulatory procedure, which changes the behavior of the vertebra as each range of motion is introduced repetitively.

GOAL OF MANIPULATION

All manipulation is designed to obtain the maximal, pain-free movement of the musculoskeletal system in postural balance. It is anticipated that by restoring maximal function there will be enhancement of normal physiology, and in musculoskeletal pain syndromes, reduction in pain. The working hypothesis is that more normal function of mechanoreceptors and nociceptors will result in more normal neurologic function. In low back pain patients the goal of manipulation is to restore maximally the function of the three joints of the bony pelvis (symphysis pubis, right and left sacroiliac joints) and the capacity of the lumbar spine to freely sidebend and rotate to opposite sides with the presence of a neutral lordosis. The ability to achieve this goal depends upon the capacity of the anatomy present.

In the treatment process, the lumbar spine is addressed first since it is used in many of the procedures to treat sacroiliac joint dysfunction. Nonneutral dysfunctions with restriction of flexion or extension are addressed prior to the treatment of group dysfunctions. Frequently the restoration of function to nonneutral lumbar dysfunctions will allow the other segments within the group to be restored to normal function.

OSTEOPATHIC MANIPULATIVE TECHNIQUES

Osteopathic manipulative procedures are classified as direct or indirect as they relate to the approach to the restriction. Direct procedures engage the restriction and attempt to move it in the direction of motion loss. Indirect procedures move away from the restriction, either to the point of maximum ease within the remaining joint range, or in the direction exactly opposite the restriction. The activating forces operative during these procedures are intrinsic or extrinsic. Extrinsic forces include physician efforts, gravity, and the use of devices such as motorized tables and traction apparatus. Intrinsic activating forces include the inherent force of the musculoskeletal system to balance itself within three-dimensional space by many intricate reflex patterns; respiration; and muscle contraction, including isometric, concentric, and eccentric isotonic. Multiple combinations of activating forces are frequently used.

Osteopathic manipulative procedures have consistently evolved since the founding of the profession by A.T. Still, M.D. They include soft tissue procedures designed to reduce muscle spasm, enhance circulation, and produce a stimulatory or inhibitory tonic effect. Direct-action articulatory procedures put a joint or series of joints through multiple ranges of motion with particular emphasis in the direction of motion loss. These procedures are also termed mobilization without impulse. Direct-action, high-velocity, low-amplitude thrust procedures (mobilization with impulse) use both long and short lever approaches to address a specific joint. A joint pop or cracking sound is frequently heard during these techniques and is attributed to the cavitation phenomenon. These procedures are probably the most widely used and well known.

The joint pop is not necessary for success. Properly done, these procedures are not forceful but require precise localization and velocity during the thrust.

Inherent force craniosacral technique and ligamentous-articular balance technique was introduced in the 1930s by W.G. Sutherland, D.O. These procedures use the principle of balance of the musculoskeletal system, primarily the cranial base and sacrum, with the activating force coming from the cranial rhythmical impulse. This inherent body rhythm is not synchronous with any other known body rhythm and is somewhat lower in rate than respiration, usually in the range of 8 to 13 per minute. These procedures are nonforceful and quite safe. Their application in low back pain patients primarily deals with restoration of function of the sacrum between the two innominates.

In the early 1950s, a functional indirect technique system was introduced and fostered by Hoover and Bowles. This system introduces a dynamic process of active and passive movement within the patient's musculoskeletal system, constantly searching for a sense of ease and bind. It places less emphasis upon the relative positions of one bone to the other and focuses more upon the behavior of one segment of the musculoskeletal system and its relationship to its surrounding parts. Functional integrity rather than bony position is important. These procedures require a high level of palpatory dexterity and are particularly useful in acute musculoskeletal conditions.

Muscle energy techniques were introduced to the osteopathic armamentarium during the 1950s by Fred L. Mitchell, Sr., D.O. These techniques are primarily direct action in their approach and use the intrinsic activating force of the patient's muscle contraction. They are particularly useful when there is a high level of segmentally related muscle hypertonicity and spasm involved with the dysfunctional segment(s). These procedures use the application of two basic muscle physiology principles. The first is the ability to stretch a hypertonic shortened muscle to a new resting length following an isometric contraction. The second is the use of the principle of reciprocal inhibition. When the agonist muscle is asked to work repetitively through an arc of motion with increasing resistance at each effort, the antagonist is relaxed by inhibition and the agonist becomes progressively stronger because of recruitment of muscle firing from increased activity. There are at least three simultaneous outcomes of the use of a muscle energy procedure: the restoration of joint motion, the improvement of muscle physiological function, and the enhancement of lymphatic and venous circulation by muscle contraction, which is useful in alleviating the passive congestion so frequently noted in the presence of somatic dysfunction.

Since the 1960s, Larry Jones, D.O., has introduced a system of release by positioning that has been described as strain-counterstrain technique. The physican monitors palpatory tender points in various locations of the musculoskeletal system and then places the patient in a position of maximum ease with reduction in the patient's pain and in the palpatory tenderness. This position is held for a variable period of time, in the order of 90 seconds or until response is felt at the palpatory trigger point. These procedures are basically nontraumatic and are quite useful in both acute as well as chronic conditions. They appear to operate through a principle of afferent reduction of abnormal mechanoreceptor and nociceptor stimulation.

In the 1970s, Robert C. Ward, D.O., introduced a refined myofascial release technique procedure. The physician applies loads to regions of the musculoskeletal system by traction and twisting, searching for areas of tightness or looseness. Included are the skin, fascia, and muscles in addition to the osseous skeleton. The traction and twist load is applied in either a direct or indirect fashion until balance of function of related areas occurs. These techniques appear to operate through two interrelated activities. The first is the response of soft tissue to biomechanical loading by deformation and the energy release of hysteresis. The second appears to be modification of neuroreflexes based upon afferent stimulus by mechanical means.

In the treatment of the patient with low back pain, the dosage of manipulation must be appropriate. Modifications are made depending upon the patient's age, physical status, acuteness or chronicity of the condition, and the status of the musculoskeletal anatomy and physiology. As a general rule, the more acute the condition, the less intense the procedure at each visit and the more frequent the treatments. Chronic conditions require more exten-

sive treatment per visit with longer spans of time between treatments to allow for functional change to occur. In the acute low back syndrome without neurological deficit, it has been shown that appropriate manipulation will reduce severity of pain and length of disability. In chronic, recurrent, and "failed back" syndromes, manipulation takes on a different dimension. The goal now is less curative and is designed more to restore maximal functional capacity so that the total rehabilitation process can occur. Regardless of whether the patient is acute or chronic, the physician must approach the total musculoskeletal system as a unit and not place emphasis only in the area of pain complaint. Contributing factors to persistence of low back pain are lower extremity problems, imbalance in muscle function, and functional abnormalities of the upper trunk, cervical spine, and upper extremities. A comprehensive approach to integrated musculoskeletal function is the goal.

LUMBAR SPINE TECHNIQUES

Diagnosis. Group Dysfunction (Type I) sidebent right rotated left (Fig. 19.6).
Position. Lateral recumbent.
Type of Manipulation. Direct action, articulatory, muscle energy, or high velocity.

1. Patient lies in the left lateral recumbent position.
2. Operator pulls inferior shoulder caudad and anteriorly, introducing sidebending left.
3. Operator's right hand introduces right rotation from above downward to dysfunctional segment.

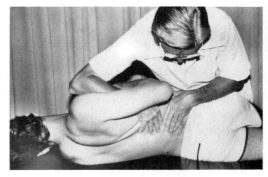

Figure 19.6. Group dysfunction (Type I) sidebent right rotated left—direct action manipulation.

4. Lower extremities taken to neutral position.
5. Operator's left arm rotates pelvis anteriorly to lock at dysfunctional segment.
6. Articulatory procedures can be done by springing of both of operator's hands in opposite directions.
7. Muscle energy activitation can be made by patient pushing right shoulder forward for 3 to 5 seconds and with three to five repetitions.
8. High-velocity activating force can be implemented by the operator's left arm in an anterior rotary thrust incorporating the left arm with the operator's body.
9. Reexamine for effectiveness of treatment.

Diagnosis: Group Dysfunction (Type I) sidebent right, rotated left (Fig. 19.7).
Position: Lateral recumbent.
Type of Manipulation: Muscle Energy.

1. Patient lies on right side in lateral recumbent position with shoulders perpendicular to the table introducing some left sidebending.
2. Operator flexes and extends lumbar spine to neutral and lifts both feet to the ceiling introducing left sidebending.
3. Operator's hand monitors group dysfunction at level of major restriction.
4. Patient attempts to pull feet down to the table against resistance offered by operator's right hand for 3 to 5 seconds and three to five repetitions.
5. Increasing left sidebending is made by lifting feet further to the ceiling and muscle energy efforts are repeated.

6. Reexamination to evaluate effectiveness of treatment.

Diagnosis: Nonneutral dysfunction (Type II) extended, sidebent left, rotated left (Fig. 19.8).
Position: Sitting.
Type of Manipulation: Muscle energy (demonstrated by Fred L. Mitchell, Sr., D.O.).

1. Patient sits on stool with left hand holding right shoulder.
2. Operator stands at left of patient controlling both shoulders with the left arm and monitoring dysfunctional segment with the right hand.
3. Operator introduces forward bending, right sidebending, and right rotation to first motion barrier.
4. Patient exerts left sidebending effort against resistance offered by operator's chestwall for 3 to 5 seconds.
5. Operator increases forward bending, right sidebending, right rotation to next resistent barrier, and patient repeats muscle energy effort.
6. Three to five repetitions of patient effort are made.
7. Reexamination to see if motion is restored.

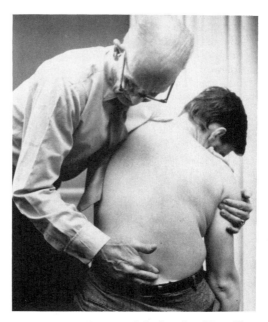

Figure 19.8. Nonneutral dysfunction (Type II) extended, sidebent left, rotated left—muscle energy manipulation.

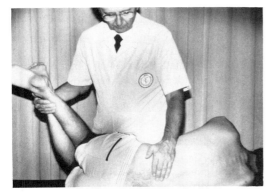

Figure 19.7. Group dysfunction (Type I) sidebent right rotated left—muscle energy manipulation.

Diagnosis: Nonneutral dysfunction (Type II) flexed, sidebent left, rotated left (Fig. 19.9).
Position: Lateral recumbent.
Type of Manipulation: Muscle energy.

1. Patient lies on left side in lateral recumbent position.
2. Operator extends bottom leg to first motion at inferior segment of dysfunction.
3. Patient introduces right sidebending and right rotation with right arm reaching down side of table.
4. Operator introduces right sidebending by lifting foot and leg to ceiling.
5. Patient exerts 3- to 5-second muscle effort by pulling right foot to table against resistance offered by operator who is monitoring at dysfunctional segment.
6. Increased sidebending and extension occur with the patient's right leg next to barrier and muscle energy repeated three to five times.
7. Reexamination.

SACROILIAC TECHNIQUES

Diagnosis: Left superior pubic dysfunction (Fig. 19.10).
Position: Supine.
Type of Manipulation: Muscle energy.

1. Patient supine on table with left leg over the side and with left posterior innominates still on table.
2. Operator controls left lower extremity between operator's knees.

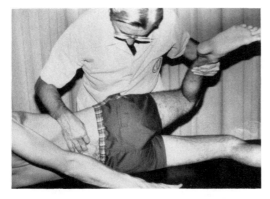

Figure 19.9. Nonneutral dysfunction (Type II) flexed, sidebent left, rotated left—muscle energy manipulation.

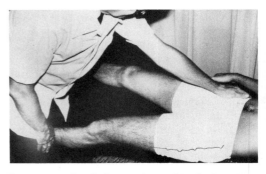

Figure 19.10. Left superior pubic dysfunction—muscle energy manipulation.

3. Operator holds right anterior superior iliac spine, stabilizing the pelvis.
4. Patient exerts an effort of lifting up the left leg to the ceiling against resistance offered by operator's hand above the patellar on distal femur. Muscle effort for 3 to 5 seconds.
5. Following muscle effort increased hip extension occurs and patient reapplies muscle energy for 3 to 5 seconds for three to five repetitions.
6. Reexamination.

Diagnosis: Right inferior pubic dysfunction (Fig. 19.11).
Position: Supine
Type of Manipulation: Muscle energy.

1. Patient supine on table with operator standing on left side.
2. Operator's left hand contacts right ischial tuberosity and puts a cephalward and medial force in the direction of the symphysis pubis.
3. Patient's hip flexed, internally rotated, and adducted to barrier.
4. Operator's right hand stabilizes anterior superior iliac spine.
5. Operator resists effort of extension of patient's right leg for 3 to 5 seconds.
6. Increased hip flexion to new barrier, followed by patient muscle effort of 3 to 5 seconds.
7. Reexamination.

Diagnosis: Sacroiliac dysfunction, left torsion on left oblique axis (Fig. 19.12).
Position: Left lateral recumbent Sims position.
Type of Manipulation: Muscle energy.

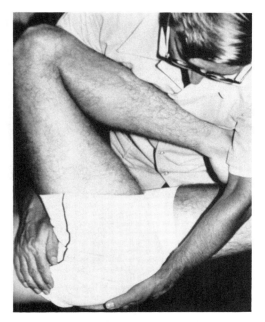

Figure 19.11. Right inferior pubic dysfunction—muscle energy manipulation.

1. Patient in left lateral Sims position with operator supporting both knees upon operator's left thigh.
2. Left rotation of L5 accomplished by operator's right hand on patient's right shoulder.

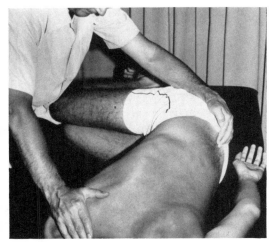

Figure 19.12. Sacroiliac dysfunction, left torsion on left oblique axis—muscle energy manipulation.

3. Patient's hips flexed until sacrum moves posteriorly.
4. Operator resists patient's effort of lifting feet to the ceiling for 3 to 5 seconds.
5. Operator increases hip flexion and rotation of L5 to the left, followed by patient's muscle energy effort for three to five repetitions.
6. Reexamination.

Diagnosis: Sacroiliac dysfunction, right sacrum extended (Fig. 19.13).
Position: Prone.
Type of Manipulation: Operator guiding and respiratory assist.

1. Patient prone on table with right lower extremity abducted to loose pack position of right sacroiliac joint.
2. Operator contacts right sacral base and stabilizes right anterior superior iliac spine.
3. Patient assumes extended trunk position.
4. Operator puts ventral and caudad pressure on sacral base as patient fully exhales.
5. Three to five repetitions of respiratory effort of forced exhalation with continuous counterforce of operator on sacral base.
6. Reexaminatin.

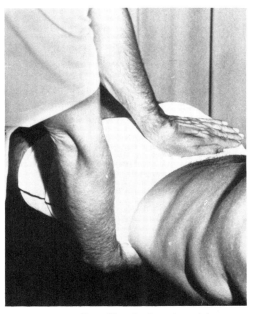

Figure 19.13. Sacroiliac dysfunction, right sacrum extended—operator guiding and respiratory assist manipulation.

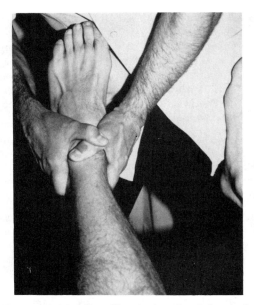

Figure 19.14. Sacroiliac dysfunction, left superior innominate shear—operator guiding and respiratory assist manipulation.

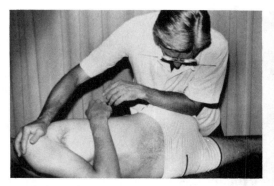

Figure 19.15. Iliosacral dysfunction, right anterior innominate—high-velocity, low-amplitude thrust manipulation.

Diagnosis: Sacroiliac dysfunction, left superior innominate shear (Fig. 19.14).
Position: Supine.
Type of Manipulation: Operator guiding and respiratory assist.

1. Patient supine on table.
2. Operator grasps left lower extremity above ankle, internally rotating left hip, extending left knee, and abducting leg to 15° resulting in loose packing of sacroiliac joint.
3. Operator stabilizes right lower extremity against thigh.
4. Operator puts long axis traction on left lower extremity while patient forcibly inhales and exhales.
5. Following three to five respiratory efforts patient coughs and operator puts long axis extension on left lower extremity.
6. Reexamination.

Diagnosis: Iliosacral dysfunction, right anterior innominate (Fig. 19.15).
Position: Left lateral recumbent.
Type of Manipulation: High-velocity, low-amplitude thrust.

1. Patient in left lateral recumbent position with operator standing in front.

2. Patient's lower shoulder pulled anterior and caudad introducing locking mechanics in neutral to the sacrum.
3. Operator's left forearm contacts right ischial tuberosity.
4. Anterior rotary thrust applied by operator's left forearm incorporated as part of operator's body.
5. Reexamination.

Diagnosis: Iliosacral dysfunction, right anterior innominate (Fig. 19.16).
Position: Prone.
Type of Manipulation: Muscle energy.

1. Patient prone on table with right lower extremity flexed, externally rotated, and abducted.
2. Operator controls right knee with right hand and places right foot against thigh.
3. Barrier to posterior innominate rotation engaged and monitored by operator's left hand.
4. Operator resists extension effort of patient's right leg for 3- to 5-second contraction.
5. Three to five repetitions of muscle effort.
6. Reexamination.

Diagnosis: Iliosacral dysfunction, right anterior innominate (Fig. 19.16).
Position: Prone.
Type of Manipulation: Muscle energy.

1. Patient prone on table.
2. Operator stands on opposite side of dysfunction and grasps distal femur with patient's knee flexed.

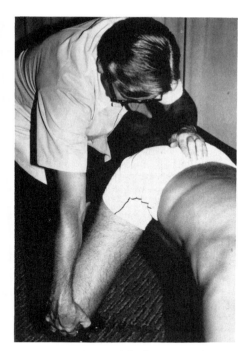

Figure 19.16. Iliosacral dysfunction, right anterior innominate—muscle energy manipulation.

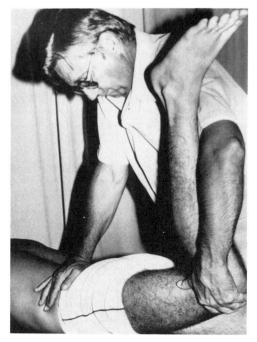

Figure 19.17. Iliosacral dysfunction, left innominate posterior—muscle energy manipulation.

3. Operator contacts left iliac crest with right hand exerting an anterior counterforce.
4. Operator resists patient's effort to pull knee to table for 3 to 5 seconds.
5. Three to five repetitions of muscle effort.
6. Reexamination.

ADJUNCTIVE THERAPY

The low back pain patient requires not only an integrated diagnostic approach but an integrated treatment plan as well. Manipulation is but one part of the treatment program. The patient must become a part of the treatment team and should be instructed in the basics of musculoskeletal anatomy and physiology and those things that enhance or detract from it. Instruction is given for appropriate body posture in the standing, sitting, and lying positions, as well as in proper means of change of position. Analysis is made of the patient's activities of daily living, particularly occupation, and appropriate instructions are given to avoid aggravation of the condition. Specific exercises are given every patient to maintain and enhance the increased function provided by the manipulation. Exercises include those to enhance range of motion, lengthen tight muscle and muscle groups, and strengthen weak muscles. Stretching exercises should always precede strengthening exercises. Of particular importance is the use of walking as an exercise, not only enhancing lumbar spine and pelvic girdle function, but also physical conditioning. A cross-pattern pep walk of 20 minutes daily is the goal.

The use of medication depends upon the patient's condition. In acute conditions, appropriate analgesic and narcotic use are in order for pain control. However, care must be used in the long-term application of narcotics since they appear to interfere with the patient's inherent pain control mechanisms. Nonsteroidal anti-inflammatory agents are quite useful in both acute and chronic conditions, particularly for the short-term posttreatment flare-up. Muscle relaxants have a limited use in acute conditions for the short term only. In the chronic low back syndrome, the use of antidepressants, particularly amitriptyline, has been found useful particularly in the restoration of a more normal sleep cycle. Short-term use of oral steroids has been found useful in the acute low back syndrome.

Injection techniques are occasionally found adjunctive and useful, particularly the injection of myofascial trigger points. Spray and stretch technique has been less useful in the chronic low back patient. Injection of steroid and local anesthetic in the posterior aspect of the sacroiliac joint and in the region of the facet joints is occasionally useful diagnostically and therapeutically.

The use of heat, cold, and physical therapy modalities is highly individualized and dependent upon tissue response. Applications of cold appear to be better for reduction of pain and muscle spasm. Application of heat for too long a period of time can overly congest the part and increase the amount of disability. If tissue heating is thought to be indicated, then the appropriate use of ultrasound can be beneficial.

External devices found most beneficial have been a cinch-type sacroiliac belt that provides circumferential tension around the bony pelvis giving stability without restriction of motion. Low back braces are seldom used and only for short periods of time during the acute phase. One of the most frequently used orthotic devices is a heel lift, or other adjustment to footwear, to balance the sacral base of the pelvis in the presence of the short leg—pelvic tilt syndrome.

SUMMARY

Osteopathic manipulative therapy can be most useful in the management of the low back pain patient. Structural diagnosis is a useful tool in the evaluation of the patient. Different techniques are more appropriate for different patients and conditions. If one only has a hammer in the toolbox, one is surprised how many things look like nails. The manipulative physician's toolbox should contain many techniques.

Manipulation is most useful in the management of low back patients but must be done within the context of total patient care. As with all treatment modalities, appropriate use and awareness of potential complications are essential.

Suggested Readings

Beal MC. Motion sense. Osteopath Assoc 1953; 53:151–153.

Beal MC. Spinal motion. Carmel, CA; Yearbook of the Academy of Applied Osteopathy. 1970; 11–16.

Bourdillon JF. Spinal manipulation. 3rd ed. East Norwalk, CT: Appleton-Century-Crofts, 1982.

Bowles CH. Functional technique: A modern perspective. J Am Osteopath Assoc 1981; 80:326–331.

Dvorak V, Dvorak V, Schneider W, eds. Manual medicine 1984. Heidelberg: Springer-Verlag, 1985.

Farfan HF. The scientific basis of manipulative procedures. Clin Rheum Dis 1980; 6(1):159.

Greenman, PE. The osteopathic concept in the second century: Is it still germane to specialty practice? J Am Osteopath Assoc 1976; 75:589–595.

Greenman, PE. Layer palpation. Mich Osteopath J 1982; 47(9):936–937.

Greenman PE, ed. Concepts and mechanisms of neuromuscular functions. Berlin: Springer-Verlag, 1984.

Greenman PE. Models and mechanisms of osteopathic manipulative medicine. Osteopath Med News 1987; 4(5):1–20.

Hoover HW. Functional technique. Carmel, CA: Yearbook of the Academy of Applied Osteopathy, 1958; 47–51.

Johnston WL, Robertson JA, Stiles EG. Finding a common denominator for the variety of manipulative techniques. Carmel, CA: Yearbook of the Academy of Applied Osteopathy, 1969; 5–15.

Jones LH. Strain and counterstrain. Colorado Springs, CO: American Academy of Osteopathy, 1981.

Kimberly PE. Formulating a prescription for osteopathic manipulative treatment. J Am Osteopath Assoc 1976; 75:486–499.

Kimberly PE, ed. Outline of osteopathic manipulative procedures. 2nd ed. Kirksville, MO: Kirksville College of Osteopathic Medicine, 1980.

Kirkaldy-Willis WH. Managing low back pain. Edinburgh: Churchill Livingstone, 1983.

Lewit K. Manipulative therapy in rehabilitation of the motor system. Stoneham, MA: Butterworth, 1985.

Magoun HI. Osteopathy in the cranial field. 2nd ed. Kirksville, MO: Journal Printing Co., 1966.

Mitchell FL Sr. Motion discordance. Carmel, CA: Yearbook of the Academy of Applied Osteopathy, 1967; 1–5.

Mitchell FL Jr, Moran PS, Pruzzo NA. An evaluation and treatment manual of osteopathic muscle energy procedures. Valley Park, MO: Mitchell, Moran, and Pruzzo, 1979.

Nicholas NS. Atlas of osteopathic techniques. Philadelphia: Philadelphia College of Osteopathic Medicine, 1974.

Northup G. Osteopathic medicine. An american reformation. 2nd ed. Chicago: American Osteopathic Association, 1979.

Northup GW, ed. Osteopathic research: Growth and development. Chicago: American Osteopathic Association, 1987.

Retzlaff EW, Mitchell FL Jr. The cranium and its sutures. Berlin: Springer-Verlag, 1987.

Stiles EG. Manipulative techniques: Four approaches. Osteopath Med 1976; 1(6):27–30.

Stoddard A. Manual of osteopathic technique. London: Hutchinson, 1959.

Stoddard A. Manual of osteopathic practice. New York: Harper & Row, 1969.

Upledger JE, Vredevoogd JD. Craniosacral therapy. Chicago: Eastland Press, 1983.

Walton WJ. Osteopathic Diagnosis and technique procedures. 2nd ed. Colorado Springs, CO: American Academy of Osteopathy, 1970.

Ward RC, Sprafka S. Glossary of osteopathic terminology. J Am Osteopath Assoc 1981; 80:552–567.

20

DIVERSIFIED APPROACH OF CHIROPRACTIC

Kelli Pearson
Tammy De Koekkoek

Chiropractic has survived and flourished as a profession since the time of its formal introduction by D.D. Palmer in 1895 (1). In this chapter, our goal is to provide a brief overview of contemporary chiropractic procedures, including some indications, contraindications, and benefits surrounding spinal manipulative techniques (SMT), which are common to the diversified approach to chiropractic. (Diversified techniques include those manipulative procedures most commonly taught by chiropractic colleges accredited in the United States by the Council on Chiropractic Education.) In tackling this large subject, we understand that the chiropractic approach to management of low back pain includes an abundance of diverse but effective protocols too numerous to describe in this setting. In this chapter, only a selection of the more commonly employed procedures as they are applied to selected clinical conditions will be described. By no means should the practice of chiropractic be construed as limited to the examples given here. Furthermore, it is difficult to treat the body effectively by addressing only joint dysfunction without taking into consideration the condition of the adjacent soft tissue structures, including ligaments, tendons, muscles, and even the dura mater. Treatment of soft tissue dysfunction is thus beyond the limited scope of this chapter. The diversified approach, however, recognizes that the treatment and rehabilitation of such structures constitutes a vital part of contemporary chiropractic practice.

ETIOLOGY OF LOW BACK PAIN RELATED TO DIAGNOSIS

Awareness of the etiologic factors in low back pain is imperative for the manipulative practitioner in that this knowledge is applied to the appropriate diagnosis and resulting prognosis. Precision of diagnosis not only helps the practitioner select the best treatment regimen but, more importantly, provides patients with proper education concerning this condition, allowing them to participate intelligently in the treatment. Continual reassessment is crucial in determining the most appropriate diagnosis and redirection of the therapy (2). Furthermore, the so-called "manipulable lesion" (to be defined in the next section as the "subluxation complex") is viewed by the chiropractor as existing within the mechanics of the lower extremity–spinal kinematic chain and thus, treatment and rehabilitation are geared toward the correction of all aspects of dysfunction, rather than the pain-producing tissue alone.

DETERMINATION OF THE SUBLUXATION COMPLEX

The decision to manipulate the spine (or related articulations) of the patient with low back pain is based upon specific observed and palpable findings. The history and review of systems place the patient in the realm of the orthopedic examination (see Table 20.1), after which a specialized examination is performed.

Table 20.1.
Two Patient Presentations

Exacerbation of Chronic Low Back Pain

1. General physical regional examination as indicated by history and review of systems.
2. Lower quarter screen (LQS) examination (includes inspection of gait and posture, functional examination of ranges of motion, muscle testing, and basic neurological examination).
3. Regional lumbopelvic examination procedures not previously performed in LQS.
4. Imaging electrodiagnostics, and other laboratory test procedures as indicated.
5. Specialized examination for the subluxation complex and its pathomechanical context.

Acute Onset Low Back Pain

1. Vital signs.
2. Pertinent regional examinations as indicated by history and review of systems (e.g., abdominal examination).
3. Regional neuromusculoskeletal lumbopelvic examination.
4. Imaging, electrodiagnostics, and other laboratory tests as indicated.
5. Specialized examination for the subluxation complex and related structural components (muscle spasm, myofascial trigger points).

The decision to manipulate, however, usually precedes this portion of the examination, and is based on the absence of contraindications and the presence of qualifying criteria.

Typically, the implied mechanical nature of certain components of the condition are sought, including, for example, restriction of intersegmental and gross ranges of motion of the affected joints. Indicators of the site, nature, and extent of such manipulative procedures (adjustments) are largely dependent on the extent of the intersegmental ranges of motion, joint play, muscular integrity, the age of the patient, chronicity of the condition, and the perception of pain.

In order to appreciate the context in which the specialized portion of the examination exists, two basic patient presentations have been selected (Table 20.1). The "subluxation complex" of chiropractic was described by Gillet as having three components: muscular, articular, and neurological; in other words, the articular

dysfunction, (be it hypomobility, hypermobility, altered structural integrity, or misalignment) has multiple causes and effects in the spinal column (3). In the patient with low back pain particularly with intermittent bouts or exacerbations of a chronic condition, the chiropractor seeks to place the articular dysfunction of the spine within the larger picture of the body as a whole. The subluxation complex exists within the greater framework of pathomechanical function of the lower extremities and trunk as a kinematic chain. To this end, postural and gait inspection constitutes a major part of the examination and dysfunction of all of the components of the lower extremities is considered in assessment and treatment for low back pain.

Following the overall examination, the patient is given a specialized examination, specific to identification of the subluxation or dysfunction, with all the related soft tissue affections. The examination consists of the following six parts:

1. posture,
2. movement inspection,
3. static palpation,
4. movement palpation,
5. muscle length assessment, and
6. muscle strength assessment.

Posture

The patient is examined for optimal alignment of the various body segments, with much attention being given to the muscular components of postural dysfunction (see below, Common Muscle Syndromes). Idiopathic scoliosis, sciatic scoliosis, and torsional asymmetries of the tibiae, femora, and pelvis are noted, along with mechanical abnormalities of the feet and knees, all of which are considered in the overall postural statics which contribute to the production of low back pain.

Movement Inspection

The patient is examined in the standing and seated positions for the six directions of spinal movement. The examiner observes active movements for symmetry of movement of articulations, such as the smooth symmetrical opening of the facets on forward bending and closure on backward bending. The capacity of all the vertebral segments to participate in each movement is inspected noting, for example, aberrant movement during lateral bending, producing a disruption in the smooth C-shaped curve that normally develops during this movement. Also noted are the patterns of muscular activity with each action. Movement patterns, such as faulty lumbopelvic rhythm (4), are observed and correlation with later palpatory findings is made.

Static Palpation

1. The pads of the fingers are used to ascertain alterations in skin texture and temperature. Temperature differences are occasionally noted at the sites of dysfunctional segments (5). Edema is felt in the paraspinal tissues at the sites of injury or inflammation. As in the case of increased local temperature, the presence of edema does not necessarily imply the presence of a subluxation warranting manipulation. On the contrary, such evidence of inflammation may, at times, be associated with hypermobility, instability, infection, or other active pathology—all contraindications to local manipulation.

2. At the next level of palpation muscle tone and texture are determined. Tone is best felt by a light prodding action. Muscle texture, i.e., fibrous bands or hypertonic bands of muscle tissue, may be felt by a gentle but firm pressure on the muscle by moving the integumentary structures over the muscle band or trigger point (6, 7).

3. Alignment and symmetry of the bony structures are also checked. Overall curvature of the spine and posteriority of the rib cage are confirmed by palpation. The bony elements of the spine are among the most anomalous components of the skeleton; thus, the apparently rotated position of one spinous process should correspond with a posteriorly palpated transverse process or apophyseal joint on the side opposite the spinous rotation. Without such correlative findings, the spinous process may be assumed to be anomalously developed, bent, or bifurcated.

Movement Palpation

Overall spinal mobility is palpated in one commonly used procedure known as the "quick scan" (8). In the seated position, overall sagittal plane joint play is felt by creating momentum in the spine in order to ascertain the areas of greatest restriction of movement. Then in the coronal plane, the examiner leans on the patient's shoulders and introduces thoracolumbar sidebending, (which of necessity is coupled with rotation) and thus assesses gross restriction of movement and joint play. These areas of major restriction are correlated with the standing and seated inspection of ranges of motion and posture, and are then palpated for specific regional intersegmental joint movement and joint play.

1. Intersegmental palpation is the evaluation of the participation of local spinal joints in the overall spinal movement accomplished; for example, the extent to which the L4-5 segment participates in thoracolumbar rotation.

2. Joint play palpation is defined by Mennell in the neutral position for the joint (9) with the term "endfeel" used by Cyriax to describe the quality of movement at the limits of passive range of motion (10). It is important to remember, however, that these qualities of movement have been largely applied to the joints of the extremities, which are relatively large and simple in movement when compared with the size and complexity of the interaction of spinal articulations. Thus, the examiner assesses endfeel by applying "overpressure" to gross ranges of spinal motion, such as seated thoracolumbar sidebending. The examiner assesses the endfeel by application of overpressure on each individual bony segment, by contacting the spinous process or other available bony prominence, such as the transverse process or posterior articular processes. Thus the chiropractor determines not only those joints that do not fully participate in a given movement and are said to be restricted or "in fixation" (3) but also the quality or nature of restriction. It is through this avenue the clinician primarily determines the site, direction, and amplitude of the manipulative procedure to be employed.

Muscle Length Assessment

The length of the muscular structures largely determines the static misalignment of various body segments at their joints. This, in turn, results in limitation of ranges of motion and incoordinated movements. One of the sequelae of such insufficiency is chronic postural strain, under which circumstances the patient may develop myofascial pain syndromes or chronically restricted movement of joints with attendant capsular fibrosis. The pain that results from these conditions causes the patient to seek care. Thus the assessment and treatment of the muscular length component of joint dysfunction, both spinal and extraspinal, is central to the comprehensive management of the low back pain patient (11). Specific postural muscle and myofascial syndromes are described below.

Muscle Strength Assessment

In traditional orthopedics, muscle strength testing has been relegated to the neurological component of the examination, and Cyriax provided us with the consideration of pain production resulting from the use of the "contractile elements" (10). There is a third aspect of muscle testing that affects the diversified approach of chiropractic, and that is the subjective assessment of muscle strength as it relates to postural statics. Lewit described the weakened phasic muscles as being the product of postural muscle antagonist inhibition (12), whereas others considered the muscle weaknesses to be the cause, rather than the effect of such postural faults, with resultant dysfunction of the joints they control (13–15). Janda demonstrated with EMG that the strength of abdominal muscles was greatly enhanced immediately following stretching of the antagonist postural muscles, namely the lumbar erector spinae (16). Thus, although muscle strength testing in clinical practice is largely a subjective tool, it nonetheless contributes to our greater understanding of the total picture of disturbed neuromusculoskeletal function.

TECHNIQUES

There are a great variety of manipulative techniques employed in treating musculoskeletal lesions. We refer to a number of these throughout this chapter. Buerger has developed a taxonomy of spinal manipulative therapy (17), taking into consideration the previous attempts to standardize the terminology (18–21). These modified classifications are listed in Table 20.2 and are described below.

1. *Thrusting short lever techniques.* Use of high-velocity, low-amplitude force to enhance joint mobility. Most commonly directed toward the spinal joints although extremity thrusting techniques are effectively employed as well.

Table 20.2.

1. Thrusting/short-lever techniques
2. Non-specific long-lever manipulation
3. Specific long-lever manipulation
4. Mobilizing or articulating techniques
5. Traction techniques
6. Muscle energy/antagonistic techniques
7. Point pressure techniques
8. Cranial techniques

2. *Nonspecific long lever techniques.* Application of force and motion through a relatively long section of the patients spine using the femur, or pelvis, shoulder or head, as lever handles. No attempt to localize the effect to one specific vertebral joint is made.

3. *Modified specific long lever techniques.* A similar approach is taken as in the previous technique. A force is applied through modified contact on the "long levers"; however, the forces are localized to specific joints by accurate palpation, and the effects are limited to these articulations by the addition of specific manual contacts.

4. *Mobilizing or articulating techniques.* Use of low-velocity, medium- to high-amplitude passive movements of one or more joints.

5. *Traction techniques.* High- or low-amplitude force is used to stretch or separate one or more joints without attempting to localize the effect. The joint is usually perpendicular to the plane of the joint.

6. *Muscle energy/antagonistic techniques.* Although Buerger makes a distinction between these two forms of SMT, they can be grossly categorized as techniques employing counter-resistive forces performed by the patient against the resistive force supplied by the doctor in order to create movement of a joint by way of muscular contraction and relaxation.

7. *Point pressure techniques.* Deep goading or application of pressure without attempting soft-tissue massage or joint movement.

8. *Cranial techniques.* The application of light forces to the skull in a precisely determined manner to normalize craniosacral motion.

The diversified approach to chiropractic may include any or all of the above techniques, depending on the clinician's experience and area of skill. However, high-velocity, short amplitude thrusting (short-lever) techniques are preferred to the nonspecific long-lever forms of manipulation, especially when a specific focal increase in intersegmental mobility at a site of joint dysfunction is desired.

Specific adjustment or correction of spinal and pelvic articular derangement remains the focus of chiropractic practice. The adjustive thrust (see Table 20.2) is characterized by a transmission of force using a combination of leverage and patient position (22). The force is delivered with controlled speed, depth and magnitude through a specific contact on a particular structure such as the spinous process, mamillary process or transverse process of a vertebra. Control of the adjustment requires practice and skill in order to deliver a thrust with exact amplitude, speed, and force. A selected manipulative procedure will usually involve manual contact on the spine, with the removal of joint slack or passive range of motion in the joint, at which point a controlled dynamic thrust will produce a specific movement of an articulation. Common mechanisms of delivery of the adjustive thrust include the recoil triceps motion, shoulder/straight arm thrust, and body drop thrust.

As we review some of the more commonly presenting low back pain syndromes, specific adjustments that illustrate the so-called diversified approach and have proven useful are described. The reader should understand that a number of different manipulative techniques exist that may be successfully utilized in treating a pathomechanical lesion. Variation of clinician experience, education, body type and clinical goals all contribute to the choice of a specific procedure to a given mechanical lesion.

CLINICAL LESIONS

The progression from joint dysfunction to instability and restabilization is a model that enables the practitioner to consider the multiple components to spinal diagnosis in manipulable patients. Table 20.3 (reproduced from Kirkaldy-Willis) categorizes the more commonly presenting syndromes with their associated phases of degeneration, a paradigm that Kirkaldy-Willis introduced to explain the natural history of progression of lumbar spine mechanical disease. The diagnosis must encompass not only the affected tissue, but also the state of degeneration in which the painful lesion exists. For example, a patient presenting with a facet syndrome in the dysfunctional phase will re-

Table 20.3.
Specific Clinical Lesions

Dysfunction	Posterior facet syndrome
	Sacroiliac syndrome
	Maigne's syndrome
	Myofascial syndromes
	Gluteus maximus
	Gluteus medius
	Gluteus minimus
	Quadratus lumborum
	Piriformis
	Tensor fasciae latae
	Hamstring
	Disc herniation
Unstable Phase	Facet and disc degeneration
	Lateral stenosis
	Central stenosis
	Disc herniation
Stabilization	Lateral stenosis
	Central stenosis
	Multilevel stenosis
	Disc herniation

Reprinted by permission from Kirkaldy-Willis, WH. The site and nature of the lesion. Kirkaldy-Willis, WH. ed. Managing low back pain, 2nd ed. New York: Churchill Livingstone, 1988; 134.

quire not only a different therapeutic approach from that occurring in the unstable phase, but will have a substantially different prognosis, necessitating specific therapeutic exercise and lifestyle changes. To further complicate the issue, it is not uncommon for a localized lesion in the spinal somatic structures to be aggravated or compounded by lesions of more peripheral structures, such as hip joint dysfunction, genu valgum, or mechanical problems of the feet. This is locally exemplified by the case of disc degeneration, in which posterior joint irritation develops secondary to the abnormal distribution of weight-bearing load, thus lending itself to facetal sclerosis and ligamentous laxity (23). It is our contention that the low back pain patient typically presents with multiple lesions that necessitate thorough diagnosis and subsequent skilled manipulation and other manual care to restore complete mechanical function. For these reasons, the provider should meticulously attempt to identify the type of tissue affected, the phase of degeneration of the lesion and the related peripheral structural abnormalities. The next section will attempt to define the more commonly presenting combined clinical syndromes listed in Table 20.4.

Table 20.4.
Common Clinical Patterns of Mechanical Stress Resulting in Multiple Lesions

1. Facet syndrome associated with disc degeneration
2. Intevertebral disc syndrome (IVD)
3. Associated sacroiliac and lumbar dysfunction
4. Maigne's syndrome and associated sacroiliac dysfunction
5. Spondylolisthesis and associated sacroiliac dysfunction and/or lumbar dysfunction
6. Postsurgical conditions associated with compensatory hypermobility
7. Common muscle syndromes
8. Extraspinal articular dysfunctions associated with low back pain

Empirically, manipulation has proven to be effective in treating these syndromes. Under scientific scrutiny, manipulation has also been demonstrated to be effective in the treatment of low back pain. However, most of the clinical trials do not differentiate the etiologies of the conditions treated (24). In addition to a brief clinical description of the syndromes listed in Table 20.4, some methods of manipulation used in chiropractic appropriate for these conditions are described and illustrated in the following sections. It should be appreciated that these descriptions are not intended to train the health care provider in these procedures, but rather to provide a concept of some of the methods used.

Facet Syndrome Associated with Disc Degeneration

The patient presenting with an acute onset of low back pain due to facet irritation may assume a forward antalgic position, and avoid any form of backward bending. Although upon digital palpation the pain may be localized to the posterior joints, the patient may report referred pain into the buttock, lateral thigh, and calf. There is typically an absence of hard neurological signs. Both Cailliet and Grieve state that the etiology is due to articular strains, in which slips of muscle tissue within the posterior joint complex fail, resulting in painful trapping of capsular material (2, 25). Frequently, manipulation can quickly reduce the dysfunction and the patient reports rapid alleviation of pain. In cases where this syndrome continues without appropriate treatment, or where the history

suggests repeated episodes, it is assumed that concomitant discal degeneration occurs, resulting in altered weight bearing and further strain. Farfan introduced the concept of the triple joint complex and showed that torsional strain affected both the facet and disc as the function of these structures is interdependent (26). Kirkaldy-Willis concurs on the familiar relationship of facet and disc lesions, and reports that most of the symptoms in the early stages of the patient's history of back pain arise from changes in the facet joints, but that as the dysfunction continues, discal degeneration is inevitable. An effective manipulation commonly used is illustrated in Figure 20.1. This demonstrates a manipulative procedure performed in the sidelying position with the goal of restoring lost motion to the L4-5 joint complex, in this case left lateral bending having been found lacking. The patient is lying on his right side while the doctor contacts the left side of the fourth lumbar. Once the tissue slack is taken up, a thrust is generated in the direction that creates left lateral bending of the patient at this level.

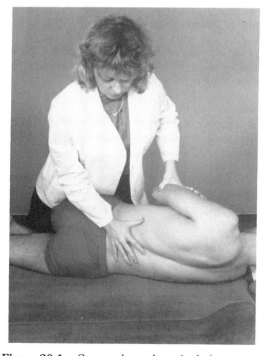

Figure 20.1. Commonly used manipulation.

Intervertebral Disc Syndrome

In the patient whose primary dysfunctional pain-producing mechanism is related to discal derangement, an entirely different approach is taken. In the acute presentation of herniation of a lumbar disc, the complaint is one of sharp low back pain with or without leg and/or buttock pain of sudden onset, usually following trivial and apparently innocuous activity. Pain is intensified with forward bending, but ranges of trunk motion are markedly diminished in all directions, with backward bending and side-bending into the side of pain typically having the most remarkable limitation. Pain may be exacerbated by coughing, sneezing, and bearing down. Irritation or compression of the nerve root is objectified by findings of impaired dural mobility limiting the straight leg raise and/or contralateral leg raise and of altered neurological functions such as altered skin sensation in the affected dermatome, diminished deep tendon reflexes, and finally, muscle weakness and atrophy.

Therapeutic approaches to the disc vary widely within chiropractic as well as physical therapy and manual medicine. Flexion-distraction is well documented (see Chapter 21) but extension procedures fare very well also (27). Extension protocols may encompass prone manipulation as described by Gonstead and Reinert, as well as passive and active extension maneuvers as described by McKenzie (28–30). Active self-correction principles are employed that reduce pain and improve the functional status of the patient rapidly. Furthermore, side-posture rotary manipulation, which has been considered taboo in the treatment of disc injury, may not be as great a culprit as previously thought (31). However, great care and experience with manipulation are needed in determining the dysfunctional segments that may be contributing to the mechanical stressors in the herniated disc condition before manipulation can be administered (32). Myofascial techniques are very helpful, possibly because they interrupt the pain-spasm-pain cycle that often appears to prolong the course of disability associated with herniation (33). Following the acute period of the condition, appropriate rehabilitative muscle lengthening and strengthening procedures are used, followed with postural, proprioceptive, and movement pattern reeducation (34). Patients who are not responsive to conservative manual care, that is, those who fail to demonstrate at least a 50% improvement in functional status and pain diminution within 3 weeks of concerted care and have evidence of hard neurological deficit, are referred for neurological consultation (35).

Associated Sacroiliac and Lumbar Dysfunctions

A commonly overlooked cause of low back pain is related to sacroiliac (SI) dysfunction (36). There has been some conflict as whether or not this joint complex enjoys sufficient mobility to result in clinical dysfunction, but the lesion has been well described (37–40). The patient with a primary SI lesion often describes unilateral dull or sharp pain over the involved SI joint and buttock that may have a radiating component into the ipsilateral groin, testicles, greater trochanter, posterior or anterior thigh, and occasionally, into the posterior or lateral calf, possibly extending into the ankle, foot, or toes (2, 23). The patient may have difficulty rolling over in bed at night, walking for a moderate distance, and getting up from a seated position. The pain may coincide with the stance phase of each gait cycle.

Examination procedures will establish marked tenderness to palpation over the affected joint, often with hypersensitivity to skin rolling in the adjacent gluteal region. In many cases, the joint will lack normal mobility to movement palpation. (It is interesting that movement restriction is occasionally noted in the contralateral joint. It may be that this alters the instantaneous axis of rotation for the sacroiliac joints as they behave in concert, placing greater stress on the mobile joint, which then becomes symptomatic.) The finding of hypomobility in isolation does not constitute the diagnosis of a primary sacroiliac lesion, since sacroiliac hypomobility is frequently implicated as a contributor to other lumbopelvic disorders. Thus, careful examination is needed to rule out primary disc or facet disease or myofascial referral. The palpation procedures diagnosing aberrant SI motion can be easily performed by the skilled manipulator. Taking into consideration that sacroiliac joint movement is governed by movement of the hips, a noted decrease of the SI joint play in the direction of extension or flexion as the hip joint extends or flexes (in the open chain situation of palpation) enables the chiropractor to decide what direction of movement the selected manipulative procedure (adjustment) should serve to restore.

To the physician who does not manipulate, SI joint dysfunction can mimic an acute disc derangement unless the practitioner is aware that treating the offending SI joint can produce dramatic pain relief and restoration of function. Norman and May treated more that 300 patients with local anesthetic over the involved SI joint, which relieved pain immediately in those patients who also had sensory changes in the involved lower extremity and an absent Achilles reflex (41). The SI lesion, particularly with a history of repeated episodes of irritation, creates an alteration in normal smooth gait. When the joint's movement is aberrant, increased compensatory bending and rotatory motion of the lumbar joint complexes and of the acetabulofemoral joints ensues, resulting in fatigue and stress with subsequent altered mobility and pain (42). The pelvic and lumbar muscles, including the multifidus, psoas, and piriformis, may undergo shortening with fibrosis and even contracture. Thus, treatment of the sacroiliac syndrome is incomplete without consideration of the dysfunctions of the lumbar, lumbosacral, and hip joint complexes. Figure 20.2 illustrates a commonly used adjustment for the case of decreased freedom of motion in the direction of extension (anterior rotation of innominate) of the superior aspect of the right sacroiliac joint. With the patient lying on the involved side, the doctor contacts the right side of the sacrum as close as possible to the joint, having first placed it in a position of sacroiliac "extension" by flexing the opposite hip, and introduces a force in a posterior to anterior direction, following the orientation of the joint plane as much as possible. When the movement is restored and pain is relieved, the diagnosis is confirmed retrospectively (2).

Maigne's Syndrome with Associated Sacroiliac Dysfunction

According to Maigne, thoracolumbar facet joint irritation is a fairly common cause of pain in the lower lumbar and lumbosacral area. Despite the patient's persistent complaints of lower lumbar, pelvic crest, and/or groin pain, the lumbar spine examination may result in

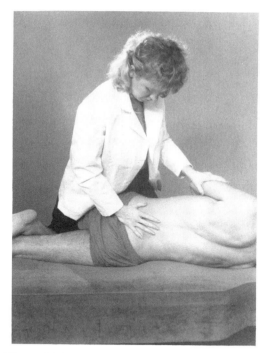

Figure 20.2. Adjustment for decreased freedom of motion.

negative findings. Maigne suggests that the pain can be the result of irritation of the iliohypogastric and ilioinguinal nerves, which exit from the first lumbar level and may refer pain to the pelvic crest and groin regions and may mimic signs of renal colic and testicular tenderness or pain (43). The patient frequently has a palpatory tenderness and increased sensitivity to skin-rolling at the pelvic crest as well as the level of the thoracolumbar posterior joints and spinous processes. Sidebending and extension may aggravate the pain referral to the low back, and motion palpation examination reveals a loss of normal motion at the thoracolumbar junction. There may be associated sacroiliac joint dysfunction on the same side serving to complicate the diagnosis (44). Figure 20.3 illustrates an effective technique used to restore flexion motion at the thoracolumbar region during treatment of this syndrome.

In this maneuver, the doctor contacts the spinous process of the involved segments with the thenar eminence of the hand. The patient is gently rolled down towards the table, and at the

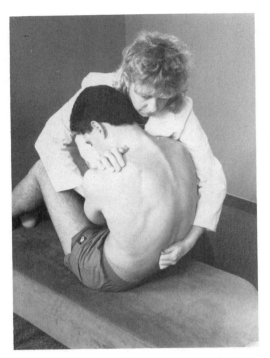

Figure 20.3.   Technique for restoring flexion.

Spondylolisthesis with Associated Sacroiliac and/or Lumbar Dysfunction

Spondylolytic spondylolisthesis is a structural defect best diagnosed on the lateral and oblique projections of a lumbar series where it is characterized by breaks in the pars interarticularis with forward translation of the vertebral body. The patient may complain of pain in the low back and leg(s). Range of motion seems most restricted due to pain with backward bending, and forward bending is often impeded due to shortened hamstrings. Physicians are often tempted to attribute the patient's pain to the defect because the radiographic changes are so obvious (45). The evidence strongly disputes this conclusion (46). The vast majority of cases of spondylolisthesis occur between 5 and 10 years of age and will continue to slip forward for 18 to 24 months after the onset of the pars defect, and once that period of time has elapsed, these segments are very stable, as established on motion radiographic studies. It has been reported that 97 to 98% of people with spondylolisthesis do not have instability of the motion segment, despite severe anterior slippage in some cases (47). Symptoms arise in patients with a spondylolisthesis because of sacroiliac syndromes, or lumbar facet or disc disorders. If the exam findings support a primary sacroiliac syndrome, conservative care should first address that dysfunction. On the other hand, strain from the spondylolisthesis is transferred to the posterior joints one or more levels higher and pain ensues from the added compression irritation (23, 35). Some practitioners have noticed effective relief from pain in these patients by treatment of posterior joint dysfunction at the thoracolumbar region (48). On rare occasions, the segment affected is found to be unstable on flexion and extension radiographs (49). The patient then should present with the history and clinical findings commensurate with instability (50), and the examiner remains aware that the clinical signs of instability are not necessarily corroborated by radiographic signs (51). In these situations, if the instability is not considered surgical, perhaps spinal stabilization may be adequately accomplished with a carefully supervised program of strengthening and stretching exercise and proprioceptive re-education (52). The grading of instabil-

moment the involved segments meet the table surface through the doctor's hand, a quick thrust is exerted, which originates from the doctor's thorax, moves through the patient's folded arms, and results in an effective separation of the spinous processes, inducing flexion.

Correctly performed, adjustments such as these provide quick results, and may be pivotal in relieving otherwise persistent undiagnosed low back pain. If sacroiliac dysfunction is also found, appropriate manipulation is performed at this level. Myofascial trigger points of the quadratus lumborum, iliocostalis lumborum, and other paraspinal muscles are commonly found in these persistent pain syndromes and will require local digital pressure or stretch and spray techniques. As in all mechanical spinal conditions, occupational and postural reeducation will be given for complete resolution of the dysfunction. Maigne's syndrome is a facet syndrome of the transitional thoracolumbar spine and is frequently missed because of the emphasis placed on the lumbosacral area during examination.

ity remains very obscure and ill-defined at this time, and the realm of non-surgical management has not been adequately explored.

Postsurgical Syndrome Associated with Compensatory Hypermobility

Although a low back postsurgical patient is not often referred to a chiropractor for follow-up care, many patients seek our services independently, as they experience the many residuals attendant to surgical intervention of the spine. It has been our experience that manipulation and flexion-distraction mobilization serve to complement rehabilitation following diverse surgical interventions. It has been observed that ankylosis or fusion of joints may result in compensatory increase of movement in adjacent articulations. Brooks examined 38 ankylosed sacroiliac joints postmortem and found that 81% showed a very free range of motion much in excess of normal at the lumbosacral joint. The remaining 19% showed ankylosis at both SI and lumbosacral joints, yet with compensatory increased mobility at the lumbar spine (53). According to Coventry, patients who have undergone fusion of L4-5 or L5-S1 segments sometimes report a different pattern of pain localized near the posterior haunch area ipsilateral to the now irritable SI joint. Previously neither irritability nor increase in mobility had been found. In some cases the compensatory mobility occurred at the L3-4 segment and not the SI joint (54). It has been theorized that stiffness produced by the fusion protects the area and subsequent strains affect the area above it with resultant spondylosis and stenosis (55).

Manipulation and soft tissue techniques may be an excellent inclusion in the treatment and rehabilitation plan for postsurgical patients when fibrosis and decreased range of motion are evident in adjacent structures.

Common Muscle Syndromes

Imbalances of muscle length and strength are not traditionally viewed as diagnostic entities in low back pain. With increasing attention being given to aberrant movements of joints and greater understanding of how these dysfunctions are produced, the diagnosis of chronic postural strain is probably highly accurate as well as common. We propose that it may be the underlying mechanical diagnosis behind the final diagnosis of record, which attempts only to identify the tissue of pain origin. The muscular components to posture were described by Kendall and Kendall (13) and Walther (14), with their attention being focused on the weakened muscles. More recently, Janda and Lewit studied the role of the postural muscles that exhibit shortness as their major pathomechanical expression. Furthermore, it has been noted that there are predictable muscle patterns that behave in this fashion. The result of their overactivity is the inhibition of the antagonist groups of muscles, resulting in their weakness. This chronic imbalance will produce altered statics, i.e., abnormal postures, and the sequelae to this are aberrant function and faulty movement patterns. Table 20.5 summarises the function, dysfunction, and treatment of muscle patterns (56).

One of the patterns of interest in the lumbopelvic region is the lower crossed syndrome of Lewit, in which the postural muscles are typically found to be shortened and tight and their antagonist phasic muscles are found to be weak (12). The following muscle groups have postural function and thus tend to be shortened: the hip flexors (rectus femoris, tensor fascia lata, and iliopsoas), the hip adductors, and the lumbar erector spinae. Those muscles with antagonist function to the above behave phasically and are the hip extensors, the hip abductors, the abdominals, and the lumbar flexors.

This clinical finding produces a static posture of increased lumbar lordosis, anteriorly tilted innominates, and protuberant abdomen

Table 20.5.
Function, Dysfunction, and Treatment of Muscle Patterns

	Postural	Phasic
Muscle type	slow	fast
Function	postural statics	active movements
Dysfunctional tendency	shortening	weakening
Results of dysfunction	inhibits antagonist	faulty movement patterns
Treatment	postisometric relaxation	remedial exercises

with ramifications continuing up the kinematic chain, producing increased thoracic kyphos and forward head carriage. In the lumbar spine, weight bearing will be transmitted via the facet articulations to a greater extent than normal, which is an established mechanism for the production of pain (see facet syndrome; 57). Thus the treatment of articular dysfunction with manipulation may become "aspirin" manipulation unless it is only a component of the comprehensive rehabilitation of the patient, which in this case clearly requires muscle relaxation techniques in order to minimize the postural strain. Treatment of such muscle imbalances has classically been to address the weakened structures by giving strengthening exercises. Janda has shown, however, that the weak muscle exhibits far less strength of contraction when it is tested prior to achieving adequate length of the postural antagonist. Thus therapy involves postisometric relaxation (or other muscle relaxation/lengthening techniques) to lengthen the short muscle and later remedial movement pattern reeducation followed by proprioceptive rehabilitation (16). Figure 20.4 demonstrates the evaluation of iliopsoas length in which position postisometric relaxation may be performed.

Extraspinal Articular Dysfunctions or Asymmetries and Their Roles in the Production of Low Back Pain

Nonspecific low back pain (pain to which tissue-specific diagnosis cannot be applied) is a common finding in the arena of low back disorders. The nagging backache is often found to be relieved by altering faulty postures, stretching postural muscles, strengthening weakened ones, and/or correcting malalignment of the lower extremities. Chiropractic views joint dysfunction in the context of dysfunction in the kinematic chain of the spine and lower extremities. Lewit coined the phrase "functional pathology of the locomotor system," which takes into account the statics of connective tissue adaptations and the ways in which these influence function, primarily locomotion (12). Indeed this concept has developed independently in many corners of the world of manual arts, including chiropractic and osteopathy.

HIP JOINT CAPSULAR TIGHTNESS

In examination of the ranges of motion at the hip joint, internal rotation is frequently found to be limited. Apparently this direction is sus-

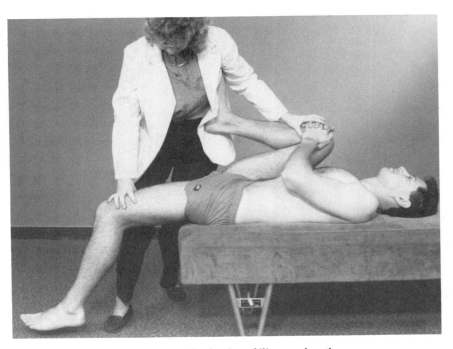

Figure 20.4.   Evaluation of iliopsoas length.

ceptible to early restriction because the piriformis muscle has a tendency to shortness because of its postural activity, resulting in limited passive internal rotation, which eventually may precipitate a loss of extensibility of the capsule and with time becomes one component in the capsular pattern described by Cyriax (10). This loss of internal rotation may affect the ability of the hip to participate fully in the rotatory function of the lower extremity during gait. In this case, the pelvis and spine will rotate excessively in the transverse plane to accommodate the needed motion with resultant aberrant movement of the spinal and pelvic articulations.

The second common example at the hip involves a loss of extension range of motion (usually as a result of hip flexor postural shortening, which in turn may produce capsular adaptations) which is commensurate with the capsular pattern. Loss of hip extension at toe-off may cause an increase in anterior tilt of the pelvis when it should have a relative posterior tilt (58). This will produce relative anterior movement of the ipsilateral lumbar spine in that phase of gait, which may result in abnormal torsional strain with attendant lumbar joint dysfunction.

Treatment of these commonly restricted ranges of hip motion includes postisometric relaxation of the affected shortened muscle, hip joint mobilization (and manipulation), and passive stretches for the home exercise program. Figure 20.5 illustrates one mobilization procedure for the hip joint. Thus the restoration of normal hip flexibility is necessary for optimal function and rehabilitation of a symptomatically expressive low back.

STRUCTURAL MALALIGNMENT OF THE LOWER EXTREMITIES

The second group of disorders that contribute to the etiology of chronic postural strain and related low back conditions may be classified as structural malalignments. These may be hereditary, congenital-developmental (e.g., excessive femoral anteversion), traumatic (fracture), the product of surgical intervention (prosthesis), physiologic-developmental (genu valgum associated with obesity), or the result of metabolic and endocrine diseases.

The most commonly seen malalignments are anatomical leg length disparity, foot and knee postural aberration, and increased femoral anteversion with increased external tibial torsion

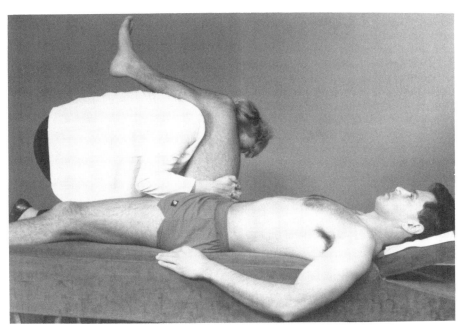

Figure 20.5.   Mobilization procedure for the hip joint.

and genu valgum. This last situation is caused by congenital torsional abnormalities of bone that are not affected by manipulative procedures or orthotic devices and thus will not be addressed in the following section.

Anatomical Leg Length Inequality

Discrepancies in actual (anatomical) leg length of 5 to 7 mm have been found in about 25 to 35% of the population (59) and correlations have been noted between the incidence of leg length inequality (LLI) and low back and hip pain (60, 61). The traditional methods of direct measurement (using bony landmarks in the supine-lying position) have been demonstrated to have no reliability for either inter- or intraexaminer observations (62). The only method that demonstrated any reliability in Woerman's study was the indirect assessment of the standing palpation of iliac crest heights. Thus, clinical suspicion of LLI is made during the postural exam where unlevel iliac crests are seen. Triano has established criteria which need to be met to determine suitability for lift therapy (63):

1. Lumbar convexity is on the side of the low iliac crest,
2. Vertebral bodies are rotated into the convexity of curve,
3. Sacral base is low on the side of the low iliac crest.

Having identified the above, the doctor examines the lower extremities for signs of correctible flexible flat foot on the side of the low iliac crest, and associated increased Q angle (formed by the axes of the patellar tendon and the quadriceps mechanism) at the knee. These should be corrected as much as possible by means of a protocol that we now use, incorporating muscle length and strength correction, proprioceptive reeducation on a rocker board, the "short foot" described by Janda (57), and manipulation of the foot and related articulations. Following a reasonable length of time with this protocol, conscientiously applied, any adaptations that are likely to occur should have taken place. The patient is reexamined for excessive pronation. Lack of response will probably necessitate the application of an orthotic device to correct the faulty foot subtalar or midtarsal joint mechanics. If this correction of the foot does not bring about sufficient correction of the unlevelling of the pelvis, and the patient's spine meets the radiographic criteria listed above, the pelvis is examined for signs of gross pelvic joint torsional asymmetry (64). If this is not a factor, the patient is now a candidate for radiographic assessment of LLI.

The plain film modified scanogram is a useful radiographic method for establishing the length and site of anatomical leg length disparity (65). The net result of this important consideration is a comprehensive management approach to chronic back pain, rather than a reductionist approach, which often creates only temporary relief.

Foot and Knee Postural Aberration

We have already acknowledged that the integrity of the base of support is necessary for optimal function of spinal articulations and associated soft tissue structures. With long-standing malalignment of the bony constituents of the lower extremities, soft tissue adaptation occurs. Acquired bilateral flexible flatfoot will usually produce an internally rotated stance of both femurs (with attendant medial knee strain) and/or increased valgus at the knee. Associated with this posture is an anterior tilt of the pelvis and increased lumbar lordosis with attendant clinical consequences. Consequently, the patient must be evaluated for aberration of foot and knee function and treated accordingly. We have already mentioned the inclusion of rocker board exercises in the treatment of the flexible flatfoot. However, in the case of so many other disorders of foot alignment, the use of orthoses may be extremely beneficial in the comprehensive approach to managing low back pain.

Contraindications

Little appears in the literature on the prevention of complication from spinal manipulative therapy (SMT), probably because the extreme situations (even fatal consequences from cervical manipulation on certain patients) are extremely rare, yet are too frequently the alibi invoked to discredit manipulation (66). Nonetheless, complications from SMT should obviously be prevented, and a rationale for that prevention may be based on understanding: (1) the causes of reported complications of SMT, (2) the contraindications to SMT, and the (3) diagnostic assessment of patients prior to SMT.

Contraindications for certain forms of SMT can be grossly classified under the six categories discussed below. It is important to note that some of the conditions necessitate less aggressive forms of SMT and, when adequately performed, can be of great benefit to the patient. Some of the conditions require referral to other branches of the health care system. The chiropractor's training enables him or her to make such decisions.

LACK OF SKILL AND DIAGNOSTIC ABILITY

Lack of skill by the practitioner may often result in aggravation or exacerbation of symptoms that would ordinarily be relieved by appropriate manipulation (66–68). Excellent diagnostic acumen does not supplant the need for manipulative skill in the application of SMT (10). Lack of proper diagnosis, when coupled with inadequate skills or rational technique, can cause considerable harm (67, 69). Doctrinal antipathy toward diagnosis, and the failure to perform a proper mechanical and physiological evaluation of the spine and thence to manipulate accordingly, have been considered potential causes of injury (70).

TUMORS AND BONY INFECTIONS

Any bone-weakening disease predisposes the patient to serious consequences if manipulation is applied without adequate evaluation. In those patients who have a suspicious history, who do not readily respond to manipulative card, whose pain is exacerbated at night, and in whom pain is not altered by different postures, further evaluation is indicated, including special imaging procedures and lab studies. Manipulation is contraindicated at the site of the lesion until any infection is managed, or local tumor is ruled out (35). Malignancy generally is not a contraindication in and of itself unless it involves the tissue in question for manipulation.

TRAUMATIC INJURIES

Major trauma resulting in the hypermobility which accompanies the severe sprain and strain of the affected tissues is clearly a contraindication for manipulation at the specific site (71).

This does not, however, rule out the appropriateness of manipulation at juxtaposed regions of hypomobility or soft tissue therapy at the specific site. Furthermore, mobilization applied early in the course of care for joints affected by mild and moderate sprain shows improved outcomes when compared with the traditional approach of immobilization and analgesics (72). Compression fractures resulting from impaction stress, may require traction techniques at the site of the lesion, and the juxtaposed dysfunctional (hypomobile) segments should be gently treated with mobilization and manipulation to aid in efficient healing (35).

METABOLIC AND ARTHRITIC DISORDERS

When patients with osteoporosis present with musculoskeletal pain, they may still be excellent candidates for gentle manipulation or mobilization that avoids aggressive rotary forces, which might otherwise increase the chance for fracture—particularly of the ribs. Patients with rheumatoid or psoriatic arthritis or ankylosing spondylitis benefit from the timely application of manipulation, but not during the inflammatory or erosive periods of the diseases (73). However, they must be carefully screened for joint instability, particularly in the upper cervical region.

DRUG THERAPY

Anticoagulant therapy and SMT are not compatible since hemmorrhage may result from trivial events, even those less forceful than manipulation (74).

VASCULAR CONSIDERATIONS

Vascular catastrophes such as abdominal aortic dissection or rupture of abdominal aortic aneurysms may not yield signs or symptoms of an impending crisis (75), but in a patient with increased vascular risks, noted palpatory pulse and auscultatory aberration and radiographic evidence of vessel dilatation, rotary or forceful posterior to anterior thrusts may be contraindicated.

NEUROLOGIC CONSIDERATIONS

Rotary side posture manipulation has been touted as disastrous in cases of disc herniation, particularly with hard neurologic findings (76, 77). There is opposition to the theory by those who think that the clinically determined herniation should properly be viewed as the end point of a series of compressive, torsional, and bending injuries, rather than a sudden result of an abnormal force such as lifting too great a load or receiving a single inappropriate manipulation (78, 79). Nonetheless, a thorough neurologic evaluation is necessary prior to initiation of manipulation to rule out the possibility of precipitating a cauda equina syndrome or disc prolapse. It is interesting to note that this is also an arbitrary restriction that has been self-imposed both by those manipulating the spine, and by those who know nothing of manipulation, although there is no conclusive evidence that these situations are, in fact, aggravated and not helped by manipulation. Cassidy reports favorable results in patients with confirmed disc herniations who have been treated with rotary side posture manipulation, throwing further into question certain suppositions previously held (31). Hard neurologic signs warrant constant monitoring but, in the absence of cauda equina symptoms, are not a reason to discontinue manipulation. Naturally, if they rapidly progress and the condition of the patient continues to deteriorate, surgical consultation is needed.

Benefits of Manipulation

Although the scope of this chapter does not allow for an expansive description of the benefits associated with manipulation, we feel that a brief mention of the major ones is essential to increase awareness of this subject.

PHYSIOLOGIC EFFECTS

The physiologic benefits from manipulation are under much study and comprise four major areas: restoration of normalized movement, relief from pain, normalization of muscle hyperactivity, and reflex effects.

In order to appreciate that manipulation (passively induced motion) may have beneficial effects on movement of the joint manipulated, consideration must first be given to the histological effects of immobilization on joints. Akeson and colleagues have demonstrated that periods of prolonged total immobilization result in an increase in collagen synthesis, with cross-linking between collagen fibrils. Fibrofatty material is formed between joint surfaces, which leads to the formation of adhesions (80). Farfan proposes the production of a "contracted capsule" that would result in loss of range of motion, which could be produced in four basic ways:

1. Scar formation of the capsule or capsular ligament does not have the same extensibility as normal ligament.
2. Scar formation may occur between 2 ligamentous bundles that need to move independently.
3. A scar formed within a ligament may increase the thickness such that its overall length is reduced.
4. In a "creeping subluxation," the outside of the capsule may become "plastered down" to the periosteum of the articular processes of the joint, resulting in fibrocartilaginous metaplasia. The sequela to this is shortening of the capsule and synovium, with resultant loss of joint excursion (81).

Farfan considered the periarticular structures to be more significant in the production of loss of range of motion than intraarticular inclusions (meniscoids) or intraarticular adhesions, although both of these have been well documented (82–84). In the spine specifically, scarring between different lamellae of the disc or between various independently moving bundles of a capsular ligament is a mechanism that results in loss of range of motion. As scar tissue will fail under a smaller deforming load than normal tissue, when a normal load is rapidly applied (as in manipulation), the scar tissue will be stretched and altered without concomitant injury to the normal tissues. Furthermore, controlled passive or active movements of joints have been shown to improve the rate of tendon repair, and the gliding function of tendon sheaths during repair. Salter demonstrated that passively induced movement promoted the healing of full-thickness defects in articular surfaces, and subsequently went on to apply this principle in clinical orthopaedics (85). Passive motion has been shown to reverse the effects on connective tissue of stress-deprivation (immobility) such as inhibition of healing, the formation of joint contractures, diminished elasticity of periarticular structures (86). These mechanisms may explain some of the effects of manipulation and mobilisation on joints with established articular or muscular restrictions.

Relief from pain is the most obvious immediate response to manipulation. Pain thresholds are apparently lowered in the presence of somatic lesions (dysfunction, subluxation complexes) and these are elevated upon the application of manipulation (87). Several mechanisms have been proposed for this phenomenon, one of which is the short-term increase in circulating plasma beta-endorphin levels, which has been noted following manipulation and not following placebo "laying on of hands" (88). Temporary analgesic effects are attributed to the endorphins, and thus long-term pain relief is not explained by this mechanism. Long-term studies are not as plentiful as their short-term counterparts; however, Cassidy has demonstrated lasting effect for both functional improvement as well as pain relief following a course of chiropractic manipulation (23).

Several studies have demonstrated short-term reduction in the muscle activity of paraspinal musculature following manipulation (89, 90) and thus some techniques of manipulation, particularly the muscle energy approach of Mitchell (91), are geared specifically to the anatomical orientation of muscle fibers and generate quick stretch as the method of increasing joint mobility (92). It is important to note, however, that there are joints in the body that are not directly individually controlled by specific muscles (namely, the sacroiliac, and acromioclavicular) that derive their movement indirectly by way of a controlling joint (such as the hip controls the SI joint) yet readily undergo dysfunction (93). Thus the mechanical effect of manipulation cannot be limited to muscle stretch alone. Furthermore, Lewit has described the persistence of articular blockage in the cervical spine of patients under general anesthesia, in whom muscle activity clearly had no influence on joint range of motion (94). Thus manipulation will have an effect on both the contractile and inert elements surrounding the joint.

Experimental evidence has demonstrated increased activity in muscles distant from the site of painful stimulus, lending credence to the clinical cycle of pain-spasm-pain (Travell). Muscle spasm is itself a source of chemically mediated pain, and may also be a source of mechanically mediated pain via nociceptors in the walls of blood vessels supplying the affected muscle (95). Thus, interruption in either the painful portion of the cycle or the muscle spasm portion may occur with manipulation. In this way, function and well-being may be restored. This exciting arena looks very promising for further investigation.

FUNCTIONAL IMPROVEMENT

Although most of the clinical trials done to date use pain alteration as their parameter for success, few studies have measured changes in function to define treatment success (96). In one such study Kirkaldy-Willis and Cassidy evaluated 171 people who had been disabled for an average of 7.6 years because of low back pain. Following a 2 to 3-week regimen of daily chiropractic manipulation, 87% returned to full function with no restriction for work or other activities. Significantly, that success rate was maintained at 12-month follow-up, and no patient was made worse (97). This study and modifications should be repeated in other clinical settings in order to help scientifically objectify the positive functional gains that chiropractors find commonplace in daily practice.

COST EFFECTIVENESS

Since 1960 there have been no fewer than eight studies concerning cost effectiveness of chiropractic in the United States. Included in those reports are two government inquiries [New Zealand, 1979 (98) and Sweden, 1987 (99)] whose results indicate that chiropractic care is not only cost effective, but is also treatment effective; increased government funding for chiropractic services was recommended in both cases. Several worker's compensation board studies have been performed [California, 1972 (100), Wisconsin, 1978 (101), and Florida, 1987 (102)], which all favor chiropractic and suggest a significant savings in health care costs for low back pain when that care is chiropractic rather than the traditional medical approach.

There is another facet to cost effectiveness that has to do with the manner in which patients are diagnosed and treatment is initiated. An initial visit to the family physician usually requires referral to a specialist (neurologist, orthopedist) with whom the clinical examination and special diagnostic studies are performed. Specialized imaging studies may follow this, and only then is a working diagnosis rendered and the patient finally referred for physical therapy. In contrast with this, the initial visit to the chiropractor usually results in an examination with plain film radiography, rendering an immediate working diagnosis (unless further imaging or electrodiagnostics are indicated) and initiation of treatment. Despite the increased number of subsequent visits necessitated by manual care over medication, the time period of care has been described as shorter when compared with medical treatment (103), and may result in the patient's returning to work earlier (104).

PATIENT PERCEPTION

The results of clinical trials investigating the effect of manipulation and low back pain indicate that the patient's perception of chiropractic treatment typically is very positive (105). In a study performed by the Center for Health Promotion at an HMO in Seattle, it was found that patients of chiropractors were more satisfied with the "overall care" they received than were patients of family physicians. Chiropractic patients were more satisfied with the "concrete positive approach to treatment and provider's understanding of the patient's concerns" (106). Although patient response is not considered as objective as the research critiques suggest, the importance of this human factor cannot be overlooked as we continue to investigate which treatment protocols are most efficacious in treating low back pain.

SUMMARY

Recent trends in treating back pain emphasize the principles of early rehabilitation to restore function over the out-dated approach that focuses on bed rest and movement restriction. Time can no longer be considered the healer, because stiffness and predisposition to injury are very real consequences of failure to intervene therapeutically and often necessitate more exhaustive care later (105). There is evidence to suggest that the pharmacological relief of pain may not be the optimal treatment of choice in low back pain management, but rather that the restoration of motion may be an alternative goal. Relief of pain with medication has not been shown to enhance the healing of spinal tissues. On the contrary, an individual who is rendered pain-free may be more apt to return to strenuous activity and thus strain soft tissues that lack extensibility and flexibility (105). All

treatments are ineffective with some patients. There will be those people who do not respond to decompression, microdiscectomy and other surgical procedures because the stenosis or disc herniation visualized on imaging is often not the source of the symptoms experienced. Many times the etiology is mechanical-postural, causing facet, sacroiliac, or muscle syndromes. Likewise, some patients will not respond to manipulation and related therapy because the etiology of their pain is not associated with subluxation complex or manipulable lesion. It is difficult to contest, however, that early therapy for low back pain patients (with the exception of cauda equina syndrome) should begin with conservative care. This consists of manipulation, mobilization, soft tissue manipulation, electrical and nonelectrical adjunctive modalities, rehabilitative exercise, and postural and proprioceptive reeducation. The benefits of manipulation in acute low back pain are well established in the literature, although randomized clinical trials designed for long-term follow-up are definitely lacking. The field is wide open and demands research to objectify the positive clinical responses the chiropractor enjoys daily in clinical practice.

References

1. Lomax E. Manipulative therapy: A historical perspective from ancient times to the modern era. In Goldstein M. Research status of spinal manipulative therapy (NINCDS No 15). Bethesda, MD: US Dept of HEW, 1975.
2. Grieve G. Common vertebral joint problems. New York: Churchill Livingstone, 1981.
3. Gillet H, Liekens M. Belgian Chiropractic Research Notes. Huntington Beach, CA: Motion Palpation Institute, 1981.
4. White AA, Panjabi MM. Clinical biomechanics of the spine. Philadelphia: JB Lippincott, 1978.
5. Korr I. The concept of facilitation and its origins. Symposium on the functional implications of segmental facilitation. J Am Osteopath Assn 1955; 54:265–268.
6. Chaitow L. Soft tissue manipulation. Wellingborough, UK: Thorsons, 1987.
7. Travell JG, Simons DG. Myofascial pain and dysfunction: The trigger point manual. Baltimore: Williams & Wilkins, 1983.
8. Schafer C, Faye LJ. Motion palpation and chiropractic technic. Principles of dynamic chiropractic. Huntington Beach, CA: Motion Palpation Institute, 1989.
9. Mennell JMcM. Joint pain. Boston: Little, Brown and Company, 1964.

10. Cyriax J. Textbook of orthopedic medicine. Vol. I, 8th ed. London: Ballière Tindall, 1982.

11. Jull GA, Janda V. Muscles and motor control in low back pain. In Twomey L, Taylor J, eds. Assessment and management in physical therapy of the low back. New York: Churchill Livingstone, 1987.

12. Lewit K. Manipulative therapy in rehabilitation of the motor system. London: Butterworth, 1985.

13. Kendall FP, McCreary EK. Muscles: Testing and function. 3rd ed. Baltimore: Williams & Wilkins, 1983.

14. Walther D. Applied kinesiology. Pueblo Colorado: The International College of Applied Kinesiology, 1981.

15. Faucret B. Lumbopelvic technique. Lecture series: Los Angeles College of Chiropractic, 1986.

16. Janda V. Muscles, central nervous motor regulation. In Korr IM, ed. The neurobiologic mechanisms in manipulative therapy. New York: Plenum Press, 1978.

17. Buerger AA. A non-redundant taxonomy of spinal manipulative techniques. Man Med 1981; 1:54-55.

18. Nwuga VC. Manipulation of the spine. Baltimore: Williams & Wilkins, 1976.

19. Neumann HD. A concept of manual medicine. Osteop Ann 1981; 9:11-13.

20. Greenland MS, Reisbord LS, Haldeman S, Buerger AA. Controlled clinical trials of manipulation. J Occup Med 1980; 22:670-676.

21. Ward R, Sprafka S. Glossary of osteopathic terminology. J Am Osteopath Assoc 1981; 80:552-567.

22. Grice A. A biomechanical approach to cervical and dorsal adjusting. In Haldeman S, ed. Modern developments in the principles and practice of chiropractic. New York: Appleton-Century-Crofts, 1980.

23. Kirkaldy-Willis WH. ed. Managing low back pain. 2nd ed. New York: Churchill Livingstone, 1988.

24. Deyo R. Conservative therapy for low back pain. JAMA 1983; 250(8):1057-1062.

25. Cailliet R. Soft tissue pain and disability. New York: FA Davis, 1977.

26. Farfan HF. Biomechanics of the lumbar spine. in Kirkaldy-Willis WH, Managing low back pain, 2nd ed. New York: Churchill Livingstone, 1988.

27. Ponte DJ, Jensen GJ, Kent BE. A preliminary report on the use of the McKenzie protocol versus Williams protocol in the treatment of low back pain. J Orthop Sports Phys Ther 1984; 6(2):130-139.

28. Reinert O. Divserified technique. Chesterfield, MO: Logan College of Chiropractic, 1982.

29. Gonstead C. Seminar notes on Gonstead technique, Mount Horeb, Wisconsin.

30. McKenzie R. Mechanical diagnosis and treatment of the lumbar spine. Upper Hutt, New Zealand: Spinal Publications, 1981.

31. Quon JA, Cassidy JD, O'Connor SM, Kirkaldy-Willis, WH. Lumbar intervertebral disc herniation: Treatment by rotational manipulation. J Manip Phys Ther 1989; 12:220-227.

32. Gitelman R. A chiropractic approach of biomechanical disorders of the lumbar spine and pelvis. In Haldeman S, ed. Modern developments in the principles and practice of chiropractic. New York: Appleton-Century-Crofts, 1980.

33. Sandoz R. Newer trends in the pathogenesis of spinal disorders. Ann Swiss Chirop Assoc 1971; 5:93.

34. Janda V. Visiting scholar's program, second annual interdisciplinary symposium. Whittier, CA: Los Angeles College of Chiropractic, 1988.

35. Cox J. Low back pain. Baltimore: Williams & Wilkins, 1985.

36. Wedge JH. Differential diagnosis in low back pain in Kirkaldy-Willis WH, ed. Managing low back pain. 2nd ed. New York: Churchill Livinstone, 1988.

37. Illi F. Sacroiliac mechanism: Keystone of spinal balance and body locomotion. Lombard, IL: National College of Chiropractic, 1940.

38. Cohen AS, McNeill IM et al. The 'normal' sacroiliac joint. Amer J Roentgenol Rad Ther Nuc Med 1967; 100:559.

39. Colachis SC, Warden RE et al. Movement of the sacroiliac joint in the adult male. Arch Phys Med Rehab 1963; 44:490.

40. Eglund N, Olsson TH, Schmid H, Selvick G. Movements in the sacroiliac joint demonstrated with roentgen stereophotogrammetry. Acta Radiol 1978; 19:883.

41. Norman GF, May A. Sacroiliac conditions simulating IVD syndrome. Western J Surg Obstet Gynecol 1956; 64:461-462.

42. Illi F. The vertebral column—life-line of the body. Lombard, IL: National College of Chiropractic, 1951.

43. Lewis T, Kellgren JH. Observations related to referred pain, viscero-motor reflexes. Clin Sci 1939; 4:47.

44. Proctor D, DuPuis. Thoracolumbar syndrome as a cause of low back pain: a report of 2 cases. J Can Chirop Assoc 1985; 29(2)71-73.

45. Yong-Hing K. Surgical Technique. In Kirkaldy-Willis WH. ed. Managing low back pain. 2nd ed. New York: Churchill Livingstone, 1988.

46. Yochum T, Rowe L. Essentials of skeletal radiology. Vol I. Baltimore: Williams & Wilkins, 1987.

47. Friberg O. Lumbar instability: A dynamic approach by traction—Compression radiography. Spine 1987; 12:(2):119-29.

48. Faye LJ. Motion palpation of the spine. Seminars by Motion Palpation Institute Huntington Beach, CA, 1981.

49. Dupuis PR, Yong-Hing K, Cassidy JD, Kirkaldy-Willis WH. Radiologic diagnosis of degenerative lumbar spinal instability. Spine 1985; 10(3):262–276.
50. Stokes IAF, Frymoyer JW. Segmental motion and instability. Spine 1987; 12:688–691.
51. Morgan MP, King T. Primary instability of lumbar vertebra as a common cause of low back pain. J Bone Joint Surg 1957; 1(39B):6–22.
52. Hubka MJ, Hubka MA. Conservative management of idiopathic hypermobility and early lumbar instability using proprioceptive rehabilitation: A report of 2 cases. J Chirop Tech 1989; 1(3):88–93.
53. Brooke R. The sacroiliac joint. J Anat 1924; 58:299.
54. Coventry MB, Taper EM. Pelvic instability. J Bone Joint Surg 1972; 54A:83.
55. Cameron AJR, Shepel LF. Psychological Assessment in Kirkaldy-Willis WH, ed. Managing low back pain. 2nd ed. New York: Churchill Livingstone, 1988.
56. Liebenson C. Active muscular relaxation techniques, Part II. (Clinical Application). J Manip Phys Ther 1990; 13(1):2–6.
57. Janda V. Lectures to Los Angeles College of Chiropractic, Whittier, CA. 1988–1989.
58. Thurston AJ, Harris JD. Normal kinematics of the lumbar spine and pelvis. Spine 1983; 8(3):199–205.
59. Banks S, Willis J. Anatomical leg length inequality—Current thinking. Literature Review 1985; 1(1):1–6.
60. Giles LGF. Leg length inequalities associated with low back pain. J Can Chirop Assoc 1976; 20:25–32.
61. Friberg O. Clinical symptoms and biomechanics of lumbar spine and hip joint in leg length inequality. Spine 1983; 8:643.
62. Woerman AL, Binder-MacLeod SA. Leg length discrepancy assessment: Accuracy and precision in five clinical methods of evaluation. J Orthop Sports Phys Ther 1984; 5:230.
63. Triano JJ. Objective electromyographic evidence for use and effects of lift therapy. J Manip Phys Ther 1983; 6:13–16.
64. Lawrence D, Pugh, J, Tasharski C, Heinze W. Evaluation of a radiographic method determining short leg mensuration. J Chiro 1984; 21:57.
65. Winterstein JF. The "short leg" syndrome. Digest Chiro Econ 1974; 16:78–82.
66. Kleynhans AM, Terrett AGJ. The prevention of complications from spinal manipulative therapy. In Glasgow EF, Twomey LT, Sculler ER, Kleynhans AM, Idczak RM, eds. Aspects of Manipulative Therapy. 2nd ed. Edinburgh: Churchill Livingstone, 1985.
67. Maigne R. Orthopedic medicine: A new approach to vertebral manipulation. Springfield, IL: Charles C Thomas, 1972.
68. Cyriax J. Textbook of orthopaedic medicine. Vol. 2. London: Ballière-Tindall, 1972.
69. Kaiser VG. The manual therapy of the spine and its indications. Orthop Traumatol 1973; 11.
70. Sandoz RM. About some problems pertaining to the choice of indications for chiropractic therapy. Ann Swiss Chirop Assoc 1965; 3:210.
71. Gatterman M. Contraindications and complications to spinal manipulative therapy. J Chiro 1981; 15:82–84.
72. Mealy K, Brennan H, Fenelon GCC. Early mobilization of acute whiplash injuries. Br Med J 1986; 292(8):656, 657.
73. Haldeman S. Spinal manipulative therapy in the management of low back pain. In Finnesson B, ed. Low back pain, 2nd ed. Philadelphia: J B Lippincott, 1980.
74. Dabbert O. Spinal meningioma hematoma warfarin therapy and chiropractic adjustment. JAMA 1970; 214:11.
75. Hadler N. Regional low back pain. N Engl J Med 1986; 315(17):1090–1091.
76. Janse J. Principles and practice of chiropractic: An anthology. Hildebrandt R, ed. Lombard, IL: National College of Chiropractic, 1976.
77. Winterstein JF. Acute lumbar disc syndrome. Lecture notes, National College of Chiropractic, Lombard IL.
78. Bogduk N, Hutton B. Lecture to the International Congress of Chiropractic, October 1988, Sydney, Australia.
79. Farfan HF. Mechanical disorders of the low back. Philadelphia: Lea and Febiger, 1973.
80. Frank C, Akeson WH, Woo SL-Y, Amiel D, Coutts RD. Physiology and therapeutic value of passive joint motion. Clin Orthop Rel Res 1984; (185):113–125.
81. Farfan HF: The scientific basis of manipulative procedures. Clin Rheum Dis 1980; 6:159–177.
82. Giles LGF: Lumbar apophyseal joint arthrography. J Manip Phys Ther 1984; 7(1):21–24.
83. Bogduk N, Engel R. The menisci of the lumbar zygapophyseal joints: A review of their anatomy and clinical significance. Spine 1984; 9(5):454–460.
84. Rahlman J. Mechanisms of intervertebral joint fixation: A literature review. J Manip Phys Ther 1987; 10(4):177–187.
85. Salter RB, Simmonds DF, Malcom BW, Rumble EJ, MacMichael D, Clements ND. The biological effect of continuous passive motion in the healing of full thickness defects in articular cartilage. J Bone Joint Surg 1980; 62A:1232.
86. Akeson WH, Amiel D, Woo SL-Y. Immobility effects on synovial joints: The pathomechanics of joint contracture. Biorheology 1980; 17:95–110.
87. Terrett AC, Vernon H. Manipulation and pain tolerance. Am J Phys Med 1984; 63:217–225.
88. Vernon HT, Dhami MSI, Howley TP, Annett R. Spinal manipulation and beta-endorphin: A

controlled study of the effect of a spinal manipulation on plasma beta-endorphin levels in normal males. J Man Phys Ther 1986; 9(2):115–123.

89. Buerger AA. Experimental models of spinal manual techniques. Man Med 1983; 1:10–17.

90. Grice AS. Muscle tonus changes following manipulation. J Can Chiro Assoc 1974; (Dec):29–31.

91. Mitchell FL, Moran PS, Pruzzo NA. Evaluation and treatment manual of osteopathic manipulative procedures. Privately printed, 1979.

92. Sandoz R. Some physical mechanisms and effects of spinal adjustments. Ann Swiss Chiro Assoc 1976; 6:91–141.

93. Lewit K. The contribution of clinical observation to neurobiological mechanisms in manipulative therapy. In Korr IM, ed. The neurobiological mechanisms in manipulative therapy. New York: Plenum Press, 1978; 4–5.

94. Lewit K. The muscular and articular factor in movement restriction. Man Med 1985; 1:83–85.

95. Roland MO: A critical review of the evidence for a pain-spasm-pain cycle in spinal disorders. Clin Biomech 1986; 1:102–109.

96. Deyo R. Conservative therapy for low back pain. JAMA 1983; 250(8):1057–62.

97. Cassidy JD, Kirkaldy-Willis WH, McGregor M. Spinal manipulation for the treatment of chronic low back pain: An observational study. In Buerger AA, Greenman PE, eds. Empirical approaches to the validation of spinal manipulation. Springfield, IL: Charles C Thomas, 1985.

98. Inglis BD. Chiropractic in New Zealand. Wellington: The New Zealand Commission on Chiropractic, 1979.

99. Commission on Alternative Medicine, Social Departementete. Legitimization for vissa kiropractorer. Stockholm: SOU (Engl. summary), 1987; 12, 13–16.

100. Wolf CR. Industrial back injuries. Internat Rev Chiro 1974; 26:6–7.

101. Duffy DJ. A study of Wisconsin industrial back injury cases. Unpublished Monograph, University of Wisconsin, 1978.

102. Wolk S. An analysis of Florida's worker's compensation medical claims for back related injuries. Arlington, VA: Foundation for Chiropractic Education and Research, 1988.

103. Kane R, Olsen D, Leymaster C, Wooley FR, Fisher FD. Manipulating the patient: A comparison of effectiveness of physician and chiropractor care. Lancet 1974; (6):1333–1336.

104. Farrell JP, Twomey LT. Manipulation in the treatment of low back pain: Comparison of two conservative treatment approaches. Med J Aust 1982; 1:160–164.

105. Brunarski D. Clinical trials of spinal manipulation: a critical appraisal and review of the literature. J Manip Phys Ther 1984; 7(4):243–249.

106. Cherkin D, MacCornack F. Patient evaluations of low back care from family physicians and chiropractors. Western J Med 1989; 150:351–355.

21

FLEXION DISTRACTION MANIPULATION OF THE LOW BACK

James M. Cox

This chapter will be devoted primarily to a particular type of chiropractic spinal manipulation developed in our low back clinic. Flexion distraction manipulation is a form of chiropractic manipulation designed to achieve the following goals: 1. Increase the intervertebral disc height to remove anular distortion in the pain-sensitive peripheral anular fibers; 2. Allow the nucleus pulposus to assume its central position within the anulus and relieve irritation of the pain-sensitive anular peripheral fibers; 3. Restore the vertebral zygapophyseal joints to their physiological relationships of motion; 4. Improve posture and locomotion while relieving pain, improving body functions, and creating a state of well-being.

CLINICAL DIAGNOSIS OF LOW BACK PAIN

Following examination of the patient in our clinic utilizing standard orthopaedic, neurological, and radiographic procedures, we divide our diagnoses of low back pain into one or a combination of 15 categories of etiology:

1. anular tear,
2. nuclear bulge,
3. nuclear protusion,
4. nuclear prolapse,
5. discogenic spondyloarthrosis,
6. facet syndrome,
7. spondylolisthesis,
8. stenosis,
9. iatrogenic back pain,
10. functional low back pain,
11. sprain/strain,
12. subluxation,

13. tropism,
14. transitional segment, and
15. other pathologies.

In this chapter we demonstrate various categories of back pain by clinical and radiographic findings and discuss the manipulative treatment of each.

MANIPULATIVE TREATMENT CONSIDERATIONS

Treatment is designed according to two patient types for manipulative care: patients with low back pain only and those with low back pain and sciatica. Figure 21.1 describes our treatment outline. We do not place zygapophyseal joints through their physiological ranges of motion when the patient has sciatic radiculopathy until the leg pain shows at least 50% relief as noted by subjective patient evaluation and objective signs of straight leg raise, range of thoracolumbar motion, Dejerine's triad, and Kemp's sign. Any patient who has only low back pain, with leg pain not extending below the knee, is treated with full physiological range of motion applied to the facet articulations. Flexion distraction is the first manipulative movement administered, followed by the remaining four normal ranges of motion to be discussed below.

Normal Joint Kinematics

The brevity of this chapter will not allow any great deal of discussion on the clinical background of spinal manipulation. However, the

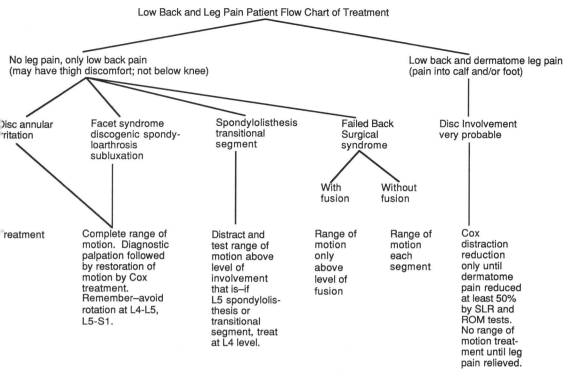

Figure 21.1. Flow chart defining treatment protocol based upon the established diagnosis and findings in the patient.

basic fact that a lumbar facet joint is capable of the movements of flexion, extension, lateral flexion, and rotation, as well as the combination of flexion and lateral flexion known as circumduction, must be considered.

Pearcy (1) measured the ranges of active flexion and extension, axial rotation, and lateral bending in the lumbar spines of normal volunteers in vivo to assess the relation between the primary and accompanying movements in the other planes. He stated that L5-S1 revealed larger movements of flexion and extension than other levels of the lumbar spine although L5-S1 did not demonstrate consistent patterns of equal movement of flexion and extension as seen at other levels of the lumbar spine. Lateral bending at L4-5 and L5-S1 was significantly less mobile than in the upper three levels.

Pearcy found lateral bending of approximately 10° occurring at the upper three lumbar levels, while there was significantly less lateral bending of 6° and 3° at L4-5 and L5-S1 respectively. In flexion and extension, accompanying axial rotation of 2° or more and lateral bending

of 3° or more occurred rarely, and larger accompanying rotation at an intervertebral joint should be considered abnormal. During twisting and sidebending, axial rotation to the right is accompanied by lateral bending to the left and vice-versa at the upper three levels. At L5-S1, axial rotation and lateral bending generally accompany each other in the same direction while L4-5 is a transitional level. During lateral bending, there is generally extension at the upper levels and flexion at L5-S1.

Painful versus Nonpainful Spinal Motion

Mayer studied the range of motion in the lumbar spine in patients with pain versus research subjects.

1. No significant differences between inclinometer techniques and radiographic ranges of motion measurements were found.
2. In normal subjects, lumbar motion accounts for 63% of gross flexion with 37% due to pelvic

motion in the range up to about 90 degrees of flexion.

3. Low back pain subjects exhibit lower gross motion than normal subjects (54%), with the ratio of lumbar flexion to gross flexion decreased (63–43%). Range of motion exercising can significantly increase functional pain-free range both in lumbar (71%) and pelvic motion (39%) over a three week period. (2)

What is Normal Lumbar Lordosis?

Hansson et al. (3) found no difference in the variation of lumbar lordosis on spinal x-rays of men denying any back pain history compared with those of patients claiming low back injury or chronic low back disability. This suggested that the shape of the lumbar lordosis as noted on survey x-ray technique is unimportant as a sign of either acute or chronic low back pain. Physicians can thus omit discussion of minor variations in the amount of lordosis on plain films of the lumbar spine.

Facet Weight Bearing: Normal and Arthritic

Yang and King (4) state that normal, nonarthritic facet joints carry 3 to 25% of the superimposed body weight. If the facet joint is arthritic, the load could be as high as 47%. The transmission of the compressive facet load occurs through contact of the tip of the inferior facet with the pars interarticularis of the vertebra below. Their data also showed that an overloaded facet joint will cause rearward rotation of the inferior facet, resulting in the stretching of the joint capsule. The finite element model predicted an increase in facet load due to a decrease in disc height. They hypothesized that excessive facet loads stretch the facet capsule and can be a cause of low back pain.

Foraminal Compression Mechanics

Rydevik (5) states that the dorsal root ganglion is usually located in the central part of the intervertebral foramen and that functional changes induced by compression of the ganglion can be a consequence of changes in nerve root microcirculation.

Rydevik also notes that there are no measurements performed in vivo on the pressure levels acting on a nerve root as, for example, by

a herniated disc. However, one could extrapolate from existing knowledge on the swelling pressure of a nucleus pulposus. It has been demonstrated in vitro that specimens of nucleus pulposus may generate pressures of several hundred millimeters of mercury if exposed to free fluid within a confined space. If a sequestered fragment of nucleus pulposus is displaced into the foramen, the nearby nerve root could be compressed at high pressure levels by the swelling disc fragment. The pain mechanism in nerve root compression of human peripheral not necessarily by mechanical fiber deformation.

Stenosis of the intervertebral foramen or vertebral canal by facet subluxation, disc protrusion or prolapse, hypertrophic changes of articular facets, ligamentum flavum hypertrophy, or posterior vertebral plate hypertrophy can be responsible for nerve root compression.

Nociceptor Origin of Low Back Pain

Wyck states that the cause of low back pain is irritation of nociceptors instigated by mechanical and/or chemical abnormalities (6). There are three morphological types of nociceptors: (1) unmyelinated fibers in interstitial tissues, (2) free naked nerve endings, and the (3) perivascular nociceptive system in the adventitial layers of unmyelinated blood vessels.

Wyck also points out that the apophyseal capsule contains unmyelinated nerve fibers. They are sensitive to both chemical and mechanical irritation, including high tensions that develop in the facets following disc degeneration and the carrying of more weight. Myogenic back pain is due to the perivascular nociceptive system in the erector muscles.

The substances that irritate these nociceptors include lactic acid, potassium ions, bradykinin, and histamine deriving from breakdown of glycosaminoglycan in the disc. These substances diffuse through the dura to the perineurium where they may produce inflammatory reactions. They can also enter dural sleeves and nerve roots.

Stenosis as a Factor in Back Pain

Stenosis of the vertebral canal is important to the manipulating physician as it determines the severity of patient symptoms and the success of treatment. Clark (7), in estimating the association between low back pain and the vertebral canal size, notes that only a 2 mm decrease in canal size separates persons with and without low back pain. He states that the frequency of small transverse vertebral canal sizes occurring with low back pain has been suggested to be 53% and that the anteroposterior diameters are most variable in the vertebral canal and most frequently associated with low back pain.

Summary of Manipulative Principles

Based upon the above citations, manipulation may be beneficial by increasing spinal range of motion, relieving nociceptor irritation, perhaps equalizing the weight bearing between the anterior weight-bearing column of the lumbar spine (made up of the vertebral body-disc-vertebral body) and the posterior column of the spine the (articular facet), and relieving the compressive forces against the nerve root within the vertebral canal and intervertebral foramen.

SPECIFIC MANIPULATIVE TREATMENT OF LOW BACK DIAGNOSES

Rules on Prior Submission of a Patient to Flexion Distraction

It is extremely important to test the patient's tolerance to distraction manipulation to determine limitations prior to its application. This is done according to rules formulated by Kramer (8).

1. If a decrease of pain can be demonstrated under distraction, traction treatment should be instituted. As a rule, the pain first changes its character. For instance, a lateral pain will be transferred centrally and a sharp lacerating root pain can turn into dull low back pain.

2. On occasion there may be an increase of pain during traction: (a) When shearing forces influence a displaced fragment and detach it completely. Pain will always be increased when the prolapse is medial and near the nerve root. (b) When a prolapse is still within the boundaries of the vertebral margins but during traction has bulged into the spinal cord. (c) When there are adhesions around the nerve root. (d) When there are adhesions in the spinal canal following surgery.

3. Traction is contraindicated in patients who have had an increase of symptoms during

a long period of relaxation such as sleeping at night when there is increase of disc volume.

4. Moreover, traction should not be used in patients with hypermobile segments and muscle insufficiency. Young people with disc degeneration experience very good results with traction treatment.

Testing Procedure Prior to Manipulative Care

In our clinic, we use the following procedure to test the patient's ability to withstand flexion distraction. With the patient lying prone on the treatment table, a thenar contact of the doctor's hand is made upon the spinous process from the first to the fifth lumbar vertebrae while the caudal section of the table is gently pressed downward no more than 1 to 2 inches. No cuffs are placed on the patient for tractive force; rather, the patient's pelvic and lower extremity weight is the only distractive force utilized as the caudal section is distracted downward (Fig. 21.2). If this amount of traction causes pain to the patient, the cuffs are not placed and this distraction technique is not used. In case of an acute low back pain, it may be hours or days before the patient will tolerate any tractive treatment. Occasionally a patient will not be able to tolerate the tractive force at all. It is necessary to test the patient's ability to withstand flexion distraction repeatedly until there is no adverse reaction. If no pain is felt using the patient's weight as a tractive force, proceed to test

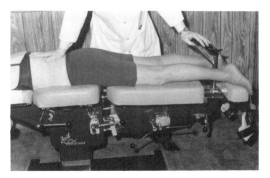

Figure 21.2. Testing patient tolerance to distraction without the ankle cuffs applied. Contact on the spinous process of the lumbar vertebrae is made while applying cephalward pressure to stabilize the vertebral segment. The caudal section is distracted downward 1 to 2 inches while patient evidence of pain or muscle spasm is documented.

lateral distraction by grasping the patient's ankle as shown in Figure 21.3 and test irritation to unilateral distraction. We feel this places stress upon the unilateral facet articulations and will reveal any latent pain probability.

LIMITATION TO DISTRACTIVE FORCE

Never distract downward more than 2 inches with the caudal section at any time in treating the lower lumbar spine. As you progress into the thoracic or cervical spine, you will go down more than 2 inches with the caudal section of the table as you dissipate the distractive force over a longer area of the spinal column.

DESCRIPTION OF A MANIPULATIVE INSTRUMENT

Prior to application of the technique, please note the movements capable with the flexion distraction table as shown. This table is made by the Williams Manufacturing Company for the manipulative procedures demonstrated in this chapter.

Figure 21.4 demonstrates the flexion application, Figure 21.5 extension, Figure 21.6 lateral flexion, and Figure 21.7 rotation by both the thoracic and lumbar section.

FACET SYNDROME

Facet syndrome is a subluxation complex of the articular processes in which increased weight bearing due to intervertebral disc narrowing and degeneration or hypertension subluxation of the superior vertebra on the inferior segment

occurs. Facet capsule irritation, stenosis of the intervertebral foramen, and arthrosis may be the result. Figure 21.8 shows the posterior narrowing of the L5-S1 intervertebral disc space and imbrication of the first sacral facet into the upper third of the intervertebral foramen of the L5-S1 resulting in vertical stenosis of the L5-S1 foramen as compared to the foramen above.

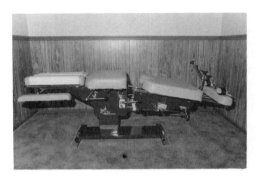

Figure 21.4. Table in the flexion position instrument.

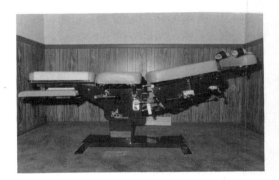

Figure 21.5. Table in the extension position.

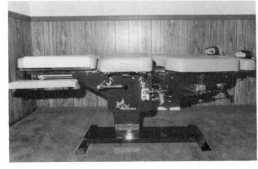

Figure 21.6. Table in the lateral flexion position.

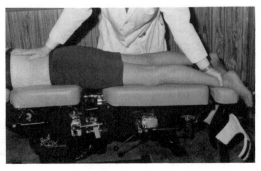

Figure 21.3. Apply unilateral distraction by grasping the ankle and placing the caudal section downward as in Figure 21.2. Again test patient reaction.

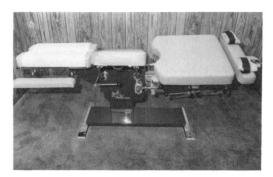

Figure 21.7. Table in the rotation maneuver position.

The radiograph in Figure 21.9 shows Macnab's lines (9) to identify the hyperextension subluxation of L5 on the sacrum with the tip of the superior facet of sacrum imbricating above the line drawn along the inferior plate of L5. The telescoping of the superior facet of sacrum

upward into the intervertebral foramen (IVF) at L5-S1 creates vertical stenosis of the IVF.

Figure 21.10 reveals a stable, normal disc space with no evidence of facet imbrication. Note that the lines drawn along the inferior and superior plate of L5 and sacrum will intersect far posterior to the lumbosacral junction. We feel that in this type of stable articulation there is weight bearing primarily on the disc body with minimal weight bearing on the articular facets at L5-S1.

Treatment

Two types of facet syndrome are identified in our clinic—stable and unstable. Figure 21.11 is a facet syndrome of a stable variety. A stable facet syndrome is determined by Van Akkerveeken (10) measurement showing less than 3 mm of translation of the posterior plates of

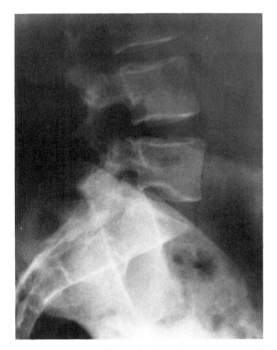

Figure 21.8. Radiograph of a facet syndrome diagnosis at L5-S1. There is posterior narrowing of the L5-S1 intervertebral disc space, with the first sacral facet stenosing the L5-S1 foramen by its vertical telescoping subluxation. Note also the nuclear disc invagination of the L5-S1 disc into the inferior vertebral body plate of L5.

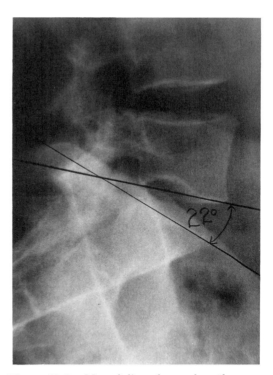

Figure 21.9. Macnab lines drawn along the superior S1 vertebral plate and inferior L5 vertebral plate show them to intersect at the level of the zygapophyseal joints instead of posterior to them. Also the S1 superior facet lies well above the line drawn along the inferior L5 body plate, indicating probable vertical stenosis at the L5-S1 intervertebral foramen. This is termed facet imbrication.

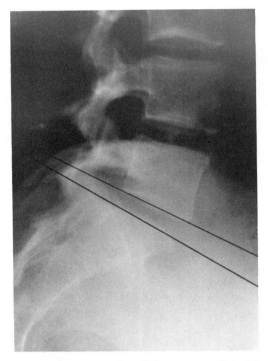

Figure 21.10. The Macnab lines are parallel with no facet imbrication as shown in Figure 21.9. This represents a stable, normal disc-facet relationship.

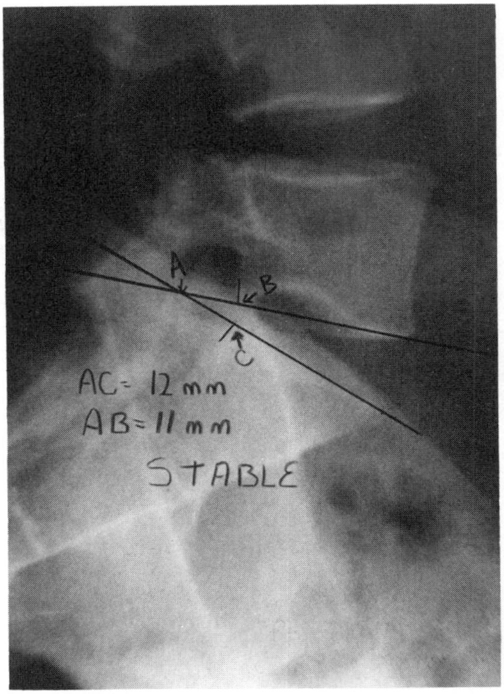

Figure 21.11. Here is a stable facet syndrome as determined by Van Akkerveeken's measurement. There is less than 3 mm of *posterior* malalignment of the L5 body plate on sacrum.

two adjacent functional spinal units on neutral or extension motion. Greater than 3 mm of posterior alignment of one vertebra upon another indicates instability by Van Akkerveeken measurement (Fig. 21.12). This would indicate that the intervertebral disc and longitudinal ligaments are unstable and not capable of holding the two functional spinal units in adjacent relationship during physiological ranges of motion.

Figures 21.13 to 21.15 show the setup for the treatment of facet syndrome. We place a small flexion pillow under the abdomen to produce a flattening of the lumbar lordotic curve in order to assist in reduction of any hyperextension subluxation of L4 on L5 or L5 on sacrum.

The first movement used in treating facet syndrome subluxation is flexion distraction applied by contacting the spinous process of the vertebra above the facet syndrome and applying flexion distraction as seen in Figure 21.14. We limit the downward flexion movement of the caudal section of the table to 2 inches or less,

and we apply this limitation to downward force when treating the lower three lumbar segments. When treating above the L3 level, we will use more downward force since we are dissipating the tractive force over several segments instead of applying it to one or two levels. Always remember to test patient tolerance prior to any manipulative maneuver. Figure 21.15 shows a sidelying maneuver to treat facet subluxation syndrome when the patient is in too much pain to lie prone.

When applying flexion distraction to facet syndrome, we utilize a push-pull pumping effect on the spinous process in order to induce an increased interspinous spacing. We feel that this allows us to open the intervertebral foramen and disc and to bring the zygapophyseal joints into an open, nonhyperextended position. With this position, we can apply lateral flexion, circumduction, and limited rotation without causing subarticular entrapment neuropathy by bringing a superior facet of the vertebra below into the lateral recess and subarticular

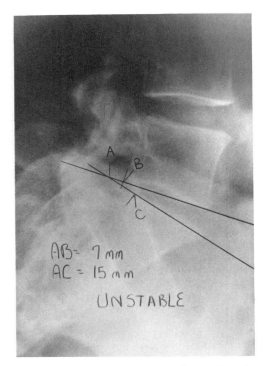

Figure 21.12. Unstable facet syndrome. Here there is 8 mm of posteriority of L5 on sacrum. This exceeds 3 mm of translation, which would be the upper limit of normal motion and would indicate stability.

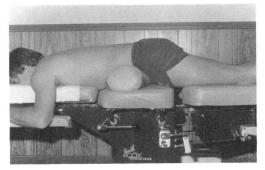

Figure 21.13. A flexion pillow is placed under the lumbosacral spine to create a flattening of the lumbar lordosis and reduction of the hyperextension of L5 on S1.

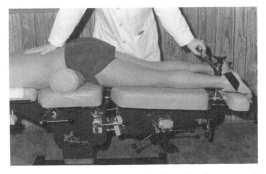

Figure 21.14. The doctor's hand's thenar eminence contacts the spinous process of L5 and flexion distraction downward motion of the table is given to approximately 2 inches of distance.

gutter where the nerve root could be compressed. In the vertical stenosis induced by facet syndrome, the nerve root can be vulnerable to more compression if we do not first flex open the facets and disc spaces prior to applying other facet movements.

MOTION PALPATION AND RANGE OF MOTION MANIPULATION

Following flexion distraction in facet syndrome, we place the articulations throughout the lumbar spine through their physiological ranges of motion. One author has found that rotation is a very limited motion at the lower two segments but is capable of being performed in the upper lumbar spine (1). We know that flexion extension is a strong movement in the lower lumbar spine. The zygapophyseal joints are capable of five normal ranges of motion with coupling combinations of these motions possible. These five motions are flexion, extension, lateral flexion, circumduction, and rotation. Figures 21.16

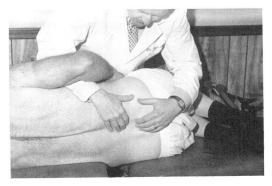

Figure 21.15. If the patient feels too much pain to lie on the abdomen for treatment, we have the patient lie on the side and lateral flex the caudal table section so as to create flexion at L5-S1. The hand contacts at the spinous processes of L5 and S1 localize and direct the tractive force.

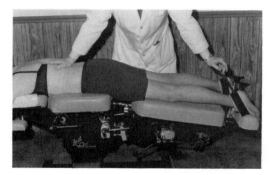

Figure 21.16. Flexion distraction is applied to the lumbar segment by contacting the spinous process above the segment to be manipulated with the thenar process of the treatment hand. The caudal section of the table is flexed until tautness of the interspinous space occurs and motion is felt between the adjacent vertebrae. This necessitates 1 to 2 inches of downward distractive force with the table section. This maneuver is repeated until the freedom of motion is felt.

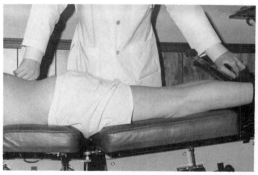

Figure 21.17. Extension is applied by contacting the spinous process of the segment to be manipulated, a downward force applied gently as the caudal table section is brought into slowly increasing extension. This maneuver is done repeatedly until freedom of motion is felt. This may be one time or several, depending on the resistance encountered.

to 21.20 provide a description of each and its application.

RETROLISTHESIS SUBLUXATION

Figure 21.21 reveals a retrolisthesis subluxation, while Figures 21.22 and 21.23 reveal two methods of spinal manipulation for the treatment of retrolisthesis. The first (Fig. 21.22) is performed with the patient prone on the instrument with hyperextension induced to the segment with the caudal section of the table. The second (Fig. 21.23) is performed with the patient lying on the table while the caudal section of the table is taken into lateral flexion to induce hyperextension of the lumbar spine. Sometimes one of these techniques causes the patient pain while the other does not.

SPONDYLOLISTHESIS

Figures 21.24 and 21.25 represent true and pseudospondylolisthesis in the lumbar spine, with the true at the L5 level and the pseudospondylolisthesis at L4.

Treatment of spondylolisthesis will involve a facet syndrome present above the level of the spondylolisthetic slip. This is because the superior facet of the spondylolisthetic vertebra will tend to move anteriorly and superiorly as the vertebral body translates anteriorly on the

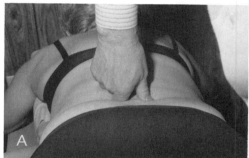

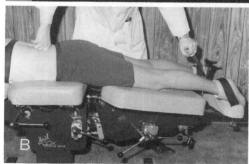

Figure 21.18. **A,** Lateral flexion is shown. The spinous process is held as shown during lateral flexion motion of the caudal section of the table. **B,** Resistance is applied to the right spinous process as the table is right flexed and to the left spinous process as left lateral flexion is applied. If the spinous process of L4 is held, the facets between L4 and L5 are tested for their ability to go through physiological motion. This movement may be sufficient to regain normal motion if hypomobility of a facet articulation is found.

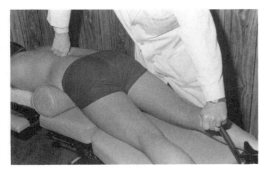

Figure 21.19. Circumduction is a combined coupled motion of flexion and lateral flexion applied at a motion segment. The spinous process is held as flexion is first applied followed by lateral flexion. This is performed in clockwise and counterclockwise motion.

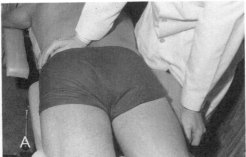

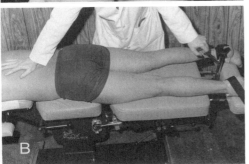

Figure 21.20. A, Rotation is applied by placing the palm of the hand on the paravertebral area of the segment to be manipulated while the thoracic section of the table is rotated under the patient. This allows the vertebra to be rotated right or left, with the needed force applied with the treating hand. **B,** Traction can be applied to the motion segment as rotation is applied to the lumbar spine. This allows coupling of two movements to single or multiple vertebral segments.

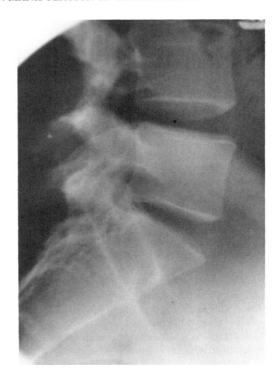

Figure 21.21. Retrolisthesis subluxation of L5 on sacrum.

vertebra below. This can induce a facet syndrome at the level above the spondylolisthetic slip. Therefore, in treating spondylolisthesis, we will place a flexion pillow under the anterior slippage vertebra, but our contact hand thenar eminence will be upon the spinous process above the spondylolisthetic slip. Figures 21.26 and 21.27 show the setup and delivery of the spinal manipulation with the patient prone. Flexion distraction with the patient lying on the side is utilized when prone distraction is painful for the patient (Fig. 21.28).

ROTATIONAL OR SCOLIOTIC SUBLUXATION CURVATURE PATTERNS

A degenerative disc disease-induced scoliosis or at least a scoliosis accompanied by degenerative disc disease is seen in Figures 21.29 and 21.30. Figure 21.31 represents a scoliotic spine in an individual who does not demonstrate the degree of degenerative disc disease seen in Figures 21.29 and 21.30. Our goal in treating these type of curves is to regain and maintain range

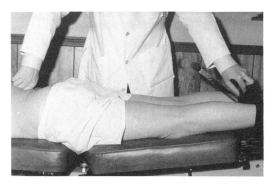

Figure 21.22. Extension manipulation is applied to the retrolisthesis subluxation as described in Figure 21.17.

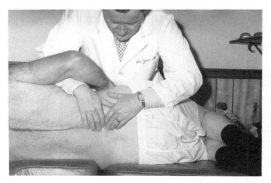

Figure 21.23. If the patient is in too much pain to lie prone for care, sidelying manipulation is applied. Pressure contact is made on the spinous process as the caudal table section is laterally flexed into extension of the lumbar spine. The hand contact controls the manipulative force and direction.

of motion for the articular facets while applying antigravitational flexion distraction manipulation to the intervertebral disc spaces. The distractive manipulative forces used in treating degenerative and idiopathic scoliosis are demonstrated in Figures 21.32 to 21.35.

MANIPULATIVE CARE OF DISC PROTRUSION

In our clinical approach, patients with sciatica are treated with only flexion distraction or extension manipulative movements.

LUMBAR DISC PROTRUSION

The diagnosis of disc protrusion is based on the presence of 3 of 5 of the following criteria (12):

1. Unilateral leg pain, especially below the knee. The leg pain should be more severe than the back pain.

2. Symptoms of specific neurologic dysfunction of a single nerve, such as numbness over a specific anatomic location or weakness of the foot.

3. A straight leg raise defect greater than 50% of normal and/or crossover pain from the unaffected leg to the symptomatic leg on straight leg raising.

4. A specific sign of peripheral neurologic dysfunction such as muscle weakness, observable sensory deficit, or reflex changes.

5. Radiographic confirmation of the neurologic dysfunction by either myelogram or CT scan.

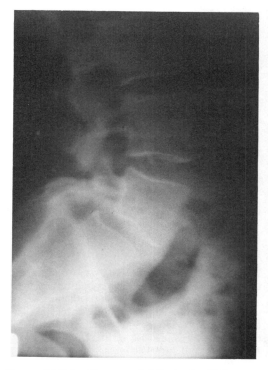

Figure 21.24. True spondylolisthesis of L5.

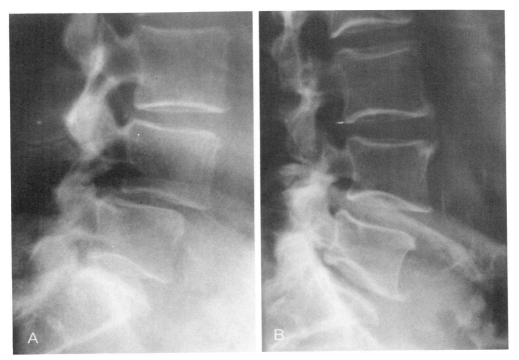

Figure 21.25. **A,** Pseudospondylolisthesis. L4 is a degenerative spondylolisthetic slip on L5 with no interruption of the pars interarticularis. **B,** Here L4 is a much less severe slippage on L5.

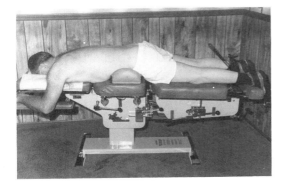

Figure 21.26. A flexion pillow is placed under the spondylolisthetic segment to flatten the lumbar lordotic curve.

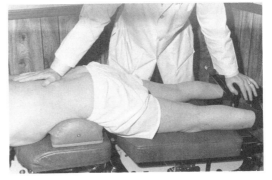

Figure 21.27. A thenar hand contact is applied to the spinous process above the slipped vertebra. A gentle downward pressure is applied with the table as cephalward pressure is applied with the treatment hand on the spinous process. We apply this manipulation until we feel the tautness and mild increase of interspinous tension. This may be repeated numerous times until free motion is elicited.

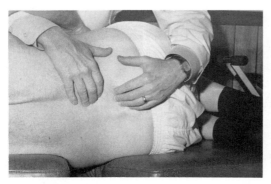

Figure 21.28. If the patient feels pain lying prone for this treatment, sidelying can create flexion. The contact hands control the interspinous process mobility during manipulation.

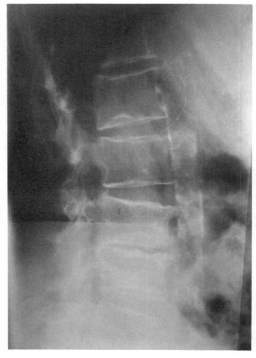

Figure 21.30. Lateral radiograph of Figure 21.29 shows advanced L3-4 degenerative disc disease with flexion subluxation of L3 on L4.

As noted above the patient must be carefully tested for ability to withstand any distraction prior to its application. If there is any pain upon testing, this procedure should not be used. We utilize physiological therapeutics instead, in the form of positive galvanism, alternating hot and cold packs to the lumbar disc and sciatic nerve, acupressure points, massage, and recumbency until such time as swelling in the disc and irritation of the nerve root subside so that the patient can tolerate distraction.

Figure 21.36 shows use of a flexion roll. This helps to maintain a slight degree of flexion that mimics the patient's entry antalgic lean. Figure 21.37 represents the treating hand contact on the spinous process above the disc to be distracted. Figure 21.38 represents the contact hand with the thenar eminence upon the spinous process directly above the protruding disc. This shows the application of distraction without ankle cuffs on, using only the patients pelvic and lower extremity weight as a tractive force, to test the patient's pain response.

Figure 21.39 and 21.40 demonstrate grasping one ankle or the other to apply unilateral dis-

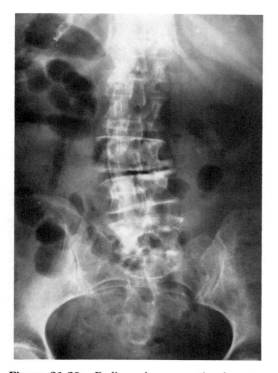

Figure 21.29. Radiograph representing levorotatory scoliosis of the lumbar spine with degenerative disc disease of the L3-4 intervertebral disc of a major degree. This unequal weight bearing of the disc and facet joints leads to advanced spondyloarthrosis on the concave side of the curve. This may have been an idiopathic adolescent scoliosis or one caused by or aggravated by degenerative disc disease.

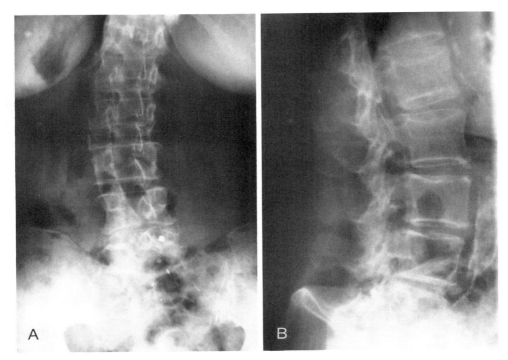

Figure 21.31. **A,** Another example of levorotatory scoliosis, but without the presence of degenerative disc disease as a factor in the etiology or progression of the scoliosis. **B,** Lateral projection shows good discal spaces compared to the scoliosis shown in Figures 21.29 and 21.30.

traction to the disc and facet joints. This allows us to test each side of the spine for aggravation of pain prior to the application of the cuff. If there should be any pain on central or lateral distractive testing, this procedure is not utilized.

Figure 21.41 shows the contact hand on the spinous process above the disc protrusion, the cuffs placed on the patient, and a very gentle downward force being applied to the intervertebral disc space. We go down with the caudal section until we feel tightening of all tissues in the lower extremity and pelvis to the point of our spinous process contact. From this taut point, we do not go down any more than 1 to 2 inches with the caudal secton of this table as we open the intervertebral space. We apply this distraction for three 20-second sessions. During each 20-second session, instead of just holding the pressure continuously, we will apply it in a milking or push-pull-pumping effect. We use 5 or 6 pumping sessions during each 20-second distractive session. This allows us to gently oscillate the vertebrae and intervertebral disc structures as opposed to just holding a sus-

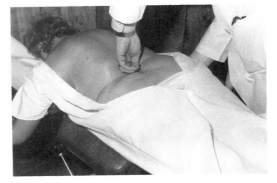

Figure 21.32. The scoliosis shown in Figure 21.29 through Figure 21.31 is treated first by derotating the rotational component of the curve as shown here. The table section under the lumbar spine is rotated so as to derotate the posterior levorotation. Pressure is applied to the left spinous process at the level to be derotated as the table is brought into derotation. In this case, the L3 spinous process is contacted.

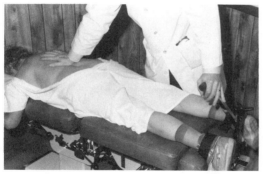

Figure 21.33. As the derotation is applied, flexion is added by downward pressure to the caudal section. The spinous process is held by the treating hand's thenar eminence and is tractioned cephalward as flexion distraction is applied.

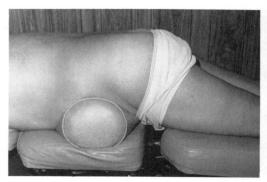

Figure 21.36. A flexion pillow is placed under the abdomen at the level of disc protrusion.

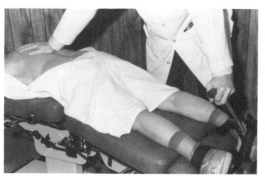

Figure 21.34. Lateral flexion into the side of levoscoliosis is added along with derotation and flexion. This combines the three motions allowing levoscoliosis reduction-derotation, flexion, and lateral flexion into the convexity of the curve. *Remember:* always carefully check the patient's ability to withstand each of these motions before applying them.

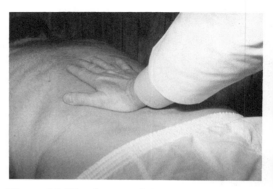

Figure 21.37. Contact of the treating thenar portion of the doctor's hand on the spinous process above the disc space to be distracted.

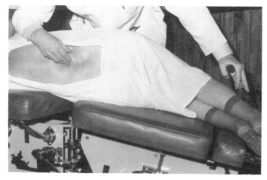

Figure 21.35. If the patient has pain when lying on the abdomen during treatment, we lay the patient on the side of convexity and use flexion to reduce the levoscoliosis, as shown here.

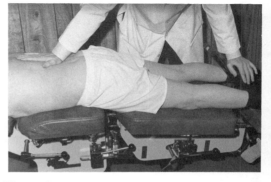

Figure 21.38. Distraction applied without ankle cuffs, using only the patient's pelvic and lower extremity weight as the tractive force. This allows testing the patient for pain at minimal amounts of force, so that if pain is elicited, further force is avoided.

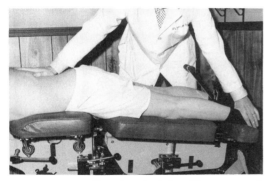

Figure 21.39. Grasping the left ankle to test unilateral tolerance of the disc and facet joints to distraction.

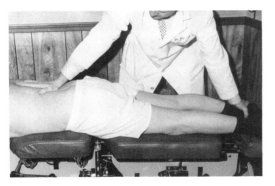

Figure 21.40. As in Figure 21.39, we test the opposite side.

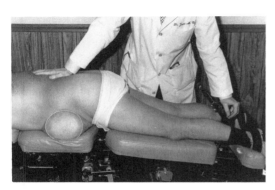

Figure 21.41. Application of distraction with the ankle cuffs in place.

tained traction. This is applied to patient tolerance.

The position shown in Figure 21.42, with the patient sidelying, is used with the patient who finds lying prone is too painful. The disc protrusion level is placed in flexion distraction while we grasp the spinous process above and below the disc lesion, applying a very gentle flexion motion.

Our clinic generally utilizes extension as soon as 50% relief of leg pain is attained as this indicates disc reduction of nerve root compression and we feel that extension can now reduce the nerve root tractive force and further enhance healing of the disc. In some cases, when flexion causes pain, extension can be tested and if it gives the patient relief, it should be the treatment modality utilized as shown in Fig. 21.43.

Following 50% relief of the low back and leg pain, we begin to place the articular facets of the disc protrusion patient through their physiological ranges of motion. These are instituted carefully, testing the patient's ability to withstand each range of motion prior to its application.

We also place our patients through Low Back Wellness School, exercise them both at home and in the clinic on Nautilus equipment, and see them periodically following attainment of maximum chiropractic improvement for manipulation to maintain this degree of relief.

DISCUSSION OF DISC TREATMENT

The determination and effects of proper distractive forces in a disc case are outlined by Cyriax (11). Some cases respond to flexion and

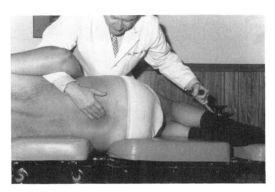

Figure 21.42. We place patients who find marked pain when lying prone, on their sides and apply flexion distraction as shown here.

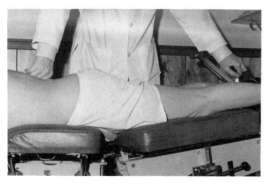

Figure 21.43. Extension is applied by contact of the spinous process, applying a gentle downward force as the table is drawn into increasing degrees of extension, as patient tolerance and benefit allow.

Chiropractic care can render relief when other procedures have failed and often in demonstrably fewer visits and less time. Further, costly institutional diagnostic procedures might well be preceded by conservative chiropractic care in cases of low back and leg pain patients who do not reveal cauda equina symptoms demanding surgical consideration, but who meet the criterion of nerve root irritation by a disc lesion as described above (12).

Lastly, instead of starting with more invasive treatments such as epidural steroid injections, manipulation could be utilized first, with more detailed procedures brought in if results are not forthcoming in a 3- to 4-week treatment period.

some to extension distraction. The following determining points are used to arrive at the flexion or extension mode of distraction.

1. If extension is pain-free and flexion hurts, traction will be comfortable if given in slight extension.

2. If both flexion and extension are painful (or neither is) distraction of the joints with the articular surfaces parallel may be tried.

3. When extension is painful and flexion pain-free, the distraction should fall mainly on the posterior part of the joint. The lumbar spine needs to be in a slight degree of flexion to achieve this.

The beneficial effects of distraction are:

Distraction. The increase in distance between the articular edges may disengage a protrusion that was just too large to shift during mere avoidance of compression in recumbency. X-rays have shown an increase of 2.5 mm in width of the joint (12).

Ligamentous Tightening. Movement apart of the vertebrae tightens the posterior longitudinal ligament, which then exerts force on a central protrusion.

Suction. A subatmospheric pressure is induced when the bones move apart, with a centripetal effect on the contents of the disc.

SUMMARY

It is often said that physicians should wait at least 2 months before recommending surgery; 90% of paitents will likely be better by then.

References

1. Pearcy MJ. Stereo-radiography of lumbar spine motion. Acta Orthop Scand (Suppl) 1985; 56(212):58–66.
2. Mayer TG, Tencer AF, Kristoferson S, Mooney V. Use of noninvasive techniques for quantification of spinal range of motion in normal subjects and chronic low back dysfunction patients. Spine 1984; 9(6):588–595.
3. Hansson T, Bigos S, Beecher P, Wortley M. The lumbar lordosis in acute and chronic low back pain. Spine 1985; 10(2):154–155.
4. Yang KH, King AI. Mechanism of facet load transmission as a hypothesis for low back pain. Spine 1984; 9(6):557–565.
5. Rydevik B. Pathoanatomy and pathophysiology of nerve root compression. Spine 1984; 9(1):557–565.
6. Wyck B. Mechanical and chemical mechanisms of pain. Paper read at Challenge of lumbar spine. New Orleans: Dec. 1984.
7. Clark GA, Panjabi MM, Wetzel FT. Can infant malnutrition cause adult vertebral stenosis? Spine 1985; 10(2):165–170.
8. Kramer J. Intervertebral disc diseases. Chicago: Year Book Publishers, 1981.
9. Macnab I. Backache. Baltimore: Williams & Wilkins, 1977; 200.
10. Van Akkerveeken PF, O'Brien JP, Park WM. Experimentally induced hypermobility in the lumbar spine. Spine 1979; 4(3):236–241.
11. Cyriax J. Textbook of orthopaedic medicine. Treatment by manipulation, massage and injection. Vol. 2. London: Ballière-Tindall, 1984; 164, 166.
12. Mooney V. The syndromes of low back disease. Orthop Clin North Am 1983; 14:500–511.

22

PHYSICAL THERAPY APPROACH TO FACET, DISC, AND SACROILIAC SYNDROMES OF THE LUMBAR SPINE

Stanley V. Paris

The lumbar spine is a complex structure subject to a number of devastating dysfunctions. These dysfunctions present as clinical syndromes enabling management to be directed at their objective findings. Foremost of these syndromes are those affecting the facet joints, the intervertebral disc, and the sacroiliac joint. Syndromes, as groups of signs and symptoms that point to a specific diagnosis, rarely exist as single entities. Most patients will present with a number of signs and symptoms so that one structure at one segmental level may appear to be the principal immediate cause of the complaint, but other structures at the same or adjacent levels will also inevitably be involved. It is well recognized that changes in the disc, for example, will affect changes in the facet, and vice versa (1). While the surgical approach may tend to focus on one diagnosis and on one procedure for correction, the physical therapy approach engages the patient's overall physical structure and function and may see the immediate cause of symptoms as but one structure in a complex whole that failed as a functional unit in the process of bodily adaptation to physical and psychosomatic stress. Thus while the therapist may direct attention to the level and the structure immediately at fault, he or she might also succeed by adopting a "whole body approach" to improve or relieve the complaint by paying attention to posture, work habits, leg length, and exercises and education.

In this chapter, discussion will be limited to the specific syndromes that relate to the facet, the disc, and the sacroiliac joint and not to the whole body approach referred to above. These are essentially nonoperative or conservative management syndromes.

FACET JOINT SYNDROMES

The term facet syndrome was first coined by Ghormely in 1933 (2). However, what he actually described was not a syndrome of the facet complete with its signs and symptoms, but rather that type of facet degeneration that would account for neurological compromise of the nerve roots. While osteopaths (3) and some medical writers wrote of the facet as a source of low back pain (4, 5), it was not until Rees in 1971 (6) claimed he could relieve 99.8% of all low back pain by ablating the nerve to the facets that the joint began to receive the attention it now commands. Mooney and Robertson in 1976 studied the reproduction of pain from the facet in patients who had chronic low back pain (7). The pain pathways they mapped conformed closely to the patients' existing pain and permitted them to detect a facilitated pathway rather than a true facet referral, which the authors were able to produce on themselves. This aspect of pain referral is of considerable significance, for it illustrates that pain reproduced from a facet injection may reproduce the pain of a disc, and that a painful discogram may reproduce the pain of a sacroiliac joint or a facet. Admittedly this clouds our ability to localize the source of pain by provocation techniques. The lumbar spine consists of many innervated structures and failure to recognize this fact may lead us to direct attention to the wrong structure.

CLINICAL ANATOMY

The facet joint consists of a synovial cavity with a superior and an inferior recess, each containing a meniscus. The superior recess which projects into the intervertebral foramen may press on the nerve root when infiltrated with contrast medium or following synovitis. Injection into the joint of more than 0.8 cc is likely to burst the recess and cause leakage into the neural foramen (8). The anterior joint capsule is made up of the ligamentum flava. The posterior joint capsule comprises a strong fibrous capsule that sweeps upwards and medially to be continuous with the interspinous ligament. The posterior capsule also lies in firm contact with a posterior cartilaginous ridge that separates the "true"

joint space from a more medial and more richly innervated posteromedial compartment, as only recently described by this author (9). This finding is considered significant since the indifferent results that have been obtained from injections into the sparsely innervated "true" joint space may be improved by utilizing a two-injection approach that would include the more extensive and richly innervated posteromedial compartment.

The multifidus muscle arises just laterally to the facet and from the capsule of the facet joint at both its level of origin and from the level above (10). Thus it is able to pull on the joint capsule during the performance of such movements as coming up to the erect position from forward bending. It appears to be particularly active during a diagonal lift.

Pathologically, the facet joint shows the usual changes that may take place in a synovial joint, including degenerative osteoarthrosis demonstrating loose bodies, surface erosions

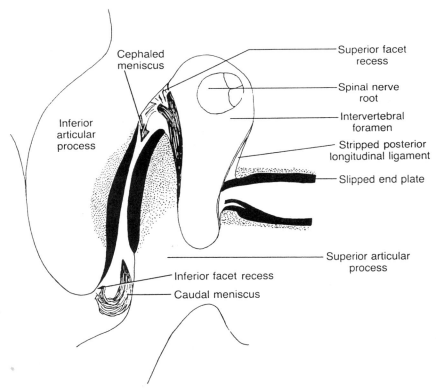

Figure 22.1. Lateral view of the facet joint showing the superior and inferior articular recesses along with their enclosed menisci. Reprinted with permission from Paris SV. Anatomy as related to function and pain. Orthop Clin North Am 1983; 14(3):479.

(11), and adhesions in the posterior medial compartment between the capsule and the lamina (12).

Clinically, this joint may demonstrate four different syndromes, comparable to those identified with the knee joint, which is also synovial and which also contains menisci.

Facet Synovitis Hemarthrosis

The cause of facet synovitis hemarthrosis is usually an awkward movement that initiates a sudden acute attack of pain. This is the familiar "crick" in the neck or "catch" of the thoracic or lumbar spine. The patient is able to straighten up immediately. The discomfort is initially localized to one side and at one level, but may soon spread as the muscles begin to offer protective guarding and, later, provide chemical irritation from the retention of metabolites.

In the clinical examination it is unfortunately not possible to distinguish between facet synovitis and a facet hemarthrosis. If it is the former, then movement may be allowed to continue at almost full range and to reach full range in 2 to 3 days. But if it is hemarthrosis, then such activities, including manipulation, may well prolong intraarticular bleeding and result in the formation of adhesions from the serum and fibrinogen, even though movement, including manipulation, may provide temporary pain relief. The result, therefore, of too early an intervention may be a chronic low back disorder with a restriction of motion.

Thus synovitis or hemarthrosis should be treated as though it were always the latter. Movement should be restricted to mid-range and activities kept light for 10 days. Treatment should consist of nothing more than heat with massage and perhaps transcutaneous electrical nerve stimulation. After 10 days the pathology should resolve into a stiff facet, and since stiff joints do not hurt, the patient should be pain free. However, if the condition is recurrent, the patient should be carefully assessed at the tenth day postinsult for the presence of segmental restrictions, and if such is found, manipulation would be indicated.

Facet Restricted Motion

It is recognized that early or moderate stiffness of joints does not cause pain. It is equally rec-ognized that such stiffness impedes nutrition and repair, may lead to further degenerative changes, reduces proprioceptive output, and offers a lowered resistance to physical insult. Additionally, stiffness at one or more levels may result in compensation and instability at other levels, usually cephalad to the restricted facet. For these reasons, stiffness, once found, should be corrected, particularly in individuals suffering from recurrent, severe, or chonic low back pain.

The treatment for facet restriction is to manipulate both adjacent muscles and the joint. The muscles may require heat, connective tissue massage, and neuromuscular facilitation techniques or prolonged stretching to restore length and flexibility. The joint restriction itself is best treated by specific manipulations directed at the direction of the stiffness and confined as much as possible to that level in order

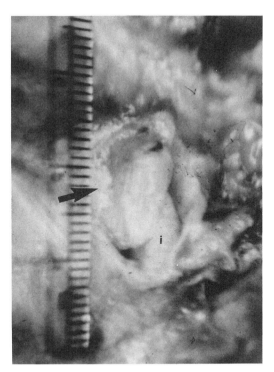

Figure 22.2. Facet joint adhesion. Adhesion within the posterior medial compartment of the right L4 facet joint is illustrated. The *arrow* points to an adhesion between the capsule and the lamina of the inferior articular process. The marker *(i)* is on the superior articular process of the vertebra below. The offset of the articular surfaces is from simulating the action of forward bending.

to reduce the stress at neighboring and possibly hypermobile segments.

Facet Mechanical Lock

Any number of synovial joints are prone to lock, especially if, like the facet, they possess menisci. These joints include the knee, the craniomandibular, the wrist, and even the elbow in some individuals. Why a frequently repeated motion should one day cause a lock is, of course, unkown. Some have speculated that the meniscus becomes jammed between the cartilaginous surfaces (13). Normally, the meniscus no doubt serves to push the capsule out of the way and thus to prevent it from being pinched to give rise to synovitis. A mechanical lock might also be due to simple jamming together of joint surfaces, especially if they have roughened through degenerative changes.

The patient's complaint is that a movement, usually involving forward bending and side-bending, resulted in the joint's becoming "stuck" and unable to straighten up. Upon early examination, the patient demonstrates good movement except for the inability to resume an upright position. A few hours in this position can produce a hydrodynamic fluid shift in the disc with a resultant inability to resume the erect position throughout the lumbar spine. This situation will then recur in the lumbar spine whenever a fixed forward bent position is adopted. Most individuals experience this postural phenomenon after activites such as a long drive with the back unsupported or working off a coffee table while sitting on a low settee.

The treatment for a joint lock is manipulation using a facet distraction technique. Figure 22.3 demonstrates a rotation to the trunk, but more specifically, a distraction to the facet. Once the facet is freed, a series of backward bending activites should be added to restore the lordosis. (See Fig. 22.4.)

Facet Painful Block

Although facet blocks are more common in the neck, the lumbar spine can on occasion give rise to a painful block. This condition is distinguished from a mechanical block in that any attempt to straighten up is painful whereas for a mechanical block it is relatively painless. The cause is thought to be entrapment of the synovial capsule.

In the cervical spine, the diagnosis is somewhat proven by the method of using an isometric contraction of multifidus to pull the capsule out and thus provide a very dramatic relief. In the lumbar spine, the multifidus is somewhat less effective and a distraction technique similar to that shown in Figure 22.5 will usually be successful provided the patient can be helped to relax sufficiently. Medication, anesthetic, or acupressure may adequately prepare the patient. Should these not succeed, then a facet injection into the joint, and particularly into the richly innervated posteromedial compartment, should confirm the diagnosis and assist with the treatment.

This author does not recommend ablation techniques directed at the facet, for these techniques are nonspecific and denervate muscles and ligaments of the lumbar spine, as well as a portion of the sacroiliac joint, in addition to the posterior facet capsule.

DISC SYNDROMES

The disc, of course can cause significant low back pain and dysfunction. But is the disc a primary cause of low back pain, or does the clinical disc result from a breakdown of function in other spinal structures such as the facet joint and the paravertebral musculature? Facet joint restrictions may inhibit disc nutrition, hasten degenerative changes in the disc at that level and then produce hypermobility at adjacent levels. Ligaments then weaken (and the most significant ligament is the outer anulus). Age and lifestyle also take their toll. At some point a tear begins at the outer anulus of the disc. Although most would consider that fissures first occur internally in the disc, the author has recently shown that although aging and degenerative changes may occur throughout the disc, tears can only begin at the periphery (14). These tears then spread into the disc. The result is a weakening of the anular "dam" and a realignment, not a detachment, of the anular rings across the surface of the cartilaginous end plate leading to an opening toward the tear. During this time the tear is vascularized from its neurovascular capsule (15; see Fig. 22.6), and since this posterior lateral aspect of the disc is richly innervated (16), it is no doubt pain

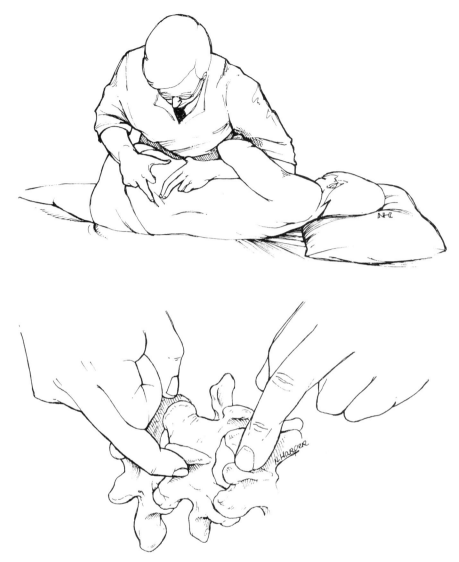

Figure 22.3. Manipulation of a midlumbar facet joint in distraction on the left side. Although the gross motion is rotation, that occurring at the facet is distraction. The patient's spine has been forward bent and rotated to the level to be manipulated.

producing from time to time. Especially is this so toward the end of the day because of creep relaxation of the disc. Eventually the nucleus will begin to herniate and finally a trivial insult may suffice for the patient to experience a prolapsed disc.

But I consider that in any surgical disc, the patient will reveal a history of low back pain, usually of increasing frequency and severity. If this is the case, then earlier intervention might well have prevented prolapse. On the basis of these observations, it appears that several stages of disc dysfunction will be encountered in low back pain patients, and that each stage can be treated conservatively with varying levels of success.

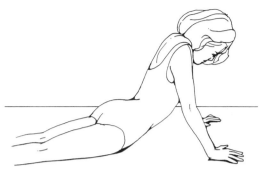

Figure 22.4. Backward bending of the midlumbar spine in order to regain the neutral lordosis. The patient performs prone push up while attempting to keep the pelvis flat on the table.

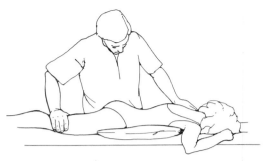

Figure 22.5. Resisted isometric contraction of the multifidus muscle to attempt to have it pull the facet capsule from between the entrapping joint surfaces. The patient lies on a soft pillow in the manner shown. Isometric resistance to the right leg will bring in the left multifidi. Should this technique not succeed, then that illustrated in Figure 22.3 should be attempted.

PREPROLAPSE

Two preprolapse patterns may be demonstrated clinically. The first and more common is that of ligamentous weakness with associated hypermobility and, perhaps, instability. The second is lumbar spine stiffness due to facet and/or muscle restrictions, which in turn increase joint load and restricted mobility and thus nutrition to the disc.

The Hypermobile Type demonstrates ligamentous weakness characterized by signs of instablity, including difficulty in sitting still for any great length of time without developing low back pain, especially later in the day. The pain is often more noticeable in the ovulation and premenstrual phases of the menstrual cycle. Muscle guarding, which is visible while standing, that disappears during lying is a reliable sign of instability, as is shaking on forward bending or experiencing more difficulty in coming up to the erect position than in going down when performing trunk forward bending. Also, the tendency to develop a lateral shift as the day goes on implies the presence of excessive creep characteristics suggestive of instability. To the author, these findings all demonstrate that the ligaments of the back, and especially the outer anulus, have weakened to the point that they do not provide segmental support as they should. Furthermore, this weakness leads to undue stress relaxation of the anular fibers and hence the firing of their rich nociceptive innervation resulting in what I have described as a neurovascular capsule (10). Treatment should

take the form of postural and other activities that decrease the load on the back. Avoidance of prolonged sitting, bending, and twisting is encouraged. Support in the form of a corset may

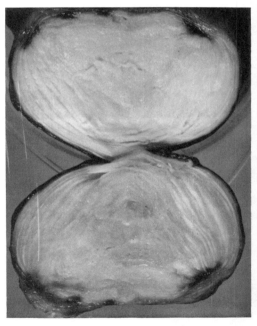

Figure 22.6. Posterior lateral rupture of the disc with resultant anular migration. The anular rings have not detached but rather "migrated" toward the posterior lateral tears, which have become vascularized—no doubt in an effort to heal.

assist initially. Manipulation other than oscillatory movements for the relief of discomfort is not indicated.

The Second Type is the opposite of hypermobility. It consists of chronic segmental stiffness due, no doubt, to pain of disc or facet origin that causes chronic muscle guarding and hence increases the load on the disc, restricts nutrition, and induces foraminal narrowing. This condition is distinguished from initial facet stiffness in that the latter causes little if any discomfort. Treatment should be directed to the muscles in the form of heat and deep massage, and to the segments with manipulation to promote motion.

In this preprolapse stage, it is essential that patients be instructed in first aid should they have an acute bout of low back pain (distinguished from their usual dull ache), especially if it is associated with a sense of a tear, rip, or giving way during a motion such as bending and twisting. These patients should be instructed that if such an event occurs they must place themselves immediately into backward bending. The theory here is that when the tear is closed down the nucleus and inner anulus will be unable to expand into it and to move in the direction of creating a prolapse.

Typically, however, patients in such a state sit down and lean away from their pain, thus further loading the disc and opening up the tear. This does not cause pain initially. Neither does pressure on the nerve root cause pain, for these are insensitive to pressure until they become ischemic, which will occur some 20 or so minutes later. Once the leg discomfort begins, any attempt to straighten up will only further narrow the neural foramen and further increase the size of the disc protrusion (7).

The lordosis must be maintained night and day for 2 weeks. During this time, adhesive tape is applied to the back both to support and provide a pointed reminder not to forward bend or rotate. Sleeping on a hard bed and sleeping prone will both maintain the lordosis, and are advocated during this stage. After 2 weeks, the back may rest flat to assist nutrition to the posterior disc, but it must not bend forward during standing. For at least 6 weeks forward bending must be avoided as the increased load and stress on the posterior anulus can still be harmful.

The 6-week period is arbitrary, but is based on my observations that the outer anulus of the disc is at least as vascular as the medial ligament at the knee, and for the latter, 6 weeks of relative immobilization is often recommended.

THE ACUTE DISC

Most acute disc injuries will not have received the benefits of the above first aid advice, and thus will have proceeded to herniation and/or prolapse. The patient is now demonstrating neurological signs and is usually unable to straighten up fully. Most patients are ambulatory, but demonstrate considerable muscle guarding and, hence, restriction of motion.

The differential diagnosis of an acute disc herniation/prolapse from an acute facet condition is not always easy in the early stages. If there has been a history of low back pain of increasing frequency and severity, then a disc should be suspected. If, on the other hand, there is no history, then the most probable cause of the low back pain is a facet lesion. If in doubt, treat conservatively with rest for 2 or 3 days. If no neurological signs emerge, then the condition may be considered a facet dysfunction, and one may proceed as outlined above.

However, if the patient presents with a history of low back pain and shows solid neurological signs, then the condition is quite obviously a disc, and must be treated as such. The patient should have as much rest as possible, preferably in bed. The injury will have caused a traumatic reaction that causes problems in a space-critical area such as the neural foramen. Every effort to reduce swelling and biochemical reactions should be undertaken. Bed rest combined with deep abdominal breathing should decrease the irritation and enhance the vascular pump. Two weeks would seem sufficient. A good result in terms of symptom relief at one week should not mislead the practitioner into thinking that the patient can resume stressful activities. The disc takes time to heal, and too early a return to activities may only result in incomplete healing and delayed recovery. Every effort should be made to avoid forward bending and rotation, but taping is often not practical as the individual is usually unable to attain a lordosis, at least initially.

After 2 weeks, moderate positional distraction may be attempted for temporary relief of nerve root pressure. This method of bed or treatment table traction seeks to open the intervertebral foramen by first forward bending to the involved level (non-weight bearing) and then sidebending away from the involved nerve root. The purpose is to open the intervertebral foramen and to draw the disc bulge somewhat straighter during the period of treatment, thereby removing pressure from the nerve root. The position needs to be comfortable so that it can be adopted for up to 40 minutes three times a day. Positional distraction before the end of the 2-week period may only further stretch the tear and worsen matters.

After 6 weeks the patient should be in a stable situation and may be able to return to work depending, of course, on the severity of the complaint. Obviously, if the neurological signs are significant and if the patient is intolerant of the pain, surgical intervention may be required.

THE CHRONIC DISC

By "chronic" is meant symptoms that have been present for 3 or more months without any improvement over the last month.

With these patients, the most important priority is to conduct a full and complete physical evaluation relying less on the history and radiologic and neurologic findings and more on the patient's general structure, function, and attitude to well-being. Only on occasion will a dramatic relief of symptoms occur in these patients, and then only if something such as a facet or sacroiliac block has been performed.

In this evaluation, the clinician should look for the possibility that several of the following may apply;

1. Improving structure and function
   • correction of leg length by heel lifts
   • correction of foot, knee and hip problems

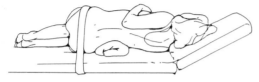

Figure 22.7. Illustration of positional distraction. The subject lies over a firm roll with the compromised neural foramen uppermost. The spine is then rotated almost to the involved level to increase the sidebending at that level. The result should be a widened neural foramen with more space for the nerve root.

   • correction of head posture and thus whole body alignment
   • stretching out of any tight lumbar and pelvic myofascia
   • improvements to gait, stance, sitting
   • improvements in physical fitness
2. Education—Back School
   • posture, work, and living habits
   • nutrition, substance abuse
   • positive mental attitude
   • work hardening
3. Psychotherapy
   • behavioral psychology
   • existentialist philosophy
   • instruction in self-care
   • ending dependence

SACROILIAC DYSFUNCTION

The sacroiliac joint is still the big enigma in the lumbar spine. It could be said that surgeons only accept the presence of a problem after they have found a surgery for it. In this way, surgeons did not accept the disc until after Mixter and Barr described a surgery (18), nor did they acknowledge the facet joint until after Rees did likewise. Sacroiliac dysfunction is accepted by almost every group, including physical therapists, osteopaths, and chiropractors. Surgeons for the most part ignore it, except for a few notable exceptions (19).

Part of the problem has no doubt been that the proponents of the sacroiliac joint as a source of low back pain have failed to present a sound balanced approach acceptable to those who already have a strong bias in favor of other causes of low back pain.

But the sacroiliac is a synovial joint capable of a number of conditions including ligamentous strain and displacement. The joint is well innervated by branches off the posterior primary rami from L4 to S3. It does not have a meniscus, nor does it have a musculature acting directly over it, although the multifidus arises from it. Essentially, more than any other joint, it is passive and depends on ligaments for support. During standing, the wedge-shaped sacrum, which contributes the medial aspects of the two sacroiliac joints, is forced downwards between the two ilia, which contribute the lateral aspects of the joints. It follows, then, that the paired ilia tend to rotate posteriorly, especially in the female, because the sacroiliac joints and the line of gravity are located behind the hip joint. The downward movement or slip of the sacrum, which is a response to body weight from above and from impact loads through the leg from below, is resisted by the deep and superficial posterior sacroiliac ligaments. Rotation is resisted principally by the sacrospinous and sacrotuberous ligaments.

Movements do occur at the sacroiliac joint and this has now been well documented (20). Displacements due to hypermobility or rupture have also been radiographed (21) and the methods of testing for passive motions (22) described.

Clinically, the natural progression of the joint is to become stiff and fibrous, or even ankylosed, especially in males. Since stiff joints do not hurt, and because innervation is only to the ligaments, then stiffness should not of itself cause pain in the sacroiliac. Rather, there may be just two clinical conditions that can give rise to pain, namely laxity (hypermobility or instability) and displacement (excluding diseases such as Padget's and ankylosing spondylitis).

Scaroiliac Laxity (Hypermobility)

Laxity is more likely to occur in females of childbearing years. The causes are several, including habitual one-legged standing, falls onto the ischial tuberosity, childbirth, and sexual intercourse strains. The pain is at first well localized over the sacroiliac joint. Thus there is no central back pain and no pain across the back. There may in addition be rather distinct ipsilateral muscle guarding of the multifidi of the sacral, lumbar, and low thoracic spines, and this will be present during and sometimes after lying. The posterior capsular ligaments are tender to touch and the pain can be reproduced by ligamentous palpation and, more significantly, by manipulative tests designed to stress the ligaments. Manual therapists and physicians can also conduct motion palpation on the joint to assess its degree of motion. Such testing does have satisfactory reliability (23).

Laxity of the ligaments does not produce continuous discomfort. Like the early stages of disc dysfunction (see above) pain is greater when the strain is greatest and therefore mostly toward the end of the day. The condition improves with rest. Stiffness is rarely complained of.

On structural examination in standing, the patient may display level iliac crests in a sacral

downslip, but with a convexity of the lumbar spine to the involved side. If an iliac rotation is present, there may again be a lumbar convexity to the same side but a more obvious lowering of the iliac crest will also be present. If in standing the pelvis is firmly squeezed or supported in a binder, thus forcing together the articular surfaces, both the scoliosis and unequal height iliac crest may temporarily disappear.

Treatment is education to reduce stress, frequent rest—preferably on a firm bed that will test to relieve the posterior rotation, and support in the form of a binder.

Sacroiliac Displacement

Displacement of the sacroiliac is uncommon and usually results in patients with the above clinical history and findings of laxity. The auricular-shaped surfaces of the joint are not mirror images of one another. It is conceivable that the two opposing articular surfaces may, if laxity is present, override an incongruency and suddenly become locked and unable to return to the neutral position. Such a displacement may now give rise to a lower level but to a more constant discomfort than that of the previous laxity and may even continue at rest.

The displacements are usually rotary but can also be one of a vertical slip of the sacrum on the ilium (downslip of the sacrum, or as some express it, upslip of the ilium). Displacements need to be manipulated to free them from their present locked position and then treated as a hypermobility, which preceded the displacement and thus needs to be treated with support.

Precise manipulative techniques work best, but nature is forgiving and any manipulative movement in the direction of correction will invariably result more in a correction than in further displacement.

SUMMARY

Three of the principal dysfunctions that cause low back pain are those that arise from the facets, the discs, and the two sacroiliacs. In each category there are more than one syndrome. Thus it is not possible to speak purely of a facet syndrome any more than it is possible to speak of a disc syndrome. They have several distinct yet at times overlapping sets of signs and symptoms. For the most part, they respond well to conservative management.

References

1. Kirkaldy-Willis WH. Managing low back pain. 2nd ed. New York: Churchill Livingstone 1988; 9

2. Ghormely RK. Low back pain with special reference to the articular facets, with the presentation of an operative procedure. JAMA 1933; 101:1773.

3. Stoddard A. Manual of osteopathic technique. 3rd ed. London: Hutchinson 1980.

4. Mennel JB. Physical treatment by movement manipulation and massage. 3rd ed. London: Churchill, 1934.

5. Mennell JMcM. Back pain. Boston: Little, Brown, 1962.

6. Rees WES. Multiple bilateral subcutaneous rhizolysis of segmental nerves in the treatment of the intervertebral disc syndrome. Ann Gen Prac 1971; 26:126.

7. Mooney V, Robertson J. The facet syndrome. Clin Orthop 1976, 115:149–156.

8. Graham-Smith A. personal communication.

9. Graham-Smith A, Paris SV. The importance of facet joint arthrography: The posteromedial compartment—A new finding. Proceedings of the International Society for the Study of the Lumbar Spine. Kyoto, Japan, May 1989.

10. Paris SV. Anatomy as related to function and pain. Symposium on evaluation and care of lumbar spine problems. Orthop Clin North Am 1983; 14(3):484–485.

11. Kirkaldy-Willis WH. Managing low back pain. 2nd ed. New York: Churchill Livingstone 1988; 56–58.

12. Paris SV. Clinical decision making in orthopaedic physical therapy. In Wolf S. ed. Clinical

13. Kraft GL, Levinthal OH. Facet synovial impingement: A new concept in the etiology of lumbar vertebral derangement. Surg Gynecol Obstet 1951; 439:443.

14. Paris SV, Nyberg R. Healing of the lumbar intervertebral disc. Proceedings of the International Society for the Study of the Lumbar Spine. Kyoto, Japan, 1989.

15. Paris SV. Functional anatomy of the lumbar spine, Ann Arbor: University Microfilms International, 1984.

16. Paris SV, Nyberg R. Innervation of the posterior lateral aspect of the lumbar intervertebral disc. Proceedings of the International Society for the study of the Lumbar Spine. Kyoto, Japan, 1989.

17. White AA, Punjabi MM. Clinical biomechanics of the spine. Philadelphia: Lippincott, 1978; 15.

18. Mixter WJ, Barr JS. Rupture of the intervertebral disc with involvement of the spinal canal. N Engl Surg Soc 1934; 2:210–215.

19. Kirkaldy-Willis WH, Hill RJ. A more precise diagnosis for low-back pain. Spine 1979; 4(2):102–109.

20. Dihlmann W. Diagnostic radiology of the sacroiliac joints. Stuttgart: Year Book Medical Publishers, 1980.

21. Paris SV. Clinical decision making in orthopaedic physical therapy. In Wolf S, ed. Clinical decision making in physical therapy. Philadelphia: FA Davis, 1985; 230.

22. Paris SV. The spinal lesion. Christchurch, New Zealand: Pegasus Press, 1965.

23. Gonnella C, Paris SV, Kutner M. Reliability in testing passive intervertebral motion. Phys Ther 1982; 62(4):436–444.

decision making in physical therapy, Philadelphia: FA Davis, 1985; 228.

PSYCHOLOGICAL AND MEDICAL DIMENSIONS

23

PREDICTORS OF LOW BACK PAIN DISABILITY

Peter B. Polatin

The cost of back injuries in the United States in 1980 came to a total of $24 billion ($8 billion for medical costs and the remainder for disability and indirect costs; 1, 2). Annual expenditure has increased since then. Various surveys show that between 60 and 90% of people will experience an episode of low back pain at some time during their lives (2–6). At any given time, 20 to 30% of the population may be symptomatic (4).

In the United States, 2% of workers suffer a job-related compensable back injury every year (7, 8). Nineteen to twenty-five per cent of all workers' compensation claims are back-related (7, 9). While 90 to 95% of acute low back pain patients will resolve their disability within 3 months of injury (10), up to 80% of the industrial medical expense is consumed by the 5 to 10% of patients who remain symptomatic and disabled after that period of time (8).

It is because of this problematic subset of low back pain patients, with lingering disability and high medical costs, that the need for predictors of disability has arisen. If these patients can be identified early, it is hypothesized, measures might be taken to prevent chronicity, thereby reducing health care expense (11). Additionally, these patients also represent a "red flag" to the spinal surgeon, since, in many cases, complex psychosocial issues make them less than optimal surgical candidates (12). A conservative course of treatment rather than surgery is justified for them.

PREDICTORS: INJURY, CHRONICITY, AND CHRONIC OUTCOME

Within the context of low back pain disability, predictors have relevance at several different levels. In the general uninjured population, certain factors (injury predictors) may serve to differentiate the subgroup at risk for a back injury. Other factors (chronicity predictors) may have relevance in evaluating a group of acute low back pain patients to delineate those five or ten percent who will go on to chronicity. Finally, another subset of predictors (chronic outcome predictors) might be meaningful in attempting to forecast the success or failure of a treatment intervention in the chronic low back pain patient. In the following discussion, I will delineate wherever possible the specificity of predictive factors.

PHYSICAL FINDINGS

The clinical presentation of a patient over the initial weeks and months after injury has been felt to give some chronicity predictive information.

Leg Pain

The presence of nerve root tension signs (13) and leg pain (6) is associated with an increased length of illness and disability. This is contrary to expectation, since a radicular component would imply better success for a surgical intervention, but these studies do not delineate a surgical versus a nonsurgical group. However, Dzioba and Doxey (12), in an investigation of candidates for first back surgery, did find leg pain predictive of successful outcome by orthopaedic assessment and patient self-report, but not of return to work, which is a more sensitive long-term outcome criterion.

Table 23.1.
Nonorganic Signs of Waddell

A finding of three or more is significant
1. Tenderness—widespread over the lumbar area
    Superficial; to light touch
    Nonanatomical; to deep palpation, not one
      structure
2. Simulation Tests—painful motion is mimicked,
      but not performed
    Axial Loading: LBP when pressure exerted
      over skull while standing
    Rotation: LBP when pelvis and shoulders
      rotated together while standing
3. Distraction
    Straight-leg raising in the sitting position
      (Flip test)
4. Regional Disturbances
    Weakness: non neurological, involving many
      adjacent muscle groups
    Sensory: "glove" or "stocking" hypesthesia
5. Overreaction—verbalization, grimacing, collaps-
      ing, etc.

Nonorganic Signs

The nonorganic signs described by Waddell (14; Table 23.1) are also chronicity predictors, both in the surgical and the nonsurgical patient (12, 15). These findings are elicited by the clinician on physical examination and their presence has been associated with such pejoratives as "hypochondriasis" and "malingering," but, in fact, should more appropriately be regarded as indicative of psychological distress, as Waddell points out. They most likely correlate with psychological predictors such as scales 1 and 3 on the Minnesota Multiphasic Personality Inventory, described later in this chapter.

Decreased Spinal Range of Motion

Several investigators have found a decreased spinal range of motion to be associated with chronicity and persistent disability (16, 17). However, other studies found that a decreasing spinal range of motion over a period of several years is correlated with improved pain and disability ratings (18), and that a good surgical prognosis is correlated with a reduced range of motion at the operated segment (19). This may suggest that decreased spinal mobility predicts disability in an acute and early chronic low back pain population, but that in a chronic

group, both surgical and nonsurgical, it is a positive outcome predictor.

Pain Self-report

Pain self-report has some relevance as a predictor of chronicity. A pain complaint that does not conform to known physiological pattern, particularly when coupled with an abnormal pain drawing (20), should probably be regarded in the same context as Waddell's nonorganic signs, indicating distress and excessive somatic concerns that may lead to a more protracted course.

Nonspecific Diagnosis

Finally, the lack of a specific anatomical-structural diagnosis is associated with a less favorable prognosis. Studies on both surgical and conservative care outcomes clearly show that an unequivocal diagnosis is associated with a better result (11), and that the "functional group" of patients has a higher incidence of psychological disturbance.

DEMOGRAPHIC FACTORS

Age, sex, and education have both injury and chronicity predictive significance.

Sex

Low back pain appears equally in males and females (2), though 80% of back injury compensation claims are filed by men (7), consistent with the fact that more men work at higher risk, heavy jobs. However, an occupationally injured female is more likely to remain disabled (12), perhaps because of child-care concerns and more work ambivalence as well as less work satisfaction or more occupational stress.

Age

The highest incidence of low back pain occurs between the ages of 30 and 50 (21), which are the most industrially productive years. Older individuals have a higher incidence of chronicity and disability, which may be reflective not only of slower healing but also of more psychosocial barriers at that age. Workers under the age of 25 have a higher risk of injury but return to work sooner (22), suggestive of less caution and experience on the one hand, but higher motivation to remain productive on the other.

Education

Finally, there is an inverse relationship between educational level and low back pain and disability (2, 17, 23), with the most pronounced incidence to be found in those individuals with the least education. Again, this is not surprising; lower education is probably associated with fewer job options, lower salary, and less work satisfaction, so that disability with some compensation will be more attractive.

ANTHROPOMETRIC FACTORS

Height/Weight

Heavy body weight alone does not appear to be an injury predictor for low back pain (3, 24, 25), but some studies have suggested that greater height may be such a predictor (3, 25). Other investigators, however, have not found this to be true (22, 24), and if such a correlation does exist, it is most likely on the basis of the different spinal configurations of taller people or of the awkward positions they may have to assume while working (3).

Conditioning

Poor physical conditioning is a definite injury predictor (17, 26). More specifically, trunk muscle strength deficits have not only injury predictive significance (16, 27), but may have chronic outcome significance as well (28), in that correction of this deconditioning leads to correction of disability.

ENVIRONMENTAL FACTORS

Compensation/Litigation

Empirically, low back pain patients receiving workers' compensation payments or who have pending litigation related to their injuries are expected to have poorer chronic and chronic outcome prognoses. Cynical clinicians regard the most relevant event in these patients' course as the settlement or "greenback poultice," after which disability usually resolves. In fact, studies have demonstrated poorer response to conservative treatment in chronic pain and back pain patients on compensation (29–31). However, other investigators have pointed out that while these patients do not do as well as a nonreinforced group, they do make significant treatment gains, but continue to have a higher self-report of pain and disability (32, 33).

The need to document illness may be more reflective of the compensation-litigation process than of underlying psychopathology in this patient group, but another study has documented a higher incidence of conversion and personality disorders in compensated chronic pain patients as compared to a noncompensated group (34). Robertson and Keeve (35), in a large survey, reported a clear trend toward increased occupational injury claims with associated sick leave after workers' compensation payments had been adjusted upwards. They hypothesize that while this may have stimulated more malingering or unjustified claims, the trend may also reflect injured workers who had previously continued to work when workers' compensation payments were insufficient to support them. One cannot avoid the conclusion that compensation and litigation do contribute to chronicity by general positive reinforcement of illness behavior or through a more specific exacerbation of regressive behavior in individuals with previous psychopathology.

A higher compensation rate was reflective of a better chronic outcome prognosis in a study of conservative care in the chronic low back pain population, possibly because of an increased incentive for these patients to return to their higher paying jobs (36).

Context of Injury

The injury event itself has a somewhat controversial prognostic value. Many occupational injury studies document that an acute event related to lifting, bending, or twisting (31, 37, 38), or an accident such as a slip or fall (39), has a negative predictive impact for chronicity. Others, however, find that a more gradual and insidious onset is not indicative of greater ongoing disability (16, 40, 41). Part of the disparity may be reflective of context. A worker in an industrial setting will more likely identify an acute precipitating event at work, which will be covered by compensation, even though the actual onset may have been more gradual (11).

JOB

Much has been written about the relationships between workplace factors and low back pain. Injury predictors include heavy manual labor, particularly in the construction, materials handling, and nursing categories (3, 23, 38, 42), vibration and driving, such as truck and heavy equipment operation (3, 5, 8, 43), heavy lifting (3, 5, 44–46), and prolonged sitting (2, 10). The probability of injury is three times greater when job lifting requirements approach or exceed the individual's functional capacity (45).

Additionally, short length of time at the job (2, 22, 23), lack of job satisfaction (46–48), higher stress level at work (46, 48), poor supervisory rating (22), and lack of availability of interim light duty work (31) all have predictive injury and chronicity relevance. We will deal with this further below.

Health Delivery

It has been suggested that inconsistent medical care may contribute to a longer duration of disability and a poorer prognosis for the injured worker. Weisel and colleagues (44, 49) applied a standardized diagnostic and treatment protocol to two industrial settings. In one, the patients were seen weekly, while in the other, they were seen only once. In both settings, the evaluation and treatment of workers with back injury were standardized according to a flow sheet made available to all health providers, and any deviation was scrutinized and corrected by the investigators. In both settings, treatment costs and disability were reduced, leading to the conclusion that consistency through the use of a standardized care algorithm may improve the prognosis for low back pain in the workplace.

MEDICAL HISTORY

Previous Low back Pain

Previous history of low back pain is the most relevant medical injury predictor of all (39, 47, 50, 51), particularly if it occurred as a previous sciatica (43). A preceding episode of low back pain makes the probability of an additional occurrence four times greater than normal (52).

Smoking

Cigarette smoking, both number per day and years of exposure, has been noted to be an in-

jury predictor (5, 25, 43, 53), perhaps because of increased intradiscal pressure exerted by frequent coughing, or perhaps because smoking is associated with a decreased diffusion of nutrients into the intravertebral disc (3, 5, 40, 29).

Poor Health

Poor previous and concurrent health are injury and chronicity predictors. Back injury claimants were characterized by multiple claims compared with claimants for injuries unrelated to the back (8). Male workers with an increased number of "sickness absence days" due to other medical problems subsequently tended to develop low back pain (42) and a higher prevalence of diseases of the respiratory and gastrointestinal systems (47). Astrand (23) noted that workers identified as complaining of low back pain had poorer health, both by self-report and clinician evaluation, than normals. Workers with diagnosed back abnormalities had an even higher poor health rating whether by themselves or by physicians. Biering-Sorenson and colleagues (43) found injury predictors to be "frequent pain in the top of the stomach" as well as previous hospitalizations and surgeries. Additionally, they found chronicity predictors in men to be intermittent claudication, lower extremity restlessness or discomfort and frequent headaches. In women the predictors were "rumbling of the stomach" and "feeling of fatigue." They suggest that even prior to a first episode of low back pain, this group of patients had poorer general health. Frymoyer and Cats-Baril (11) note a three to four times greater than normal incidence of headaches, ulcers, and other psychosomatic complaints in the chronically disabled low back pain population.

MENTAL HEALTH

Stress

The association between emotional and physical health has long been known, and the possibility of using stress as a predictor of future illness is well documented. This has particular relevance in the workplace. In a study of air-traffic controllers, high scores on self-report measures of work-related life change distress, other life changes outside of the work setting, type A behavioral patterns, and dissatisfaction with management were predictive of future rates of injury and of physician-diagnosed illness episodes, though not necessarily of low back pain (48). Magora (46) has documented that individuals dissatisfied with their jobs or social status who felt stressed at work and were tense and fatigued after work had a higher incidence of low back pain than did a comparable group showing lower self-report scores on these issues.

Psychopathology

Psychopathology, whether preexistent or subsequent to a back injury, has important relevance for predicting a chronic outcome.

Preexistent conversion and personality disorders in chronic pain patients occur in higher than expected levels as preinjury pathology that clearly affects the course of treatment (34). Personality disorders themselves are refractory to psychotherapy and may be the limiting factor in recovery. Westrin (47), in his epidemiological evaluation of psychological symptoms in chronic low back pain, has commented on the higher incidence of "mental trouble of a cerebrolesional type," "social instability," and "social insufficiency" in this group, which is suggestive of psychiatric illness.

Psychological disturbance in the chronic low back pain population, as manifested by depression, anxiety, somatization, pessimism, despair, and social alienation (23, 43, 54, 55), is reflective most often of the impact of the back pain, but will clearly affect outcome if not treated concurrently. This can be done relatively well within a short period of time with psychotherapy, education, and appropriate medication. It is the "functional" group of chronic low back pain patients, with no structural diagnosis, who appear to exhibit the highest incidence of "psychological disturbance" (56) and psychiatric illness, particularly depression (57). Here again, which came first, the psychopathology or the diagnostic uncertainty, is unclear, but the psychopathology, nevertheless, has predictive significance.

Depression has been documented at a very high incidence in chronic low back pain. Krishnan and co-workers (58) found that 56 out of 71 consecutive chronic low back pain patients admitted to an inpatient service had significant depression. Lindsey and Wycoff (59) have documented an 87% incidence of depression in chronic pain. Other studies have been confirmatory (60, 61). In fact, it has been suggested that the best prediction of treatment response might be achieved by dividing chronic pain patients into a depressed versus a nondepressed group, since their outcomes are predicted by a different pattern of variables (62).

Krishnan and colleagues (63) also document an increased incidence of anxiety in the chronic low back pain group, accompanied by somatization and particularly associated with major depression. Again, if this disturbing symptom cannot be controlled, treatment outcome will be adversely affected.

Alcoholism and Drug Abuse

Alcoholism has been found in up to 40% of chronic pain patients (61). Sandstrom et al (64) comment on its high incidence in the back pain group, and warn that it can adversely affect rehabilitation unless it is treated concurrently, in which case the prognosis can be significantly improved.

Similarly, drug abuse is particularly high in this population (4), frequently iatrogenically induced, and becomes a negative chronic outcome predictor unless treated specifically.

Psychological Testing

Psychological testing has been found to be of both chronicity and chronic outcome predictive value. The MMPI, perhaps the most standardized of all psychological tests, has been noted in patients with chronic pain to show particular pathologic profiles characterized by elevations on scales 1 (hypochondriasis), 2 (depression), and 3 (hysteria) (55, 56, 65–70). Frymoyer, Rosen, and co-workers (66) have noted that patients with elevations on scales 1 and 3 were more likely to experience increased disability as manifested by a reduced range of spinal motion, decreased trunk muscle strength, and greater limitations of straight-leg raising. Love and Peck (69), in their extensive review of the MMPI in chronic low back pain, point out the pitfalls of a single-minded approach to the use of this instrument. They discuss distinctive profiles characterizing different types of psychological response to chronic low back pain, different pain-related behaviors, and perhaps differing responses to various treatment interventions.

The MMPI does change both for the better and for the worse, so that at any given time it is reflective of the patient's psychological state at that moment. Hendler (71) points out that pain has an effect on mental health, even in the pre-

Table 23.2.
Stages of Pain (Hendler)

Acute stage (0–2 months)
   expects to get well
   not depressed
   normal MMPI
Subacute stage (2–6 months)
   the first doubts
   emergence of hypochondriacal concerns
   MMPI: elevations of 1 and 3
Chronic stage (6 months—8 years)
   realization that pain is permanent
   clinical depression
   MMPI: elevations of 1, 2, and 3, especially 2
Subchronic stage (3–12 years)
   adjustment
   decline in depression
   MMPI: "conversion V" (high 1 and 3, low 2)

viously well-adjusted individual, so that some caution must be exercised in interpreting psychological findings to make statements about personality and psychopathology in the chronic pain patient. He delineates the "stages of pain" (Table 23.2) and discusses MMPI changes which might be seen in each, even in a patient with a premorbidly normal MMPI.

Because the MMPI is such a lengthy test to administer and complete, some investigators have attempted to develop abbreviated forms that may have the same predictive value for the low back pain patient, such as the Faschingbauer abbreviated MMPI (41, 72). Others have explored the particularly responsive scales, 1 and 3, to understand more clearly what these evaluations mean in the chronic low back pain patient (68).

The Millon Behavioral Health Inventory has recently been found to be a possible chronic outcome predictor for conservative care. Gatchel and colleagues (73) report that success and drop-out groups of chronic low back pain patients differed in the profiles on a number of scales taken together. Barnes and co-workers (36) found, in a similar group of patients, "success" and "failure" profiles of some consistency.

Family

Studies have documented an increased incidence of depression, alcoholism, psychosomatic disorders, and chronic pain in the families of chronic pain patients (61, 74). One particular study of low back pain patients with and without depression found a significantly higher oc-

currence of depression, alcoholism, and chronic back pain in the first-degree relatives of both groups, but depression occurred at a higher rate in the families of depressed chronic low back pain patients (75). Therefore, family history has clear chronicity predictive significance, though the epidemiological studies thus far have been retrospective, based upon already identified chronic groups with psychiatric symptoms.

SUMMARY

As we have documented, extensive research has already been devoted to identifying predictors of back injury and resultant disability (see Table 23.3). The economic and social impact of chronic low back pain continues to escalate. Our ability to contain this health problem in the future will be contingent upon increased understanding of the biological, psychological, social, and economic factors involved in perpetuating this condition in the modern world. Prevention of disabling and costly complications will require our ability to use an understanding of predictors to alter the course of the disease by changing attitudes, patterns of response, and reinforcers.

References

1. Benica JJ. The nature of the problem. In Caron H, McLaughlin RR. eds. Management of low back pain. Boston: John Wright, 1982; 1–15.
2. Deyo RA, Tsui-Wu Y. Descriptive epidemiology of low back pain and its related medical care in the U.S. Spine 1987; 12(3):264–268.
3. Kelsey JL, Golden AL. Occupational and workplace factors associated with low back pain. Occup Med 1988; 3(1):7–15.
4. Cassidiy JD, Wedge JH; The epidemiology and natural history of low back pain and spinal degeneration. In Kirkaldy-Willis WH. ed. Managing low back pain (2nd ed.) New York: Churchill Livingston. 1988; 3–14.
5. Frymoyer JW, Pope MH, Clements JH, Wilder DG et al. Risk factors in low back pain. J Bone Joint Surg 1983; 65A(2):184–213.
6. Biering-Sorensen F. A prospective study of low back pain in a general population. Scand J Rehab Med 1983; 15:81–88.
7. Klein BP, Jensen RC, Sanderson LM. Assessment of workers' compensation claims for back strains/sprains. J Occup Med 1984; 26(6):443–448.
8. Spengler DM, Bigos SJ, Martin MA et al. Back injuries in industry: A retrospective study. I.

Table 23.3.
Predictors in Low Back Pain

	Preinjury	Prechronicity	Chronic outcome
Physical Examination and Medical Evaluation		leg pain nonorganic signs decreased spinal range of motion (?) nonphysiological pain self report lack of specific diagnosis	
Demographic	working male under age 25 low education	working female older low education	
Anthropometric	taller (?) poor conditioning weak trunk muscles	poor conditioning	weak trunk muscles
Environmental	acute vs gradual onset (?) heavy manual labor vibration/driving heavy lifting (over 25 lbs freq.) prolonged sitting (?) short time on job poor job satisfaction high work stress poor supervisory rating	compensation ligation lack of light duty inconsistent medical care	compensation litigation
Health	previous LBP smoking poor general health	poor general health	poor general health
Mental Health	stress	"psych. disturbance" depression anxiety alcoholism drug abuse MMPI HSC BPCS Oswestry	depression anxiety alcoholism drug abuse MMPI MBHI (Millon)
Family History		family history of depression chronic pain alcoholism	

Overview and cost analysis. Spine 1986; 11(13):241–245.

9. Morris A. Identifying workers at risk to back injury is not guesswork. Occup Health Safety Dec. 1985; 16–20.

10. Andersson GBH. Epidemiological aspects of low back pain in industry. Spine 1981; 6:53.

11. Frymoyer JW, Cats-Baril W. Predictors of low back pain disability. Clin Orthop 1987; 221:89–98.

12. Dzioba RB, Doxey NC. A prospective investigation into the orthopedic and psychological predictors of outcome of first lumbar surgery following industrial injury. Spine 1984; 9(6):614–623.

13. Troup JDG. Straight-leg-raising (SLR) and the qualifying tests for increased root tension: Their predictive value after back and sciatic pain. Spine 1981; 6(5):526–527.

14. Waddell G, McCullough JA, Kummel EG, Venner RM. Nonorganic physical signs in low back pain. Spine 1980; 3:117–125.

15. Waddell G, Main CJ. Assessment of severity in low back disorders. Spine 1984; 9(2):204–208.

16. Biering-Sorenson F. Physical measurements as risk indicators for low back trouble over a one-year period. Spine 9(2):106.

17. Magora A, Taustein I. An investigation of the problem of sick leave in the patient suffering from low back pain. Ind Med 1969; 38(11):80–90.

18. Lankhorst GJ, Van De Satdt RJ, Van der Korst JK. The natural history of idiopathic low back pain. Scand J Rehab Med 1985; 17:1–4.

19. Froning EC, Frohman B. Motion of the lumbosacral spine after laminectomy and spine fusion. J Bone Joint Surg 1968; 50A(5):897–918.

20. Kirkaldy-Willis WH. The clinical picture—introduction. In: Kirkaldy-Willis WH. ed. Managing low back pain. 2nd ed. New York: Churchill Livingstone, 1988.

21. Frymoyer JW. Back pain and sciatica. N Engl J Med 1988; 318(5):291–300.

22. Bigos SJ, Spengler DM, Martin NA et al. Back injuries in industry: A retrospective study. III. Employee-related factors. Spine 1986; 11(3):252–256.

23. Astrand NE. Medical, psychological, and social factors associated with back abnormalities and self-reported back pain. Br J Indust Med 1987; 44:327–336.

24. Dehlin O, Hedenrud B, Horal J. Back symptoms in nursing aides in a geriatric hospital. Scand J Rehab Med 1976; 8–47.

25. Gyntelberg F. One year incidence of low back pain among male residents of Copenhagen age 40–59. Dan Med Bull 1974; 21:30.

26. Cady LD, Bischoll DP, O'Connell ER et al. Strength and fitness and subsequent back injuries in fire fighters, J Occup Med 1979; 21:269.

27. Leino P, Aro S, Hasan J. Trunk muscle function and low back disorders: A ten-year follow-up study. J Chron Dis 1987; 40(4):289–296.

28. Mayer TG, Gatchel RJ, Kishino N et al. Objective assessment of spine function following industrial injury, Spine 1985; 10(6):482–492.

29. Hammonds W, Brena SF, Unikel IP. Compensation for work-related injuries and rehabilitation of patients with chronic pain. South Med J 1978; 71(6):664–666.

30. Block AR, Kremer E, Gaylor M. Behavioral treatment of chronic pain variables affecting treatment efficacy; Pain 1980; 8:367–375.

31. White AWM. Low back pain in men receiving workmens' compensation. Can Med Assoc J 1966; 95:50–56.

32. Leavitt F, Garron DC, McNeill TW, Whisler WW. Organic status, psychological disturbance, and pain report chracteristics in low back pain patients on compensation. Spine 1982; 7(4):398–402.

33. Trief P, Stein N. Pending litigation and rehabilitation outcome of chronic back pain. Arch Phys Med Rehab 1985; 66:95–99.

34. Fishbain DA, Goldberg M, Labbe E, Steele R, Rosomoff H. Compensation and non-compensation chronic pain patients compared for DSM-III operational diagnoses. Pain 1988; 32:197–206.

35. Robertson LS, Keeve JP. Worker injuries: The effects of workers' compensation and OSHA inspections. J Health Politics Policy Law 1983; 8(3):581–597.

36. Barnes D, Smith D, Gatchel R, Mayer T. Psychosocioeconomic predictors of treatment success/failure with chronic low back pain patients. Presented at the ISSLS meeting in Rome, April, 1987.

37. Venning PJ, Walter SD, Stitt LW. Personal and job-related factors as determinants of incidence of back injuries among nursing personnel. Occup Med 1987; 29(10):820–825.

38. Bigos SJ, Spengler DM, Martin NA et al. Back injuries in industry: A retrospective study. II. Injury factors. Spine 1986; 11(3):246–251.

39. Troup JDG, Martin JW, Lloyd DCEF. Back pain in industry: A prospective survey. Spine 1981; 6:61–69.

40. Weber H. Lumbar disc herniation: A controlled, prospective study with ten years of observation. Spine 1983; 8(2):131–140.

41. Roland M, Morris R. A study of the natural history of low back pain. Part II. Development of guidelines for trials of treatment in primary care. Spine 1983; 8:145–150.

42. Svensson HO. Low back pain in forty to forty-seven-year-old men. II. Socio-economic factors and previous sickness absence. Scand J Rehab Med 1982; 14:55–60.

43. Biering-Sorensen F, Thomsen C. Medical, social and occupational history as risk indicators for low back trouble in a general population. Spine 1986; 11(7):720-725.

44. Lonstein, MB, Weisel, SW. Standardized approaches to the evaluation and treatment of industrial low back pain. Occup Med 1988; 3(1):147.

45. Snook S. Approaches to the control of back pain in industry: job design, job placement and education/training. Occup Med State of the Art Reviews 1988; 3(1):45-59.

46. Magora A. Investigation of the relationship between low back pain and occupation. Scand J Rehab Med 1973; 5:191-196.

47. Westrin C, Hirsch C, Lindegard B. The personality of the back patient. Clin Ortho 1972; 87:209-216.

48. Niemcryk S, Jenkins CD, Rose RM, Hurst MW. The prospective impact of psychosocial variables on rates of illness and injury in professional employees. J Occup Med 1987; 29(8):645-652.

49. Weisel SW, Feffer HL, Rothman RH. Industrial low back pain—a prospective evaluation of a standardized diagnostic and treatment protocol. Spine 1984; 9(2):199-204.

50. Buckle P, Kember P, Wood A et al. Factors influencing low back pain. J Occup Med 1971; 13:376-478.

51. Rowe M. Low back pain in industry—a position paper. J Occup Med 1969; 11:161-169.

52. Dillane JD, Fry J, Kalton G. Acute back syndrome—a study from general practice. Br Med J 1966; 2:82.

53. Kelsey JL, Githens PB, O'Connor T et al. Acute prolapsed lumbar intervertebral disc: An epidemiological study with special reference to driving automobiles and cigarette smoking. Spine 1984; 9:608.

54. Merskey H, Lau CL, Russell ES et al. Screening for psychiatric morbidity. The pattern of psychological illness and premorbid characteristics in four chronic pain populations. Pain 1987; 30:141-157.

55. Trief PM, Elliott DJ, Stein N, Frederickson BE. Functional vs organic pain: A meaningful distinction? J Clin Psychol 1987; 43(2):219-226.

56. Leavitt F, Garron DC. Validity of a back pain classification scale for detecting psychological disturbance as measured by the MMPI. J Clin Psychol 1980; 36(1):186-189.

57. Magni G, Merskey H: A simple examination of the relationships between pain, organic lesions and psychiatric illness. Pain 1987; 29:295-300.

58. Krishnan KRR, France RD, Pelton S, McCann UD et al. Chronic pain and depression. I. Classification of depression in chronic low back pain patients. Pain 1985; 22:279-287.

59. Lindsey PG, Wyckoff M. The depression-pain syndrome and its response to antidepressants. Psychosomatics 1981; 22(7):571-577.

60. Bradley JJ. Severe localized pain associated with the depressive syndrome. Br J Psychiat 1963; 109:741-745.

61. Katon W, Egan K, Miller D. Chronic pain: Lifetime psychiatric diagnosis and family history. Am J Psychiat 1985; 142(10):1156-1160.

62. Dworkin RH, Richlin DM, Handlin DS, Brand L. Predicting treatment response in depressed and non-depressed chronic pain patients. Pain 1986; 24:343-353.

63. Krishnan KRR, France RD, Pelton S, McCann UD et al. Chronic pain and depression. II. Symptoms of anxiety in chronic low back pain patients and their relationship to subtypes of depression. Pain 1985; 22:289-294.

64. Sandstrom JS, Andersson GB, Wallerstedt S. The role of alcohol abuse in working disability in patients with low back pain. Scand J Rehab Med 1984; 16:147-149.

65. Lawlis GF, McCoy CE. Psychological evaluation: Patients with chronic pain. In Evaluation and care of lumbar spine problems. Orthop Clin N. Am 1983; 14:3,527-538.

66. Frymoyer JW, Rosen JC, Clements J, Pope MH. Psychologic factors in low back pain disability; Clin Orthop 1985; 195:178-184.

67. Costello RM, Hulsey TL, Schoenfeld LS, Ramamurthy S. P-A-I-N: A four-cluster MMPI typology for chronic pain. Pain 1987; 30:199-209.

68. Schmidt JP, Wallace RW. Factorial analysis of the MMPI profiles of low back pain patients. J Pers Assess 1982; 46(4):366-369.

69. Love AW, Peck CL. The MMPI and psychological factors in chronic low back pain: A review. Pain 1987; 28:1-12.

70. Cairns LD, Mooney V, Crane P. Spinal pain rehabilitation: Inpatient and outpatient treatment results and development of predictors for outcome. Spine 1984; 9(1):91-95.

71. Hendler N. Depression caused by chronic pain. J Clin Psychiat 1984; 45(3, sec 2):30-36.

72. Rosen JR, Johnson C, Frymoyer JW. Identification of excessive back disability with the Faschingbauer Abbreviated MMPI. J Clin Psychol 1983; 39(1):71-74.

73. Gatchel RJ, Mayer TG, Capra P, Barnett J, Diamond P. Millon behavioral health inventory: Its utility in predicting physical function in patients with low back pain. Arch Phys Med Rehab 1986; 67:878-882.

74. Chatarvedi SK. Family morbidity in chronic pain patients. Pain 1987; 30:159-168.

75. Krishnan KRR, France RD, Houpt JL. Chronic low back pain and depression. Psychosomatics 1985; 26(4):299-304.

24

PSYCHIATRIC ASPECTS OF SPINE DISEASE

David J. Anderson
Michael H. Moskowitz

The spine is an unknown organ system to the average American. To most it isn't even considered a physical system. It qualifies as such, however, via its specific function and its specific utilization of elements from several other organ systems, as well as its vulnerability to specific illnesses and physical trauma. Most people pay little attention to this part of their body, which is always behind them, until they develop back or neck disease. It is when they find their entire lifestyle coming to a grinding halt that they tend to discover the spine's importance as a frustrating reality. While care is necessarily focussed upon the discovery of the peripheral stimulus and its subsequent treatment, it is often true that the greatest contribution to chronic problems is a psychological one. The scope of psychological stressors assaulting the psychic balance point in the spine-injured patient is truly a vast one. Perhaps simplest to understand is the obvious fact that pain so inhibits function that it causes a dramatic change in self-image and loss of self-esteem. These changes increase exponentially with chronicity of illness, incomplete physical diagnosis, and inadequate treatment. This mounting uncertainty is complicated by lack of knowledge regarding potential future damage, conflicting medical information, adversarial relationships with caregivers, goals incompatible with the medicolegal system, family disruption, financial and occupational disaster, loss of social context, prior psychological problems, substance abuse, and subsequent psychosocial problems.

The general philosophy of medical treatment espouses the duality of mind and body. A few proselytize about the unity, but they are either voices in the wilderness or captives in the ivory towers of academia. The message rarely penetrates the real world of medicine. While many spine surgeons refer "problem cases" out to other specialists, including psychiatrists, for consultation, programs that integrate total psychiatric evaluation and treatment into a multidisciplinary model of care for the spine-injured patient, are quite unusual. In the San Francisco Bay Area, this type of approach arose as an evolutionary phase out of a desire to develop and deliver the highest quality of care to patients with spine disease. This chapter is devoted to describing the theoretical underpinnings, evaluative tools, treatment procedures, and clinical efficacy of this approach to the treatment of the patient with spine disease.

THEORY

Physiologic homeostatic mechanisms have been the focus of somatic medical treatment for many years. Initially, medical scientists of the Renaissance responded to the devastation of the bubonic plague by rejecting the treatment of disease as a spiritual problem, replacing that notion with the scientific method. Clinical observation of objectifiable phenomena became the cornerstone of allopathic medicine, and the hegemony of this approach gave rise to our technologically driven system of rigorous application of the scientific method. Walter Cannon, considered by most as the father of modern physiology, wrote a book in 1932 called *The Wisdom of the Body*. There he described the intricate connections between the various systems in the body and how they helped to maintain a flexible but constant balance called homeostasis (1). Followers of Cannon, including Weiner and Lowne (2, 3) have diligently brought the psychophysiologic approach to understanding such varied issues as sudden death, peptic ulcer disease, asthma, and headache.

While Cannon was developing his homeostatic theory, many of Freud's theories about the mind and its unconscious content were gaining widespread acceptance in Europe and the United States (4). From the psychoanalytic school there emerged several theoreticians who focussed upon the area of psychosomatics, particularly Franz Alexander (4). Alexander developed a theory of psychogenesis regarding what was long known as the "holy seven psychosomatic illnesses." He spent his life defining the psychological basis of these illnesses. This theory, known as organ specificity, gained widespread acceptance for a number of years, but fell apart under scientific scrutiny. Alexander's real contribution was to further the understanding and acceptance of the psyche as a major factor among the various ones that affect illness and its outcome.

Helen Flanders Dunbar developed a theory regarding personality specificity and various illnesses (5–7). This theory also has not held up to the test of time, except in one very important area that has spawned a massive amount of research, including what may be the most impressive series of prospective studies ever embarked upon in modern medicine. This is clinically confirmed type "A" personality and its relationship to cardiovascular disease (8–10). Interestingly, many have found the pursuit of this theory to be more broadly applicable to all stress-related illnesses (3, 11–14). The link here appears to relate not so much to a particular achievement-oriented personality style, but specifically to the aggressive, angry, multimodal, and time-pressured behavior found in many personality types, especially when under a good deal of stress.

The Type A observations link with the theories developed by another giant in the field of psychosomatics, Pavlov. He is considered to be the founder of the behavioral school of medicine and his Nobel Prize winning work showing the connections of learned behavior to physiologic change has had a very broad application to medicine in general and to psychosomatics, in

particular (15). His successors, H.G. Wolfe, Stuart Wolf, and Hans Selye, have done a remarkable job of linking specific environmental and psychological stressors to physiologic changes and disease processes (15, 16).

Into this melange of theories comes the more unifying biopsychosocial model of illness proposed by George Engel (11, 12, 17, 18). He is a prodigious author and outstanding teacher who drew a link between all illness and its tripartite etiology. For Engel it was never enough to look at a patient as having a biological lesion; instead, the scope of the problem and its appropriate treatment could only be understood in the context of the patient's psychological makeup and reaction to his illness, as well as the specific social and cultural setting within which the illness existed.

It is the purpose of the authors of this chapter to examine the relationship of the balance of the human mind with the physical function of the body and the social context of the patient's life. It is this balance, which is the psychological correlate to physiologic homeostasis, that ultimately determines the patient's response to disease and its treatment. This is particularly important to the patient with spine disease, because successful outcome of treatment is rarely complete restoration of premorbid comfort and function. The patient's psychological adaptation will determine success or failure. The patient who requires complete restoration will invariably experience spine treatment outcome as equivocal at best. People who are psychologically able to redefine themselves within the context of their limitations will be better able to push these limitations to maximal function and to perceive appropriate interventions as success. If we can assume that a person becomes a patient with both a mind and body present as part of a unified whole, then it is reasonable to assume that a major loss of physical homeostasis will be reflected in an adjustment and loss of psychic homeostasis, as well. This would be little more than an interesting phenomenon, if the converse were not also true. Loss of psychic balance will feed back upon the physically disrupted system to prevent homeostatic adjustment. This process continues ad infinitum, resulting in poor outcomes in the face of excellent care. If we place spine-injured patients with an underlying, driven, impulsive personality organization in a social context that is used to having them give orders and produce results, we find ourselves with a set-up for treatment failure. It is likely that these individuals will become involved with physically strenuous activities without proper use of stabilization or body mechanics. The all too frequent result is to extend the scope of the injury or to break down surgical repair. Also, it is highly unlikely that people who state that they are terrified of "becoming a cripple," but who have comfortably withdrawn into a social system that constantly reinforces pain behavior will allow conservative or surgical intervention to alter the course of disability.

If one examines spine disease in the light of these ideas one sees a clearcut connection between the amount of suffering a person with an injured spine experiences and the psychological and social upheaval present in that person's life. In turn, the stress generated by this upheaval crosses the psychological barrier back to the physical problem, wreaking havoc upon the adaptational ability of the injured patient. Patients often finds themselves in completely alien territory regarding the expectations placed upon them about their truthfulness, diligence, motivation to heal, and willingness to settle. Primary physicians are frequently frustrated by their own sense that they are fighting against the increasing demands of their patient, the patient's attorney, the patient's insurance company, and deleterious effects of medications. The psychiatrist is usually called into the case to verify that the chronically ill spine patient not responding to treatment is really no longer a spine case, but is more appropriately a psychiatric case. More often than not, the unfortunate classification of the patient as psychologically impaired is used as an excuse by all to diminish care, instead of to enhance it. To gain some comprehension of this complex interrelated picture, the physician needs appreciation of the inherent psychological forces with which patients facing chronic spine pain and their families must reckon.

THE NATURAL COURSE OF DISABLING LOWER BACK PAIN: A PSYCHOLOGICAL PERSPECTIVE

In the literature on the psychology of back pain many attempts are made to describe methods for predicting which individuals are at significant risk of failure to respond to either conservative and/or surgical care. In the author's experience, the current models have not helped to predict either who will get better, who will need help, or what kind of help will be required. To our knowledge, none of these approaches have studied the natural course of the psychological challenges and demands during recovery from chronic disabling lumbar spine pain. Rather, the focus has been on the patient's personality, family structure and dynamics, work history, litigation, and other factors with little mention of the psychological challenges facing the patient. The outcome of this omission has been a collection of data about the patient, but no increased understanding of how the patient became that way. Indeed the approaches are somewhat like attempting to predict the outcome of a disease by laboratory tests and x-rays, but without having ever examined the unique pathophysiology of the specific illness itself. Without such a context, the data are rather meaningless and clinically less than useful. The authors have performed psychiatric evaluations on over 1500 patients with disabling chronic back pain since 1982 and followed prospectively two-thirds from a single follow-up visit to biweekly visits for up to 3 years. Recurrent patterns and themes emerging from these evaluations and follow-ups form the three phases of the illness process of disabling low back pain. At any time a patient will be found in any one of the phases with a varying level of disability. Many of the more intractable situations are mired in one phase and require some form of outside intervention if change is to occur.

Though highly variable in intensity and degree of disruption, the demands to be met for a sustained recovery spare few, if any, patients. The process is cyclical and involves three distinct phases. We have named them the threat, the pit, and the renewal. Full recovery often requires several passages through the process, but usually the first is the most arduous and the one that most often requires professional help. Highly successful spine surgeries can forestall this process for years. However, unless the challenges are met by the patient, the pain will return, often in a more malignant form.

The particularly unique position of the lumbar spine in the human psyche must be appreciated. After all it is the lumbar spine that supports the human species' upright posture, which in part makes our species unique. In fact, this very upright posture that most individuals acquire between ten and fourteen months of life is threatened by the back pain. With the threat comes a state of enforced dependency that few individuals have experienced in such an open ended fashion since that time before language function was available. Thus, in many ways, that experience is beyond words and beyond verbal communication. That which is available in everyday metaphoric language is rather disparaging. Someone is accused of being "spineless" to suggest a cowardly avoidance of responsibility. People need "more backbone" to define themselves more independently. We "break our backs" when we work diligently under burdensome circumstances especially when it involves a martyred sense of duty. Thus, an ominous threat of potentially humiliating, indescribable dependency descends upon the patient disabled by back pain. As this descent occurs, the first phase begins.

The first phase is the one in which we find most of our patients. It occurs after the reality of the chronic state of torment becomes evident. The injury is no longer acute and self-limited but chronic, and relentless. It isn't going to go away on its own. A battle has become a war without any evident resolution. The patient is threatened with a state of profound helplessness and consequential loss of autonomy, control, and power by mysterious, destructive, invisible forces well beyond his or her control. The condition frequently literally brings patients to their knees. Patients' entire external material and emotional life can be under threat of dissolution by a torturous pain. The feelings of persecution, humiliation, and terrifying danger that accompany this phase are aggravated by the absence of an accurate diagnosis. Without a name, the suffering feels unauthentic. It is in their heads, which means they must be crazy. Patients attempt to defend themselves against this dangerous threat by myriad methods. Repeated attempts are made to extract themselves from this state using all the coping skills they know, but often these only lead to further frustration and increased pain. Most commonly, there is a denial of the seriousness of the problem, narcotic and sedative use, and an insistence on surgery as a magical solution

to avoid the frightening and mysterious unknown of the continued threat.

Buffeted by helplessness and humiliation, patients struggle to assert some kind of sense of individual power, competency, and real existence in a world that has become increasingly limited and restricted. Patients strongly appeal to the primary physician's desires to rescue them in some heroic fashion that is quite gratifying and indeed rarely necessary or possible. The patient cajoles, intimidates, pleads, bargains, and uses various and sundry ways of inducing guilt in the caregivers so that they will somehow slay the monster and remove the threat: "Take it away so that preinjury life can be resuscitated and the dreaded loss will not occur." This phase is riddled with feelings of rage, persecution, self-doubt, helplessness, social isolation, and intermittent embarrassment because of the loss of autonomy and function. Physically the struggle has taken its toll with disturbed sleep, appetite, weight loss or gain, loss of sexual interest and energy. The patient becomes progressively socially withdrawn and often drug and/or alcohol dependent. Inevitable social isolation (i.e., "No one knows the trouble I've seen!") occurs despite any and all attempts to empathize. The pain and its suffering are so personal that no one can really understand. The patient is close to giving up. When voluntary, this giving up actually takes the form of a withdrawal into a predictable and relatively safe world to await arrival of relief. More often, it is an involuntary form of withdrawal and depression envelops the patient in a cloak of apathy, indifference, and despair of recovery. Another form that this giving up takes is the entrenched chronic pain syndrome. In this state, the patient becomes a caricature of the acute pain patient. It can become a rigid fortress against the threatened loss and all attempts to intervene are thwarted. For others, even this fortress is inadequate and the depression deepens and suicidal ideation and impulses emerge. For the caregiver this phase can be the most taxing because of uncertainty as to whether the patient will survive. The caregiver can feel frustrated, angry, and quietly hopeful of getting rid of the patient. The patient's family is frequently in crisis at this time and it is frequently from them the panicked telephone calls are received. "Doctor, **you** must **do** something." Surgery at this time is frequently only temporarily restorative. It is at this point that the second phase can emerge if it is allowed.

The second phase rarely occurs without outside help. The help need not be professional, but it must be facilitating and tolerant of the uncertain consequences. This phase is usually brief relative to the first and third phases. It can last for a few moments or for up to a month. We have named it the pit because of the profound state of pervasive despair that marks its presence. It is a period of confusion, chaos, and emotional flux. These patients have surrendered to the pull of forces beyond their control and allowed their previous lives to collapse without any hope of return. The struggle is over; the defeat, the loss, the death are certain. The patient may experience suicidal thoughts and occasionally hospitalization is required. For the caregiver, this phase can be the most taxing because of the uncertainty as to whether the patient will survive the descent into the pit.

Slowly the patient emerges from this confusion. The circumstances are seen with a clarity and from a perspective of completely new understanding. Disordered priorities and distorted perceptions of limitations are called into question.

At this point the third phase, the renewal, begins. With collapse of the old world and the death of its ways of living, new solutions previously ignored become apparent and are entertained tentatively and cautiously. Gradually a new sense of purpose and direction emerges. The pain is frequently still present but is less of a tormenting enemy. The future is brighter, with patients displaying some hope of a return to being functional and of value to themselves, their family, and society. Flare-ups, impatience with the tediously slow pace of recovery, vocational uncertainty, and unraveling family support all threaten the survival of the emergence. It is at this point that we frequently are tempted to release patients from our care and expect that they can manage the rest of the recovery on their own. For many around the patient, the person that emerges is extremely difficult to recognize and accept no matter how much the caregivers find that person acceptable and often more admirable and respectable than the preinjury person. Family members, rather than being enthusiastic about the recovery, are disappointed that the old person hasn't returned and may actually reject the new priorities and perspectives to which the patient has adapted.

For most patients, this process has to be repeated several times. Fortunately for most, the subsequent pass-throughs are not nearly as grueling as the initial one. For many, the process is not necessarily noticeable to anyone but the most intimate loved ones. It is extremely rare for it not to occur at all in patients who recover completely.

EVALUATIVE TOOLS

The psychiatric evaluation is the cornerstone upon which the psychological understanding of the patient is developed. Many programs either start or stop their psychological assessment of the patient solely for medicolegal purposes or attempt to short-circuit the need for a psychiatric evaluation by using computer graded psychological testing. It is our experience that these are inadequate methods of evaluating the complexities of a patient's cognitive, emotional, and personality based processes in the context of spine injury.

The capacity to endure and master the challenges of the previously described three phase process is significantly affected by critical events and traumas during early psychological stages of development, current developmental stressors, and particular psychosocial factors. The central psychological theoretical basis of our assessment is attachment theory. During the last 15 years, a great deal has been learned in human development research about the importance for physical and mental health of the quality of the emotional connection known as attachment (Ainsworth, Bowlby, Mahler; 19–22). Ainsworth showed in her seminal study of infants in a strange situation that the presence of a secure or insecure (anxious) attachment can be demonstrated at one year of age (19). Such attachments are a measure of the relationship between an infant and the primary caregiver and form the template for the way in which the child will relate in other significant relationships over the course of its life. The central focus of the evaluation model is the attachment history of the patient and the particular disturbances that have occurred in it. Although statistical analysis is not yet available, initial clinical impressions indicate that the back-injured patient's ability to overcome disabling chronic pain can be assigned relative risks by assessment of the developmental history coupled with assessment of the way in which patient relates to current caregivers. During recovery from disabling back pain, the strength and resilience of the earlier template is severely tested. The physician and the medical care system become the primary caregiver, and the patient establishes a relationship consistent with this early template. Developmental history consistent with insecure attachment can be correlated with a history of physical and/or sexual abuse, neglect, and/or early loss of the caregiver. Lack of available caregivers, as might be seen in chronic disabilities, is associated with negative outcome, such as the development of chronic pain in the absence of an organic basis, or pain grossly out of proportion to the peripheral stimulus. These factors are obtained through a semistructured psychiatric interview and review of records. Also assessed in the interview is the patient's current attachment as judged by the stability of interpersonal relationships, as well as the capacity to relate to an empathic interviewer. Current attachment patterns are usually consistent with the developmental history. A problematic or an absent ability to form consoling relationships with family and friends or an empathic interviewer also represents a risk of negative outcome.

Our experiences with chronic back pain are consistent with the recent findings of Adler and colleagues in their retrospective, controlled study highly correlating developmental psychosocial experiences with psychogenic pain (23). While an understanding of predictors for negative outcome may be useful in avoiding surgery in those patients whose peripheral stimulus is minimal, the greater challenge is to help those patients who, despite being at risk for negative outcome, will likely come to surgical intervention. In such cases, psychiatric treatment is crucial. The evaluation should be in the format of a typical psychiatric assessment with the history focussed also upon the patient's injury, its course of diagnosis and treatment, alterations in the patient's mood, and specific psychological symptoms. A current history of medications and their pattern of use is of great importance. Past medical history, past psychiatric history, social history, and family history must all be carefully assessed. An objective description of the patient's mental status should

then be clearly delineated. Assessment of the patient must place into context all of the above elements and should be a narrative description evaluating the patient's general character organization, psychological adjustment to injury, extent of psychopathology, relationship of psychopathology to the patient's pre- and postinjured condition, ability of the patient psychologically to manage conservative or surgical care, risk of treatment failure, changes in the patient's social system, and ability of the patient to maintain or return to work. In certain instances, such as medicolegal evaluations or in patients exhibiting severe psychopathology, a DSM IIIR diagnostic assessment should be done. Finally, a section of recommendations must be made. It is important to keep these and the assessment section as jargon free as possible. The recommendations should be numbered, specific, addressed to issues discussed in the assessment section, and directed toward answers to specific questions from the consultee. It is important here to get a clear idea, prior to assessment, of what the consultee wishes to clarify. A final and often neglected step in the evaluation is to discuss findings with the consultee(s).

Psychiatric Evaluation

In our view, it is of critical importance to have a psychiatric evaluation done for patients in the following categories.

a. Patients who show obvious psychological problems of significant depression, severe anxiety, psychosis, phobic reactions to diagnostic tests, inconsistency of organic findings, emotional lability, suicidal ideation/attempt, or significant inconsistency of history;

b. Patient who have a great deal of difficulty with follow-through on conservative treatment plans;

c. Patients with severe intercurrent life stressors;

d. Patients being considered for a functional restoration/chronic pain program;

e. Patients considered to have a functional versus organic problem;

f. Patients suspected of malingering or factitious disorders;

g. Patients with clinical pictures complicated enough to be evaluated by the multidisciplinary team;

h. Patients being considered for back surgery;

i. Patients who exhibit postoperative psychological complications;
j. Patients who do poorly despite adequate treatment;
k. Medicolegal cases.

Hypnotherapy Evaluation

Evaluations for hypnotherapy should be done prior to starting treatment in hypnotherapy or biofeedback. These must share many of the elements of a psychiatric evaluation, unless a recent assessment has already been done. Of particular importance is any past history of abuse or severe psychological trauma. One should be aware of this or unusual areas of memory dysfunction that often represent profound levels of repressive psychological defense. The patient may experience an abreaction in hypnotherapeutic trance and these can be quite frightening. These types of problems do not rule out the use of hypnotherapy, but patients should be forewarned of their possibility. Additionally, these types of trauma may play a specific role in the patient's current complex of psychological symptoms and may point the direction of hypnotherapeutic treatment. The physically abused and abandoned patient, for example, is one whose hypnotherapeutic work must stress pain relief in the context of consistency and commitment on the part of the therapist and treatment team. All images should focus upon safe, trusting, and secure situations. Assessment of the patient's past experience with hypnosis, biofeedback, meditation, and visualization and relaxation techniques should be directed at understanding what has worked and not worked in the past. Often this experience will not be related to pain, but the patient will be expert at achieving trance. When evaluation is complete, a specific treatment plan, within the context of the patient's overall treatment plan, should be delineated. These specifics should be spelled out and should be geared toward a time-limited approach directed at clear goals and focussed upon teaching mastery through self-hypnotic techniques. Patient passivity should be discouraged.

Follow-Up

Follow-up is extremely important in the evaluation of the psychiatric status of the spine-injured patient. Although it may appear to be more of an issue in treatment, one must be willing to use ongoing follow-up as a way to change and hone the psychiatric diagnostic issues. This is extremely important in assessing psychopharmacologic and hypnotherapeutic interventions, but is also important in the patient who is assessed as not needing direct psychiatric follow-up. While this may appear to be a contradiction, it actually is quite practical if the evaluating psychiatrist solicits the input of the rest of the treatment team in evaluating the progress of the patient. If predictions of risk and outcome do not appear to be in line with the original assessment, a reformulation or fresh evaluation may be in order. Psychiatrists are all too used to the notion that they do their work in private. This often leads to the isolation of the psychiatric aspects of the case from the physical progression. Hence, the psychiatrist can become the unwitting facilitator of the mind/body split. An effective way of managing follow-up in cases that do not require ongoing psychotherapy is to arrange an afternoon per month to see follow-up cases with the primary care physician.

Psychological Testing

Our experience has not shown standardized psychological tests, including the Minnesota Multiphasic Personality Inventory or the Millon Behavioral Index, to be adequate in the assessment of the psychological functioning of spine injured patients. To the contrary, we have found these evaluations to be expensive and inadequate substitutes for a thorough psychiatric evaluation. These tests are done too routinely, and rarely add to a thorough assessment. They may be helpful in rare, specific cases where diagnostic issues remain perplexing. All too often, conclusions drawn from supposedly objective tests are used to disqualify patients from needed care. It is the opinion of the authors that the clinician assessing the spine-injured patient needs to have a medically sophisticated understanding of spine injuries. This certainly does not reflect the current standard of care, but, in our opinion, it is critical to the independence, usefulness, and reliability of psychiatric assessment of spine-injured patients. At times, neuropsychometric testing may be helpful, as may projective tests. In any case, the use of testing should be dictated by clinical efficacy and need, as determined by the evaluator. It should not be approached as a standard to be applied to all patients receiving psychiatic evaluations.

We have developed a series of 90 questions subsumed under the broad topics of present history, attachment behaviors, abuse history, family history, medical/psychiatric history, vocational history, and legal history. The questions selected have come from our experience in evaluating spine-injured patients. We are now in the stage of doing a retrospective study revolving around these questions and successful or unsuccessful outcome for back surgery and conservative care patients. We will attempt to demonstrate which specific responses and clusters of responses relate to high risk of treatment failure. We hope through future prospective studies eventually to have an objective tool to measure outcome risks for various treatment modalities of spine injured patients.

Multidisciplinary Evaluation

The opinions of the rest of the multidisciplinary team are very important in the psychiatric assessment. The psychiatrist will spend a few hours with the patient, but the rest of the team has totaled a great deal more in exposure to this person. Anxiety level, pain behavior, reactions to testing, frustration tolerance, affective lability, inconsistency of symptoms, truthfulness, exaggeration of symptoms, ability to follow directions, degree of helplessness, spousal relationship, and relationship with third party payees may be more directly accessible to the treatment team. It is a mistake for the psychiatric consultant to formulate opinions without the rest of the team's advice. The ideal consultation is at multidisciplinary conference, but prior to this, informal discussion are helpful.

Psychiatric Meaning of Illness

Understanding the psychological meaning of illness for the individual patient is an area of critical importance in assessing the overall psychiatric status. Spine disease, in the vast majority of cases, is seen as an intrusive, destructive tormenter, launching a sneak attack aimed at undermining the victim's life. Choices are ultimately made by the patient either to remain a helpless, powerless victim, or to make life work within the limits of the illness. Cases involved in compensation and the medicolegal process complicate this set of choices, which are made largely on an unconscious basis. Past psychiatric history and character organization also play a predominant role, as does the success or failure of prior medical treatment. Surgery is often sought as the relief to suffering and, in many cases, it is just that. However, all too often the expectation of surgery is an unrealistic one, based upon the belief that removal of the pain generator will completely restore the premorbid psychosocial condition. Often, the damage to psyche and social system is so extensive that by the time surgical correction is effected, the patient has embraced the role of victim in a death grip. Positive surgical outcome is best predicted by the patient exhibiting an adaptive presurgical style that is already adjusting to make life livable, regardless of medical outcome.

For other patients, the meaning of spine disease is that of escape from overwhelming responsibility into a role of illness requiring support from those people previously supported by the patient. The implications here regarding chronicity and the direction of treatment toward the support system are somewhat obvious. Others see chronic illness not merely as a crisis, but as an opportunity to change their lives. This can be quite positive, but also can be dangerous if the patient does not resolve the underlying issues at the time of definitive treatment of the physical problems. Again, it is important to understand the unconscious nature of these issues. The patient is not volunteering for illness and is operating at a psychological level beyond conscious control. Often patients stuck in the cycle of poor recovery despite effective treatment are blamed for treatment failure by their physicians or third party carriers, as if they were willingly and consciously perpetuating their condition. In fact, only a very small number of patients consciously manipulate their treating doctors and insurance carriers in order to receive payment, drugs, disability status, or the sick role.

Case example 1. The patient comes to treatment upon a routine presurgical evaluation to resolve disc herniation in her neck. During the initial psychiatric evaluation, she describes her relationship with her workaholic husband as unsatisfactory and largely unsupportive. She goes on to describe a sexually abusive father and a mother who chose to ignore the abuse. The patient has compensated for the lack of attention in her relationship with her husband by conducting a series of affairs and complaining to her friends about her husband. She goes into surgery admitting that she wants to end the relationship, but is frightened at the idea of being a single parent, although that has been her virtual situation for years. Although hand weakness improves, postoperative pain is severe. In follow-up therapy, the patient admits to feeling trapped, much as she did with her own father. She has used extramarital relationships to escape her sense of being boxed in, much as she used the relationship with her husband to leave home permanently. It seems clear to her that when her husband ignores her needs, her neck and head pain is far worse. The patient is confronted with the idea that she is afraid to live her life without a sense of being trapped and she acknowledges that the next obvious trap is perpetuating her neck pain.

Case example 2. A patient with a large series of charts and prior multidisciplinary evaluations presents to the multidisciplinary team with instructions from his insurance company to determine whether lumbar surgery was indicated. All reviewers had an uncomfortable feeling about inconsistencies in the patient's history. A review of records showed blatant distortions and lies, multiple hospitalizations, and numerous changes of state residencies. The purpose of all this was aimed at achieving and maintaining the status of patient.

TREATMENT

Psychotherapy Aimed at the Three Phases of Spine Pain

The focus of the interventions is to facilitate the successful movement through the particular phase in which the treating physician finds the patient. The treatment may utilize adjunctive antidepressant therapy, hypnotherapy, behavioral therapy, strategic therapy, insight oriented therapy, supportive therapy, couples or family therapy. The formation of a consoling relationship with such patients does, in our experience, improve outcome and is the central recurrent theme of the work. Thus, repeated surgical failures can be potentially avoided. This model of focused psychiatric intervention is important in helping the patient endure and master the demands of recovery. Such interven-

tions can both prevent and treat the chronic pain syndrome.

Strategic and Ordeal Therapy

Strategic therapy is a concept elaborated upon by Jay Haley (24, 25) secondary to his work with Milton Erikson. It is defined as any therapy in which the therapist attempts actively to influence people. This type of therapy is closely linked to hypnotherapy and has been refined into ordeal therapy. In ordeal therapy, the patients are given directives to involve themselves in a series of activities more onerous than the symptoms. They must first make a firm contract to follow through with these directives and should be held accountable by the therapist to do so. A caveat with all strategic and ordeal therapies is that the therapists must constantly be aware of and avoid their own sadistic impulses.

Erickson's understanding of hypnosis was that it was a special form of communication between people, which established motivation for change in the patient through direct action of the therapist. "The hypnotist directs a person to spontaneously change his behavior" (25). The voluntary action leads to the involuntary response. Resistance was to be expected, as with any form of psychotherapy, and Erickson developed many ways of dealing with resistance:

1. *Encouraging resistance.* The therapist observes the resistance, then sides with it. Of course you must continue to fight, but you can learn to fight to lose.
2. *Providing a worse alternative.* To encourage autonomy, the therapist selects the overall class of resistant behaviors and asks the patient to do something within that class of behaviors that is more unpleasant than overcoming his symptom. For example, exercise at 2:00 AM on days that the symptom is worse than the patient wishes it to be.
3. *Causing change by communicating in metaphor.* Do not directly address the overt problem, but discuss a metaphorical situation, distracting the patient from an attempt to directly approach the stated problem. For example, describe differences in dining preferences between a married couple with sexual dysfunction, followed by a prescription of pleasant dinner. This sets the stage for a later pleasant sexual encounter. This method re-

quires the therapist to avoid making direct interpretations.

4. *Encouraging a relapse.* The patient who improves too quickly is given the directive to relapse, creating a situation of either continuing to follow the directive of the therapist or resisting the directive by not relapsing. This is a "no lose" situation for the patient. Of course the symptom will return, so why don't we bring it back and see what it tells us?

5. *Encouraging a response by frustrating it.* Cut off a partial, inadequate response, later returning to it. For example encourage the silent family member to continue to be quiet if he attempts to speak up, usually followed by provocative statements that demand he respond.

6. *Using space and position.* This disrupts the regular patterns of interaction by arbitrarily shifting seating arrangements asking family members to leave the room or change seats in the middle of a session.

7. *Emphasizing the positive.* Find the positive aspect the symptoms play in a person's life and enlarge upon this aspect. Your symptom gives you the chance to say no to your parents; perhaps we can find another way.

8. *Seeding ideas.* Initial use of ideas that may be emphasized later in therapy.

9. *Amplifying a deviation.* Seek a small change from the static norm and encourage it. Induction of a small change in a family system leads to a mild crisis, which is then encouraged until the system must change to deal with it.

10. *Avoiding self-exploration.* Avoidance of intellectualizing symptoms.

By expecting resistances and making them the focus of the therapy, the strategic or ordeal therapist uses the inevitable to bring on change. Instead of responding to the patient's resistance with frustration and rejection of the patient, the therapist moves the patient in the direction of the resistance to effect shifts in the patient's maladaptive behavior. This type of therapy is best used with the group of patients who have been unable to receive help from other caregivers.

Behavioral Therapy

Behavioral therapy is often viewed as the cornerstone of treatment of chronic back pain. Since pain is a problem that has been particularly refractory to more traditional psychotherapeutic techniques, behavioral models have been readily applied. Sternbach (26) states that behavioral therapy has not proven to be of any long-term benefit in the treatment of chronic pain. While in isolation this may be an accurate statement, if behavioral treatment is integrated into an overall treatment plan, it can be quite effective. Operant techniques recommended by Fordyce (27) have been useful in pain programs. Since operants are behaviors that involve involuntary muscles, pain behavior is often an operant condition. Reinforcers powerfully establish operant behavior. The focus here is on extinguishing pain behavior by eliminating positive reinforcers. Basically, pain complaints, both direct and indirect, are ignored. Stress in these program is placed upon increased function and strength, with clear positive reinforcement for accomplishments in these endeavors. Family treatment is critical since much operant reinforcement of pain behavior occurs in the family or social milieu. When combined with cognitive learning techniques, behavioral treatments are quite valuable. In a sense, the patient must be reeducated to eliminate false beliefs about pain as a degenerative illness process, while pain behavior is ignored and return to physical function is reinforced via appropriate physical activity.

Pharmacotherapy

Pharmocotherapy with spine-injured patients can be quite challenging. Many of the patients present to the physician with chronic pain exacerbated by chronic use of opiate analgesics. Often the treating physician is uncomfortable with the ever-escalating dose of opiates, but feels helpless about stemming the tide in the face of escalating pain. The irony is that it is clear that pain tolerance diminishes with long-term use of opiates and resultant increased opiate tolerance. Patients must be withdrawn from these types of medication if they are to progress with their chronic pain problems. These drugs do have a use with posttraumatic or postoperative acute pain. Psychotropic drugs of significant value are the nonaddictive class of medications known as antidepressants. These are useful in lower doses for pain, sleep disturbance, stress, and irritability. In higher doses, they can effectively treat the depression that often develops with unremitting pain. A relatively new antidepressant, fluoxitene, has a significantly different pharmacologic and side-effect profile than older antidepressants. It is quite attractive as a treatment modality due to its lack of sedation, weight gain, anticholinergic, or drug hangover side effects. It also has a rather uniform dose-with-treatment efficacy in a broad range of depressive problems. Use of anxiolytics should be approached with caution. The benzodiazepines are addictive and can cause the same problems as opiates regarding tolerance and the need for increasing doses. Additionally, they often deepen preexisting depressions. These drugs are particularly troublesome when used as hypnotics. We prefer to use lower doses of antidepressants for sleep disturbances in spine-injured patients. Although antipsychotics have been studied and shown to be useful in pain management, we feel their use should be reserved for psychotic patients, because of the potentially devastating long-term side effects of this class of drugs.

Chemical Dependency Treatment

Not uncommonly, the patient with chronically disabling spine pain has developed a serious alcohol or chemical dependency. Often this problem had little predisability significance and has developed at least in part by inadequate medical management or denial by well-intentioned physicians. Without specific detoxification and vigorous treatment, any psychiatric intervention is marginally effective. Frank confrontation of the patient with dependency by the physician is essential and either inpatient or outpatient treatment specifically focused on the chemical dependency leads to the most salutary results.

Family/Couples Therapy

Because of the major disruptive consequences on the patient's social life, interventions aimed at the couple or family unit can be extremely effective. The mobilization of corrective and helpful support by family members is often essential if the patient is to move through the phases of recovery as quickly as possible. If this perspective is ignored, frequently well-planned and executed interventions at the personal level fall short. Indeed, the destructive effects of divorce and other domestic disruption can severely stall any potential recovery.

Hypnotherapy

Hypnotherapy is misunderstood and often maligned as "hocus pocus." The reality is that there have been a multitude of studies that show the efficacy of this treatment (26, 28–30). Perhaps a great deal of the problem with accepting this treatment comes from the stage hypnotists' dramatic and often embarrassing use of the hypnotic state to entertain an audience. Even the roots of the clinical application of this phenomenon rest with a controversial progenitor, Franz Mezmer, who established his theory of animal magnetism. Mezmer himself was quite a showman, treating his patients while he was dressed in a bejeweled robe as they rested in a bathtub filled with iron filings. Although the theory of magnetic forces at play was a false one, Mezmer is credited with having discovered the clinical application of hypnosis. This was a dubious distinction at best, hypnosis having been rejected by the majority of medical and psychiatric practitioners until its resurgence following World War II. Currently, it is considered an effective treatment modality for dissociative psychiatric conditions, recovery of repressed memory, habit control, sleep disturbance, stress reduction, and pain control. The last three clinical applications are particularly important to back pain patients. It is important to add to these a sense of mastery over one's symptoms.

The technique of hypnosis we use with spine pain patients is that of teaching them self-hypnosis to control their pain. Hilgard sites several studies done at Stanford that show pain control and the hypnotic state to be directly related to the hypnotizability of the patient. While this has paralleled our own clinical experience, we have found that increased hypnotizability is something that can be taught. People have an innate skill level at self-hypnosis, but almost all can be taught to improve this level. Exceptions may be those people with attention deficit disorders and severe depressive or anxiety states. It is our impression that even many of these patients may improve their ability to achieve deeper hypnotic trance. Part of the logic here is that the hypnotic state is neither the exclusive purview of the skilled clinician or slick stage hypnotist. Rather, it is one of the usual states of consciousness seen in people and animals. People are in and out of self-induced trance states on a daily basis. It is the state of consciousness used prior to sleep, while reading a good novel, when daydreaming, during sexual activity, and in any other set of behaviors requiring focussed attention. In the clinical setting of pain control, it is our opinion that by teaching the patient how to use trance in a stepwise manner of increasingly rapid, self-directed inductions, a tool for pain control is combined with a sense of increased mastery over previously demoralizing symptoms. We approach this by teaching self-directed induction techniques, followed by trance deepening techniques, pain reduction metaphors, dissociative visualizations, age regression techniques, and posthypnotic suggestion. This approach is then supplemented with several weeks of practice at home by the patient. It is followed up with reinforcement of techniques that work for the patient and rapid (less than one minute) trance induction techniques. The patient is instructed to use the longer techniques at the end of the day and the more rapid, stress reducing techniques throughout the day. Additionally, we integrate hypnotherapy into the rest of the patient's treatment plan, with distinct approaches developed for the surgical patient, chronic pain patient, and functional restoration patient. Tapes should be used with caution. It is important for all hypnotherapeutic work to stress practice of the honing of *self-hypnotic* techniques. It is all too easy for the patient to develop a passive attitude regarding hypnotherapy and, and in our experience, this is anathema to successful use of this technique.

Biofeedback

Biofeedback is actually quite similar to hypnotherapy. Basically, biofeedback uses hypnotic trance induction to alter a measurable physiologic function such as striated muscle tension, skin temperature, or blood pressure, while feeding back the changes via sound and/or light impulses to the patient and the therapist. Almost all of the patients who suffer chronic pain have difficulty with handling life stresses. Many have initial difficulty with the idea of hypnotherapy, feeling that it represents a loss of control and a submission to someone else. This opinion is also held by many of the physicians referring patients for psychiatric care. Although this is not the case, it is often more palatable for patients and their primary

physicians to enter into this type of work via the more technologically driven route of biofeedback. For patients it gives some objective evidence of the mind/body connection and in particular the mind's ability to influence physiologic processes. In treating spine-injured patients for their pain, it is important for biofeedback to be aimed at weaning the patients off the biofeedback machines and tapes into a routine of self-hyponosis. We have found that by utilizing the two methods in tandem, especially in patients with chronic pain, the best clinical results can be effected. Some patients do better with the biofeedback approach and others do better with self-hypnosis. Biofeedback is a particularly useful method in the somatically preoccupied patient with a purely mechanistic view of spine disease. One of the main functions of using this method is to educate the patient to the undeniable connection between mind and body. By using biofeedback with this group, much time spent dealing with resistance can be saved. A complete program of stress and pain reduction treatment should include a time-limited number of biofeedback and hypnotic sessions combined with self-hypnotic practice. These treatments are usually pleasant and relaxing and it is easy for patient and therapist to continue them in an open-ended manner, thus unwittingly encouraging dependency on the part of the patient. Since our entire approach is to emphasize independence, our strong recommendation is to keep them time-limited with occasional reinforcement, as clinically indicated.

Functional Restoration Program

Chapter 34 below is dedicated to the functional restoration program. Of emphasis here is the role of the psychotherapist. The patient placed in the functional restoration program is usually one for whom surgery is not a viable option. If surgery is a possibility, it is clear to the surgeon that the patient needs to overcome the physical and psychological blocks to positive outcome by training to capacity in both areas prior to consideration of the rigors of surgical treatment and its recovery process. These patients are usually the most complex people we treat and have most often been "treatment failures" with other methods. Psychologically, they are most often in an extreme position regarding mood changes, social disorganization, somatic preoccupation, identity changes, helplessness, and a sense of being overwhelmed. Psychiatric intervention must include time-limited and focussed individual psychotherapy, hypnotherapeutic and biofeedback stress and pain management, and focussed group therapy. Often, pharmacotherapy and family therapy must also be included. The advantage here is of having the patients in one place and among peers for the intensive treatment of their spine-mediated dysfunction. Treatment needs to be integrated into the overall team approach, with avoidance of isolation of the psychiatric treatment. While issues of confidentiality need to be respected, splitting of treatment staff by patients demanding complete separation of psychiatric problems from physical issues should be discouraged. The psychiatrist must take a leadership role with the rest of the treatment team, communicating frequently with trainers, occupational therapists, physical therapists, and other physicians involved in the patient's care. A psychiatric treatment plan should be developed early in the patient's care, with the focus upon mastery of dysfunctional behavior.

Working with the Third Party Payer

Working with the third party payer is an area of care that is often either ignored or overemphasized. It is a fact that the third party payers have a right to be involved in overall treatment planning, because the care of the patient is being funded by them. This means that the treating psychiatrist must make an effort to explain clearly the indication for ongoing care following the initial evaluation. Insurance companies do not relish the notion of long-term psychotherapy on an open-ended basis. This is especially problematic in the area of workers' compensation, when it is clear that most people requiring long-standing psychiatric care have had preexisting problems. It is critical, therefore, for the psychotherapist to be well versed in short-term therapy and to assess fairly the apportionment between work injury and preexisting condition. Since not all original assessments can be done accurately, a close communication with the carrier is in order. Recommendations should be made on the best estimate of the amount of time required to treat the work-related condition. It is often baffling to the individual case manager how psychiatric care relates to spine-injured patients. Again, it is the job of the psychotherapist to communicate the need clearly. If the worker is having difficulty, a conference with the supervisor can be quite helpful.

Psychiatry is an area where special attention to the rules of confidentiality must be followed. It is essential that the psychiatrist talk to the patient about the need to include the third party payer in treatment planning and to provide the payer with updated progress reports. If patients balk at this, they can be offered the option of paying for their psychotherapy with other insurance or, in the rare instance of independent wealth, on their own. It is also often the case that the patient and the third party carrier have a less than satisfactory relationship. The psychiatrist often sympathizes with the patient. The patient's feelings must be explored to help deal with the psychological injuries experienced by the patient in a system often felt as dehumanizing and abusive. Unfortunately, it is not unusual for patients to be quite correct in their assessment. Here, the job of the therapist is a tricky one. While supporting the patient, the psychiatrist must try to maintain therapeutic neutrality. Again, it is important to communicate with third party payers as clearly as possible to try to defuse these potentially destructive and litigious situations. At times, the third party payer is already in a hostile posture with the patient, and it is here that the psychiatrist may need to become more directly involved with the patient's advocates, most often attorneys involved in litigation.

On the other side of the fence is the insurance-carrier-funded second opinion. Psychiatrists and psychologists are no more ignorant than the rest of the medical field about who pays the bill. Often individual practitioners develop a fairly sizable amount of their practice doing evaluations. Insurance carriers also know which psychotherapists give the most economically favorable opinons. This can lead to rather cynical and destructive issues with patients and it is in the best interest of all involved to try to avoid these predetermined evaluation outcomes. Much of the time the conclusions drawn from these evaluations merely reflect a difference of opinion between evaluators. Unfortunately, the legal process involved does not lend itself to resolving these differences in a collegial way, frequently resulting in further psychological injury to the patient. The other side of the coin is also in need of examination. It is not uncommon for defense attorneys to rely upon their own "experts" to perform the type of evaluations that support their own cases. Again the potential harm to the patient is quite high, with people placing all of their psychological energy into the legal struggle, leaving little for the healing process. Compromise and resolution are the best tactics, and it is here that the evaluating psychiatrist can do the most good. It is our opinion that a significant part of the evaluation should assess the patient's relationship with third party payers and the medicolegal system. This should be viewed as another psychosocial stressor and it should be dealt with accordingly in any evaluation. Psychiatrists who do this type of work must strive to evaluate cases from a purely clinical standpoint. Although they are not responsible for follow-up care, the "do not harm" ethic remains an important cornerstone of professional integrity.

CONCLUSIONS

One aspect of chronic disabling spine pain that is both stimulating and challenging is that, despite all the literature, very little is known about the psychology of spine pain. What appears to help someone overcome the disability will cripple the next person. More intensive study of those that do get well in a timely manner with long-term follow-up is extremely important to avoid the bias of a disability based model. The role of social expectations of the family, the work environment, the medical profession, and the third party payers toward the person with spine pain needs further investigation. A more comprehensive model of those actually at risk for chronic disability is extremely important. The model needs to be tested by therapeutic interventions consistent with the model's theory.

Other areas for further research include more thorough controlled study on the use of hypnotherapy and biofeedback in nonsurgical and surgical treatment of spine pain. While ther is good experimental research showing the efficacy of hypnosis in the control of pain, there is little decent clinical research into this area. Further study should also be done on how to teach patients deeper hypnotizability. Research in the area of pharmacology regarding use of new antidepressants needs to be established. Of particular interest here is fluoxetine, because of its low side-effect profile, broad-based clinical efficacy, energizing properties, weight reduction properties, and ability to help people stop smoking. It needs to be compared with longer standing antidepressant treatments already judged to be efficacious in the treatment of pain.

As suggested above, we know much less than we need to know to adequately comprehend spine pain and intercede therapeutically. Spine pain quickly becomes a somatopsychic disorder with potentially devastating consequences. Many of the consequences are in the form of lost or wasted potential, prolonged suspension of a productive living, hardship on family, and extraordinary economics of lost time and medical costs. Psychiatric intervention is freqently too little too late, and split off from the main treatment. We have tried to delineate in this chapter a methodical psychological approach to understanding, evaluating, and treating chronic spine pain. It is our strong recommendation that this be carried out by experienced psychiatrists who have a broad-based understanding of the physical, psychological, and social issues involved in the care of the spine-injured patient. Awareness of the concept of psychological homeostatic mechanisms is essential if treatment is to be effective. The phenomenology of the patient's experience must be understood, so that a natural unfolding of the illness process can be approached in a clinically efficacious, nonpunitive manner. The patient's developmental history, especially as it relates to past and present attachment behavior, should be explored. The meaning of illness to each individual patient must be examined to help with acceptance and adaptation during and after the healing process. The psychiatrist has to be an active part of the overall multidisciplinary treatment team, not allowing the patient to be dismissed as "a psychiatric case." Finally, treatment has to be tailored to the needs of the patient. The therapeutic approach should be a truly eclectic effort directed toward disruption of the homeostatic balance point of chronic pain, in an active attempt to propel the patient towards health, function, and fulfillment.

References

1. Cannon WB. The wisdom of the body. New York: Norton, 1932.
2. Weiner H, et al, Etiology of Duodenal Ulcer: I.

Relation of specific psychological characteristics to rate of gastric secretion (serum pepsinogen). Psychosom Med 1957; XIX (1).

3. Lown et al. Psychophysiologic factors in sudden cardiac death, Am J Psychiat 1980; 137 (11):1325–1334.

4. Alexander F. Psychosomatic medicine: Its principles and applications. New York: Norton, 1950.

5. Dunbar HF. Emotions and bodily changes: A survey of literature on psychosomatic interrelationships: 1910–1953. 4th ed. New York: Columbia UP, 1954.

6. Powel RC. Helen Flanders Dunbar (1902–1959) and a holoistic approach to psychosomatic problems. I. The rise and fall of a medical philosophy. Psychiat Q 1977; 49(2):133–148.

7. Westrin, C-G, Hirsch C, Lindegard B. The personality of the back patient, Clin Orthop 1972; No. 87.

8. Friedman M, Rosenman, R. Association of specific overt behavior pattern with blood and cardiovascular findings: blood cholesterol level, blood clotting time, incidence of arcus senilis, and clinical coronary artery disease, JAMA 1959; 169(12):1286–1296.

9. Friedman M, Rosenman R et al. Coronary-prone individuals (type A behavior pattern): Some biochemical characteristics. JAMA 1970; 212 (6):1030–1037.

10. Rosenman R, Friedman M et al. Coronary heart disease in western collabortive group study: Final follow-up experience of 8½ years. JAMA 233 (8):872–877.

11. Engel G. The clinical application of the biopsychosocial model. Am J Psychiat May, 1980; 137(5):535–544.

12. Engel G. The need for a new medical model: The challenge for biomedicine. Science 1977; 196:129–136.

13. Frymoyer JW, Rosen JC et al. Psychologic factors in low-back pain disability. Clin Orthop 1985; 195:178–184.

14. Lipowski Z. Psychosocial aspects of disease. Ann Int Med 1979; 71(6):1197–1206.

15. Lipowski ZJ. Psychosomatic medicine in the seventies: An overview. Psychiatry 1977; 196:129–136.

16. Wolfe HG. Sress and Disease. Springfield, IL: Charles C Thomas, 1964.

17. Engel G. "Psychogenic" pain and the pain-prone patient. Am J Med 1959; 26:899–918.

18. Engel G. Sudden and rapid death during psychological stress: Folklore or folk wisdom? Ann Int Med 1971; 74:771–782.

19. Ainsworth MDS. The development of infant-mother attachment. In Caldwell BM, Riccuiti HN, eds. Review of child development research. vol 3. New York: Russell Sage Foundation, 1972.

20. Bowlby J. Attachment. New York: Basic Books, 1972.

21. Bowlby J. Loss. New York: Basic Books, 1980.

22. Bowlby J. Separation. New York: Basic Books, 1973.

23. Adler RH, Zlot S et al. Engel's Psychogenic pain and the pain-prone patient: A retrospective, controlled clinical study. Psychosom Med 1989; 51:87–101.

24. Haley J. Ordeal therapy. San Francisco: Jossey-Bass, 1984.

25. Haley J. Uncommon therapy. New York: WW Norton, 1975.

26. Sternbach RA ed. The psychology of pain. New York: Raven Press, 1986.

27. Fordyce WE. Behavioral methods for chronic pain and illness, St. Louis, Mosby, 1976.

28. Barber TX. The effects of Hypnosis on pain: A critical review of experimental and clinical findings. Psychosom Med 1982; 65:411–418.

29. Hilgard ER. Neodissociation interpretation of pain reduction in hypnosis, Psychol Rev 1976; 180:396–411.

30. Orne MT. Hypnotic control of pain: Toward a clarification of the different psychological processes involved. Pain 1980; 155–172.

25

THE PSYCHOLOGIST'S CONTRIBUTION TO SPINE CARE

Richard E. Hunt
Ross E. Goldstein

Sixty to eighty per cent of the population will experience symptoms of low back pain at some point in their lives (1, 2). Nearly seven million Americans are treated every day for low back pain (2). But all too often, the outcomes of surgery and other more conservative treatments are less than satisfactory. Some statistics rate the success rate of surgery as low as 10% (3). A study of low back pain patients by White suggests that surgical intervention may be effective for a greater proportion of the target population, but reveals that only 39.5% of the patients treated by surgery were able to return to a type of work comparable to their preinjury employment within the 4 years following this intervention (4).

The rather high failure rates for surgery and other treatment modalities can, in part, be attributed to the failure to address the complexities of the pain phenomenon. Traditionally, pain has been understood to be a somatosensory experience. In this mechanistic model, pain is considered to be a reflection of neurons firing in a fashion proportionate to the amount of tissue damage sustained. However, the frequent instances of pain with little or no physical damage, and the converse, physical damage without pain, have pointed out the inadequacies of this perspective.

Increasingly, health care professionals are adopting a broader, less mechanistic view of pain. The biopsychosocial perspective of pain acknowledges the ways in which an individual's pain experience is determined by the interaction of variables arising from three major spheres of the patient's life: the biological ("pure sensory input" resulting from tissue damage), the psychological (processing and interpretation of the input, "internal" individual response), and the social (overt reaction to input, social reinforcements, and subsequent revision of the interpretation of input). The impetus for adopting this more holistic perspective on pain comes from the work of Melzack and Wall on the "gate control" theory of pain (5). This seminal theory postulated that a host of variables play important roles in shaping a patient's experience of pain (including psychological, situational, and cognitive factors), and research exploring the predictions made by this theory has demonstrated that physiological mechanisms of pain are both afferent and efferent (4).

While the literature arising from the gate control theory has clearly indicated the need for approaching pain from the more holistic biopsychosocial framework, some professionals have been slow to jump on the bandwagon. For some, the biopsychosocial perspective may appear to be more obfuscating than illuminating. They may feel that the net effect of adopting this perspective is the introduction of new, imprecisely defined variables into an area that is already cloudy and ambiguous. Since physiologic and structural factors may be readily apparent and easily understood, it is seductive to look no further and to avoid the difficulties that arise from struggling with less tangible variables. However, experience has proven that back pain is rarely, if ever, all in the patient's back, nor is it often found to be exclusively psychogenic in its origin. This is why working from within the biopsychosocial perspective has proven to be cost-effective and clinically useful (in terms of increasing the efficacy of treatments provided, enhancing patient satisfaction, providing a framework for increasing the functioning and quality of life of patients previously considered to be intractible), and why most health care professionals have moved towards acceptance of this broader conceptualization of pain.

PSYCHOLOGICAL FACTORS INVOLVED IN BACK PAIN

Nowhere is the complex interaction of pain factors more evident than in back pain (6). Following is a brief overview of the psychosocial variables that have come to be recognized as being significant parts of the back pain gestalt.

Situational Factors. Situational factors often play a central role in the sculpture of a pain problem. Situational features that are considered to be "stressful" (virtually any significant life change, including legal problems, financial difficulties, a change of residence, death of a loved one) have been shown to be related to the development and continuation of back pain (7–9). Stressful events also appear to play a role in many symptomatic exacerbations of mechanically based back and neck problems. The wide range of body functions that are affected by stress can be taken as presumptive evidence that stressful events affect postsurgical healing. And stressful events can disrupt compliance with prescribed regimens in patients who would otherwise be compliant. Finally, situational factors such as secondary financial gain are often critically important to understanding the development and maintenance of pain complaints and disaiblity (10).

Personality Factors. The patient's personality acts as a template through which the pain experience is processed. Thus, it stands to reason that a patient's personality and character are important determinants of the pain experience. At a minimum, personality factors affect a patient's willingness to disclose the presence of pain, as well as shape the way in which disclosures about pain are presented to the physician. Maximally, personality factors may actually amplify discomfort and/or prompt an individual to invoke unpleasant sensory

stimulation as a justification for lifestyle adaptations that actually stem from psychological conflicts.

Personality traits and states, such as hypochondriasis, somatic preoccupation, histrionic tendencies, and depression have been found to be associated with back pain in a host of studies, and such factors appear to influence patient response to treatment (4, 11–15). Such factors exert an influence on a patient's experience of pain even when they are not of an intensity to produce actual psychopathology (15). For patients manifesting bonafide psychopathology, personality factors can be the primary determinant of pain. For example, it is not uncommon for elderly patients to present with complaints of pain that are later found to be primarily rooted in a clinically significant depression that has been mislabeled or misperceived by the patient (16). Severe histrionic tendencies can be the most significant pain factor for some patients.

Even when personality factors do not directly affect the experience of pain, they can still exert a profound influence upon the course of treatment and the patient's adaptation to the presence of pain. Some personality features, such as rebelliousness or impulsivity, will hold important implications for the patient's ability to comply with treatment prescriptions and/or successfully manage a painful condition. And patients who manifest psychopathology that does not directly affect the pain experience will still display decreased frustration tolerance and behavioral inflexibility, which tends to have a negative impact upon the patient's clinical course, his or her ability to comply with treatment recommendations, and upon physician-patient interactions.

Social System Factors. The pain patient lives in a social milieu that either reinforces or discourages the expression of pain behaviors and the patient's efforts to adapt to a painful condition. In fact, some theorists argue that the actual experience of pain may be affected by the response of others, because pain and pain behavior are so inextricably intertwined as to be effectively synonymous. The effects of the patient's social system can be construed in several ways. An interactional view suggests that pain behavior increases in frequency when this behavior elicits responses from others that are experienced as rewarding by the pain patient. A typical interactive cycle is: Person A complains about pain; Person B expresses concern, excuses A from onerous responsibilities; in the future, the frequency of Person A's pain complaints increases in order to secure further "rewards."

A transactional view of social system effects pays less attention to the individuals involved and the particular nature of social interactions. Instead, the transactional view postulates that social systems have a life of their own, and that the behavior of the individual members of a system is greatly determined by system principles and dynamics (such as the tendency of a system to maintain an established homeostasis, or the need of every system to have a scapegoat). A transactional view would suggest that an individual responds to a pain problem in a "maladaptive" way in order to meet some need existing in a social system, such as the nuclear family. For example, the crisis of having a system member incapacitated by pain may increase family cohesiveness and provide a feeling of emotional closeness (and hence, security) that would otherwise be absent. The thrust of the transactional view is that "maladaptive" responses are actually adaptive to a larger context, and this implies the need to change system functioning to produce a change in individual behavior.

ROLE OF THE PSYCHOLOGIST

The psychologist who works as a part of the multidisciplinary pain team can occupy a number of roles. In many team settings, the psychologist serves as a treatment specialist and psychological liaison to the treatment team. The psychologist is well-suited to this role, because she or he brings a thorough familiarity of behavior change technology (which is the basis of virtually all stress management and pain management interventions), knowledge of several theories of interpersonal interaction (which inform work with families, couples, psychotherapy groups, and other social systems), and thorough exposure to the many theories that can guide work with individual problems and psychopathology. As psychological liaisons, psychologists draw on their training to guide other treatment professionals to approach patients in ways that are likely to produce compliance and reduce other frustrating interactions. The psychologist can also help other professionals to appreciate the psychological limiting factors

that some patients carry into their treatment, thus decreasing the psychological frustration and burnout experienced by these fellow professionals.

The psychologist has also received extensive training in research design, test construction, and statistical analysis. Hence, the psychologist can serve as a researcher (either independently, or in concert with epidemiologists, and other researchers) in systems that are inclined to conduct research on treatment efficacy, prediction of outcome, and identification of mediating variables.

The psychologist's traditional role in mental health systems has been that of evaluation specialist, in part because the psychologist is the only mental health professional who has a thorough knowledge of psychological tests and testing issues. The psychologist is also trained in the gathering and analysis of behavioral data. The remainder of this chapter will address some of the major issues related to the psychological evaluation of the pain patient.

PSYCHOLOGICAL EVALUATION OF A PAIN PROBLEM

The psychological evaluation of a pain problem is a delicate undertaking at best. A referral to a psychologist or a psychiatrist is often taken by the pain patient as insinuating madness or badness in the patient's character. Even enlightened individuals are inclined to view the mental health professional as representing an obstacle that stands between them and a desired outcome, whether it be securing a place on the surgery schedule or obtaining a prescription for narcotic analgesics, and such a perception does not always markedly diverge from the truth of the matter. When the psychologist is working as part of a multidisciplinary team, some of these perceptions can be side-stepped, as the psychological evaluation becomes routine, being merely one facet of the multidisciplinary evaluation.

Clinical Interview

Even in a multidisciplinary setting, the psychologist will typically begin the clinical interview by exploring the patient's understanding of why she or he has been referred to a psychologist; any mistaken impressions, fantasies of magical cures, or unwarranted anxieties can be identified and addressed near the outset of the interaction. Such an opening also provides the opportunity for the interviewer to indulge in some self-disclosure in response to the patient's declarations, a process that simply and quickly defines the relationship as interactive in nature. Not only does such an exchange tend to reduce patient anxiety, it also begins to delineate the evaluator from stereotypic images of the "shrink" who wants to talk about dreams, free associations, and early childhood experiences.

From this beginning, the interview will continue to blend one part relationship definition (building a relationship that emphasizes a nonjudgmental examination of the patient's pain problem, the demands for change that accompany its persistence, and the emotional repercussions that result) to several parts information gathering (regarding the patient's response to pain, the response of significant others to the patient's pain, and the information bearing upon the patient's coping capacity) as the psychologist strives to develop a better understanding of the person who is the experiencer of the back pain.

Most patients find their time with the psychologist to be, at worst, benign. At its best, the psychological evaluation proves to be rather reassuring and comforting. Many patients cherish the opportunity to talk in a relatively unhurried way to a member of the treatment team (an opportunity that rarely presents itself in the course of standard medical care), and this interaction fosters the perception that the patient has an ally and confidant who is part of the inner circle of professionals. Further, the psychologist can often give the patient some important feedback regarding coping successes, psychological strengths and weaknesses, and potential trouble spots that may loom ahead. In so doing, the psychologist can 1) draw the patient's attention to the unfolding process of coping with pain, 2) increase the patient's sense of self-efficacy, 3) minimize the patient's anxiety regarding the challenges of the future, and 4) encourage the patient to engage in anticipatory rehearsal of his or her response to stressful events related to the pain problem. If the patient is open to accepting feedback, the process can reframe the pain problem in a way that makes it more tolerable and less defeating.

The exact form of the assessment interview will vary greatly as a function of the personality and theoretical orientation of the professional conducting the interview. Some interviewers will focus primarily upon sequences of behavior, while others will spend more time exploring the patient's coping history. Still others will spend more time asking about the patient's family. Regardless of the particular interviewing style or theoretical orientation employed by an evaluator, the data derived from the patient interview will be markedly incomplete. There are always significant gaps in the information base, and the quality and nature of the data will vary from one interview to the next. While there is no substitute for a well-conducted interview, it is typically necessary and prudent to use psychological testing to insure a complete body of assessment data.

PSYCHOLOGICAL TESTS

A number of psychological tests have been used in the evaluation of pain patients. Yet there is widespread disenchantment with psychological testing among many professionals who deal with pain patients, especially nonpsychologists. In part, this is a result of a failure to perceive psychological testing in its proper light. Succinctly, a psychological test is nothing more (and nothing less) than another source of data about the patient's psychological functioning, personality, and perception of his or her predicament. The primary advantages of psychological test data are that 1) they are derived from a consistent input to the patient (tests and test instructions do not change over time the way interviewer behaviors can), and 2) results obtained from one patient can be objectively compared to results obtained from others, and interpreted actuarially.

The data derived from psychological tests may corroborate impressions gleaned from an interview, thereby greatly increasing the confidence assigned to that impression. And, when psychological testing does not serve to corroborate the interview data, the perspective suggested by the testing can be treated as an hypothesis that can be explored in posttesting interviews. Seeking convergent validity and entertaining hypotheses that may not be apparent during the course of an interview are central to the generation of an adequate evaluation.

Much of the criticism of psychological testing stems from expectations that psychological tests should be able to 1) distinguish between "functional" and "organic" pain, 2) predict who will have a positive surgical outcome, or 3) determine which patients are malingering. Given the complexity of the pain phenomenon, it seems unrealistic to hold such expectations of any one person or procedure. Further, such expectations are typically rooted in the types of false dichotomies that the biopsychosocial approach has sought to overthrow.

Below is a brief review of some of the psychological tests that are often used in the evaluation of a pain problem.

The Minnesota Multiphasic Personality Inventory (MMPI) is the psychological test that is most often used in the evaluation of low back pain (17). It is a self-administered inventory of 566 true-false questions, and it provides information about the patient's degree of emotional distress, certain personality traits, the patient's social adaptation, and the patient's coping style. Research suggests that the MMPI is useful in predicting treatment outcome. The primary drawbacks of the MMPI are that 1) the items on this test address the full range of personality functioning and psychopathology, hence patients sometimes feel that being asked to complete the test represents a questioning of their authenticity or stability, and 2) it is a lengthy test, typically taking 2 hours or more for the patient to complete.

The Chronic Illness Problem Inventory (CIPI) was developed by Naliboff and Kames, and it addresses the fuctional manifestations of a pain problem (18). The patient rates the degree to which 62 statements accurately describe aspects of his or her life (finances, sleep, socializing). The results give a fine summary of the patient's sense of the impact that pain has had upon his or her life. Patients' scores can be compared to norms for pain patients, which can provide some indication of any catastrophizing, minimizing, and the presence of secondary gain issues. The data derived nicely augment the personality and psychopathology data obtained from the MMPI.

The McGill Pain Questionnaire (MPQ), developed by Richard Melzack, is a self-administered instrument consisting of 20 adjectives describing pain (19). The patient indicates which descriptors apply to his or her pain. The patient also completes a pain drawing, a line drawing of a human figure that allows the patient to indicate the distribution, character, and intensity, and temporal constancy of the pain. The MPQ objectifies the pain experience, and provides the patient with a means of clearly communicating the elusive and difficult to describe sensations that are discomfiting. The MPQ can indicate the gross exaggeration of complaints and can distinguish patients whose pain does not follow anatomically appropriate patterns. Its best application may be the documentation of changes in the pain experience as a function of treatment, time, or other elements.

The Psychosocial Pain Inventory (PSPI) is a structured interview that evaluates psychosocial factors related to chronic pain (20). The patient's answers to questions regarding medical history, secondary gain, pain behavior, stressful events, and interpersonal relationships are scored according to norms derived from a sample of pain patients. The summation of these scores yields an objective indication of the degree to which the various factors are involved in the pain presentation. Perhaps the greatest strength of this instrument is its structured assessment of secondary gain.

The Back Pain Classification Scale (BPCS) is a self-administered test that appears to be of greatest utility as an early screening device for psychological disturbance (21). It consists of 103 pain terms (nagging, sickening, throbbing) that are presented in three columns. The words presented have been shown to be useful in delineating psychologically disturbed patients from "organic" pain patients. By using the discriminant weights assigned to each word the patient endorses, the clinician can derive a fairly accurate preliminary categorization of the patient as potentially disturbed (though a determination of the specific nature of the disturbance must be made by other means).

The Millon Behavioral Health Inventory (MBHI) is a 150 item, true-false inventory that has been designed to assess the psychological functioning of medical patients (22). Computer scoring provides an actuarially based report that discusses personality traits relevant to the illness experience, the patient's perception of the current level of stress, some emotional factors relevant to psychosomatic illnesses, and a general prediction of the patient's prognosis (23). The computer-generated report is clear, concise, and directive. The chief weakness of this instrument is its limited scope.

Fruits of the Psychological Evaluation

A thorough psychological evaluation of a pain patient often includes: 1) an MMPI or other personality measure, 2) an interview with the patient, 3) an interview with both the patient and the patient's spouse (and, occasionally, other family members), and 4) a review of behavioral data, such as activity diaries, gathered by the patient. Many evaluators choose to include a second psychological test designed to objectively assess complaints or problems that the patient ascribes specifically to pain (e.g., the CIPI). After assembling all the data that have been generated from all facets of the evaluation, the psychologist should have information bearing upon all of the following questons.

1. What are the environmental consequences that follow expressions of pain (whether verbal or nonverbal), claims of disability, and lifestyle changes precipitated by the pain problem? This is always important information; as the success of behaviorally based interventions for pain problems attests, the situation or "stimulus field" shapes the topography of a pain problem quite dramatically (3, 4, 6, 24). Sometimes, the variables that might shape pain behavior can be rather elusive. For example, Fordyce has described a case in which disabling pain appears to have enabled a patient to avoid confronting the fact that she had accrued cortical deficits as a sequela of encephalitis (16). In other instances, the environmental influences are relatively easy to identify, as when prominent verbalization of pain is intended to elicit a prescription for narcotic medication.

2. What is the patient's understanding of his or her condition? The patient who does not have a reasonably sophisticated understanding of the nature of the condition and the process by which this produces discomfort will undoubtedly have greater difficulty adjusting to chronicity. The uninformed patient is also more likely to seek magical cures and/or to hold unrealistic expectations.

3. What is the patient's emotional response to the pain? Even patients who have an adequate factual understanding of their condition will have an emotional response to their pain. Some feelings will be of relatively brief duration and of an intensity that is in proportion to the many lifestyle changes and stresses that arise from any significant pain problem. Such feelings simply reflect the fact that the development of a pain problem represents a psychological crisis, which means that most patients will experience the successive emotional stages that characterize the crisis response: denial, anger, bargaining, depression, and accep-

tance. Some patients will also experience other, more intense and/or long-lasting emotions, often because the patient assigns some type of meaning to the pain experienced (e.g., pain equals punishment from God, pain equals personal inadequacy, pain equals unacceptable vulnerability). The presence of pain may also restimulate feelings associated with other trauma or unpleasant experiences. The clinician must assess whether the patient has been successful in negotiating the various stages of the crisis response, determine the extent to which any lingering crisis reaction shapes the patient's overall presentation, and identify the roots of feelings that are not strictly related to the crisis response.

4. How does the patient's pain problem effect his or her ability to accomplish developmental tasks? The pain patient in the late teens faces a very different set of challenges than the pain patient who is nearing fifty. The former may have trouble negotiating age-appropriate individuation and may be more likely to have problems with compliance; the latter may have trouble acting on the fruits of stage-appropriate life review, and might be more vulnerable to feeling unsupported and isolated than is typical of pain patients.

5. How does the patient's family respond to the pain problem? What are the family system dynamics; how flexible is the system? From a systems perspective, the patient's pain problem represents input that the family system must process and respond to. A system that is fairly flexible and not experiencing other destabilizing influences can alter role definitions, develop new and appropriate alignments of power, and otherwise alter system patterns to make an adequate adaptation to the new input. The result is a system that encourages the pain patient to develop an appropriate blend of striving, acceptance, and lifestyle modification. A less functional system may be mired in rigid roles or maladaptive power alignments, or it may have limited adaptive resources. Hence, the system may be overtaxed by the new input of a pain problem, and respond in inadequate or stereotyped ways that stultify the process of adaptation. The result may be a system that locks the patient into a role that she or he cannot fulfill, which insures the persistence of anxious seeking after a "magic bullet." Alternatively, the family system may make an initial adaptation to the pain problem but, owing to limited adap-

tive resources, be all too ready to persist in this early response, thus harboring ongoing disability and underfunctioning.

6. What is the meaning assigned to the patient's pain problem by the extrafamilial network (i.e., friends, co-workers)? Clearly, some social systems are more likely to imbue the existence of a pain problem with negative meanings than are other social systems. The psychologist or physical therapist with back pain may have to deal with more insinuations of psychopathology; the professional athlete may be more likely to be labeled "a wimp"; the factory worker more often subjected to allegations of malingering. Some responses by the patient's social network may make it more difficult to respond effectively to the painful condition, and may produce feelings of anxious alienation from peers. Amplification of maladaptive responses can occur, and system intolerance of appropriate lifestyle modifications can exacerbate stress for the patient.

7. What is the patient's preferred coping response, and what is the range of coping responses available in his or her repertoire? Many people have a preferred coping response that they tend to apply as widely as possible (e.g., taking the tension or upset that derives from passive psychological conflicts and channeling it into active pursuits such as vigorous exercise, housecleaning). Even the most accomplished and adaptable people use only a small proportion of the total number of coping responses that are available in any situation. The breadth of a person's coping repertoire and the particular nature of the responses that are most often used is a central concern. For example, the patient who relies primarily upon the passive into active response outlined above is a poor candidate for back surgery until some new responses are incorporated into the repertoire. Otherwise, the patient may well be up and cleaning the house 3 weeks postoperatively.

8. What are the important personality traits and dynamics? The psychologist must identify cross-situational consistencies in the patient's behavior and use this knowledge to predict future behavior. Typically, the psychologist focuses attention upon the likelihood of psychological decompensation under continued stress, characteristic responses to other individuals (e.g., "nobody really cares about me"; "nobody tells me what to do"), passivity, dependency, and impulsivity.

9. What are the situational factors influencing the patient's response to pain or to treatment? Stressful events are not an uncommon part of life, and this is especially true for people besieged by pain. Identifying stress factors and helping the patient to deal with stress effectively enhances treatment success. Situational factors that will not soon remit (e.g., financial problems) should be explored to insure that the patient has not chosen to ignore impending crises, that might blossom and effectively sabotage a planned intervention. The ways in which stress might alter the patient's presentation must also be evaluated.

10. What types of psychological interventions should be included in the patient's multidisciplinary treatment plan to address the patient's problem areas, weaknesses, or (if it is present) psychopathology? How much participation will be required of the psychologist in order to effect an optimal outcome? The range of options include inpatient pain programs, outpatient pain programs, outpatient psychotherapy as an adjunct to other treatments, provision of psychological support, and referral to a pain support group, among others.

SUMMARY

Pain is a complex phenomenon and, as a result, the treatment of pain problems is fraught with difficulties, frustrations, and challenges. And nowhere is the Hydra-like nature of pain more apparent than in cases involving the lower back. Hence, professionals who treat pain problems have found it necessary to renounce the convenience and ease of working from traditional modes of thinking that ignore the interaction of mind and body, or that treat this elegant dance as if it were as rudimentary as the hokey-pokey. Increasingly, health care professionals are guiding their work from a biopsychosocial map, and they are striving to become truly holistic in their formulations of their patients' pain.

An attempt has been made in this chapter to outline the ways in which psychological and social factors shape the pain experience, and to describe the psychologist's methods, techniques, and thinking as she or he approaches the pain phenomenon. The orthopaedist need not (and should not) become an expert on psychological factors in pain. The orthopaedist only need know when it is time to consult a psychologist and be willing to take the information that is offered and use it to build a fuller, more holistic understanding of the patient.

The type of interchange that is required among the representatives of several disciplines (internal medicine, occupational therapy, orthopaedics, psychology, physiatry, physical therapy, radiology) implies that pain patients are best treated in a team setting. Further, it suggests that the relationships among these professionals must transcend the typical consultation interactions and actually foster an atmosphere of teamwork: each individual bringing unique talents to bear upon the construction of a whole. The extent to which this ideal is realized will be reflected in enhanced treatment outcomes, increased patient satisfaction, and decreased frustration and burnout among the treatment professionals.

References

1. Pope MH, Rosen JC, Wilder DG et al. The relation between biomechanical and psychological factors in patients with low-back pain. Spine 1980; 5:173–148.
2. Ranga Rama Krishna K, Prance RD, Pelton S, et al. Chronic pain and depression: I. Classification of depression in chronic low back pain patients. Pain 1985; 22:279–287.
3. Gottlieb H, Strite LC, Koller R et al. Comprehensive rehabilitation of patients having chronic low back pain. Arch Phys Med Rehab 1977; 58:101–108.
4. Turk DC, Flor H. Etiological theories and treatments for chronic back pain. II. Psychological models and interventions. Pain 1984; 19:209–233.
5. Melzack R, Wall PD. Pain mechanisms: A new theory. Science 1965; 150:971–979.
6. Fordyce WE, Lansky D, Calsyn JD et al. Pain measurement and pain behavior. Pain 1984; 18:53–69.
7. Feuerstein M, Sult S, Houle M. Environmental stressors and chronic low back pain: Life events, family and work environment. Pain 1985; 22:295–307.
8. Holmes TH, Rahe RH. The social readjustment scale. J Psychosomat Res 1967; 11:213–218.
9. Murray JB. Psychological aspects of low back pain: Summary. Psychol Rep 1982; 50:343–351.
10. Mendelson G. Compensation, pain complaints, and psychological disturbance. Pain 1984; 20:169–177.
11. Frymoyer JW, Rosen JC, Clements J et al. Psychologic factors in low-back pain disability. Clin Orthop 1985; 195:178–184.
12. McCreary C. Empirically derived MMPI profile clusters and characteristics of low back pain patients. J Consult Clin Psychol 1985; 53:558–560.
13. Sternbach RA, Wolff SR, Murphy RW et al. Traits of pain patients: The low back "loser." Psychosomatics 1973; 14:234–239.
14. Wilfling BA, Klonoff H, Kokan P. Psychological, demographic and orthopaedic factors associated with prediction of outcome of spinal fusion. Clin Orthop 1973; 90:153–160.
15. Strassberg SS, Reimherr RF, Ward M et al. The MMPI and chronic pain. J Consult Clin Psychol 1981; 49:220–226.
16. Fordyce WE. Clinical notes on the MMPI, Number 3. Nutley, NJ: Hoffmann-LaRoche Inc. 1979.
17. Hathaway SR, McKinley JC. Minnesota multiphasic personality inventory manual. rev ed. New York: Psychological Corporation, 1951.
18. Kames LD, Naliboff BD, Heinrich RL, Schag CC. The chronic illness problem inventory: Problem-oriented psychosocial assessment of patients with chronic illness. Int J Psychiat Med 1984; 14(1):65–75.
19. Melzack R. The McGill pain questionnaire. In Melzack R. ed. Pain measurement and assessment. New York: Raven Press, 1983.
20. Heaton RK, Getto CJ, Lehman RAW, et al. A standardized evaluation of psychosocial factors in chronic pain. Pain 1982; 12:165–174.
21. Southwick SM, White AA. The use of psychological tests in the evaluation of low-back pain. J Bone Joint Surg 1983; 65A:560–565.
21. Leavitt F, Garron DC. The detection of psychological disturbance in patients with low back pain. J Psychosomat Res 1979; 23:149–154.
22. Millon T, Green C, Meagher R. The Millon behavioral health inventory manual. Minneapolis: Interpretive Scoring Systems, 1982.
23. Millon T, Green C, Meahger R. The MBHI: A new inventory for the psychodiagnostician in medical settings. Professional Psychol 1979; 10:529–539.
24. Fordyce WE, Roberts AH, Sternback RA. The behavioral management of chronic pain: A response to critics. Pain 1985; 22:113–125.

26

MAKING PAIN CLINICS WORK

Jerome Schofferman

Back pain affects a large segment of the population. Fortunately, most patients recover with conservative care. Others with more severe pathology may require surgery. However, despite excellent treatment, a significant number of patients do not improve and are referred to a pain clinic. The short-term success rates reported from most pain management programs are impressive but, unfortunately, long-term results are less gratifying. It is the goal of this chapter to look at chronic pain patients and pain clinics to determine the factors that make pain clinics work.

The hallmark of chronic pain patients is that pain and disability appear out of proportion to the known peripheral stimulus. It is commonly assumed that the problem is primarily psychological. Although it is true that most chronic pain patients have a psychological component to their problems, most have a peripheral stimulus present as well (1). There may be residual painful degenerative disc(s), instability, scar tissue, spinal stenosis, and/or muscle deconditioning. Successful treatment requires attention to both physical and psychological problems. Many patients can manage the somatic component if they are trained to a high level of strength and flexibility and in body mechanics. Psychotherapy must help the patient manage the psychological and social components that impede return to function.

There are two basic treatment approaches. One is psychologically based with an active but nonspecific exercise program and basic back school (2). The other emphasizes functional restoration while also addressing the psychological factors that contribute to disability (3).

It is not appropriate to place all chronic back pain patients into one category when, in fact, they may be quite different. The nature of the pathology will influence treatment outcome and future medical care. One type of patient has significant organic pathology that is no longer directly treatable. This patient may or may not have significant psychological problems as well. In others, only a minimal peripheral stimulus can be identified and the disability appears primarily psychological. Still others suffer from surgically correctable disease, but with training may be able to obtain a decrease in pain and an increase in function that will obviate the need for an operation. Finally, there are patients with significant spinal pathology whose psychological problems make successful surgical intervention unlikely.

CHRONIC PAIN AND CHRONIC PAIN PATIENTS

Pain is the most common reason patients come to health care providers. Pain is "an unpleasant sensory and emotional experience associated with actual or potential tissue damage, or described in terms of such damage" (4).

Chronic pain and acute pain are different (5). Most clinicians are trained to treat acute pain, but treating a chronic pain patient with an acute pain model will fail. Acute pain has a well-defined onset and a clear etiology, and is expected to resolve in a predictable period of time. It is well localized, clearly described, and may be associated with signs of sympathetic overactivity such as tachycardia, dilated pupils, or increased blood pressure. Acute pain serves the purpose of preventing use of the injured part until healing occurs and therefore rest may be appropriate.

Chronic pain may be arbitrarily defined as pain that has been present for several months or more. The pain serves no useful purpose nor indicates ongoing tissue damage. Rest and disuse are deleterious and lead to further disability. There is adaptation of the autonomic nervous system. Sympathetic overactivity is replaced by vegetative symptoms such as sleep disturbance, appetite change, weight change, and decreased libido.

Many patients become depressed and irritable. They feel helpless and eventually lose hope. These psychological changes may lead to family and social problems. Patients feel isolated and alone, yet at the same time they become dependent on others and assume the "sick role." Family members do not know how to react and by behaving in a manner appropriate for acute pain, they inadvertently perpetuate the patient's dysfunction and abnormal pain behavior.

A person who is not psychologically equipped to deal with life's stressors may readily assume the sick role. The care and attention received because of pain might not be there if the person were well. The sick role may provide temporary escape from problems and an unconscious excuse to avoid even more unpleasant or difficult problems than the pain as such. In this way, the pain has psychological value for the patient.

GOALS OF TREATMENT

Even among professionals, there is a greal deal of misunderstanding about the goal of "pain clinics," which is to change a chronic pain patient into a person with chronic pain. This requires restoring function and decreasing disability, not necessarily eliminating pain. The experienced clinician realizes that although *excess* pain may be lessened and flares may be reduced in frequency, intensity and duration, eliminating the pain may not be possible (5). If the patient becomes functional, learns to cope, improves psychologically, and feels less disabled, or if strength, conditioning, and body mechanics can alter the peripheral stimulus sufficiently, pain reduction may occur.

The patient's goal, however, is usually quite different. It is relief of pain. The patient knows only an acute pain model in which pain means tissue damage and therefore continuing pain means continuing damage. The different goals may lead to disappointment and misunderstanding unless they are clarified at the onset of treatment. Providing realistic expectations is a major step towards making pain clinics work.

EVALUATION OF THE PATIENT

Evaluation of the Peripheral Stimulus. Adequate diagnosis of the peripheral problem is essential to specific treatment. There are two major components to assessing the peripheral stimulus. The first is an accurate diagnosis of the spinal pathology using state of the art means (6). This may only require a detailed history, physical examination, and review of records and radiological studies. However, in selected cases, additional testing may be necessary.

The second is an analysis of physical capacity and function to provide objective data in order to identify specific weaknesses for intervention (3, 7). The strength of muscles of the trunk and upper and lower extremities must be tested and compared to specified norms. Testing of range of motion, aerobic capacity, position tolerances, and body mechanics should also be included.

Psychological Evaluation. It is clear that different people react differently to similar peripheral stimuli. Part of the difference is due to psychological processes that modify the perception of the sensory component and reduce, amplify, or modify the final sensation. The role of the psychological assessment is to evaluate the influence of psychological and social factors in the perception and perpetuation of pain and disability (8–10).

The psychological evaluation is based on the interview. Psychological testing may be used to supplement the interview. The assessment must examine the affective, behavioral, cognitive, and social components of the person with pain (9). An accurate psychological diagnosis must identify affective disorders, behavioral factors, cognitive distortions, and developmental disorders in order to design specific therapeutic interventions.

The relationship between chronic pain and depression is complex, but it is clear that there is a high incidence of depression in chronic pain. Most often, the depression is a result of the pain rather than the cause, although an underlying major depression may be present in a significant number of patients. Evaluation should include an assessment of the psychological status before the pain was present, current mood, drug use, and a screening for vegetative symptoms.

Generalized anxiety disorders and situational anxiety are common and may be overlooked if symptoms are attributed solely to the pain. In addition, the patient must be evaluated for panic disorder and posttraumatic stress disorder.

The role of behavioral factors is often misunderstood. Pain behaviors in chronic pain may be abnormal and result in further dysfunction, or they may be neutral. It is unlikely that behavior alters pain directly, but the consequences of pain behavior influence the degree of disability (9, 10).

Behavioral analysis is based on the theory that communication of pain requires behavior (2, 10). These behaviors can be influenced by their consequences and are more likely to recur if they are reinforced by positive consequences or if they allow avoidance of unpleasantness. A behavioral analysis seeks to identify stimuli that either reinforce or elicit pain behavior and to determine which of these behaviors may respond to behavioral treatment (9). Obvious reinforcers include workers' compensation payments that are nearly equal to prior income, upcoming litigation, increased attention from family or friends, and the avoidance of unpleasant work or personal situations. Less obvious are the use of pain to control family or sexual dynamics.

Cognitive theory stresses that the response to pain is influenced by the meaning of the pain to the patient (9, 11). Dysfunctional reaction to pain may result from distorted interpretations of the meaning of the pain, unrealistic images of the spinal pathology, beliefs about future pain, and quality of life issues.

It is our impression that there is a disproportionate number of chronic pain patients who have had severely dysfunctional childhoods. The patient may have had alcoholic parents or may have been the victim of physical, sexual, or psychological abuse. Unresolved aspects of early childhood development may predispose a person to chronic pain.

MEDICATIONS: USE AND MISUSE

Improper use of medications can contribute to dysfunction and disability by causing adverse physiological and behavioral effects (12). Patients are usually unaware of the injurious effects of chronic use of opioids, benzodiazepines, or "muscle relaxants." Patients with previous chemical or alcohol dependency may be especially at risk.

Tolerance occurs in most patients who use opioids regularly over a long period of time. Tolerance has developed when the patient needs larger quantities of the opioid to obtain the same relief. Frequently, the duration of analgesia is shorter as well. The patient consequently uses more opioid at shorter intervals and may interpret this to mean his back is getting worse.

When tolerance occurs, patients may experience subtle withdrawal periods throughout the day and night (13). There may be increased pain (which can be quite focal), anxiety, malaise, irritability, and/or sleep disturbance. Many patients who take opioids remark that they only take the edge off. The edge is withdrawal. The patient feels better after taking opioids and attributes the improvement to analgesia rather than the amelioration of the abstinence syndrome. This reinforces further drug use and dependence.

Exogenous opioids apparently suppress the endogenous opioid (endorphin) system. The quantity and duration of opioid use necessary to suppress endorphins have not been established (14). There is a period of 3 to 6 weeks after stopping opioids when the patient has neither exogenous nor endogenous opioids and may feel ill and in more pain.

Subtle psychological abnormalities may occur when patients take opioids chronically. Some of the changes are nonspecific, but depression, mood swings, and irritability are frequent. It is only when a patient has been opioid free for weeks that he or she can identify the changes retrospectively. Patients usually state that their pain is the same but they can deal with it better. A spouse will comment that the patient's old personality is back.

Patients have difficulty learning body mechanics or retaining educational materials when they are taking opioids, even if the dose is being tapered. Therefore, opioids should be eliminated before beginning training. If this is not possible, a rapid withdrawal regimen is preferred (12).

Hypnotics can cause depression, dependence and tolerance and there is an abstinence syndrome when they are discontinued. There is also evidence of cognitive impairment that interferes with learning (14). Patients who take both benzodiazepines and opioids show more pain behavior, more down time, time in bed, on a recliner or lying on the floor or couch and increased use of medical care, and carry less weight than patients with similar pathology but no drugs (16). Alcohol must also be considered a drug of abuse in chronic pain patients if it used as an analgesic or for sleep.

Even when properly used, analgesics play only an ancillary role in chronic back pain. Useful medications include the peripheral acting agents acetaminophen (APAP), aspirin, and other nonsteroidal anti-inflammatory drugs (NSAID). Unfortunately, there is little data regarding their effectiveness in chronic nonmalignant pain (17).

Analgesics can be administered in either a pain-contingent dosing schedule in which the analgesic is taken for flares, or a time-contingent schedule in which the analgesic is taken on a regular schedule. For chronic pain, time-contingent dosing should be tried to see if pain is reduced. If not, medication can be reserved for flares (12).

Aspirin has been shown to be effective for mild to moderate acute pain. There is increasing analgesia with increasing dose until a ceiling effect at 600 to 900 mg. At 600 mg, the duration of analgesia is about 4 hours, but at 900 mg analgesia lasts for 6 hours. At doses of 4 grams per day, a substantial minority of patients suffer gastrointestinal side effects and/or salicylism (17).

APAP is useful for mild to moderate pain and has a dose response curve similar to aspirin. Complications are rare except in patients who consume large amounts of alcohol or take an overdose. APAP does not produce dependence or tolerance. There are no significant hematological or gastrointestinal side effects.

The shallow dose response curves and low ceiling for aspirin and APAP led to the investigation of other NSAID as analgesics. Several NSAID are efficacious but, again, data in chronic nonmalignant pain are insufficient (17). The NSAID are generally better tolerated than aspirin when used chronically. Neither tolerance nor dependence occur. The ceiling effect is substantially higher than with aspirin or APAP. Ibuprofen 400 mg is more effective than aspirin 650 mg or codeine 60 mg in postsurgical dental pain, and has an analgesic duration of 6 hours. Naproxen sodium 550 mg is also more effective than aspirin or codeine and provides 8 hours of analgesia in most patients (17).

The cyclic antidepressants have assumed a prominent role in treating chronic low back pain. Their effectiveness in reducing pain has not been demonstrated definitively in nondepressed patients with low back pain, but improved sleep and reduction of anxiety have been noted (15, 18, 20). Doxepin, amitriptyline, desipramine, and imipramine may reduce pain in patients with both low back pain and depression (19).

FUNCTIONAL RESTORATION

Functional restoration is the prototype model for treating chronic back pain (3, 7). Treatment stresses rehabilitation using a sports medicine model. Specific deficits in strength, flexibility, and aerobic conditioning are identified, and treatment is directed to the specific objective deficits. There is concomitant psychological treatment to address stress, depression, and factors that perpetuate disability. Individual and family therapy are included to provide strategies for successful return to work and family life (3). In addition, reconditioning should be accompanied by basic back school and advanced body mechanics training followed by work hardening when the patient reaches fitness goals.

During functional restoration, patients should learn first aid for flares. The experience of a flare while the patient is in a supportive environment helps the patient overcome the fear of flare by providing an opportunity to practice first aid while remaining active. Various techniques may be helpful and each patient should experiment with topical ice, ice massage, or transcutaneous electrical nerve stimulator (TNS). Flares are a good time to use NSAID and also to learn that opioids are not necessary. Stretching in spine-safe positions may relieve muscle pain. Relaxation may ease primary or secondary muscle pain or anxiety. If other measures are not successful, a maximum of 2 days of rest may be necessary. In severe, persistent flares, therapeutic injections can be employed.

PSYCHOLOGICAL THERAPIES

Sternbach correctly summarizes psychological therapy for chronic pain when he states:

The somatic therapies, when they work, may abolish pain, but the psychologic therapies do so seldom. The psychologic therapies are designed to treat excess pain and disability, to teach patients to live and cope better, and to live well despite their pain—a goal that is in the tradition of rehabilitation, as Fordyce et al. have pointed out. Only incidentally is pain reduced in severity, although this does occur (5).

Several types of psychological treatment models have evolved (2, 5, 8, 9, 11, 22). Although different in theoretical framework, all approaches share certain elements. Behavior modification programs seek to reduce maladaptive behavior and thereby reduce dysfunction. Treatment reinforces well behavior and, by not reinforcing abnormal pain behavior, seeks to extinguish it (2, 10). Graduated and progressive exercise and tasks are emphasized (11). Gains are promoted by behavioral strategies such as goal setting and reinforcement of successes. Individual and group psychotherapy are also options, as is basic back school, but much of the exercise and aerobic reconditioning is nonspecific.

Cognitive therapy attempts to modify the patient's perception, interpretation, and dysfunctional reaction to the pain (11, 22). Through education, information, and reconceptualization, the meaning of the pain is changed to help promote functional and effective coping strategies. Most cognitive programs are in fact cognitive-behavioral in that they also use progressive physical reconditioning and reinforcement techniques (11).

Depression must be treated. Patients with both chronic back pain and depression may respond to cyclic antidepressants (15, 19). Doxepin and amitriptyline are used most often, but other drugs may be effective if the former are not tolerated. Either may be started at 10 to 25 mg at night and the dose increased every third night until the patient sleeps well or side effects occur. Individual psychotherapy is essential and must accompany medication.

Relaxation training has been shown to be effective for pain reduction in some patients (11). Theoretically, relaxation serves to quiet the arousal, irritability, and nervousness of the painful state. There are no convincing data to support any individual technique.

OUTCOME ASSESSMENT

Despite many articles that address the outcomes of pain clinics, controversy remains (23, 24). There are no unified criteria for definition

of success. Reports of outcome lump together back patients with a wide spectrum of psychological and physical problems. In addition, patients start treatment at different levels of pain and disability. Therefore, the relative improvement may be more meaningful than the discharge scores (24).

There are subjective and objective criteria of success. Subjective criteria include pain reduction, satisfaction with quality of life, and improvement in mood and feeling of well-being. It is interesting that pain reduction is the outcome considered least meaningful by researchers, although it is the most important to the patient.

Objective criteria include improvement in strength, flexibility, and aerobic capacity; reduction in medication intake; change in pain behavior; and return to work (3, 10). Insurers are concerned with reduction in future disability payments, health care costs, and prevention of reinjury (25).

EXISTENTIAL ISSUES

It is too easy to discuss chronic pain patients in an impersonal or general manner. However, in clinical practice, we must deal with real people whose lives have been altered significantly by the effects of chronic pain (26). For an individual, success means quality of life, not statistics. Patients who feel they have succeeded share certain features that have helped them decrease their suffering and carry on irrespective of pain relief.

Patients who accept the realities of their condition at a deep personal level feel better. Those who accept that they will never have a normal back and make plans to cope effectively do better than those who continue to search for magical relief. It is as if the burden has been lifted and the person can now carry on. But acceptance does not mean giving up. It means making a deep philosophical readjustment. Successful patients have learned to make the most of the physical, psychological, family, and social strengths that they have in order to compensate for what they do not have.

Many patients suffer overwhelming loss of self-esteem. People who were active and productive have been reduced to being weak, ineffective, and at times unable to provide adequately for their families. Those who are able to acknowledge these feelings and work with them in psychotherapy appear to do better.

Patients who overcome their fears also do better. They fear that activity will worsen pain, but at the same time they fear the adverse consequences of inactivity. In a pain program, they learn from experience that it is not *what* you do that causes pain, but *how* you do it. Many successful patients say that one of the most beneficial things they have learned is that they can be active and live, work, and exercise in a spine-safe manner without flaring. If they do flare, they learn that they can still remain active and, as a result, the flare will often be shorter and less intense than when they *went to bed* for an acute exacerbation.

Patients who learn that their persistent pain does not mean ongoing tissue damage and that flares do not mean further injury do better. They accept that their signals are crossed and that their previous experience with acute pain has little relationship to their chronic pain.

Patients learn that they are not alone. The group interaction introduces others who are experiencing similar pain and suffering. This interaction with people who understand is helpful.

Patients learn to set reasonable, specific, and timely goals, not goals that are vague or that depend on pain relief. There should be short-term goals that are readily within reach as well as intermediate and long-term goals that are appropriate for that individual.

Finally, there are some patients who just have to hit rock bottom before they can recover. Life must become intolerable before certain patients can take responsibility for getting better. An outside observer cannot assume that the patient is at the bottom, no matter how bad the patient's condition seems. Those who are fortunate enough to respond to treatment when they hit bottom may recover and do unexpectedly well.

References

1. Zucherman J, Schofferman J. Pathology of failed back surgery syndrome. Spine: State of Art Reviews 1986; 1:1–12.
2. Fordyce WE. Behavioral methods for chronic pain and illness. St Louis: Mosby, 1976.
3. Mayer TG, Gatchel RJ, Mayer H et al. A prospective two-year study of functional restoration in industrial low back injury. An objective assessment procedure. JAMA 1987; 258:1763–1767.
4. Merskey H. Pain terms: A list with definitions and notes on usage. Recommended by the IASP Subcommittee on Taxonomy. Pain 1979; 6:249.
5. Sternbach RA. Clinical aspects of pain. In Fordyce WE. ed. Behavioral methods for chronic pain and illness. St. Louis: Mosby, 1976; 223–240.
6. Zucherman J, Schofferman J. Diagnostic and therapeutic strategies. Spine: State of the Art Reviews 1986; 1:159–175.
7. Mayer T, Mayer H. Functional restoration: New concepts in spinal rehabilitation. In Kirkaldy-Willis WH. ed. Managing low back pain. New York: Churchill Livingstone, 1988.
8. Aronoff, GM, Evans WO. Evaluation and treatment of chronic pain at the Boston Pain Center. In Aronoff GM. ed. Evaluation and treatment of chronic pain. Baltimore: Urban and Schwarzenberg, 1986; 495–502.
9. Romano JM, Turner JA, Moore JE. Psychological evaluation. In Tollison CD. ed. Handbook of chronic pain management. Baltimore: Williams & Wilkins, 1989; 38–51.
10. Fordyce WE, Roberts AH, Sternbach RA. The behavioral management of chronic pain: A response to critics. Pain 1985; 22:113–125.
11. Sternbach RA. Specific therapeutic techniques in pain management. In IASP refresher course on pain management. Book of Abstracts. 1987; 107–112.
12. Schofferman J. The use of medications in failed back surgery. Spine: State of the Art Reviews 1986; 1:129–138.
13. Brodner RA, Taub A. Chronic pain exacerbated by long term narcotic use in patients with nonmalignant disease: Clinical syndrome and its treatment. Mt Sinai J Med 1978; 45:233–237.
14. Gold MS, Pattash AL, Extein I et al. Evidence for an endorphin dysfunction in methadone addicts: Lack of ACTH response to naloxone. Drug Alcohol Dependence 1981; 8:257–262.
15. Atkinson JH. Psychopharmacologic agents in the treatment of pain syndromes. In Tollison CD. ed. Handbook of chronic pain management. Baltimore: Williams & Wilkins, 1989; 69–103.
16. Turner JA, Calsyn DA, Fordyce WE et al. Drug utilization patterns in chronic pain patients. Pain 1982; 12:327–363.
17. Beaver WT. Maximizing the benefits of weaker analgesics. In IASP refresher course on pain management. Book of Abstracts. 1987; 1–25.
18. Alcoff J, Jones E, Rust P, Newman R. Controlled trial of imipramine for chronic low back pain. J Fam Practice 1982; 14:841–846.
19. Ward NG. Tricyclic antidepressants for chronic low-back pain. Mechanisms of action and predictors of response. Spine 1986; 11:661–665.
20. Merskey H. Psychotropic drugs as analgesics. In Tollison CD. ed. Handbook of chronic pain management. Baltimore: Williams & Wilkins 1989; 41–50.

21. Feinmann C. Pain relief by antidepressants: Possible modes of action. Pain 1985; 23:1–8.

22. Turk DC, Meichenbaum D. A cognitive-behavioural approach to pain management. In Wall PD, Melzack R. eds. Textbook of pain. New York: Churchill Livingstone, 1984.

23. Aronoff GM, Evans WO, Enders PL. A review of follow-up studies of multidisciplinary pain units. In Aronoff GM. ed. Evaluation and treatment of chronic pain. Baltimore: Urban and Schwarzenberg, 1985.

24. Kleinke CL, Spangler AS. Predicting treatment outcome of chronic back pain patients in a multidisciplinary pain clinic: Methodological issues and treatment implications. Pain 1988; 33:41–48.

25. Simmons JW, Avant WS, Demski J, Parisher D. Determining successful pain clinic treatment through validation of cost effectiveness. Spine 1988; 13:342–344.

26. Fordyce WH. Pain and suffering. American Psychologist 1988; 43:276–283.

27

BACK PAIN COMPLICATED BY AN ASSOCIATED DISABILITY

Gerald P. Keane

The presence of associated physical impairments or disabilities adds a further challenge to the conservative approach to low back pain. These associated factors may often reinforce the need to manage such patients conservatively. The medical plan for treatment must often emphasize a management, rather than a curative, model. The focus of the program should be on improving the patient's level of functional activity as much as on pain relief. Many of the common methods used in patient management are often ineffective, counterproductive, or even risky, when such associated factors are at play. The back pain patient with secondary medical factors at issue needs a strong educational program as well. The assistance of health professionals less commonly involved in management of back pain, such as occupational therapists, social service workers, or nutritionists, may be of great value. Involvement of spouse, family members, or friends may also be helpful. Enlisting their support may often tip the balance in favor of a positive outcome.

The decision to elect various forms of treatment for back pain in patients with associated medical issues requires the ability to evaluate the patient holistically. Avoiding patient frustration because of inability to make progress or even carry out the recommended treatment will allow a program of steady gains and feelings of success to result. Realistic goals should be set, and encouragement must be a continual part of the treatment program.

This chapter will look at some of the more common factors of associated disability that must often be addressed, with a focus upon their impact on a conservative approach to back pain managment (1–4).

HIP PAIN

Hip pain may have multiple etiologies. Hip pain referred from the low back can often be quite difficult to sort out from intrinsic hip pain. When such pain is determined to be a separate process, it may often have a major impact on the program for back pain management. The goal in many of the aggressive back strengthening and stabilization programs, as well as in body mechanics training, is to place increased demand on areas away from the spine. The hips are a central locus of stress redistribution. A hip problem, then, can interfere with body mechanics training and back stabilization programs. Gait, when disturbed by hip abnormalities, will often place increased stress on the lumbar spine. Many patients with chronic back pain will develop secondary hip bursitis or iliotibial band problems from compensatory changes in their gaits.

Those patients with soft tissue problems, such as ligamentous or muscular restrictions, or bursitis, must have a concomitant active therapy approach that addresses these problems. Such techniques as psoas or iliotibial band stretching, ultrasound, local heat or ice, body mechanics, and gait training, as well as strengthening programs, can be helpful. Hip pain of this type, if recognized and treated, will not usually interfere with a back rehabilitation program.

Hip pain of a more serious etiology, such as aseptic necrosis or degenerative joint disease, often presents a greater challenge. Individuals with such problems require additional approaches beyond the previously discussed treatments. Assistive devices to reduce weight bearing on the joint, or even surgical treatment, should be considered. The patient who is facing lumbar surgery and who has associated hip disease of a surgical nature will probably be best served by hip surgery first. This will allow further gains with conservative back care, and perhaps even avoidance of lumbar surgical treatment. Those patients requiring both surgeries seem to do better when the hip surgery is done first (Kenneth Hsu, M.D., personal communication).

KNEE PAIN

One of the primary admonitions of the back school approach is to "use your knees." Again, the transference of stress and movement from the spine and through the pelvis, hips, and legs is one of the key points of such training. Patients with knee pain, from whatever cause, face added difficulties in a back training program. The key is to focus on an active, aggressive approach to the source of the knee pain. The issues of flexibility, muscle weakness, joint involvement or instability must all be addressed. Commonly, for example, imbalance exists between strong lateral and weaker medial thigh musculature. Patellofemoral syndromes can often be improved by addressing such imbalances. The use of medication for inflammation, local injections, modality therapy, supportive braces during back training exercises, and modification of exercises to reduce knee stress can all be of value. Surgical treatment of refractory knee problems, particularly in problems amenable to arthroscopic treatment, should also be considered. The overriding goal should be to avoid lumbar surgery that might be required if the conservative low back program were ineffective because of knee pain.

CARDIOPULMONARY DISEASE

One of the more common problems in back rehabilitation, particularly in an elderly population, is limitation due to cardiopulmonary disease. Here greater modification of the program, setting of more limited and realistic goals, and constant encouragement are required. Many such patients are in any case limited to conservative back care approaches because of the risk of surgical approaches, and so even greater conservative care efforts are required.

Exercise programs must often be monitored from a cardiac standpoint, and interaction with the physician responsible fro the primary medical care should be part of the treatment. Aerobic exercises remain important but must be modified to allow continued participation in the back exercise program. The inability to sustain a functional level of aerobic activity will cause major difficulties in building the strength and endurance required for back stabilization during normal daily tasks. During the initial period of training, monitoring is begun and patients are taught to monitor their own heart rates and recovery responses. This facilitates independence and self-confidence in maintaining a program of independent exercise.

ARTHRITIS

The treatment of the patient with the sequelae of the various rheumatologic diseases requires enormous patience. Attempts at accomplishing physical goals rapidly will often lead to increased pain and further disability. This is especially true for individuals whose back pain must be managed along with other areas of limitation.

Exercises should be designed to minimize stress on other involved joints. Starting programs in a low-impact fashion is advisable. Pool exercises designed to improve strength, endurance, and flexibility often provide a good starting point. Warm pools can be particularly helpful in improving activity tolerance. Back strengthening exercises should be done isometrically where possible to minimize joint stress. Gentle warm-up exercises should be encouraged, and programs are best divided into two or three times per day sessions. Training in lifestyle modification and in the activities of daily living should be undertaken. Energy conservation principles should be stressed during therapy sessions. Joints should be placed through full pain-free range of motion several times per day to minimize progressive range-of-motion loss and then stabilized, with movement kept to a minimum. Those patients limited by pain should be managed by experienced practitioners. The long-term use of corticosteroids and narcotics must be avoided whenever possible. Management of the associated areas of involvement will frequently allow a conservative back program to progress. Patients with ankylosing spondylitis should be given exercises to maintain vital capacity, and chest musculature stretching exercises should be taught. Prolonged periods of rest can be particularly devastating to the rest of the musculoskeletal system, and should be avoided at all costs. Rest often initiates a downhill slide from which a patient's function activity levels never quite recover. Manipulative treatments should also be approached cautiously due to joint injury potential.

COGNITIVE IMPAIRMENTS

Many older people face difficulty in undertaking what is largely an educational process, i.e., the process of learning to manage one's own back pain. Short-term memory difficulties, fatigue, limitations of vision, impaired hearing, and habit patterns can all play a role. These problems with learning can lead to frustration and a sense of resignation to "old age." This can be overcome by an encouraging environment, the use of written instruction programs, and a frequent repetition of basic concepts. Spousal and family support can be a key to success in long-term follow through.

Those patients with more serious cognitive impairments, such as head injury or stroke, require even more concentrated effort. Presentation of new information should be based on a clear understanding of the patient's capabilities. Many patients with such impairments, will learn quite dramatically through either visual or auditory input, but not through both. Careful repetition, slow presentation, and ample demonstration of what is being requested are essential. Longer term follow-up and a slower progression to independence than usual are the goal. Patients often have difficulty expressing their thoughts and feelings, so an attentive ear may often be their best support. To the observer, the associated disabilities may often appear overwhelming as compared to the back pain. However, it may be the interaction with the back problem that finally tipped the patient's lifestyle from manageable to miserable, and for this reason, it needs to be seriously addressed.

PROGRESSIVE NEUROLOGIC DISORDERS

A number of common neurologic processes, separate from the radiculopathies, impact on a back management program. They require some understanding to allow modification of the management plan in an appropriate manner.

Peripheral neuropathies, in general, lead to a greater level of impairment when they coexist with radicular involvement. Electrodiagnostic testing should include screening for such neuropathies. Patients often do no respond as dramatically to surgical decompression in terms of overall recovery. When severe, impairment of proprioceptive feedback from the lower extremities may seriously affect exercise and body mechanics training. Repetition of training and treatment designed to manage the underlying process, such as alcohol treatment programs or diabetic care, should be included in the overall plan.

Multiple sclerosis typically results in early fatigability and requires exercise programs that take this into account. Heat tolerance is often poor, and treatment plans incorporating local heat use or ultrasound, should be approached with caution. Recognition of the associated psychological stressors related to the multiple sclerosis itself, as with many of the other diseases that have been discussed, is important. Psychiatric referral in such instances may be essential as part of an overall recovery program for a back problem. Stress management, counseling and psychiatric support care provide substantial benefit to many individuals with low back pain, particularly in instances of associated disability.

Parkinson's disease and other disorders affecting gait and coordination require modifications in exercise programs. Gait training, gentle strengthening and flexibility exercises, and proper body mechanics are all of benefit. Goals should be realistic. Adaptive devices such as braces and ambulatory supports may be needed to reduce physical stress on the spine while encouraging activity.

POSTPOLIO SYNDROME

The late sequelae of poliomyelities have been increasingly recognized for their impact on a population once thought to have reached a stable level of impairment. Problems related to postpolio include increasing complaints of fatigue with routine activity, loss of endurance, and increased weakness.

Postpolio patients with associated low back pain often find that their back symptoms increase as their postpolio syndrome becomes more apparent clinically. This is due in part to the need to use lumbar motion to compensate for pelvic and lower extremity weakness. Thus, the postpolio syndrome can lead to progression of the degenerative changes occurring in the lumbar spine and in, many cases, can result in increased low back symptoms. Loss of ability to use the muscles of lumbar stabilization to adapt to spinal abnormalities complicates the treatment of such patients. Lumbar CT and MRI studies often reveal significant loss of paraspinal musculature.

The rehabilitation plan should emphasize endurance training, low-intensity strengthening programs, and energy conservation. The use of exercise intended to fatigue muscles and to promote increased strength should be avoided. Swimming programs and pool exercise in general are often well tolerated. Selective bracing for instability may be necessary. Contractures should be addressed, as decreased activity and muscle imbalance tends to perpetuate loss of functional range of motion.

The primary emphasis should be toward maintaining a functional activity level, promoting endurance while encouraging selective rest, and avoiding heavy muscular demand that may worsen the underlying condition. Referral of patients to educational resources and peer support groups can be of tremendous benefit.

AMPUTEES

The etiology of back pain in many individuals with lower extremity amputations is often related to the effects of the amputation itself. Low back pain is a common complaint for many amputees. The cause is usually related to one of two factors: either alteration of normal gait with increased low back stress on a mechanical basis or problems with the prosthetic fit itself. Ill-fitting prosthetic devices lead to pain, alteration of normal gait, and increased demand on the lumbar spine. The evaluation of such patients must, therefore, center on a thorough gait and prosthetic evaluation. Identification and correction of these underlying factors will often lead to improvement of the back complaints.

Strengthening programs designed to correct underlying muscle imbalance are also beneficial in many cases, as are basic exercises. Muscle imbalance is the result of traumatic or surgical alteration of the affected limb. Such imbalance, increases low back stress.

LOWER EXTREMITY AND FOOT DISORDERS

Leg length discrepancies, neuromas, plantar fascitis, arch abnormalities, and other common foot and lower extremity disorders can contribute significantly to low back pain. Correction or treatment of the underlying problem may often provide significant low back pain relief. Anatomic leg length discrepancies should be corrected slowly over the course of weeks. Usually, correction of one-half of the length discrepancy is the optimal goal.

Arch supports, particularly in runners with low back pain, are often beneficial. Heel cups, shock absorbent inserts, and proper shoes will often allow the low back pain patient to improve activity level, at least in terms of comfort, even if a true "cure" has not been achieved.

SUMMARY

The presence of associated impairments combined with back pain may often impact significantly on the outcome of managing back problems. An understanding of how these factors interact can often lead to improved results, both in terms of improving the health of the back and of limiting disability associated with these other impairments. In the final analysis, diagnosis and the design of a treatment plan will only be complete if the low back disorder is evaluated as part of the often complex realities that can characterize the individual patient as a totality.

References

1. DeLisa JA. ed. Rehabilitation medicine—principles and practice: Philidelphia: JB Lippincott, 1988.
2. Basmajian JV. Therapeutic exercise, 4th ed. Baltimore: Williams & Wilkins, 1984.
3. Saal JA. ed. Rehabilitation of sports injuries. Rehab State-of-the-Art Reviews 1987; 1(4):1–683.
4. Kottke FJ, Stillwell GK, Lehmann FJ. eds. Krusen's Handbook of Physical Medicine and Rehabilitation, 3rd ed. Philadelphia: W.B. Saunders, 1982.

PREVENTION IN THE WORK PLACE

28

PREEMPLOYMENT SCREENING

Nikki L. Burrous

There's something funny here. There must be. This is an unusual chapter because it is written by someone other than an M.D., D.C., or P.T. But when you stop to think about it, we are talking about employment. Employment is a business contract, not a clinical situation. Since the corporate world is where preemployment screening takes place, maybe looking at it from that perspective makes sense after all.

This reminds me of a recent symposium I attended. The first morning, a physical therapist introduced himself and was shocked when he found I was the only stowaway, nonclinician in attendance. He said, "but this is a scientific meeting—it has nothing to do with practicality!" Perhaps we can turn that around and consider this subject an attempt at the practical and not the scientific.

If this is to be a helpful, how-to-do-it guide, I will have to describe how we are doing it at Safeway. First, however, you should know something about our employment picture. In the United States and Canada, 30% of our 131,000 employees are full-time, and 70% part-time. Although a few years ago it was the opposite, 24-hour stores have increased the need for shift flexibility. This balance of part-time to full-time directly affects our exposure to back injuries—more people in the same number of hours are exposed to the repetitive lifting inherent in most jobs.

In the grocery business, almost every job calls for moving merchandise from one place to another. This merchandise is of varied weights, sizes, and shapes and is often moved from floor to shoulder height. To further challenge the body mechanics, the lift usually moves the merchandise from one side to the other.

It is not only ethical, it makes good business sense to do everything possible to engineer out such physical hazards. However, until our industry progresses further into the use of robotics, we will continue to have people move merchandise. Where engineering leaves off, it is the employer's responsibility to train around the lifting challenges that remain. With an increasing number of part-timers creating a revolving door through the store, training is like walking up a down escalator. The more people we have to train, and the higher the attrition rate of those who have been trained, the easier it is to reach the conclusion that to hire more potentially bad backs would only continue to make matters worse.

Putting someone to work who is destined to have a back injury is cruel and unfair and should be discouraged. Hiring someone with a predictably bad back is inheriting a costly worker's compensation claim and low or no productivity, and is poor risk management.

Yes, it is easy to reach the conclusion that preemployment screening is a desirable goal. However, to reach that goal we must work through a maze of clinical and legal restrictions and detours. Even then, the road is often bumpy and fraught with danger. Let's have a closer look.

EMPLOYER RESPONSIBILITY

As dictated by most state workers' compensation laws, employers accept employees "as they are" and are responsible for their health and safety while on the job.

"As they are" calls for some explanation. In essence, workers' compensation laws hold that employers should assume the costs of occupational disabilities without regard to any fault involved. A basic objective of workers' compensation is to provide compensation for work-related injuries and diseases. Note that workers' compensation does not seek to cover all worker health problems. To make the distinction, fairly uniform statutory definitions and tests have been adopted in each state. Typically, the statutes limit the compensation benefits to "personal injury caused by accidents arising out of and in the course of employment." Although the test is fairly uniform, its interpretation has not resulted in completely uniform coverage of injuries and diseases. Injuries no longer must arise out of an accident or specific incident. The cumulative effects of repetition can be considered compensable. Likewise, the aggravation or recurrence of an old injury is compensable.

In *McAllister V. Workers' Compensation Appeals Board* in California in 1968, the court held "an employer takes an employee as he finds him. The fact that a healthier individual could withstand an exposure without sustaining disability will not bar a finding of compensability for a person with a weaker constitution."

In another case a judge noted "an employer takes an employee as he or she is with all the employee's preexisting weaknesses and predispositions, and the employment need only contribute to the injury."

LEGAL RESTRAINTS

Preemployment screening is a difficult subject involving inevitable tension between an employer's obviously well-founded operational interest in screening out applicants who are not physically suited to perform the available work, and the applicable legal standards that limit an employer's right to deny employment to an individual based upon medical evidence of a predisposition for injury.

Under federal law and, to my knowledge, all state physical handicap laws, an employer is entitled to require that prospective employees undergo a preemployment physical examination. For most physically demanding jobs, such a physical typically includes a back examination, either by means of an x-ray and/or testing procedures. While these tests legally may be administered, the generally applicable rule of law is that an otherwise qualified applicant may be denied employment because of the results of preemployment examination only if denial is based on individual consideration of that particular applicant's condition and the physical requirements of the available position, and it can be determined that the applicant's performance of the job would pose an imminent and substantial risk of injury.

Imminent and Substantial Risk Standard

The fact that an applicant for employment may be diagnosed with a back condition that renders the applicant predisposed to injury after performing physical labor may not suffice to meet the imminent and substantial risk standard. For example, a doctor who conducts the preemployment physical and recommends against hiring because of the risk that *at some point,* performing the job requirements of repeated lifting, bending, and stooping *could* result in serious back injury, does not meet the imminent, substantial standard.

The problem with defending such a decision not to hire these applicants is that it is very difficult for the doctor to quantify the degree of risk involved. The doctor has acknowledged that any one of these individuals *might* be able to perform the full range of a laborer's job duties for many years without incident.

Individual Consideration of Applicants

Individual consideration must be given to measure the impact of the person's specific condition upon the ability to perform the specific functions of the available job and to other factors, such as the applicant's prior work history.

Reasonable Accommodation of Physical Handicaps

Even if we clear all the hurdles of showing that an applicant's specific back condition renders that applicant unable to perform the job, or places a substantial risk of injury if the job is performed, handicap discrimination laws force us to consider whether reasonable accommodation can be made to permit employment. For example, if a person applies for a job that normally entails lifting weights up to 80 lbs, and that person is determined to be subject to a 50-lb lifting restriction, the issue then becomes one of "reasonable accommodation." A written job analysis that identifies the extent and frequency of the physical and mental demands of a particular job can be of tremendous assistance in determining the extent to which reasonable accommodation of handicaps can be made.

CLINICAL INDICATORS

Clearly, we need to avail ourselves of all technical and medical expertise that will assist us in making the most of the opportunity to reduce the incidence of back-related workers' compensation claims without running afoul of applicable physical handicap discrimination laws.

It would be wonderful if the computerized evaluation equipment now on the market had reached the state of technology that would indeed objectively measure "imminent and substantial" risk of back injury. It would then be a key part of the preemployment screening process. A green light would mean go and a red light would mean no. As useful as the equipment may be for evaluation, it is still of little use as a preemployment screen.

A predictor must have accuracy, sensitivity, and specificity. Accuracy means it will give a true measure of a variable that is job specific. Sensitivity means it would measure a certain condition, and specificity means it measures people who do not have a specific condition as well as those who do. One computerized motion analysis system uses a video camera to record actual jobs and could potentially meet these criteria.

BLENDING THE CLINICAL AND THE LEGAL

About 10 years ago, our company began working on a test battery that would identify applicants able to do an order selector's job in our warehouses. We looked at all aspects of the job and identified the specific skills needed. It took a number of years to work through the validation process. This means that a particular skill or the measurement of a particular skill had to be tested with our current workforce. If, in fact, any number of current employees failed a part of the test while at the same time carrying out

the job description appropriately, that particular test had to be thrown out. It could not be verified as specific, sensitive, and accurate, or necessary to do the job. After a good deal of patience and perserverance, we now have a three-part test battery consisting of 1) hand-to-eye dexterity, 2) a mock order selection, and 3) flexibility or body mechanics. At present, about 35% of all applicants (in recent sample, $N = 815$) are unable to pass the test battery. Those who do pass ($N = 533$) the order selector test battery are interviewed. Thirty-two per cent are screened out at this stage. Those who pass the interview ($N = 362$) are given a drug-alcohol test, which a further 14% fail. Those passing the drug screen ($N = 311$) go for a preemployment physical and x-ray where 7% are screened out. In the end, 65% of those originally applying fail various stages for various reasons.

How have we managed to get where we are today? In 1977, it was our good fortune to meet Arthur H. White, M.D., spine surgeon and medical director of the San Francisco Spine Institute and Spine Care at Seton Medical Center. He became our advisor in developing our back injury prevention program called Professional Weightlifting, and continues as our mentor to this day. He is currently clinically guiding our preemployment screening refinement program for predictable back injuries.

In order to bring the clinical and the legal into focus we brought Dr. White and his clinicians together with our legal staff. Having both sides present avoided the need for translation and reduced misinterpretation. Our only condition for the meeting was that no one could leave until we identified all areas of harmony. The clinical message was that epidemiologically there are certain predictors of back injury. It is a business decision, not a medical decision, to hire or not to hire an individual with statistically high risk factors. However, the legal risk must also be considered in that business decision. The legal question is whether a test can show indirectly or directly that an individual will have immediate and substantial injury. According to Dr. White and the literature, the answer is yes. Our attorneys think that, if the clinical experts say the predictors are valid, then the predictors are helpful and can be used as a preemployment screen.

Dr. White reported that a task force of spinal disability specialists reviewed all of the literature on spinal disability to date and most of the disability ratings now in existence. From that study, certain factors were developed that these experts believe can be substantiated by the literature and by the collective experience of hundreds of qualified spinal disability specialists. It is these substantiated factors that we intend to follow in our preemployment screen. Although there are certain questions that will be included in the interview, and some indicators will be apparent during the order selector test battery, our legal advisors think we would be on thin ice if a rejection for employment were based solely on a potential for back injury and that rejection were made by anyone but a physician. With all of this in mind, here is how the selections process would work.

The Order Selector Test Battery for Warehouse and Plant Employees. Since flexibility and strength are integrated into the physical tasks of each part of the test battery, our hiring representatives will be trained to note aspects pertinent to back injury predictors.

Job Interview. The hiring representative interviewing a job applicant will ask questions which give information on abdominals, gluteals, athletic activities, flexibility, previous back pain, what was done about the back pain, how long it lasted, whether the applicant smokes, and the kind of work previously done. Since if the imminent and substantial risk of injury judgment determination is made by a layperson, it could doom us from a legal point of view, this information will be noted and passed along to the screening physician for use during the physical examination.

Physical Examination. We have shared the 21 factors in predicting back injury provided by Dr. White with the physicians currently giving our physical examinations. By improving training of and communication among our hiring reps, our occupational health nurses, and our preemployment physicians, we anticipate accelerated, refined, and defendable results in screening predictably bad backs.

CONCLUSIONS

Those of us in industry are most fortunate. If we recognize our business, legal, and ethical responsibilities and match up the areas that overlap, we can accomplish a great deal.

It is often said that with enough energy we can solve any problem. Today we have access to the best scientific minds, the technology of the 21st century, keen business tenacity, and a powerful, involved, and often vociferous workforce. If each element is allowed—or better yet, encouraged—to function and contribute to the fullest, the results can advance everyone's lot.

It is too early to measure the results of our refined preemployment screening program. We anticipate, however, that those people hired to work for our company will have far less risk of back injury, that our company will have happier, more productive employees, and spend fewer dollars on workers' compensation; and that our scientific advisors will have a control group to further measure the success of their predictors. Good business is that in which everyone wins.

29

INDUSTRIAL BACK SCHOOL

Sigmund Miller

A look at the statistics for work-related injuries reveals a need for back school programs tailored specifically for the industrial arena. Nationally, a full 25% of workers' compensation claims are made for back injuries. The outlays for these claims account for 33% of total annual expenditures (1). In 1984, the State of California Division of Labor Statistics showed that the back was the most frequently injured body part, accounting for 21% of all lost-time injuries. In the same year, 42% of all workers injured on the job had been employed in a particular capacity for less than a year (2). This positive correlation between a lack of experience and a work-related injury implies that an organized training program, such as back school, ought to significantly reduce the incidence of injury.

The best argument for increasing the implementation of back school programs is the success that has resulted from past programs. The Chelsea Back Program helped American Biltrite, Inc. reduce its annual back-injury expenditures from $215,000 to less than $2,000 in only two years (3). In one year, California Back School saved Southern Pacific Transportation Company $1,000,000 in expenditures while reducing injuries by 22% and lost-work by 43% (4). The Lockheed Corporation also profited; each dollar spent on the Back Dynamics Institute program saved the company $6.50 in injury costs (5). As these results demonstrate, back school can be both efficacious and cost effective.

The curriculum is designed with two groups in mind: 1) workers already suffering from back pain, and 2) people whose activities place them in a high-risk category for future back problems. Prevention, self-care, and back-awareness are the main themes, with special attention

paid to proper body dynamics, body mechanics, posture, and therapeutic exercise. Much of the class time is spent in active participation and the repetition of techniques.

The primary goal of industrial back school is to teach workers to perform their jobs as correctly as possible. Toward this end, I find it is helpful before scheduling classes to do some background work by touring the work-site, performing various employee tasks, identifying high-risk areas, and taking pictures to aid in illustrating particular points during the class. I also review company records, looking through injury reports, injury expenditure records, and job descriptions for the insights these may provide as to why employees are hurting their backs. I then meet with the supervisors, safety officers, and other key personnel to obtain their advice and to enlist their support.

The class curriculum focuses on the following areas:

1. The basic anatomy and function of the spine,
2. The effects of the aging process on the spine,
3. The causes and effects of neck and back pain,
4. The principles of body mechanics as they apply to everyday tasks, for example, reaching, lifting, carrying, bending, sitting, lying down, pushing, and pulling,
5. Postures that can aggravate or relieve pain,
6. Adjustments in daily living that need to be made in order to minimize back pain,
7. First aid for back pain,
8. Exercises for muscle strengthening and stretching,
9. The role of stress in chronic spine syndromes.

The necessitiy of ongoing self-care and continual back-awareness is a constant theme throughout the class.

Lectures, demonstrations, slides, workbooks, and other visual aids are all used to help convey these concepts. I have found, however, that the most effective teaching strategy is to have participants try out and then repeat each technique as it is presented. Participants are also encouraged to ask about problems particular to their lifestyles or work situations. I then help them to devise strategies for minimizing the strain on their backs.

Classes are given on-site. They usually last 60 to 90 minutes, with 20 to 25 people per class. Employees performing similar work tasks are grouped in the same class so that instruction can be geared to their particular problems. To simulate these problems, I arrange for the use of work stations or of work-station models. Supervisors are asked to be present in order to encourage worker participation, and also to learn the techniques themselves, thereby ensuring that employees will implement what they have learned after they are back on the job. (In my experience, back school generally improves management-employee relations because the workers see management as having hired a professional to present ideas that are beneficial to their health.) Completing the class is not the final step. I set aside several hours per month to revisit the work-site and reinforce concepts. Occasionally, I also schedule another class for new employees and for recently injured workers.

References

1. Benson JD. Control of low back pain using ergonomic task analysis redesign technique. Professional Safety 1987; 32(9):21–25.
2. State of California, Division of Labor Statistics and Research: California work injuries and illnesses annual report, 1984.
3. Sate of California, Occupational health and safety report, February, 1982.
4. White AH. Back school and other conservative approaches to low back pain. St. Louis: Mosby, 1983.
5. Tomer GM, Olson CN, Lepore B. Preventive measures: Back injury preventive training makes dollars and sense. National Safety News 1984; 129(1):36-39.

30

ERGONOMICS

David A. Thompson

ERGONOMICS

The basic principles of ergonomics and human factors engineering are here outlined as an aid to undertanding corrective job and workplace design measures suggested in other chapters. This chapter is not intended to be a complete treatment of ergonomics; it emphasizes particular areas of knowledge that have specific applicability to the health and safety of the lower back.

The term "ergonomics" is drawn from the Greek *ergon* meaning "to work," and *nomikos* meaning "the study of." Ergonomics is the application of the human physical and behavioral sciences together with the engineering sciences in the study of humans working with machines and tools. The purpose of ergonomic analysis is to make human/machine cooperation a safe, healthy, accurate, and efficient means toward accomplishment of personal and organizational goals.

Technologies Involved in Ergonomics

Within the general area of ergonomics the individual professional technologies cited below all bring to bear valuable techniques for analyzing and improving job design and enhancing job health and safety. Each of these techniques will be incorporated in the job design and lifting recommendations of this chapter to the extent that each is relevant. The professional practitioner in each of these areas should be consulted when relevant job designs and modifications are required.

METHODS ENGINEERING

This technique generally related to the design of the hand motion pattern used by the worker, the machines and tools utilized on the job, and the design of the workplace layout, including location of tools, parts, jigs, and fixtures. Methods engineering grew out of motion and time study and is a well-developed technique practiced by most industrial and production engineers.

BIOMECHANICS

The science of biomechanics deals with the anthropometric size, muscular strength, and postural positions of workers performing their activities. This discipline has received significant attention recently as a result of research into manual materials handling. Recent developments in biomechanical models permit fairly accurate estimates of the upper limits on handling loads for any particular lifting geometry, and estimates of the compressive force on the lower back that occurs during lifting. See Chapter 6 for a full treatment of this subject.

ASSESSMENT OF PHYSIOLOGICAL CAPACITY

This area of job analysis involves the study of the application of musculoskeletal forces over time by manual materials handlers, including estimates of aerobic and anaerobic performance. Upper limits to physiological performance are determined by local muscle fatigue and by heart rate limits.

317

ASSESSMENT OF PSYCHOPHYSICAL CAPACITY

This approach involves estimates of potential weights to be lifted by the manual materials handlers in terms of their own perceived strength and endurance capacities. It generally involves load handling on a test basis for a short period of time, which is used as the basis for estimating long-term handling capacity. This allows a manual materials handler to estimate what his or her upper limits are for handling a specific weight as a function of the lifting geometry and work pace.

Approach to Ergonomic Modification of Jobs

The principal responsibility of safety engineers and managers is to improve the design of jobs that appear unsafe. The health profession (including physicians, chiropractors, nurses, physical and occupational therapists, physiologists, and related professionals) plays a role in ensuring that jobs that have been involved in an injury are no longer unsafe when the healed worker returns. The design principles discussed here apply to both of these situations, but will be emphasized from the point of view of the health professional.

Ergonomic principles of job design and modification are relevant to both the office and the factory floor, and examples are drawn from both. Specific examples of poor designs that may cause the back to be strained or injured will be listed, as well as the physical conditions and injuries themselves. Suggestions for redesign to alleviate those problems will be made. The health professional concerned with determining ways to prevent back injury should review those sections of this chapter that discuss the physical problems related to specific job design anomalies.

Preventive Activities

It is most certainly true that a poorly designed job is an accident waiting to happen. Whenever the opportunity arises, health professionals should tour the work areas for which they are responsible to evaluate the health and safety of the job designs, job performances, and working conditions. The concepts and suggestions of this and related chapters should be kept in mind during this tour, and questionable areas or activities should be noted for later study and possible correction. Such tours, or rounds, should occur at least quarterly, with particular emphasis on those work areas where injuries are most often reported.

In addition to the redesign of unsafe and unhealthy jobs, consideration might be given to job restructuring. The skill level might be reduced or enhanced, the mechanization level increased or decreased, or the tasks performed made more or less variable. The aid of an ergonomist or an industrial engineer will often be necessary in this redesign. These professionals are concerned with employee health and safety as well as productivity, since they are strongly interrelated.

There should be a health and safety review committee within the organization to act as a focal point for planning health and safety reviews and the follow-up activities involved. It would serve as a resource to management and be of benefit to safety engineers and human resources and risk management personnel who are also involved in health and safety.

Cost Effectiveness of Preventive Activities

The health budget is becoming very large in most organizations, and the health and safety committee can advise on the competent management of these funds. The health professionals within an organization can plan programs (including supervisory training in ergonomics) that have been shown to reduce injury costs and workers' compensation insurance premiums dramatically. They can also save money by showing that it is not cost effective to supply employees with minimum-cost tools and equipment, poorly designed workspace layouts, ineffective job instructions, and overcrowded and otherwise stressful conditions.

DESIGN OF JOBS TO PREVENT BACK PAIN
Minimizing Reaches

Two types of reaches may be unsafe for workers with respect to possible lower back discomfort. The first is the upward stretch to a high shelf.

Supporting a load being placed on or removed from the high shelf may result in an asymmetry of the lumbar region of the spine. In addition to the extension involved in high reaches, the physically awkward position of an unstable load could cause a strain or an imbalance resulting in a possible accident.

The second type of unsafe reach is the outward reach, away from the center of gravity of the body. Because of lifting forces and the weight of the upper body, the most critical joint in the spine is the junction between the fifth lumbar vertebra and the first sacral vertebra (referred to as L5-S1). Far reaches move the weight of the shoulders, arms, hands, and load some significant horizontal distance from the L5-S1 joint, resulting in excessive compressive pressure on that joint and excessive tension on the lower back muscles. Whenever unsafe postures such as stretching while reaching or ducking under an overhang are observed, corrective action should be taken to change these postures.

General Examples of Materials Lifting Design

Generally, jobs should be designed so that lifting loads is avoided. When lifting does become necessary, the loads handled should be 1) light, 2) close to the body, 3) lifted at the general height of the hips, 4) grasped by both hands (with handles), and 5) handled in front of the body. Loads should preferably be moved 1) only a short vertical distance (less than 10 inches), 2) to a position close to and in front of the body (no twisting to one side or the other), 3) to a position hip high (no bending or stooping), and 4) infrequently (less often than once a minute).

To the extent that lifting can be within this prescribed geometry and satisfying these constraints, the back is not likely to be injured. Generally, these constraints will result in an upright posture during the move, which will minimize the compressive forces on the back. For example, 99% of all males and 75% of all females can safely lift a single 40 kg weight whose center of gravity is close to the body, from hip height to waist height; 95% of all males and half of all females can safely lift a 70 kg load under similar conditions. However, only half of all

males and only 5% of all females can safely lift 14 kg from the floor at a horizontal distance of 32″ from their own center of gravity. (See below for calculations.)

Effects of Lifting Frequency

CUMULATIVE EFFECTS OF LIFTING INJURIES

There has been a growing awareness recently of the effect of continuing stress on the body over long periods of work. Newly identified syndromes take on names such as "repetitive motion injury," "cumulative motion trauma," "repetitive strain syndrome," and "overuse syndrome." In any event, the continuing frequent repetitive use of the same joints and muscles, even with light loads or low levels of force, is being increasingly identified as unsafe behavior. This is sometimes referred to as the "straw that broke the camel's back" syndrome. Clearly, when one experiences lower back pain from lifting a 2 kg load from the floor when this is the 501st 2 kg load lifted that day, it may be the preceding 1,000 kg of weight lifted (2 kg at a time) that is the true culprit.

Lower back pain builds up relatively slowly during the cumulative handling of relatively small loads or the exerting of relatively light forces. In fact, the first time a worker notices lower back pain, it may be occurring relatively infrequently and would probably not be reported as an injury. Eventually, however, the cumulative effect of lifting even light loads would result in a continuously increasing experience of lower back pain, eventually resulting in the worker reporting the trauma as an industrial accident and probably ascribing it to the most recently lifted load or force exerted. Similarly, entering text or data with a computer keyboard for extended periods of time, even though each key stroke requires only a few ounces of pressure, can result in cumulative repetitive motion trauma when the job involves 60,000–75,000 keystrokes in a day.

Ways to prevent these types of injuries include reducing the frequency of handling a load with any particular pattern of movement or body member (e.g., by lifting at times with the left hand and at other times with the right hand), rotating jobs, and enlarging the job scope.

ENDURANCE EFFECTS

Endurance also plays a role in total lifting capacity when the weights are handled more often than once a minute. The general upper limit for materials handling varies from 12 to 18 times a minute, depending on the total length of time worked and the lifting posture involved. For example, someone lifting all day long in a bent or stooped position should not exceed 12 lifts per minute, but someone working for short periods of time from hip height or above could lift as often as 18 times a minute. However, as will be seen in the subsequent discussion, the weights that may be safely handled decrease dramatically as lifting frequency increases.

Effect of Body Posture While Lifting and Carrying

Generally, the further the horizontal distance between the center of gravity of the load lifted and the center of gravity of the lifter, the greater is the moment arm of the load and, consequently, the lifting torque on the lower back. To compensate for this increased torque, it is necessary for the back muscles (particularly the erector spinae) to contract strongly, compressing the lumbar vertebrae (especially the L5-S1 joint). Many lifting injuries seem to occur in this region.

It is easier to minimize this horizontal distance by keeping loads close to the body while standing. Bending and stooping postures generally require the center of gravity of the load to be further from the center of gravity of the body. If the back is kept relatively erect while lifting from the ground or floor, then bulky loads have to be handled at some distance from the center of gravity of the body in order to avoid hitting the knees. Consequently, if the load must be lifted from the ground or floor, good lifting practice would suggest that the load be pulled as close to the body as possible (probably partially between the legs) prior to lifting and then lifted with a relatively straight back. This puts more strain on the legs than on the back and, unless the materials handler has some leg pathology, generally results in greater lifting safety than does a bent lifting posture.

There is still some controversy over preferred lifting methods. The forces on the base of the spine as a consequence of two different methods of lifting a load are illustrated in Figure 30.1. When lifting is done with the legs relatively straight ("stooped" position), the forces acting on the base of the spine (L5-S1) are a shear force of 500 newtons (N) and a spinal compression of 1800 N. When the lifting is accomplished from a "squat" position, the L5-S1 shear forces are only 340 N but the spinal compression force is 2700 N. (This assumes that the load of 150 N is too bulky to fit between the knees—as is often the case in practice.)

Generally, the stooped lifting posture requires less effort expenditure and, although it may be a greater source of lower back injury, it unfortunately tends to be preferred more often by manual materials handlers. In fact, there is, as yet, no clear biomechanical rationale for recommending either lifting posture as being safer (6, 7).

When carrying loads, the ideal alignment is with the center of gravity of the load directly above the center of gravity of the body. In some cultures, this is accomplished by carrying the load on the head or on both ends of a shoulder yoke. Although these carrying postures are safer for loads of similar weight, they are generally not utilized in the United States; consequently, the common option is to carry the load in front of the materials handler and as close to the body as possible.

Effect of Load Characteristics

In general, to avoid lifting injuries, materials handlers should:

1. Reduce load to below personal strength limits for occasional lifting, and below 50% of personal strength limits for routine lifting;
2. Refer to the Acceptable Load and Maximum Permissible Load formulas for various types of lifting limits (see below);
3. Minimize twisting with a load; when twisting is necessary, rotate pelvis and step around;
4. Keep loads close to the body;
5. Exercise caution in slippery or cluttered areas.

In addition to these primary principles, other suggestions for safe and healthy lifting practices are illustrated in Figure 30.2.

Estimating General Strength Limits

When setting general lifting limits for a group of materials handlers, one should be guided by the following: most workers (99% of men and

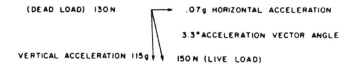

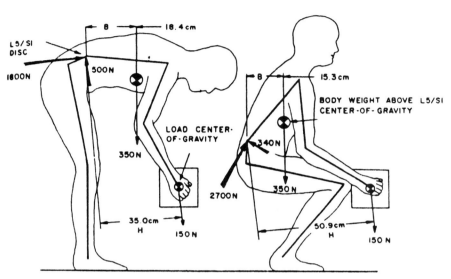

Figure 30.1. Compressive and shear forces at the base of the spine. (Reproduced by permission from Park KS, Chaffin DB. A biomechanical evaluation of the methods of manual load lifting. Am Inst Indus Eng Trans 1974; 6(2):105–113.)

75% of women) should be able to lift loads no greater than that defined by the following formula:

$$AL = 40 \ (15/H)(1-(0.004|V-75|))(0.7 + 7.5/D)(1-F/F_{max})$$

where AL = Action limit, the maximum weight lifting value (in kg) above which management action must be taken to reduce lifting parameters or simplify the job;

H = Horizontal lever arm of load [horizontal distance (cm) from load center of mass at the origin of the vertical lift to the midpoint of the ankles]; between 15 and 80 cm.

V = Height of load at beginning of lift (vertical distance [cm] from floor to load center of mass); between 0 and 175 cm. $|V-75|$ represents the absolute value of V–75.

D = Vertical travel distance of load; between 25 cm and 200-V cm.

F = Average frequency of lifting (lifts/min); between 0.2 and F_{max} period and body position when lifting. For 1-hour work

period: F_{max} is 18 when standing and 15 when stooped. For 8-hour work period, F_{max} is 15 when standing and 12 when stooped. (8)

The above equation assumes smooth, two-handed lifting in the sagital plane of moderate-width objects that are relatively easy to hold (not sharp, hot, or slippery). Moreover, it assumes that there are no physical barriers to a direct origin-to-destination lift, that the floor is uncluttered and not slippery, and that there are favorable temperature conditions in the work area. Any departure from these assumptions will lessen the effective lifting ability below the Action Limit by some appropriate amount. Chaffin and Anderson present analysis techniques to evaluate the effect of nonstandard job conditions on work difficulty (6). An Ergonomic Lifting Calculator cardboard slide rule and personal computer software are available from the National Safety Council to compute these lifting limits rapidly.

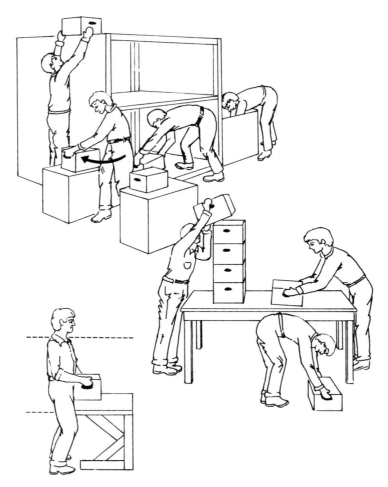

Figure 30.2. Suggestions for safe and healthy lifting. Avoid stretching to lift, twisting while lifting, lifting within constricted spaces, lifts out of a deep bin, lifting with horizonal extension, and lifting off floor. Generally, lifting should be within the shoulder (130 cm) to waist (65 cm) vertical range.

The Action Limit is intended to protect most workers from injury, including physical strain and overexertion. Calculation of the Action Limit is based on limiting the L5/S1 disc compression forces to 3400 N, which biomechanical studies indicate can be tolerated by most (but not all) people. The Action Limit also assumes the average metabolic energy requirement would be no more than 3.5 kcal/min, which most workers can sustain for reasonable periods of time.

In addition to Action Limit, NIOSH defines a Maximum Permissible Limit, equal to three times the Action Limit, above which lifting is not considered safe. Between the Action Limit and the Maximum Permissible Limit, admin-

istrative controls must be enforced, involving improved worker selection and job placement and improved worker training.

When materials handlers work at the Maximum Permissible Limit, they experience L5/S1 disc compression forces of about 6400 N, the highest value that most workers can tolerate without injury. They are also exerting energy on the job of at least 5 kcal/min, more than most workers can tolerate for very long. In general, only about 25% of men and less than 1% of women can work at or above the Maximum Permissible Limit. Lifting tasks above the Maximum Permissible Limit are clearly unacceptable for most workers, and the tasks should be redesigned. The relationship between the Ac-

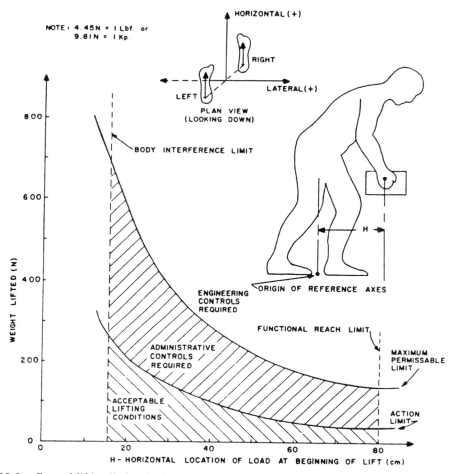

Figure 30.3. General lifting limits. Action limit and maximum permissible limit for different horizontal location of loads lifted from floor (V = 15 cm) to knuckle height (D = 60 cm) on an infrequent basis (F < 0.2). (Reproduced by permission from Chaffin DB, Andersson G. Occupational biomechanics. New York: John Wiley & Sons, 1984.)

ion Limit and the Maximum Permissible Limit is shown in Figure 30.3.

Measuring Personal Strength Limits

The most relevant lifting limits for a specific worker are those established directly from that worker's strength and endurance. As long as the worker lifts correctly within the limits thus established by his or her own ability (within a safe environment—no slippery floors, unguarded moving machinery) he or she should be relatively safe from injury. However, one must choose among several strength measuring approaches available. Static strength of localized

muscles (as in lifting with the elbow-shoulder system) is most often used. At the other extreme, dynamic whole-body strength (as in pushing a cart, or lifting to a high shelf) is generally considered more realistic and predictive of lifting ability, but harder to determine and standardize.

STATIC STRENGTH MEASURES

Standardized tests of the static strength of specific muscle groups generally are conducted in three body positions as illustrated in Figure 30.4. Each test pull lasts 4 to 6 seconds from a standardized posture, with adequate rest be-

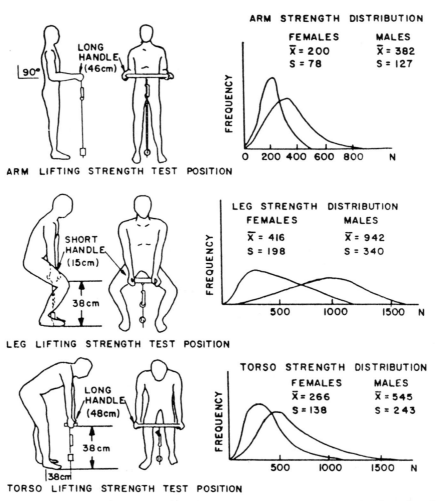

Figure 30.4. Static strength test postures. Static strength test postures and results for 443 male and 108 female workers employed in four different industries. (Reproduced by permission from Chaffin DB, Herrin GD, Keyserling WM. Preemployment strength testing. J Occup Med 1978; 20(6):403–408.)

tween pulls, and with subject encouragement without coercion (6, 8).

Table 30.1 shows the frequency distributions of male and female static strengths in each of these three positions, plus strengths in a variety of other postures and activities.

PSYCHOPHYSICAL MEASURES OF STRENGTH

The most thoroughly investigated technique of measuring voluntary whole-body dynamic strength is the Psychophysical Strength Method. Work capacity norms are elicited from

lished experimental protocol and then tested for realism over a given period of work. The result is a load value that a representative population of materials handlers is willing to lift at a specific frequency from one particular height to another height (e.g., lifting from floor to shoulder height once a minute).

Representative values for psychophysical loads that workers are willing to lift repeatedly are shown in Table 30.2 as a function of the sex of the worker, the origin and destination heights, and the depth of the load (which determines the minimum load center of gravity displacement from the spine; 9).

Table 30.1.
Static Strengths Demonstrated by Workers when Lifting, Pushing, and Pulling with Both Hands on a Handle Placed at Different Locations Relative to the Midpoint Between the Ankles on Floor.

Test description	Handle location (cm)[a]		Male strengths (N)			Female strengths (N)		
	Vertical	Horizontal	Sample size	Mean	SD	Sample size	Mean	SD
Lift—leg partial squat	38	0	673	903	325	165	427	187
Lift—torso stooped over	38	38	1141	480	205	246	271	125
Lift—arms flexed	114	38	1276	383	125	234	214	93
Lift—shoulder high & arms out	152	51	309	227	71	35	129	36
Lift—shoulder high & arms flexed	152	38	119	529	222	20	240	84
Lift—shoulder high & arms close	152	25	309	538	156	35	285	102
Lift—floor level-close (squat)	15	25	309	890	245	35	547	182
Lift—floor level-out (stoop)	15	38	170	320	125	20	200	71
Push down—waist level	118	38	309	432	93	35	325	71
Pull down—above shoulders	178	33	309	605	102	35	449	107
Pull in—shoulder level-arms out	157	33	309	311	80	35	244	53
Pull in—shoulder level-arms in	140	0	205	253	62	52	209	62
Push-out—waist level-stand erect	101	35	54	311	195	27	226	76
Push-out—chest level-stand erect	124	25	309	303	76	35	214	49
Push-out—shoulder level-lean forward	140	64	205	418	178	52	276	120

[a]Handle locations are measured in mid-sagittal plane, vertical from floor and horizontal from mid-point between ankles.
Note: 4.45 N = 1 lbf or 9.81 N = 1 kgf = 1 Kp.
(Reproduced by permission from Chaffin DB, Andersson G. Occupational biomechanics. New York: John Wiley & Sons, 1984.)

INTERPRETING STRENGTH MEASURES

Comparing the static strength measures (Fig. 30.4) with psychophysical measures of dynamic load limits (Table 30.2), one finds that the voluntary static strength of a particular muscle group (e.g., elbow-shoulder) is about 50% higher than the comparable dynamic strength (e.g.,

knuckle-shoulder lift), and may even be double the comparable dynamic strength. The reason for this is that dynamic strength involves musculature over a range of joint efficiencies, and the dynamic lifting involves ovvercoming the inertia of the load in its upward acceleration, as well as lifting its weight.

For this reason, "strength" as measured by

Table 30.2.
Psychophysical Lifting Limits.

Height of lift (cm)	Sagittal plane box dimensions (cm)	Male mean (N)	Female mean (N)
Floor to knuckle height when erect	30.5	296	194
	45.7	261	171
	61.0	236	152
Knuckle to shoulder height when erect	30.5	263	141
	45.7	233	129
	61.0	205	127
Shoulder to reach height when erect	30.5	221	120
	45.7	204	110
	61.0	195	112

The values represent acceptable lifting limits (N) based on lifting frequency of once per minute sustained for 8 hours.
Reproduced by permission from Chaffin DB, Andersson G. Occupational biomechanics. New York: John Wiley & Sons, 1984.)

the standardized static strength tests, cannot be used directly to predict the weight of loads that may be safely lifted by the person tested. Comparison of standard measures of static strengths with loads actually handled has shown that whenever the actual load is much more than 50% of the relevant static strength measure, the likelihood of injury increases dramatically (8).

Consequently, if standardized static strength testing is incorporated in a job screening program, the results must be discounted to approximately one-half of their measured values when used to estimate safe load-handling

capabilities by the tested muscle groups; and, if possible, they should be used in conjunction with dynamic strength tests (6, 10, 11)

Pushing and Pulling

The forces involved in pushing and pulling loads are illustrated in Figure 30.5. As is shown, pulling loads is much more strenuous on the lower back for the same-hand forces (Fp) than pushing loads. Pulling a 350 N force (resulting from the weight of the cart times its coefficient of rolling friction) at a height of 66 cm above the floor causes a compressive force on the lower

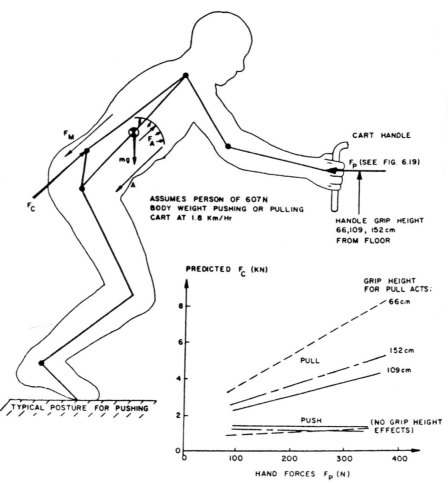

Figure 30.5.   Pushing and pulling forces on the lower back. Predicted peak L5-S1 compression forces, F_c, is in Newtons. Abdominal forces, F_A, back muscle forces, F_M, and the location of the center of gravity are also shown. (Reproduced by permission from Chaffin DB, Andersson G. Occupational biomechanics. New York: John Wiley & Sons, 1984.)

spine of about 8000 N, substantially above the 6400 N that most workers can tolerate without injury (6, 8, 10).

Seating and Posture

The ideal working posture is to be standing or seated with the back erect and the head balanced comfortably on the top of the spine. The forearms may be outstretched, but the upper arms should hang comfortably at the sides. To the extent that this ideal posture is not utilized

in one's job, fatigue and muscular soreness may occur. Figure 30.6 illustrates some postures that are likely to cause difficulty for those performing the jobs shown.

The general posture problems illustrated in Figure 30.6 are all caused by the lack of correspondence between the workers' anthropometrics and the workplace geometry, and the *failure to bring the two into registration* so that the workplace dimensions supplement those of the worker.

Guidelines for the design of seating and

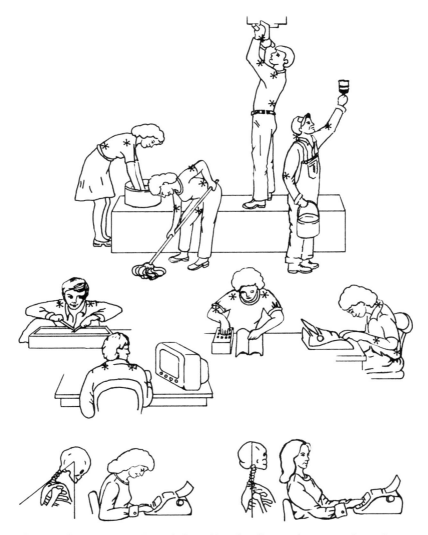

Figure 30.6. Poor working postures. Extended reaching, bending, and asymmetric static postures are illustrated as examples of causes of musculoskeletal stress, discomfort, and possible distress. The effect of cervical flexion is illustrated for typists and VDT operations. (Stars indicate general areas of stress.)

workplace design, particularly relevant to the office, have recently become available (12). These guidelines presently have the generally accepted industrial agreement of standards, but do not yet have the force of regulations. They are an excellent aid to providing a comfortable, efficient, and healthy workplace, particularly for workers using visual display terminals or similar equipment.

SEATING COMFORT

The primary purpose of a chair is to comfortably support the weight of the body without restricting circulation. The seat pan should comfortably support the thighs, and the chair back should support some of the weight of the torso, arms, and head, reducing the pressure on the lower spine (6).

Changes in posture permit different portions of the anatomy to support the body weight while other parts enjoy increased circulation. Leaning to one side, crossing the legs, slouching, are postures that allow posterior circulation. Chair design should be adjustable and flexible enough to accommodate these postural variations and movements.

Chair design also affects blood circulation in the legs. If the seat pan is too long (>16"), it cuts off circulation at the popliteus, particularly for short women. It is also helpful if the edge of the seat under the knees is smoothly curved and rounded to eliminate pressure points. The chair seat should be soft enough to be comfortable but not so soft that changing posture or standing up is difficult. The seat pan should be relatively flat, rather than concave, so that the thighs do not roll inward for heavier people. An exception to the flat seat pan principle is the kneeling chair, discussed below.

Another important aspect of seat design is lumbar support for 1) maintaining a comfortable degree of lordosis of the spine, and 2) assisting in support of the weight of the back. A chair should be easily adjustable from a sitting position to conform to the full range of back curvatures, lumbar heights, and buttock sizes. Without such support, general fatigue is much more likely, added muscular stress in the upper back tends to occur, and lower back pain may result.

Other aspects of safe and comfortable chair design are that it have five legs (to reduce the likelihood of tipping over for someone leaning backwards) and that the texture of the back and seat material be rough or nubby so that a small amount of air circulation can occur between the material and the body. Chair arms, if used, should be short enough so as not to strike the work table or bench during normal chair movements.

SEATING DIMENSIONS

Seated Posture

Workers need to be instructed in the proper use of chairs to maintain a healthy posture. The bottom of Figure 30.6 illustrates the upper back and neck stress that may occur from poor posture. Once it has been determined that undesirable job factors (e.g., poor visibility, no copy holder) have been eliminated, users with poor posture should be reminded to keep the upper back and neck in a vertical alignment.

Kneeling Chairs

Recently, several new types of chairs have come on the market that have forward-sloping seats with knee rests, but no back. Occasionally, they find a satisfied user whose physiognomy is suited to this seating convention. However, most users find that these chairs have three distinct disadvantages:

1. Support of a substantial amount of the user's weight on the knees causes pressure that cuts off circulation to the lower legs. This makes arising and walking difficult.
2. There is no satisfactory position for the toes; they are either flexed or hyperextended, both of which are uncomfortable for long periods.
3. It is not possible to change sitting positions from time to time, as one does in a normal chair to permit circulation selectively to different parts of the posterior. There is only the "correct" position, with no comfortable alternatives.

A variety of new chair designs is currently becoming available; some chairs have forward-sloping seats and backrests, but without knee-pads to support the legs. Many such designs may hold promise for various classes of jobs and preferences of users.

Neutral Body Posture Chairs

Neutral body posture chairs have seats that adjust from a rearward slope to a forward slope.

They are especially advantageous when the user has to be very close to, or up over, the work. This is the case for some repair people, air traffic controllers, dentists, surgeons, and anyone observed sitting on the edge of a seat. The degree of slope should be easily adjustable (in addition to adjustable height and back position) and should provide for some additional support to prevent slipping out of the chair (seat pan contouring, "saddle" or "tractor seat" shaping (4, 5, 13, 14).

Sit-Stand Option

A sit-stand seating option consists of an elevated workplace and a high stool. This allows workers to do their jobs comfortably while standing, and also provides for comfortable sitting. Generally, a sit-stand workbench or work desk is 36 to 38 inches high, rather than the 27- to 29-inch height of the normal office desk. The high stool provided workers in this case allows them to sit with their torsos at about the same elevation as they would be if they were standing at their workplace. The stool should also provide some footrest such as a circular foot ring near the bottom, which should probably be supplemented by a normal footrest of appropriate height.

This sitting option is particularly helpful where worker mobility is required; that is, the job requires frequent moving from one work area to another. The sit-stand option relieves the person from sitting down and standing up repeatedly in moves from work area to work area, reducing fatigue and compression on the spine.

A second work condition that makes the sit-stand option desirable exists when mobility is severely restricted by physical movement and reposturing are desired by the worker. This sitting option allows the worker to slide off the stool to a standing position without any work interruption, or slide back onto the stool from a standing position in the same manner. While standing, the worker is able to enhance lordosis and increase circulation in the pelvic region and the legs. Sliding back on the high stool while continuing to work allows the legs and feet to relax.

In some cases, each worker may be provided with a sit-stand option. In other work situations, where most workers prefer normal sitting, a limited number of sit-stand alternative work areas may be provided for workers who choose

to avail themselves of this option. This works effectively in situations such as that of telephone directory assistance operators who can unplug from their normally used low (29") desk and plug into the high (38") desk using a high stool, with an identical visual display terminal.

SEATING CHOICE

There are many types and models of chairs available today that meet all or most of the requirements discussed above. A reasonable manner of selecting the "best" of those available is to obtain a sample of two or three appropriate chairs (with or without arms) that meet the above requirements and let employees who will be using the chairs try them out for at least a week. Their opinion should be carefully considered when a supply of new chairs is ordered; if opinion is divided, order some of each.

A *brief* chair testing is usually not sufficient. Initial impressions have often been found to be somewhat different from long-term (e.g., all day) test opinions.

SEATING SUMMARY

Musculoskeletal complaints from a seated worker may be related to chair characteristics. But discomfort may be attributed to chair variables that instead is due to other factors such as the lack of wrist rests (to take weight off the shoulders), visual discomfort (radiating down the neck to the back), lack of exercise, and supervisory stress. Other sections of this chapter deal with these other factors.

Work Breaks

For most jobs, a 15-minute rest break after about 2 hours of work is standard, unless the work is excessively difficult physically or there are adverse environmental conditions (abnormal temperature or humidity; 15).

The purpose of the break, of course, is to overcome fatigue. For physically demanding jobs, the 15-minute break is probably well used in resting. Sedentary workers, however, require some physical activity to relieve the musculoskeletal stress that has accumulated from being in a rigid posture for most of the previous 2 hours. Their break time might be better used by taking one 10-minute break with several micro-breaks interspersed within the 2-hour time period. The micro-break, lasting about 10 to 15 seconds, can be used to stretch a particular body area that is tense—for example, by doing a head roll, arm and leg stretch, or shoulder rolls. Deep breathing can also relieve tension and rejuvenate the brain. In this manner, 5 minutes of exercise during micro-breaks and 10 minutes of rest during the regular break would probably reduce musculoskeletal stress far more than just a 15-minute rest break. This happens because the micro-break relieves musculoskeletal stress and tension as it builds up, preventing a painful level of stress before it is noticed and given attention.

Teaching workers appropriate exercises to perform puts healing tools in their hands to use as they feel appropriate and gives them the ability and the responsibility to relieve much of their own musculoskeletal stress. These brief exercises, of course, should not be seen as a substitute for general stress reduction in the environment but they may help alleviate it (16, 17).

Employees should be encouraged to spend more of their normal break time, lunch hour, or personal time before and after work in exercise activities to the extent they find them beneficial or enjoyable. Many companies make it easy for their employees to do this by offering on-site exercise classes and facilities, as well as special interest group activities such as walking, running, or biking.

REDESIGNING JOBS

Need for Job Redesign

The initial design of jobs comes out of immediate necessity or tradition. Jobs are then often modified as worker experience or product design changes suggest. However, specific reasons for job redesign occur in each of the following situations and may be used as an opportunity to reevaluate in a more formal manner the way in which tasks are performed.

INSPECTION TOURS

It is the responsibility of management to ensure that safe working conditions exist for all personnel. To do this, managers should tour their own facilities from time to time, looking for violations of promulgated safety rules. They should also have safety professionals tour the facilities and perform a safety audit of all work areas, products handled, and tools utilized.

The safety professionals can be those from the organization's own staff or outside consultants. If the organization is large enough to justify the use of in-house staff for this purpose, these staff members should become quite familiar with the specific needs and demands of the organization's products and services. Even with an in-house safety department, specialized outside consultants are often helpful in such specialty areas as hazardous waste control or asbestos removal. In any event, complete tours of all work facilities should be made on a timely (at least monthly) and on a nonroutine basis. All violations of standard safety procedures or regulations should be noted and documented.

REDUCTION OF INJURIES

The inspection tours described in the previous section should remove as many of the safety hazards from the workplace as possible. However, when injuries do occur, analysis should focus on any residual unsafe conditions, practices, or equipment that should also be evaluated.

Where the same type of accident occurs under similar conditions or in a certain area of the organization over time, the accident report should specify the particulars of the accident so that statistical similarities of accident characteristics will assist in pinpointing these unsafe areas.

WORKER FEEDBACK

The workers in an organization should feel free to report unsafe conditions themselves in some formal manner. In addition, worker grievances, absences, tardiness, and turnover also may be safety related and should be evaluated. If it is suspected that these worker characteristics are safety related, follow-up interviews by appropriate organization safety professionals should be conducted to determine job redesign alternatives.

OSHA CITATIONS

Occasionally, job redesign is necessitated by an inspection by a representative of the Occupational Safety and Health Association (OSHA). In the event that a formal citation is issued for violation of safety regulations, appropriate safety professionals need to advise on redesigning the affected jobs in order to bring them into compliance with OSHA regulations.

The citation often results in specification of the unsafe activities, conditions, or equipment and allows the organization time to eliminate the safety hazards. Occasionally, however, the unsafe conditions are so significant or widespread that an outside safety professional, agreed upon by OSHA and the company, must be brought in to solve the safety problems and suggest job redesigns.

ACCOMMODATE LIGHT DUTY

Finally, jobs may be redesigned on a temporary basis or modified on a continuing basis in order to accommodate injured workers who are returning to work on a limited-duty basis. If the physical stresses and strains of the job are reduced, previously injured workers may be able to perform them competently without reinjuring themselves. At times, the modified-duty work is accompanied by physical rehabilitation and work hardening. These latter techniques should reflect the physical demands of the redesigned job for the modified-duty worker.

Reducing Weight and Force Components of Job

REDUCING WEIGHT

Because of the possible injurious and even debilitating effects of weight lifted by materials handlers, it is important to reduce its effect whenever possible. Two principal ways of doing this are to repackage the product or object handled or to provide an assistive device to the materials handler.

Repackaging

Repackaging generally involves using smaller modules of weight when shipping products or packaging items. For short lifts it is possible to move two modules at a time but, for longer lifts or lifts from the floor, it then becomes safer to move only one of the modules at a time.

For example, newspapers can be in bundles of 30 rather than 50, flour or sugar can be in 25-pound rather than 50-pound bags. The ease of handling and the improved safety for employees, delivery personnel, sales personnel, and

customers more than make up for the slight increase in packaging costs.

Lifting Aids

If it is not feasible to reduce the size of a product lifted (for example, items such as refrigerators or motors) assistance when lifting should be provided to the materials handler.

Lifting aids now come in a variety of configurations and generally consist of this basic design: A rope sling, grappling hook, or suction cup typically provides the fastening device between the lifting aid and the item being handled. Once control of the item has been established, movement of the device (either electrically or pneumatically) is accomplished with fingertip controls on a guidance handle. In this manner, control over a very heavy object is accomplished by a materials handler exerting a few pounds on a guidance handle. In several applications of this technique in a California electronics company, the increase in efficiency and productivity of the materials handler more than made up for the added cost of the lifting aid.

It is clear that such lifting aids, particularly in the face of the need to handle heavy objects, enhance safety in general and reduce back injury in particular. They also increase morale considerably because they tend to upgrade the status and "control power" of the employee.

CHANGING HEIGHT OF LIFT

The effort involved in lifting (in terms of the amount lifted) varies as a function of how close to 75 cm is the initial height of the load lifted. This is approximately waist high for the average worker, and indicates that the more one has to bend over, or the more one has to raise the load with one's arms while holding the torso rigid, the less safe is the lift.

Consequently, loads should be stored as close as possible to waist level and not lifted to heights much above this. Such waist-high storage is easily accomplished with spring-loaded devices that keep the top of a stack of materials level as items are removed from the stack. Lifting and positioning equipment and systems are commercially available in a number of models and styles. They will keep a load of steel sheets or pans or heavy bales at waist level until the stack is exhausted. They may also be used in reverse, that is, they may be continuously loaded at waist level, in a spring-loaded vertical stack.

The principal visual cues of unsafe manual handling is bending and stooping to reach for or place an object. Well-designed lifting aids may virtually eliminate routine bending and stooping in many situations.

INCREASED EASE OF HANDLING

Difficulty in grasping and holding objects to be moved may lead to the objects' instability and require more difficult handling postures. Handling can be improved by providing handles or convenient corners to grasp during lifting. An alternative is to provide lifting cartons, cups, or trays with appropriately designed handles into which the objects may be placed.

An example of a poorly designed object to be lifted is a 50- to 60-pound sack of dog food or rice in a loose, slippery sack. Another example of a difficult-to-lift object is a small refrigerator carton in which the motor is on the side away from the person doing the lifting. This results in an off-balance center of gravity away from the lifter, causing extra back strain in the attempt to accomplish lifting stability.

An ideal object to lift would be a simple plastic bin no more than 12 inches deep and 18 inches wide with easily grasped, comfortable handles. Such "tote bins" actually make up a large number of industrial product carriers.

PUSH/PULL

Pushing and pulling large objects or heavy vehicles can result in large forces on the lower back. In general, to prevent injuries when pushing or pulling heavy loads, the following guidelines are suggested.

1. Ensure that the area ahead of the load is level and clear of obstacles. If not level, some system of braking should be available.
2. Push the load rather than pull it. Spinal loading will be reduced, and forward visibility will be improved (unless the load is high).
3. Be careful of foot traction. Foot-slip potential is very high whenever pushing or pulling, and a fall could result in an impact injury. The coefficient of friction between the floor and the sole of the shoes should be at least 0.8, if possible, wherever heavy loads are moved.
4. When starting to push a load, brace one foot and use the back rather than the hands to apply force.

5. If a load does not start to move when a reasonable force is applied, get help from a co-worker or utilize a powered vehicle.
6. Pushing or pulling is easier when the handles are about hip height (91–114 cm for males) than at shoulder height or above. Handles lower than the hips result in unsafe postures.

REDUCING BENDING AND STOOPING

It is safer to lift weights from waist level than from floor or near-floor level. In general, bending and stooping are to be avoided even for relatively light loads. Even though the load lifted may be, perhaps, only five pounds, bending over to lift it involves rotation of the full weight of the trunk, arms, and head about the lower back, requiring back muscle forces sufficient to rotate perhaps more than 100 pounds. The pulling forces of the back muscles produce compression on the lower spine and, in addition, the weight of the torso, arms, and head results in some shear forces at the L5-S1 juncture. Stooping involves raising and lowering the torso, arms, and head plus partial raising of the legs, resulting in a lesser lower back strain but increased compressive forces on the lower back.

The resulting safety rules for lifting from lower levels are:

1. Lift with the back relatively straight and upright whenever possible.
2. Keep the weight lifted as close to the body as possible, generally by pulling the object between the knees before lifting.
3. Ensure a good grip on the load prior to lifting so as to maintain positive control over the load at all times.
4. Ensure a stable stance while lifting. One may verify this by doing a small, short preliminary lift prior to the main lift to determine whether or not the load and the body's own weight are in balance.
5. Ensure that the floor area is not slippery or cluttered in a way which will impede movement in the lifting area.
6. Do not twist while lifting. If it is necessary to change direction, step around with one foot while keeping the pelvis and the shoulder generally aligned with one another.
7. Whenever the load to be lifted exceeds safe lifting limits use a lifting aid or get assistance from a fellow employee.

The lower back is in its most vulnerable configuration during bending and stooping, and materials handlers are well advised to protect their own health by scrupulously following safety guidelines.

REDUCING REACHING AND STRETCHING

Oftentimes, one of the easiest ways to modify a workplace design so as to improve lower back safety is to tighten up the dimensions of the work area in order to reduce reaching and stretching. This generally is easier and more feasible than attempting to reduce the weight of the product or parts handled, or changing the tasks performed on the product.

Reducing the range of reaching decreases the horizontal distance between the center of the load (including the body's own weight) and the base of the spine. This, in turn, reduces the tension on the lower back muscles required to counteract the weights involved and reduces the compressive stress on the lower back.

The general approach to workplace design, in this instance, is to store (and work on) all parts and products as close to the immediate vicinity of the work area as possible. The ideal situation would be to reach no further than the length of one's forearm to obtain or position a part or product. The worst situation would involve reaching as far as one can possibly stretch to obtain or position a part or product, as when getting an object off a shelf or placing it on a conveyor belt. Reaches and moves with such extreme stretching can be more harmful on the lower back, even for light loads, than bending and stooping to pick the same weight off the floor.

REDUCING THE EFFECTS OF STANDING

Occasionally, jobs require extensive standing and walking during a day's work. High stools can reduce some of the standing stress. When the sit-stand option is not feasible, thick rubber pads should be used to cushion the worker's movements in the area within which mobility is required. If the mobility area is extensive and walking pads are not feasible, the worker should then wear durable shoes with thick, soft soles.

The sit-stand stool, rubber mat, and cushioned shoes all act as shock absorbers for the lower back from the jolts of walking, moving, carrying, and working in general. In bipedal locomotion, the weights of the torso, arms, and head plus any load carried continuously compress the lower spine as each step is taken. On hard surfaces, such as steel or concrete, this continual jolting of the spine can result in exceptional fatigue and lower back discomfort even in healthy workers. Intervertebral disks in the lumbar spine cannot absorb all of the shock of the weight of the body above it, particularly for older workers whose disks have less resiliency.

References

1. Woodson WE. Human factors design handbook. New York: McGraw-Hill, 1981.
2. Bailey RW. Human performance engineering: A guide for system designers. Englewood Cliffs, NJ: Prentice-Hall, 1982.
3. Alexander DC, Pulat BM. Industrial ergonomics, A practitioner's guide. Norcross GA: Industrial Engineering and Management Press, 1985.
4. Eastman Kodak Company, Human Factors Section, Health Safety and Human Factors Laboratory. Ergonomic design for people at work, vol. 1. Belmont, CA: Lifetime Learning Publications, 1983.
5. Grandjean E. ed. Ergonomics and health in modern offices. In Proceedings of the international scientific conference on ergonomics and health aspects in modern offices. November 7–9, 1983, Turin, Italy. London: Taylor & Francis, 1984.
6. Chaffin DB, Andersson G. Occupational biomechanics. New York: John Wiley & Sons, 1984.
7. Garg A, Herrin GD. Stoop or squat: a biomechanical and metabolic evaluation. Am Inst Indus Eng Trans 1979; 11(4):293–302.
8. National Institute for Occupational Safety and Health, Division of Biomechanical and Behavioral Science. Work practices guide for manual lifting (PB82-178948). Springfield, VA: National Technical Information Service, 1981.
9. Snook SH. The design of manual handling tasks. Ergonomics 1978; 21:963–985.
10. Astrand PO, Rodahl K. Textbook of work physiology, physiological bases of exercise. San Francisco: McGraw-Hill, 1977.
11. Konz S. Work design. Columbus: Grid Publishing, 1979.
12. American national standard for human factors engineering of visual display terminal workstations (ANSI/HFS Standard No. 100-1988). Santa Monica, CA: The Human Factors Society, Inc., 1988.
13. Kvalseth TO. Ergonomics of workstation design. Boston: Butterworth, 1983.
14. Mandal AC. The seated man. Copenhagen: Dafnia Publications, 1985.

15. Eastman Kodak Company, Ergonomics Group, Health Environment Laboratories. Ergonomic design for people at work, vol. 2. New York: Van Nostrand Reinhold, 1986.

16. Ross A. Office exercises for sedentary jobs. San Francisco: Pacific Bell Corporate Health Services, 1988.

17. Gore A, Tasker D. Pause gymnastics, improving comfort and health at work. Sydney: CCH Australia, 1986.

31

BACK INJURY PREVENTION: ROLE OF STRENGTH AND FLEXIBILITY EXERCISES

H. Duane Saunders

Companies can play an active part in reducing both the incidence and severity of back injuries. More and more evidence shows that industry can take positive steps effectively to prevent and manage this costly epidemic that has plagued industry for the past several decades (1–12).

For the concept of back injury prevention to make sense, it is important to understand that back problems are seldom caused by a single traumatic injury. With few exceptions, back disorders are the result of the cumulative effects of months or even years of poor posture, faulty body mechanics, stressful living and working habits, loss of strength and flexibility, and a general lack of physical fitness. With these factors in mind, let's look at what a company can do to prevent problems. Generally speaking, a comprehensive preventive program includes four main goals:

1. Redesign or modify the worksite—eliminate the task or make the job less stressful.
2. Require proper body mechanics—teach employees to use good lifting, pushing, pulling, and moving methods.
3. Compensate for stressful activities—allow workers to change positions frequently, pace stressful tasks throughout the day, and utilize team lifting techniques.
4. Make sure workers are physically fit—encourage employees to maintain an acceptable level of strength, flexibility, and physical fitness.

To accomplish these goals, five specific phases should be included in a back injury prevention program:

1. Worksite evaluation and modification/redesign,
2. Training program for workers,
3. Training program for supervisors and management,
4. Strength, flexibility, and fitness assessment,
5. Participation in an exercise program.

This chapter will deal specifically with strength and flexibility assessment and exercise training for the industrial worker.

Loss of flexibility, not only of the ligaments, joint capsules and discs, but of the muscles as well, contributes to back injury. Experiments with laboratory animals show that immobilization and lack of exercise soon causes muscle tissue to be replaced by connective tissue (13). The discs and facet joint surfaces do not have blood supplies. Nutrition is received through movement of body fluids into the disc and the movement of synovial fluid within the facet joints. Thus, if flexibility is lost, the nutritional supply is decreased to these structures, which permits weakening and makes them vulnerable to injury (13).

It is important to emphasize that many work situations are like athletic events in that they require a certain level of physical fitness, strength, and flexibility. Many people attempt to work at jobs that require considerable physical labor and involve stressful positions, but they make little or no effort to keep their bodies in the physical condition required to do these jobs.

There is considerable evidence to indicate that people who are in poor physical condition (strength, flexibility, and cardiovascular fitness) are at greater risk of back injury (14–18). Therefore, it seems logical that one important aspect of a back injury prevention program would be to identify those who have strength, flexibility, and fitness deficiencies and attempt to help them improve their level of physical condition, thus reducing their risk of injury.

Strength and flexibility assessment is an informational tool to show the worker particular strengths and weaknesses. The worker is provided with an objective determination of risk level and given the necessary knowledge and responsibility to correct any problem that may be found.

In addition, strength and flexibility assessment may be used to determine if an applicant is to be hired or to determine job placement. If assessment is used in this way it becomes controversial, since some say that it may be used unfairly to discriminate against weaker or less flexible workers. It is this author's opinion that physical testing to determine work qualification should test specific physical skills necessary to do a particular job. General strength and flexibility assessment can be used as a preemployment or preplacement exam, if it has been validated to the specific job in question. Validation requires a longitudinal study that shows that individuals with certain strength and flexibility deficiencies do indeed have significantly greater back injuries in a specific job than their stronger and more flexible counterparts (19). On the other hand, the primary purpose of general strength and flexibility assessment is to determine potential risk of injury and to provide those who are at risk with a means of correcting their deficiencies.

If we are to get widespread acceptance of back strength and flexibility assessment and exercise training programs, they must be practical, easy to use, and affordable. The program described in this chapter can be done at the work site, requiring only 1 hour of the workers' time away from work. One therapist can assess and train six to eight people per hour and no expensive equipment is involved.

Another requirement of a back strength and flexibility assessment and exercise training program is that it be comprehensive enough to involve several areas of strength and flexibility. It is common to find people who are strong and/or flexible in one direction, yet weak and/or stiff in

another. These strengths and weaknesses are usually job related or may even be related to the type of exercise program in which an individual is participating (i.e., too many low back flexion activities and not enough emphasis on extension strength and flexibility). Back testing protocols that test only one or two movements will usually miss these out-of-balance individuals. In addition, if deficits are found, each assessment test should convert easily into a corrective exercise that is easy to perform.

Above all, a back strength and flexibility assessment and training program should be functional and biomechanically sound. Many back testing devices or machines are promoted as more objective or "scientifically based" than the simple assessment exams advocated here. One must be wary, however, of devices that assess strength and range of motion in nonfunctional or unacceptable biochemical positions. For example, measuring gross flexion/extension range of motion is of little value since many people will have excess mobility in one direction (e.g., flexion) and limited mobility in the other direction (e.g., extension). Such people would score "normal" on a machine that only measures gross range of motion. Lifting with the legs straight and the back in a forward bent position is biomechanically unsound. To test trunk flexion strength in the standing or sitting position requiring a concentric contraction of the abdominals when functionally trunk flexion requires an eccentric contraction of the back muscles is also unsound. We should not, therefore, be testing industrial workers in this manner. Even if strength deficiencies were found using these testing methods, we would certainly not advocate exercising in this manner to correct them. Not only because it is biomechanically unsound, but because such machines are prohibitively expensive for use with large groups of industrial clients.

I recognize that, in some cases, there are more objective methods of measuring strength and flexibility than the assessment presented in this chapter. For example, the use of an inclinometer to measure forward, backward, and sidebending (Fig. 31.1; 20, 21), the modified Schober test to measure forward bending (Fig. 31.2; 22), and the measurement of rotation with the client seated (Fig. 31.3), are all more objective methods. I use these more objective measurement methods clinically but choose to use the assessment methods presented in this

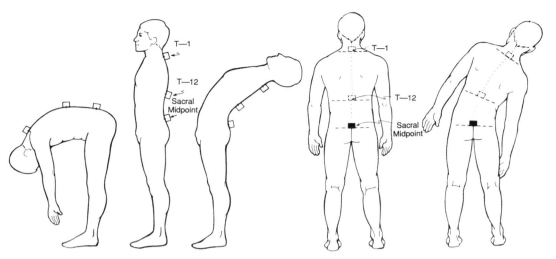

Figure 31.1. Range of motion of flexion, extension, and sidebending of the lumbar and thoracic spine can be calculated by taking inclinometer measurements as shown above.

chapter with industrial clients because they are more efficient and practical to do with groups and because the testing procedures convert easily and quickly to the exercise training that is a part of this program.

I also recognize that, regardless of the specific method of measurement we are using, scientific studies to establish normal standards for the industrial populations we assess are lacking, and that opinion varies as to what consistutes normal and abnormal range of motion and strength. Some opinions are based on scientific studies, while others are based on experience and the particular bias of a practitioner's philosophy. In this assessment program, an effort has been made to objectify acceptable levels of flexibility and strength without becoming too technical.

Figure 31.2. The modified Schober Test measures forward bending flexibility of the back.

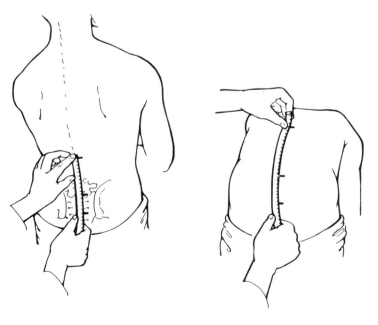

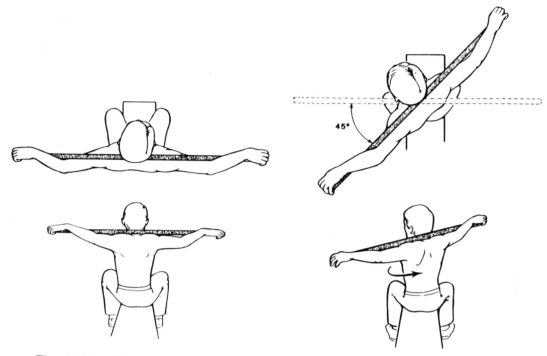

Figure 31.3.   Objective method of measuring rotation range of motion of the thorocolumbar spine.

STRENGTH AND FLEXIBILITY ASSESSMENT *

The following tests are included in the strength and flexibility assessment exam:

Forward Bending Flexibility of the Back

Procedure

1. Client sits on floor with legs extended.
2. Client bends forward as far as possible.

Scoring

1. Low back flattens to neutral = Satisfactory (Fig. 31.4**A**).
2. Very slight lordotic curve remains in low back = Marginal Stiffness (Fig. 31.4**B**).
3. Lordotic curve remains in low back = Unsatisfactory Stiffness (Fig.31.4**C**).
4. Low back flexes into kyphosis = Hyperflexible (Fig. 31.4**D**).

---

*Reprinted with permission from Saunders H. Assessing flexibility and strength in industrial workers. Minneapolis: Educational Opportunities, 1989.

Note: Since this procedure involves both lower back and hip (hamstring) flexibility, it is important for the examiner to assess the quality of the lower back curve rather than the distance the client can reach toward his or her toes. The importance of this test as an assessment of hamstring flexibility is secondary.

In Figure 31.4, each hamstring length is the same. In most cases, inability to touch the toes is due to tight hamstring muscles, not restriction in the lower back. In such a case, the person may not be able to touch toes, but may score satisfactory or even hyperflexible on the back flexion flexibility test (Fig. 31.5; 23).

Backward Bending Flexibility of the Back

Procedure   (similar to push-up)

1. Client lies prone on floor with hands directly under the shoulders.
2. Client lifts the body with arms, letting the lower back "sag."
3. The back and abdominal muscles must remain relaxed.

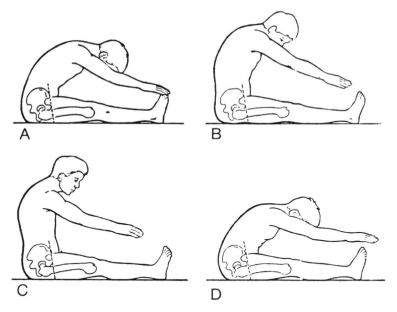

Figure 31.4.   Forward bending flexibility of the back.

4. If the client appears to be hyperflexible, test him or her standing. Measure the angle formed by the thoracic spine with the femur.

Scoring

1. Anterior superior iliac spine (asis) of the pelvis remains within 2 inches of the floor. The thoracic spine should straighten and the lumbar spine should extend. The lower lumbar spine should extend the most = Satisfactory (Fig. 31.6**A**).
2. Asis is 2–4 inches from the floor and the lower back extends slightly = Marginal Stiffness (Fig. 31.6**B**).
3. Asis is 4 or more inches from the floor and considerable limitation of back extension is observed = Unsatisfactory Stiffness (Fig. 31.6**C**).
4. If the angle formed by the thoracic spine with the femur is greater than 70° = Hyperflexible (Fig. 31.6**D**).

Rotation Flexibility of the Back

Procedure

1. Client lies supine with knees and hips bent and the feet on the floor approximately one foot from the buttocks. The knees and feet are held together and the arms are abducted to 90°.
2. Client turns the head one direction as he or she rotates the legs and pelvis in the opposite direction.

3. Examiner should be certain that the client keeps feet and knees together and that the hips and knees to do not extend.
4. Client's shoulders should maintain contact with the floor at all times.

Scoring

1. Knee contacts floor as opposite shoulder maintains contact with floor = Satisfactory (Fig. 31.7**A**).
2. Knee is within 4 inches of floor as opposite shoulder maintains contact with floor = Marginal (Fig. 31.7**B**).
3. Client is unable to get knee to within 4 inches of floor as the opposite shoulder maintains contact with floor = Unsatisfactory (Fig. 31.7**C**).

Note: Hip and pelvis flexibility may affect the results of this test.

Hamstring Muscle Flexibility

Procedure (unilateral straight leg raise)

1. Client lies supine on floor, legs straight.
2. Client raises one leg as far as able, keeping the knee extended.
3. Repeat procedure for the other leg.
4. Low back should remain flat on the floor and the pelvis should not rotate during test.

Scoring (measured in degrees from the floor) Each leg is scored separately.

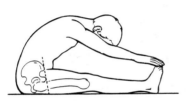

Normal back flexion and hamstring flexibility.

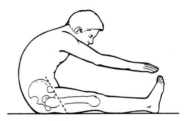

Excessive back flexion and short hamstrings.

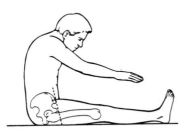

Excessive upper back flexion, limitation of flexion in back and hamstrings.

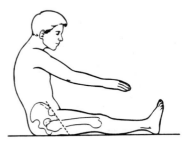

Normal upper back flexion, moderate limitation of back flexion and short hamstrings.

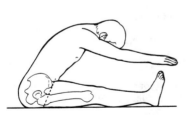

Flexion slightly limited in lower back and excessive length of hamstrings.

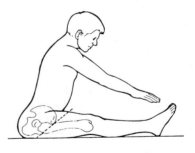

Normal flexion of upper back considerable limitation of lower back flexion and excessive length of hamstrings.

Figure 31.5. Variations in back flexion. (Adapted and reproduced by permission from Kendall R, McCreary E. Muscles: Testing and function. 3rd ed. Baltimore: Williams & Wilkins, © 1983, p. 232.)

1. Able to raise leg 80–110° from floor = Satisfactory (Fig. 31.8**A**).
2. Able to raise leg 60–80° from floor = Marginal Stiffness (Fig. 31.8**B**).
3. Able to raise leg less than 60° from floor = Unsatisfactory Stiffness (Fig. 31.8**C**).
4. Able to raise leg more than 110° from floor = Hyperflexible (Fig. 31.8**D**).

Hip Flexor Muscle Flexibility

Procedure

1. Client lies supine on table with lower leg extending over end of table.

2. Client flexes opposite knee and hip and brings knee toward chest until lower back is flat against table.
3. Repeat procedure for other leg.

Scoring

1. Client's thigh stays on table and knee flexes to at least 80° = Satisfactory (Fig. 31.9**A**).
2. Client's hip flexes no more than 10° off table and knee flexes to at least 70° = Marginal (Fig. 31.9**B**).
3. Client's hip flexes 10° or more off table and/or knee does not flex to at least 70° = Unsatisfactory (Fig. 31.9**C**).

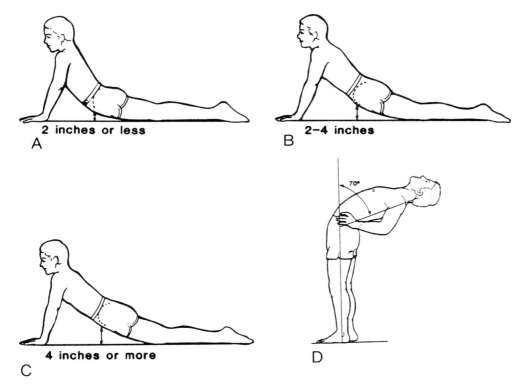

Figure 31.6. Backward bending flexibility of the back.

Note: If the thigh raises off the table, it is an indication of tightness of the iliopsoas muscle. If the knee will not flex fully, it is an indication of tightness of the rectus femoris. If you do not have a table, this test an be done on the floor. If this is the case, however, only the iliopsoas is being tested.

Hip Joint Flexion Flexibility

Procedure

1. Client lies supine on floor with legs straight.
2. Client uses arms to pull one knee and hip toward chest.
3. Low back should remain flat on table and the pelvis should not rotate during this test.
4. Repeat procedure for other leg.

Scoring

1. Client is able to flex hip to at least 125° = Satisfactory (Fig. 31.10A).
2. Client is able to flex hip 115–125° = Marginal (Fig. 31.10B).
3. Client is unable to flex hip to at least 115° = Unsatisfactory (Fig. 31.10C).

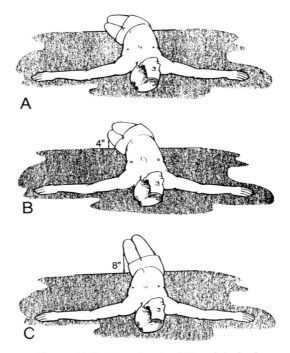

Figure 31.7. Rotation flexibility of the back.

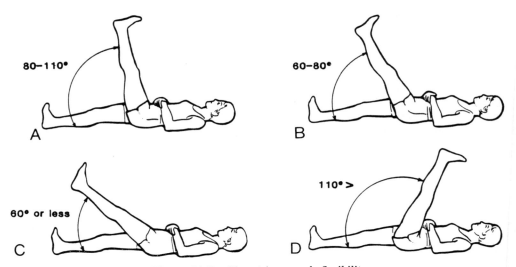

Figure 31.8. Hamstring muscle flexibility.

Figure 31.9. Hip flexor muscle flexibility.

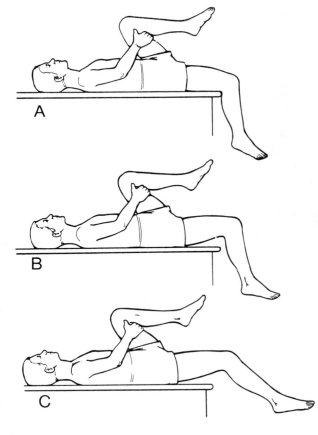

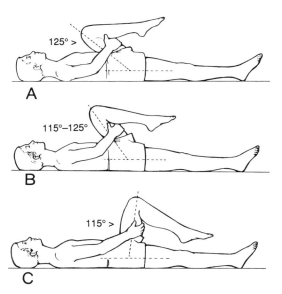

Figure 31.10. Hip joint flexion flexibility.

Squat to Stand Strength and Flexibility

Procedure

1. Client stands with feet 18″ to 24″ apart with one foot slightly ahead of the other.
2. Client squats down until he or she touches the floor with fingertips. Client must do this while maintaining a proper lumbar lordosis, keeping the head, shoulders and back upright.
3. Client rises from the squatting position while maintaining a proper lumbar lordosis; center of gravity must not fall forward.
4. Client repeats the squatting maneuver 10 times, using correct technique.

Scoring

1. Client is able to perform squat technique correctly 10 times = Satisfactory (Fig. 31.11).
2. Client is able to perform squat technique correctly but is unable to perform it 10 times = Marginal.
3. Client is unable to perform squat technique correctly = Unsatisfactory (Fig. 31.12).

Note: Inability to perform the deep squat technique correctly is often due to lack of practice. Marginal or unsatisfactory scores may be due either to lack of practice or to range of motion or strength deficits in any of the lower extremity or lower back muscles or joints. The evaluator must consider the scores of the other tests in this chapter, especially hip flexion mobility, back extension mobility, and quadriceps strength.

Shoulder Girdle and Shoulder Flexion Strength and Flexibility

Procedure

1. Client lies prone with the forehead supported on the floor. The arms are positioned overhead, with the elbows extended. The straight arms are held close to the head.
2. The client grasps stick, hands at shoulder width, elbows straight and raises arms straight up toward the celing as far as possible. The forehead should remain on the floor and the trunk should not move. Wrists remain neutral.

Scoring

1. Able to raise stick 9″ from floor (flexibility) and hold 30 seconds (strength) = Satisfactory (Fig. 31.13A).

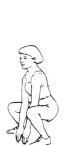
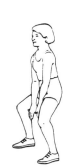
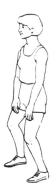
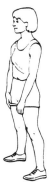

Figure 31.11. Squat-to-stand strength and flexibility.

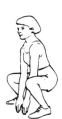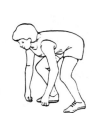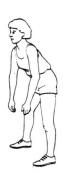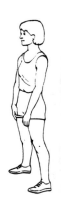

Figure 31.12. Squat-to-stand strength and flexibility.

2. Able to raise stick 6″ to 9″ off floor (flexibility) and hold 30 seconds (strength) = Marginal (Fig. 31.13**B**).
3. Unable to raise stick 6″ off floor (flexibility) and hold 30 seconds (strength) = Unsatisfactory (Fig. 31.13**C**).

Note: Inability to perform this test can be due to either weakness or stiffness. Therefore, if the client cannot raise the stick, the examiner should assist by helping lift the stick. If the client is able to raise the stick with the examiner's assistance, any deficiency is due to muscle weakness, not flexibility. Score the test for both strength and flexibility.

Back and Hip Extension Strength

Procedure

1. Client lies prone on floor with arms overhead.
2. Client lifts chest, arm and legs off floor.
3. Client holds the above position as long as able, for a maximum of 60 seconds.

Scoring

1. Client can hold position for 60 seconds = Satisfactory (Fig. 31.14).
2. Client can assume position, and hold for 30–60 seconds = Marginal.
3. Client cannot hold for 30 seconds = Unsatisfactory.

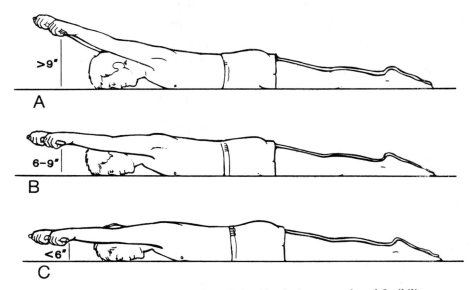

Figure 31.13. Shoulder girdle and shoulder flexion strength and flexibility.

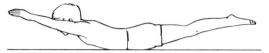

Figure 31.14.   Back and hip extension strength.

Note: Extreme stiffness of back and hip extension may make this test difficult or impossible for a few clients. The examiner should consider the client's back extension flexibility and use the alternate back strength test when necessary.

Back and Hip Extension Strength (Alternate Method)

Procedure

1. Client lies prone in "jack knife" position over edge of table, with examiner holding legs securely against table (Fig. 31.15A).
2. Client raises head, arms and trunk parallel to floor (Fig. 31.15B).
3. Client holds above position as long as able, for a maximum of 60 seconds.

Scoring

1. Client can hold position 60 seconds = Satisfactory.
2. Client can assume position and hold 30 seconds = Marginal.
3. Client cannot hold position correctly for 30 seconds = Unsatisfactory.

Abdominal Strength (Upper)

Procedure

1. Client lies supine with knees and hips bent and feet flat on floor.
2. Client reaches toward knees with arms extended, flexing the neck and trunk. The scapulae rise off the floor, and the trunk is flexed until the lower lumbar spine is off the floor. No lumbar lordosis is allowed except in the case where inability to flex the lumbar spine is due to stiffness.
3. Client repeats above test with a slight twist to the right, touching left fingertips to the outside of the right knee. Client then repeats with a slight twist to the left, touching right fingertips to the outside of the left knee.
4. Client holds each position as long as able, for a maximum of 10 seconds.

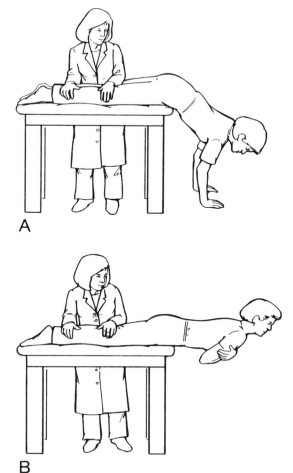

Figure 31.15.   Back and hip extension strength (alternative method).

Scoring

1. Client can hold each of the three positions 10 seconds = Satisfactory (Fig. 31.16A).
2. Client can assume positions but cannot hold for 10 seconds = Marginal.
3. Client cannot assume position correctly = Unsatisfactory. All drawings in Figure 31.16B are examples of incorrect positioning.

Abdominal Strength (Lower)

Procedure

1. Client lies supine with legs held straight up, knees straight.

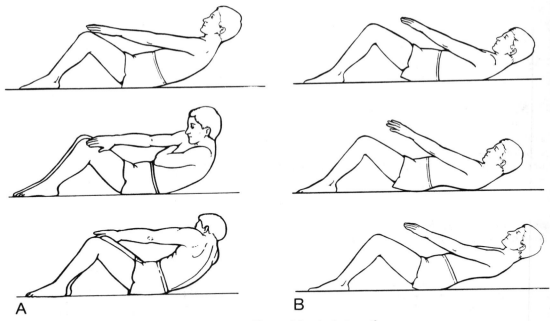

Figure 31.16. Upper abdominal strength.

2. Client flattens lower back against the floor by contracting abdominal muscles (Fig. 31.17).
3. Client bilaterally lowers the legs to within 6″ of the floor, keeping the back flat on the floor.
4. Client holds the above position as long as able, for a maximum of 10 seconds.

Scoring

1. Client can assume and hold position with feet 6″ from the floor for 10 seconds = Satisfactory (Fig. 31.18A).
2. Client can assume and hold position with knees bent to 90° and feet 6″ from the floor for 10 seconds = Marginal (Fig. 31.18B).

3. Client is unable to hold any correct position = Unsatisfactory. All drawings in Figure 31.19 show examples of failure. Note that the lower back must stay flat on the floor to pass.

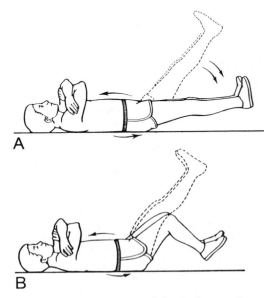

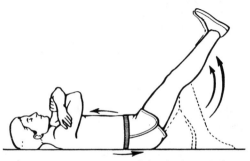

Figure 31.17. Lower abdominal strength.

Figure 31.18. Lower abdominal strength.

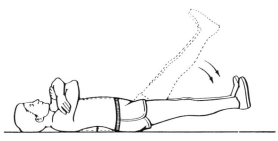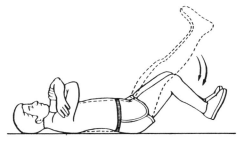

Figure 31.19.   Lower abdominal strength.

Note: Many experts consider that bilateral leg lowering tests the "lower" abdominal muscles, while the partial sit-up tests the "upper" abdominal muscles. While the upper and lower abdominal muscles actually have no anatomical differentiation, the two tests both have merit because the functional origin and insertion of the abdominal musculature is different in each test.

Anterior Thigh Strength

Procedure

1. Client stands with back against wall and feet 12–18″ from wall (Fig. 31.20**A**).

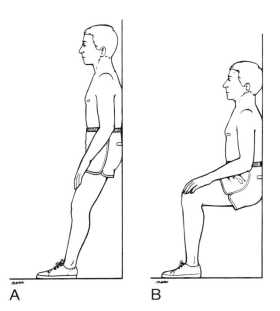

A   B

Figure 31.20.   Anterior thigh strength.

2. Client slides back down the wall by flexing hips and knees until hips and knees are bent to 90° (Fig. 31.20**B**).
3. Client holds the above position as long as able, for a maximum of 60 seconds.

Scoring

1. Able to hold position for at least 60 seconds = Satisfactory.
2. Able to assume position and hold for 30–60 seconds = Marginal.
3. Unable to hold position for 30 seconds or unable to assume position = Unsatisfactory.

When the assessment exam is completed, the examiner should inform the client of the results of the tests and demonstrate and have the client practice exercises to correct the deficiencies found. Clients who have significant deficiencies should be reassessed in 3 to 6 months or should be placed in a controlled corrective exercise program.

Corrective Exercise Programs

Basic rules for the exercises presented here are:

1. Exercises should be done regularly.
2. Always start out mildly and increase gradually.
3. A little discomfort with certain exercises is usually normal, but exercise should not cause pain that lingers after exercising, and exercises for the neck or back should not cause arm or leg pain after one stops.

Ideally, following the assessment exam, clients are shown and given the opportunity to practice the exercises they need to correct any deficiencies found. Clients are then encouraged to exercise 10 to 20 minutes a day, working on the exercises most important for them. This author has found that a certain number of clients will indeed be motivated to exercise on a regular basis and reassessment will show significant improvements in some people. Realistically, however, one certainly cannot expect that all clients will be motivated emough to participate on their own in an ongoing exercise program. Therefore, consideration should be given to establishing on-the-job exercise programs in some form.

On-the-job exercise programs as a component of back injury prevention programs are just beginning to create interest in industry. There are various ways companies can implement on-the-job exercise programs. Interest in establishing programs is often generated in the training sessions or may become a natural extension of the strength and flexibility assessment program.

Many companies start by offering assistance in getting voluntary programs started. In such cases, the company may provide a place to exercise and hire an instructor to organize and lead the exercise sessions. Once a group gets started, participants from the group often volunteer to lead the sessions and the paid instructor is no longer needed. Voluntary exercise classes are usually offered before and/or after working hours or during break times. Exercise classes during the lunch hour are often very popular, and companies sometimes extend break times or the lunch hour a few minutes longer for participants.

Mandatory exercise during work time is attracting some interest at this time. Companies are trying mandatory exercise programs on a limited or experimental basis. If these programs prove to be effective, it is this author's belief that mandatory exercise during working hours will become a popular and effective way to reduce back injuries. The obvious advantage to mandatory exercise is that those who are in poor physical condition and lack motivation to exercise on their own can be required to participate. It is often easier to get these people to participate willingly after they have attended the training sessions and/or gone through the strength and flexibility assessment program.

Perhaps one of the most effective uses of mandatory exercise is to require those who have had previous back problems and/or those who score poorly on strength and flexibility assessment tests to participate in a mandatory exercise program. Mandatory exercise programs

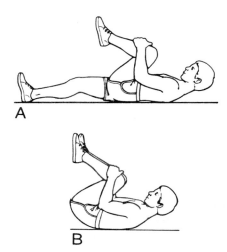

Figure 31.21. Exercises to increase forward bending flexibility.

may prove to be a major step toward solving the back injury dilemma.

On-the-job strength and flexibility exercise programs are offered three to five times per week and require only 10 to 20 minutes for each session.

CORRECTIVE EXERCISE*

Corrective exercises for each of the strength and flexibility tests are as follows:

---

*Reprinted with permission from Saunders H. For your back. Minneapolis: Educational Opportunities, 1990.

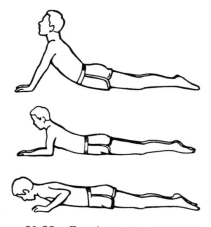

Figure 31.22. Exercises to increase backward bending flexibility.

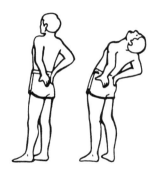

Figure 31.23. Exercises to increase backward bending flexibility.

To Increase Forward Bending Flexibility.

Single knee-to-chest exercises are done alternatively (Fig. 31.21**A**). One should hold 10 to 15 seconds with the knee flexed as close to the chest as possible. The double knee-to-chest exercise is also done with a 5- to 10-second hold (Fig. 31.21**B**). One should do 10 to 15 of each of these as often as necessary to keep the back flexible.

To Increase Backward Bending Flexibility. The press-up exercise is done by pushing up with the arms while the back and abdominal muscles are relaxed. This causes a passive stretch on the low back (Fig. 31.22). The backward bending stretch is also done standing (Fig. 31.23). These exercises should be done 5 to 10 times each occasionally throughout the day, especially after one has been sitting or forward bending and lifting.

To Increase Rotation Flexibility. If one flexes the hips and knees and brings the thighs toward the chest when doing the rotation flexibility exercises, the mid-back area will stretch (Fig. 31.24**A**). If the knees and hips are bent with the feet on the floor, the stretch is more effective for the lower back area (Fig. 31.24**B**). If one leg is raised straight overhead or crossed over the other when doing the rotation exercise, it is a more advanced stretch. Note that the head is rotated to the opposite direction with all of these exercises (Fig. 31.24**C**). Hold each stretch 10 to 15 seconds.

To Increase Hamstring Flexibility. The hamstring stretch is done as shown in Fig. 31.25. Simply hold the leg extended as straight as possible for 5 to 10 seconds. Repeat the exercise 5 to 10 times, 1 or 2 sessions per day.

To Increase Hip Flexor Flexibility. Tight hip flexors can be stretched by using the methods shown in Figure 31.26. Hold each stretched position for several seconds, making sure the lower back is as flat as possible. Repeat this exercise several times a day.

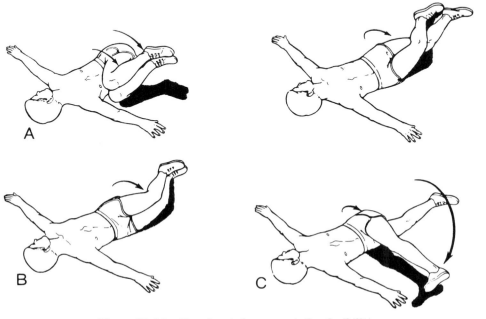

Figure 31.24. Exercises to increase rotation flexibility.

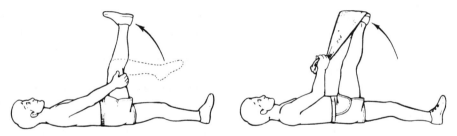

Figure 31.25. Exercises to increase hamstring flexibility.

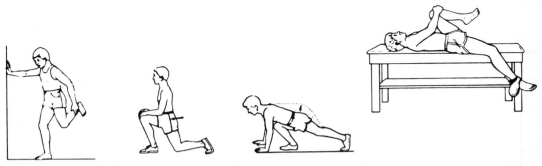

Figure 31.26. Exercises to increase hip flexor flexibility.

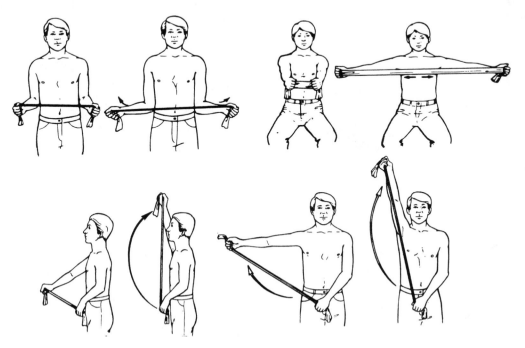

Figure 31.27. Exercises to strengthen the upper back and shoulders.

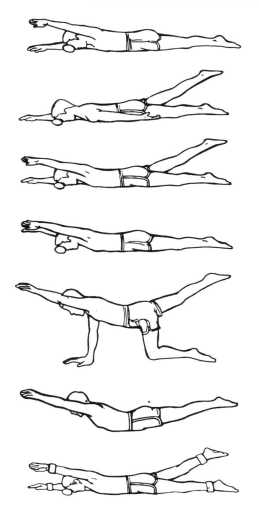

Figure 31.28. Exercises to increase back and shoulder girdle flexibility and to strengthen the back, shoulder girdle, and hip extensor muscles.

To Stregthen the Upper Back and Shoulders. Strengthening exercises for forward head, slumped sitting, and round shoulder posture and/or weakness of the muscles in the neck, upper back, and shoulders are shown in Figure 31.27. These exercises should be done once or twice daily, starting with a few of each and gradually increasing the number as tolerated.

To Increase Back and Shoulder Girdle Flexibility and to Strengthen the Back, Shoulder Girdle, and Hip Extensor Muscles. These exercises should be started gradually and done once or twice a day. Small ankle and wrist weights can be added to make these exercises more advanced (Fig. 31.28).

To Strengthen the Abdominal Muscles. The pelvic tilt is done by tightening the abdominal muscles and the buttock muscles at the same time. This pulls the pelvis up and forward in the front and down and backward in the back (Fig. 31.29). Partial sit-ups are done correctly with the hips and knees slightly bent. One should raise the arms, head, and shoulders off the floor as shown in Figure 31.30A. The position is held for 5 to 10 seconds. One should never rise until the lower back is lifted from the floor. This causes too much pressure on the disc and is unnecessary for abdominal muscle strengthening. The feet should not be stabilized; stabilizing the feet will allow the hip flexor muscles to do the work, resulting in the opposite effect desired from this exercise. It is important that the pelvis be tilted in order to keep the lower back flat on the floor throughout the exercise.

The partial sit-up should be done with a slight right and left twist to strengthen the oblique muscles of the abdomen (Fig. 31.30**B**). Strengthening exercises such as this should be started mildly and gradually increased in number as the muscles get stronger. They should be done once or twice a day.

To Strengthen the Lower Abdominals. The double straight-leg raise is done correctly by first doing a pelvic tilt to press the lower back against the floor, then raising the legs a few inches and holding 5 to 10 seconds (Fig. 31.31A). If the lower back can't be held against the floor as the legs are raised, the abdominal muscles are weak and this exercise

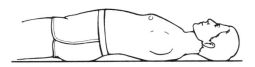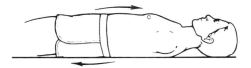

Figure 31.29. Exercises to strengthen the upper abdominal muscles.

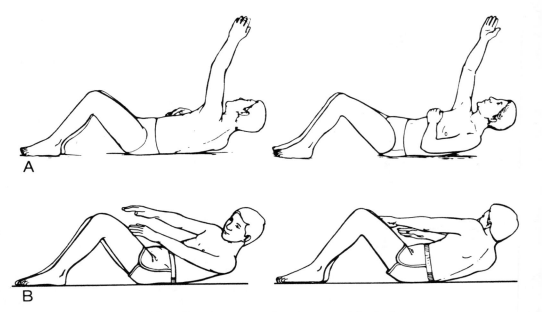

Figure 31.30. Exercise to strengthen the upper abdominal muscles.

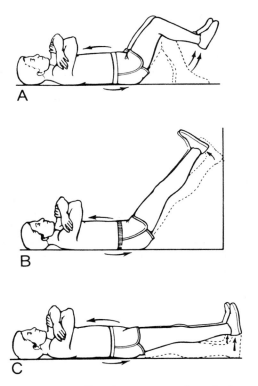

should be started with the knees bent or with the feet against the wall as shown in Figure 31.31**B.** As you become stronger, gradually advance toward the flat double straight-leg raise, which is the most advanced way to do this exercise (Fig. 31.31**C**).

To Strengthen Quadriceps. To strengthen the quadriceps muscles, stand with feet together approximately 18" from the wall (Fig. 31.32**A**), lean against the wall and slide the back down the wall until hips and knees are bent (Fig. 31.32**B**). Hold this position for 15 to 30 seconds. As you become stronger, slide further until the hips and knees are at 90° angles (Fig. 31.32**C**). As you become stronger, the hold time can also be increased.

Figure 31.31. Exercises to strengthen the lower abdominal muscles.

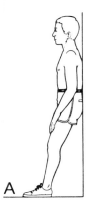 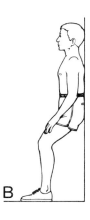 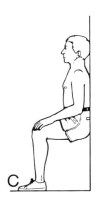

A   B   C

Figure 31.2. The modified Schober Test measures forward bending flexibility of the back.

References

1. Snook S. Approaches to the control of back pain in industry: Job design, job placement and education training. Professional Safety 1988; 33:23–31.
2. Cady L et al. Program for increasing health and physical fitness of firefighters. J Occup Med 1985; 27:111–114.
3. Palmer B. Firms try to crack back problems. USA Today, July 22, 1985.
4. Owen B. Posture, exercise can help prevent low back injuries. Occup Health Safety 1986; 55:33–37.
5. Morris A. Program compliance key to preventing low back injuries. Occup Health Safety 1984; 53:44–47.
6. Greenwood J. Back injuries can be reduced with worker training reinforcement. Occup Health Safety 1986; 55:26–29.
7. Melton B. Back injury prevention means education. Occup Health Safety 1983; 52:20–23.
8. Seater S. PT emerging as a partner in the corporate fight to contain health care costs. Phys Ther For 1986; 5:1–4.
9. Badger D. Wellness meets corporate America. Progress Report-APTA, July–August 1985.
10. Lepore B et al. The dollars and sense of occupational back injury. Clin Man 1984; 4:38–41.
11. Fitzler S, Berger R. Attitudinal change: The Chelsea back program. Occup Health Safety 1982; 51:24–26.
12. Fitzler S, Berger R. Chelsea back program: One year later. Occup Health Safety 1983; 52:52–54.
13. Kirkaldy-Willis W. Managing low back pain. 2nd ed. New York: Churchill Livingstone, 1988.
14. Cady L et al. Strength and fitness and subsequent back injuries in firefighters. J Occup Med 1979; 21:269–272.
15. Biering-Sorensen F. Physical measurements as risk indicators for low back trouble over a one-year period. Spine 1984; 9:106–119.
16. Kobasa S et al. Effectiveness of hardiness, exercise and social support as resources against illness. J Psychosom Res 1985; 29:525–533.
17. Chaffin D. Human strength capability and low back pain. Occup Med 1974; 16:248–254.
18. Anderson G. Epidemiologic aspects of low back pain in industry. Spine 1981; 6:53–58.
19. Anderson C. Pre-placement screening: Survival of the fittest RISK management 1987; 44–46.
20. Engelberg A. Guides to the evaluation of permanent impairment. 3rd ed. Chicago: AMA, 1988.
21. Mayer T, Gatchel R. Functional restoration for spinal disorders: The sports medicine approach. Philadelphia: Lea and Febiger, 1988.
22. Macrae I, Wright V. Measurement of back movement. Ann Rheum Dis 1969; 28:584–589.
23. Kendall R, McCreary E. Muscles: Testing and function. 3rd ed. Baltimore: Williams & Wilkins, 1983.

Section VIII:

RECONDITIONING THE INJURED WORKER

32

MANAGEMENT OF THE PATIENT WITH ACUTE INJURY

Robert D. Mootz

This chapter will consider a number of topics, beginning with a discussion of what constitutes an acute patient. A brief review of connective tissue repair and the influence of mobility on that process follows. The discussion continues with a description of potential pain sources in the low back and a presentation of diagnostic strategies that can be employed by the clinician to effect a higher likelihood of treatment success. Finally a management chronology is provided for the kinds of procedures that should be implemented during the first few weeks of care for acute back patients.

UNDERSTANDING "ACUTE"

It is often said that the acute low back injury is to the practitioner of conservative spinal care what the myocardial infarction is to the cardiologist. Although it is rarely life threatening, few other acquired conditions are so potentially disruptive of so many lives as significant back injury. The social and financial consequences of industrial back injuries have been well documented (1–3). Of greatest concern to the practicing doctor however, is what to do when the acute low back attack strikes. Numerous authors have defined "acute" chronologically, as ranging from 1 to 8 weeks (4–6). Within this time frame it is quite possible to determine the effectiveness of the conservative regimen. However, certain conditions and perpetuating circumstances may require clinical attention beyond this time frame.

Acute low back pain may develop with or without an apparent causative event. The repetitive postural activities of daily living and typical occupations lead many to the development of chronically deconditioned spines without an identifiable triggering traumatic episode. Physicians frequently hear a complaint like "I only bent over to pick up a pencil." Figure 32.1 illustrates the sequelae of both etiologies in the development of back pain.

An understanding of the mechanisms of injury, along with an appreciation of the nature of connective tissue damage and repair, can assist the clinician in appropriate management of an acute injury to the thoracolumbar spine, pelvic girdle, and their supporting structures. As with any injury to a joint and/or its associated soft tissues, trauma to the low back has the likely effect of causing tearing of muscle, tendon, ligament and other myofascial elements, leading to hemorrhage, edema, inflammatory reactions, and the subsequent cascade of tissue regeneration processes.

A complicating aspect of trauma to the spinal column and adjacent structures is that the location where the patient feels the pain, paresthesia, or weakness may be unrelated to the location of the injured tissue or system responsible for its creation. This can be explained by the variety of radicular, scleratomal, and musculotendinous radiation patterns that are associated with the lumbar spine. It is essential for the clinician to make detailed historical note of the exact mechanism of a problem's onset. The biomechanics of injury may provide insight into which tissues have been compromised.

Acute LBP onsets and sequelae

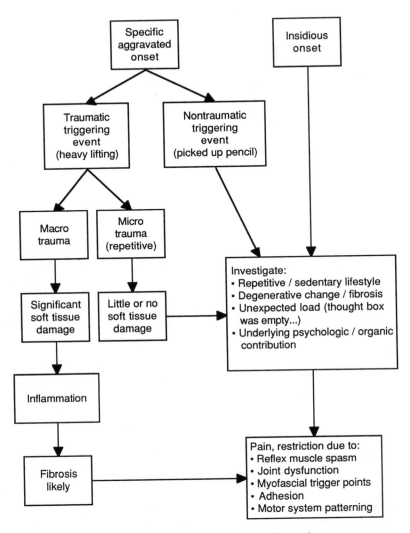

Figure 32.1. Acute LBP onsets and sequelae.

In like manner, the patient who presents with an insidious onset warrants an in-depth investigation into the nature of any previous episodes, occupational behaviors, lifestyle patterns (e.g., exercise, postural and resting habits) and other health historical data. This, followed by careful clinical and mechanical assessment, will yield the best possible treatment options. Despite the urgency of finding relief for the patient, providing no more than first aid, analgesia and rest only delay appropriate care. Rehabilitation and education are necessary to ensure proper healing and to minimize the chances for subsequent occurrences.

When patients experience their first episode of back pain, the doctor has an unique opportunity to initiate a treatment program and the training that is most likely to prevent or minimize recurrences. This kind of education is best begun while the patient is still experiencing discomfort, because those who do not hurt often do not comply with extensive lifestyle modification. Compliance in the long term seems to be a bit easier to achieve in those who have experienced multiple previous episodes. These people may be more psychologically prepared to make the commitment required for an effective rehabilitation program.

Symptomatology in acute back patients is usually self-limiting (7–9). The doctor's or therapist's role, therefore, is to maximize the efficiency and speed of recovery, enhance the quality of life during the process, and educate the patient on how to prevent future occurrences.

Although it is essential that the clinician be as specific and accurate as possible in assessing the causative elements and precise tissues affected in acute back pain, the realities of practice unfortunately still require a certain degree of diagnosis by means of a conservative therapeutic trial. A few weeks of appropriately applied conservative care is likely to be more cost effective in the majority of patients than thousands of dollars spent for CT and MRI imaging, electrodiagnostics, and a workup by a team of specialists to help ensure an accurate and specific diagnosis. High-priced and high-technology procedures become valuable for the refractory patient and for those whose clinical presentation suggests severe, organic, and/or psychogenic complicating factors.

CONNECTIVE TISSUE DAMAGE AND REPAIR

The Inflammatory Process

Damage to connective tissue is implied by definition in the diagnosis of sprain and strain. Although this is perhaps the single most misused diagnosis in low back pain syndromes, when lumbar loading is severe and rapid enough, tissue rupture may occur to various myofascial elements, particularly the periosteal attachments of tendons and ligaments. In the chronic state, this is often observed radiographically as a traction spur. But in the acute scenario, soft tissue inflammation may result.

The inflammatory response has several complex aspects. Once tissue is damaged or irritated, three general kinds of reactions take place. All tend to be interrelated and influenced by the others.

1. Hemodynamic and permeability changes lead to altered fluid exchange, which promotes edema.
2. White blood cells go through various metabolic changes that increase their activity in preparation for phagocytosis of tissue and inflammatory debris.
3. Numerous chemical mediators sustain and modify the inflammatory process over time.

Figure 32.2 illustrates key general elements in the inflammatory process.

The initial chemical mediators of inflammation are of three kinds. Histamine and serotonin are vasoactive amines and tend to increase tissue permeability, dilate the smaller vascular elements (initially the arterioles and venules and later the capillary beds), and constrict the larger veins (10). A number of plasma proteases are also instrumental in sustaining and altering vascular and capillary permeability, leukocyte chemotaxis (attraction of white cell to injured tissues), and antibody stimulation. The kinin compounds, another of the plasma proteases, contribute to increased pain sensation as well as initiate arteriole dilation and are thought to encourage margination of leukocytes in the area (11). Arachidonic acid metabolites are another group of substrates. These compounds are fatty acids that include prostaglandins and leukotrienes. They are though to be involved in a number of body processes and are the topic of much research (10). They too contribute to hemodynamics, vascular permeability, and leukocyte activity.

Soon after tissue injury, the damaged region becomes hypersensitive and edematous. Immediate swelling suggests the probability of significant hemorrhage. Swelling in and of itself distorts tissue and interplanar contours. In addition to the chemical mediation of inflammatory pain, swelling may stretch tissue mechanoreceptors leading to altered proprioception, reflex muscle splinting, and pain. This gradual development of the inflammatory process may contribute to a delay in the onset of symptoms. This matches the common clinical presentation of a patient waking up with pain on the day after a seemingly nonproblematic activity or injury.

With the extracellular accumulation of inflammatory exudate and blood, cellular debris of RBC breakdown releases hemoglobin. Platelets release thrombin, which converts fibrinogen into fibrin. Eventually, organization into collagenous scar tissue takes place, which manifests clinically as the interplanar adhesions of myofibrosis (10).

The resultant decrease in fascial plane mobility and developing joint restrictions may sig-

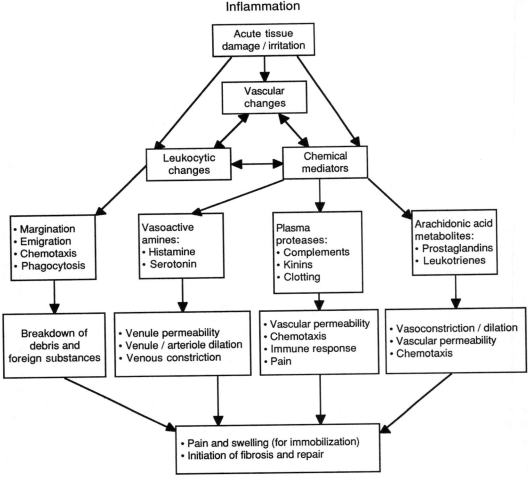

Figure 32.2.   Inflammation.

nificantly prolong recovery and/or predispose the affected area to future injury as well as contribute to a persistent functional limitation. Appropriate and timely rehabilitation can therefore be important in even relatively minor acute low back conditions.

Tissue Regeneration

Ongoing regeneration of tissue cells occurs in the labile epithelium, such as that of damaged blood vessels. The more stable mesenchymal and parenchymal cells, which are normally dormant, begin regenerative activity following injury, as when fibroblasts, chondroblasts, and osteoblasts become active (10). Various glandular cells also are stimulated into mitosis.

Lymph glands may be damaged as well in some injuries, but the labile lymph vessel epithelium, rather than actual glandular tissue, is more likely to be damaged in sprain/strain injuries. Other permanent tissues, such as nerves, will not replicate. However, the axons of nerve fibers may repair completely, provided injury does not exceed Sunderland's (12) stage 2 axonotmesis, in which the axons are compressed without complete trunk impairment. More severely damaged nerves may recover, but usually with residual deficits.

The regenerative process is most active during the first 3 weeks following injury (13). An appropriate balance of activity and immobilization should be applied to maximize muscle and connective tissue healing so that newly regenerated elements will be mechanically functional and strong enough to handle the return to previous levels of tension. Specific therapeutic guidelines are suggested in the section on chronologic management protocols. It is generally accepted that damaged muscle fibers can regenerate (14–16). Although granulation tissue develops faster with immobilization, prolonged inactivity contributes to poor scar organization and weaker muscle tissue (16). Regeneration with mobilization has been shown to speed the resorption of hematoma and cellular debris. Tension applied to healing muscle tissue has also been shown to result in a faster and stronger recovery (14, 15).

EFFECTS OF IMMOBILITY ON JOINT AND SOFT TISSUE

Immobilization of synovial joints and supporting tissues leads to other kinds of tissue restrictions. Various investigators have demonstrated that extensibility of connective tissue is due to the infusion of water between proteoglycan molecules that hold the fibers apart (17, 18). The presence of water molecules tends to arrange the fibers in a more parallel configuration, which allows more stretch and pliability of the tissue. With prolonged immobilization, the proteoglycan molecules release water, allowing the molecular strands to move closer together, thereby developing adhesive cross-linkages (19, 20). As a further complication to normal function, fatty adhesions may develop within synovial joints, adhering to joint cartilage (21).

When initial inflammation leads to pain and guarding postures, the body's natural response is to immobilize. New collagen deposition resulting from tissue trauma superimposed on the restrictions incurred from immobilization can initiate and sustain a vicious clinical cycle. The injured patient will voluntarily and subconsciously restrict activity. This in turn promotes disorganized fibrosis, dehydration restrictions, and possible joint dysfunction. Tissues so influenced can become painful upon use, thereby encouraging further immobilization. Despite intuition to the contrary, early activity (within days of the instigating trauma) should be initiated unless more serious complications are evident.

The passive therapies—those done by the practitioner—may encourage needed tissue movement and allow the patient to function with reduced discomfort. Faster, more appropriate healing is promoted. Frequently employed passive therapies include chiropractic adjustive approaches, manipulation and mobilization, soft tissue techniques, and passive stretch. Although passive therapies often provide rapid palliation and improved mobility, the doctor must avoid treatment dependency. Early involvement of the patient in the rehabilitation proceess, even with minimum actual mechanical benefit, will set the psychologic stage for the self-care and conditioning that is essential for long-term rehabilitation and education. Clinical experience suggests that going beyond a week or two without specific directed patient involvement may evolve into therapeutic dependancy that only becomes more difficult to escape from as time goes on.

POTENTIAL SOURCES OF PAIN IN LOW BACK INJURIES

Diagnosing pathoanatomic lesions in back pain can be a frustrating clinical experience. Patients' backs have not read the clinical textbooks or the insurance industry's Diagnostic Related Groupings (DRGs). Despite the more than 150 diagnostic entities the doctor has to choose from, only a small precentage of examinations yield a specific anatomic diagnosis (22). Still, there are numerous potential pain sources in the lower back, and an appreciation of them can help the clinician select the best route of care early on.

Complex Conditions: Organic

Perhaps the first thing the doctor must clarify is whether an acute episode of low back pain is actually referred from an organic pathology. Some of the more complex or life-threatening problems that must be ruled out include abdominal aortic or femoral aneurysms, spinal canal space occupying lesions, renal disease, hepatic and gallbladder disease, and referral from other abdominal viscera. A thorough history and physical examination must be a part of any acute low back work-up. The leading clue to an underlying nonmechanical pain source is the inability to exacerbate the symptomatology by mechanical means. If no rational explanation of the problem is forthcoming, specialist consults are in order right away.

Complex Conditions: Pathomechanical

In the pathomechanical domain, a minority of acute low back complaints stem from the more problematic conditions. These shall be defined as those kinds of mechanical low back problems that can be potentially aggravated during one or more phases of an aggressive conservative rehabilitation protocol. Figure 32.3 identifies mechanical sources of back pain and differentiates those tissues that are likely to produce pain.

The richly innervated periosteum is frequently damaged. At one extreme, a frank rupture or fracture can result from spinal trauma, but this is a more frequent suspicion in cervical spine injuries than in the low back (23). However, microevulsion may be present in a significant number of acute back pain patients who report traumatic triggering events. This condition is identifiable clinically by extremely localized tenderness to palpation at tendonous attachment sites. When present, this will slowly progress and require caution for 2 to 4 weeks in the application of muscle tension. Repetitive microtrauma may eventually become evident indirectly with the appearance on x-ray of a traction spur. Like so many structural alterations seen on x-rays, traction spurs in and of

themselves may not be a source of pain but, if the mechanics of onset suggest trauma or traction to a region with spurring, this region may be acutely inflamed and will need to be included in the differential diagnosis. Pars and transverse process fractures (24) are perhaps the most common complete fractures in the lumbar spine. Their management involves initial immobilization and support. Soft tissue trauma is a concurrent concern. Provided that such fractures are stable, they may be managed similarly to other connective tissue strains and sprains. Since separations of this type are either not weight bearing, or are under mechanical distraction, they usually heal as pseudoarticulations.

Disc herniation is frequently found in acute low back patients. Like sprain and strain, this term is often misused. Intervertebral disc bulges, herniations, and extrusions are space occupying lesions that may produce pain by noxious irritation, by mechanical distortion of anular nerve endings (25, 26), or by mass effects in the spinal canal (27). Disc bulging is also commonly identified in asymptomatic patients. One needs to have clinical corroboration with radicular involvement before accepting this differential as causative. Numerous texts are available that outline clinical diagnostic indi-

1. **Complicating conditions:** seen in a minority of patients.
   - fracture
   - disc herniation (anular tear, endplate fracture, disc extrusion)
   - dislocations

2. **Soft tissues contributing to pain:** seen in the majority of patients.
   - muscle and tendon tears
   - ligament tears
   - periosteal evulsion
   - fascial tears
   - vascular inflammation and ischemia
   - edema causing stretch of mechanoreceptors
   - muscle spasm and myofascial trigger points
   - altered structural mechanics (joint dysfunction)

3. **Tissues likely to be pain sources** (in order of most to least sensitive)
   - periosteum, ligament, joint capsule, tendon, fascia, bursa, muscle
   - **Note** peripheral nerves and the autonomic system are not likely to be direct sources of pain.

Figure 32.3. Mechanical sources of back pain.

cators for this syndrome (28, 29). More information is presented in chapters 11, 21, and 22 as well.

In addition to disc extrusion and anular tear, endplate fracture from compressive excesses may need to be considered. The clues here are a history that reveals compressive trauma (e.g., in the extreme case, involving onset following skydiving). Endplate fractures are frequently difficult to assess radiographically but are readily suspected in vertebral compressions. Loss of the vertebral body's vertical trabeculation pattern is the most likely radiographic finding. The pain from this may be related to that typically associated with bone trauma and often presents with a characteristic deep ache that is minimally affected mechanically (as compared to an inflamed facet or posterior disc bulge).

Posterior joint dislocation is rare in the lumbar spine and usually requires a severe enough trauma to have created an acute injury that would more appropriately be seen in the emergency room. Like vertebral fracture, dislocations are a more likely differential in cervical spine traumas, where it is not unheard of for a patient to present to a conservative practitioner (23).

All of the conditions mentioned to this point may tend to require longer periods of immobilization and, in certain situations, warrant orthopaedic or neurologic consultation. All of them also are likely to progress to mechanical back syndromes and can be helped by conservative care and education. Traumatized tissue is more prone to degenerative change and fibrosis. Many of these patients may be spared more lengthy and costly programs down the road if management includes early appraisal and treatment by a chiropractor or other neuromusculoskeletal specialist.

Joint Dysfunction Myofascitis, and Myospasm

By far the majority of acute episodes of low back pain will be related to soft tissue conditions and motion segment dysfunctions. These are termed mechanical back problems and, when acute, are readily amenable to a conservative approach. The more chronic problems are often slower to respond or may even become refractory. Although the precise role spinal adjusting or manipulation plays in chronic conditions is not yet as quantified as it is in acute problems, some think manipulation may be valuable if applied intensely at the onset of care (30). Management options in chronic care are discussed in more depth in chapters 3, 9, 11, 26.

CLINICAL ASSESSMENT OF THE ACUTE RESPONSIVE MECHANICAL LOW BACK PATIENT

The skills required for this assessment and conservative management of back pain patients are many. Because of the anatomic proximity of varied specialized tissues, low back pain and spasm are usually due to multiple etiologies. This complicates and confounds efforts to diagnose and care for people with this condition. Development of appropriate clinical skills requires observation, discussion and hands-on practice. Much of the empirical chiropractic clinical knowledge has come from the course work of practitioners and educators such as Drs. Richard Stonebrink, James Cox, Henri Gillette, Raymond Sandoz, and Joseph Janse. The osteopathic and manual medicine fields have had mentors as well. Drs. John Mennell, Phillip Greenman, Stanley Paris, and James Cyriax have provided guidance and inspiration in nonsurgical manual care over the years. Their collective experience and educational efforts have contributed much to the way conservative manual care is practiced today.

History

Previous sections have emphasized the importance a detailed clinical history and complete physical examination play in addressing the acute low back pain patient. Common objectives of thorough history taking for mechanical back problems include detailing the chronology of symptom onset and progression. Previous occurrences, provoking factors of the current and past episodes and, particularly, the kinds of repetitive postural activities the patient must endure frequently set the stage for pursuit of pertinent examination clues. Other useful historical information is what past treatment (self-provided as well as clinically sought) has provided relief.

Understanding and detailing the nature and character of the pain will also yield vital information. The goal of mechanical assessment is to differentiate between various origins of pain:

viscerogenic, psychogenic, radicular, myogenic, and sclerogenic. Viscerogenic pain often follows predictable referral patterns and is not mechanically exacerbated. It is often achy and unremitting, with little or no relief with rest. Any general or internal medicine text will provide details of specific renal, cardiac, gallbladder, and intestinal referral patterns.

In similar fashion, the role of the central nervous system, learned behaviors, and emotional make-up may also contribute psychological overlays in back pain patients. These factors can become particularly significant with chronic pain.

Pain of radicular origin usually has an electrical or shooting character. On examination, it is readily reproduced by spinal movements that stretch or compress the offending root and the pain or paresthesia tends to reproducibly follow dermatomal distribution. Nerve entrapments outside the spine refer along the distribution of the involved nerve, often crossing over dermatomes. Myogenic pain is characteristically achy and often presents in radiation patterns that follow anatomic musculotendinous distributions (31). It may be exacerbated by use of the involved muscle and can range in intensity from very mild to excruciating.

Sclerogenic pain is another great imposter in musculoskeletal disorders. It is similar to visceral referral in that the site of pain is not necessarily the source of pain. The pattern of radiation tends to follow somatosomatic reflex distributions. The puzzling aspect of this kind of radiation is that it frequently resembles visceral referral rather than radicular or musulotendinous distributions. Likewise, it may not be exacerbated by mechanical means in the local region of referral. However, mechanical exacerbation can usually be elicited at the source of the aberrant reflex. Fortunately for the clinician, the source is frequently painful itself.

Thoracolumbar syndrome can serve as an example. This may present as back pain in the region of the sacroiliac joint and pelvic crest. It is thought to originate from facetal irritation in the thoracolumbar spine that is perceived as pain from cluneal nerve distribution (32). It is unresponsive to therapy localized to the lower lumbar and pelvic region. However, manipulation applied to the thoracolumbar junction has been reported to alleviate the problem (33). Pain can be exacerbated by mechanical stress to the thoracolumbar facets (33). Sclerodermal

referral syndromes can frustrate patient and physician alike and illustrate the need for a thorough mechanical assessment of areas that may not be initially perceived as a problem source. The nature and specific biomechanics of onset provide the best clues of which regions to investigate.

An often neglected but vital aspect of history taking is the doctor-patient bonding that occurs. The history should never entail only questionnaire or assistant-obtained data. The treating physician must develop an understanding of the person he or she is to be working with, and the patient must be comfortable with the doctor or therapist. The conservative therapies, particularly the passive ones, involve much hands-on contact and conscious interaction. Rarely, if ever, are present the barriers of sterility and anesthesia that permit purely analytical and technical therapeusis. The clinical intuition afforded by understanding the kind of person a patient is often provides the doctor with the means of investing the patient in his or her own treatment plan. This may very well be a part of the process needed to achieve high patient satisfaction (34). Too often, clinical teaching assumes that the value of this encounter is to gain the doctor insight to the psychology of the patient (35). We must never forget that, more importantly, this is the time the patient gains psychological insight about the doctor.

Mechanical Assessment

The first step in any mechanical assessment involves observation of the patient in function. Guarding postures, gait, asymmetries, deformities, and tissue contours can all be suggestive of various mechanical myofascial dysfunctions. Static and motion palpation also can reveal characteristics of tissue texture, contractility, tenderness, joint function, swelling, and thermal alterations. This encounter may be the first time the clinician "invades" the patient's personal space. It is important that doctors be sensitive to this, particularly with the acute and painful injuries. The well-trained practitioner will use broad, gentle but secure contacts that convey sensitivity, security, and confidence. There is no place for rushed, jabby examinations in musculoskeletal pain patients. Awareness of the altered facial expression, involuntary muscle contraction, or altered breathing pattern can convey just as much clinical insight as the verbal response or recoil from pain. Do not forget that cessation of palpation and return to neutral position are often as uncomfortable or more painful than the initial contacts. Move slowly and securely.

Cyriax teaches the importance of making sure mechanical reproduction of pain causes the exact kind of pain the patient complains of (38). Careful application of mechanical tension in different directions to particular tissues will help delineate the anatomic site of the lesion. Active movement on the part of the patient requres involvement of both contractile and noncontractile soft tissue elements. Therefore, pain on active movement may be due to injury in either type of tissue. Pain on passive motion, minimizing the role played by the contractile muscles and their tendons, suggests the pain source is a joint or ligament. Pain on both active and opposing passive movements implicates muscle, tendon, and periosteal attachments. More confirmatory will be resisted contraction. One must also consider the mechanical stresses such movement places on tissues in the anatomic proximity. Inflamed bursas, evulsions, frank bony fractures, irritated vascular and lymphatic elements, as well as soft tissue cysts or abscesses may also produce pain under stress.

The specifics and exact nature of soft tissue and joint diagnoses are the province of well-trained chiropractic doctors, orthopaedic physical therapists and other neuromusculoskeletal specialists and are beyond the scope of an introductory text such as this. Like the skills and tools of the surgeon, extensive evaluation for and implementation of the passive therapies are best left to those with extensive training and experience. Iatrogenic complications from inappropriately applied passive therapies such as spinal manipulation are rare but are more common in the hands of the untrained or weekend seminar crowd than those with the years of training and residency required of chiropractors, manipulative specialists in osteopathy, physical therapy, and other specialists (36).

CHRONOLOGIC MANAGEMENT GUIDELINES

In the acute patient with a mechanical etiology, a conservative management protocol can be very helpful. Each patient may present with a different degree of inflammation, tissue injury,

muscle spasm, joint dysfunction, and pain. Tailoring the appropriate care to the needs of the patient is the challenge of the clinical art. The following guidelines will serve as that only and should not be construed to be a "recipe" for all acute low backs. Agian, it must be emphasized that nonmechanical (organic) and more complex conditions must be ruled out and managed accordingly.

Obviously, the kinds of conservative care, exercises, and particular supports utilized will depend on the nature of the problem and the particular tissues thought to be responsible. Following the initial work-up and implementation of a given conservative care regimen, there are some basic common home care protocols that acute mechanical back pain patients should follow in the first few days. These are discussed below and summarized in Figure 32.4. Guidelines for care during the first several weeks follow and are outlined in Figure 32.5.

Initial General Care and Home Instructions: The First 1–5 Days

The objective of the first phase of care in acute back patients is to decrease any inflammation that might be present, allow time for the necessary diagnostic tests to rule out serious complications, and provide the patient with initial education about expectations with back pain and various treatment options. During this time, brief periods of rest and immobilization interspersed with mild amounts of low stress activity are quite beneficial. Nonsteroidal anti-inflammatory medications may be useful in some patients if local application of cryotherapy is inadequate. The duration of this phase depends on the severity of any initiating trauma and the degree of muscle spasm and joint dysfunction present. If the condition is relieved with rest, this should be a clue to permit that for a day or two.

Helping the patient find a comfortable spine and pelvic position is usually an important first step. Pillows and rolled up towels are good, cheap home care items that can be used by the patient to determine the right amount of lordosis needed to minimize discomfort. Unlike more expensive premade support cushions, these common, easily modifiable items allow considerable flexibility for the patient initially. As the condition changes over time, the need for

1. **Minimize excessive inflammation pain**
   - Cryotherapy
   - Analgesic balms
   - Nonsteroidal anti-inflammatory medication
   (If local cryotherapy is inadequate)

2. **Brief period of immobilization**
   - Rest
   - Simple postural support (pillows, rolled-up towels, elastic supports, etc.)

3. **Acute back education**
   - Common activities: sitting/standing, head and arm movement, driving, pelvic tilt, gradual and repeated initiation of body movements
   - Use of chairs and beds
   - Avoid startled wake-ups/movements
   - Morning "warm-up" walks

Figure 32.4.   Initial general care and home instructions for 1 to 5 days.

replacing cushions when they "aren't comfortable anymore" is minimized. As a patient becomes more stable, the better made, longer lasting professional support cushions may be more appropriate, but emphasis on the inherent muscle strengthening and support should be the method of first resort.

Brief periods of immobilization initially may serve to break the cycle of repeated irritation of inflamed tissue. Many of the low back elastic support belts can serve to remind the patient subconsciously to maintain the most neutral position and move slowly. The additional proprioceptive input provided by the support may tend to allow muscles to contract and guard differently than without it. The belts' value in physical restriction of motion, however, is questionable. Several brands have metal stays or rigid inserts available. A piece of cardboard may be cut to fit inside the belt to help add stability. There are a few custom-made rigid and semirigid supports available but, as with cushions, the acute back will probably change over time and the more expensive items should be considered when the clinical course becomes more stable. Often the hourglass shape of the female torso complicates matters. It is difficult to get most generic support belts to position properly. The kind with large internal straps and small outer cinching straps may be helpful in some women, but experience suggests that elastic supports may not be quite as valuable

with the female as they are with the straighter male build.

It is the doctor's responsibility to make sure the acute patient is instructed in the proper methods of common activities. Be sure the patient can maintain a proper neutral posture while moving from seated to upright positions and back. Be sure the patient is taught how to turn and flex the head while maintaining posture. This first becomes important when getting back into the car after an office visit. Many physical therapists and chiropractors have experienced a patient undoing an entire session of manual care while getting back into the driver's seat.

Have the patient sit in hard chairs with arm rests at home. A few practice movements should be implemented before actually standing up or sitting down. Pelvic tilt movements and going only part way a few times will help speed the neuromuscular reeducation needed for long-term recovery. The patient should repeat the stand and return movement several times before leaving the office and should continue it at home before going on to the next activity. Teach the back sufferer to stay away from soft chairs and sofas, and to avoid looking down or flexing.

Analgesic balms following a hot shower before bedtime may be helpful if there is no great likelihood of inflammation. Stimulation of various nerve endings has been thought to assist

3–7 days:
- Soft tissue manipulation (gentle, slow, gradual)
- Low intensity muscle stimulation, ultrasound)
- Consider gentle distraction manipulation
- Passive assisted movements

1–2 weeks:
- Isometric and resisted exercise
- More aggressive spinal and extremity manipulation
- Deeper and more aggressive soft tissue manipulation
- Gradual increase in activity level
- Muscle stimulation, ultrasound, etc.
- Consider more formal education such as back school

2–4 weeks:
- Intermittent traction
- Manual traction (e.g., flexion-distraction procedures)
- Aggressive spinal manipulation
- Deep tissue myofascial work
- Continue education (or institute if not yet started)
- Aggressive conditioning exercise

Figure 32.5. Management protocols. Exact chronology and protocols vary with severity.

by reflex relaxation of spastic musculature and inhibiting pain (37, 38). As there are numerous sensory endings in the skin and subcutaneous fascia (39), cutaneous thermal and nociceptive stimulation may work in a similar fashion. Fair-skinned people may be more sensitive and should avoid heating the area first. Balms should be applied in small amounts to the thoracolumbar junction, the iliac crests, and buttocks bilaterally. This is aimed at altering the activity in somatosensory receptors and need not be applied topically in the painful region. Have the patient wear an old T-shirt to bed, as some balms may stain nightclothes and linen. With significant trauma and suspected inflammation, rest, cryotherapy, and support should be continued until inflammation is reduced.

Avoid a startled wake-up. This means waking without an alarm clock. Before getting out of bed, the patient should gradually move toes, bend the knees and hips, and do some recumbent pelvic tilt movements, then wait 5 to 10 minutes before attempting any flexion (including sitting on the toilet, brushing teeth at the sink).

The patient should walk around and let the back have plenty of time to wake up before being asked to engage in excessive or prolonged flexion. The patient should wait 20 to 30 minutes to sit and be sure that sitting for breakfast is done in a straight-backed chair.

The extremely acute patient should be instructed to report progress. Additional conservative intervention can be arranged if necessary. It may be important to support the patient psychologically, particularly in first-time back sufferers. Such a show of genuine interest contributes to a strong doctor-patient relationship that will lend itself to better compliance with essential active rehabilitation later.

Becoming Mobile
3 to 7 Days after Onset

During this time, gentle passive therapies will tend to speed along mobility. Passive assisted motions by the doctor, therapist, or carefully instructed cohabitant can help the patient's joints and tisues experience pain-free motion and teach the patient early that movement can feel good. Encourage patient-mediated motion as soon as possible to avoid dependancy. Such other procedures as soft tissue manipulation, including gentle massage, low-intensity pulsed muscle stimulation, and ultrasound can help aid in phagocytosis, reduce muscle spasm, and promote circulation and lymphatic drainage (39). This is extremely important in conditions with traumatic onsets. The duration of this phase will tend to be decreased in the more insidious cases.

Distraction-based manipulative care may be initiated as inflammation decreases. Various kinds of reflex muscle relaxation procedures and modalities such as acupuncture and proprioceptive neuromuscular facilitation exercise may help speed recovery and provide relief. At this point, the passive therapies are likely to assist this process with less chance of the pain production and irritation that may attend too aggressive active exercise, particularly when periosteal attachments have been irritated.

Early Subacute Period: Weeks 1 to 2

As inflammation is brought under control and the major activities in connective tissue repair and adhesion formation are under way, the more aggressive manual therapies have much to offer. In the normally progressing patient, this time frame is also appropriate for considering more formal education and training such as back school. Isometric and resistive exercise can be beneficial in reducing muscle spasm, increasing mobility, and rehabilitating neuromuscular coordination (40, 41). Numerous physiotherapy modalities such as electrical muscle stimulation, ultrasound, contrast baths, stretch and spray, and the like may further these goals (40). Some patients may benefit from procedures such as acupuncture.

Restoring joint motion to pain-free ranges should expedite and assist the patient to engage in the exercises needed for long-term stability. Translocation movements and slightly more aggressive mobilization and manipulation can begin. When the back pain is sore and achy in character, manipulation should be postponed. As the condition becomes more sharp and "catchy," manipulation can be better tolerated by the patient and is less likely to aggravate edematous tissue.

If the condition is severe enough to warrant disability, this time frame is appropriate to begin a gradual increase in normal activities and return to light-work duty. The objective of care during this stage is to allow soft tissue injuries to heal in an organized fashion under nearly moderate stress and tension levels. In this way, normal tissue function and joint range of motion can be achieved when the injury is fully healed. It is important to monitor and accommodate the structural and functional changes that ensue in order to prevent regression on return to normal activity.

Aggressive Passive and Transition to Active Care: 2 to 4 Weeks

The various gentle passive therapies will help to reduce muscle spasm and make it easier to define any primary complicating factors in the patient's condition. In the insidious and acute aggravations of chronic mechanical back pain patients, the doctor will need to differentiate between chronic biomechanical dysfunctions with fibrosis and acute muscle spasm. Acute aggravations are often accompanied by joint restriction, local tenderness, and tightness and respond quickly to manipulation. The fibrotic and degenerative situations may be more amenable to stretch of tissue mechanoreceptors for pain reduction via the pain-gate mechanism (38, 39).

The primary objectives in this phase of care are to set the most beneficial environment for the deposition of new connective tissue. Special attention to postural and lifestyle changes is essential. Back school or other aggressive educational efforts should be started if not begun sooner. Aggressive spinal manipulation, manual and mechanical distraction, deep myofascial and trigger point work can constitute the passive therapies. Active stretching and strengthening exercises need to be instituted and repeatedly emphasized if recurrence is to be avoided.

SUMMARY

All health care practitioners are likely to be confronted with acute low back pain patients. Proper attention to some basics will usually provide the patient with the best opportunity for successful resolution. Early attention to mobility, appropriately applied passive therapies with careful attention to prevention of dependance, and rapid involvement in active education, home care, and exercise appear to achieve the greatest degree of success in the shortest amount of time. Patient care and referral decisions must be made on the basis of the patient's need and abilities of the various members of the health care team. Although different disciplines may continue to battle over credentials, economics, and politics, such trivialities can impede the cooperation and progress essential for providing our patients with the best, most cost effective care possible.

References

1. Kelsey JL. Epidemiology of musculoskeletal disorders. New York: Oxford University Press, 1982.
2. Cassidy JD, Wedge JH. The epidemiology and natural history of low back pain and spinal degeneration. In Kirkaldy-Willis WH, ed. Managing low back pain, 2nd ed. New York: Churchill Livingstone, 1988; 3–14.
3. Spengler DM, Bigos SJ et al. Back injuries in industry: A retrospective study. Part 1. Overview and cost analysis. Spine 1986; 11:241.
4. Leblanc F, ed. Scientific approach to the assessment and management of activity related spinal disorders. Spine 1987; 12(Suppl):1–59.
5. Mayer T, Gatchel R. Functional restoration for spinal disorders: A sports medicine approach. Philadelphia: Lea and Febiger, 1988.
6. Frymoyer J. Back pain and sciatica. JAMA 1988; 318:291–300.
7. Nachemson AL. The natural course of low back pain. In White A, Gordon S, eds. Idiopathic low back pain. St. Louis: Mosby, 1982.
8. Berquist-Ullman M, Larsson U. Acute low back pain in industry. Acta Orthop Scand 1977; 170(Suppl):1–112.
9. Roland M, Morris R. A study of the natural history of back pain. Parts I, II. Spine 1983; 8:141–150.
10. Robbins SL, Cotran, RS, Kumar V. Inflammation and repair. In: Pathologic basis of disease. Philadelphia: Saunders, 1984; 40–84.
11. Movat HZ. Kinins and the kinin system as inflammatory mediators. In Weissmann G et al. eds. Chemical messengers of inflammation, Vol 1. Amsterdam: Elsevier, 1979; 47–112.
12. Sunderland S. Nerves and nerve injuries, 2nd ed. Edinburgh: Churchill Livingstone, 1978.
13. Lehto M, Jarvinin M, Nelimarkka O. Scar formation after skeletal muscle injury: A histological and radiographical study in rats. Arch Orthop Trauma Surg 1986; 104(6):366–370.
14. Denny-Brown D. The influence of tension and innervation on the regeneration of skeletal muscle. J Neuropathol Exp Neurol 1951; 10:94–96.
15. Jarvinen M. Healing of crush injury in rat striated muscle. Act Pathol Microbiol Scand 1975; 83:269–282.
16. Allbrook D, Baker W, Kirkaldy-Willis W. Muscle regeneration in experimental animals and in man. J Bone Joint Surg 1966; 48B(1):151–169.
17. La Vigne A, Watkins P. Preliminary results on immobilization induced stiffness on monkey knee joints and posterior capsule: Perspectives in biomedical engineering. Proceedings of symposium of biomedical engineering society, University of Glasgow. Baltimore: University Park Press, 1973.
18. Neuberger A, Slack H. The metabolism of collagen from liver, bones, skin and tendon in normal rat. Biochem J 1953; 53:47.
19. Akeson WD, Amiel D, Woo S. Immobility effects of synovial joints: The pathomechanics of joint contracture. Biorheology 1980; 17:95.
20. Akeson WD, Amiel D, Mechanic GL et al. Collagen crosslinking alterations in joint contractures: Changes in reducible crosslinks in periarticular connective tissue after nine weeks immobilization. Connective Tissue Res 1977; 5:5.
21. Emmeking W, Horowitz M. The intra-articular effects of immobilization on the human knee. J Bone Joint Surg 1972; 54A:973.
22. Frymoyer J: Back pain and sciatica. JAMA 1988; 318:291–300.
23. Foreman SM, Croft AC. Whiplash injuries: The cervical accleration/deceleration syndrome. Baltimore: Williams & Wilkins, 1988.
24. Yochum T, Rowe L. Essentials of skeletal radiology. Baltimore: Williams & Wilkins, 1987.
25. Bogduk N, Tynan W, Wilson AS. The nerve supply to the human lumbar intervertebral discs. J Anat 1981; 132:39–56.
26. Bogduk N, Twomey LT. Clinical Anatomy of the lumbar spine. Melbourne: Churchill Livinstone, 1987; 100–102.
27. Finneson BE. Low back pain, 2nd ed. Philadelphia: JB Lippincott, 1980.
28. Cox JM. Low back pain: Mechanism, diagnosis and treatment, 4th ed. Baltimore: Williams & Wilkins, 1985.
29. Magee DJ. Orthopedic physical assessment. Philadelphia: WB Saunders, 1987.
30. Cassidy JD, Kirkaldy-Willis WH, McGregor M. Spinal manipulation for the treatment of low back pain: An observational trial. In Buerger AA, Greenman PE eds. Empirical approaches to the validation of manipulative therapy. Springfield, IL: Charles C Thomas, 1985.
31. Simons D. Myofascial pain syndromes due to trigger points: Principles, diagnosis and perpetuating factors. Manual Med 1985; 1:67.
32. Maigne R. Low back pain of thoracolumbar origin. Arch Phys Med Rehabil 1980; 61:389–395.
33. Proctor D, Dupuis P, Cassidy JD. Thoracolumbar syndrome as a cause of low back pain: A report of two cases. J Can Chiro Assoc 1985; 29(2):71–73.

34. Cherkin DC, MacCornack FA, Berg AO. Managing low back pain—A comparison of the beliefs and behavior of family physicians and chiropractors. Western J Med 1988; 149(4):475–480.

35. Cyriax J. Textbook of orthopaedic medicine, Vol 1. Diagnosis of soft tissue lesions, 7th ed. London: Ballière-Tindall, 1978; 64–103.

36. Kleynhans AM. Complications and contraindications to spinal manipulative therapy. In Haldeman S ed. Modern Developments in the Principles and Practice of Chiropractic. New York: Appleton Century Crofts, 1979.

37. Coote JH. Somatic sources of afferent input as factors in aberrant autonomic, sensory, and motor function. In Korr TM ed. Neurobiologic mechanisms in manipulative therapy. New York: Plenum Press, 1978.

38. Wyke BD. Articular neurology and manipulative therapy. In Glasgow EF, et al. eds. Aspects of manipulative therapy, 2nd ed. Melbourne: Churchill Livingstone, 1985.

39. Gillette RG. A speculative argument for the coactivation of diverse somatic receptor populations by a chiropractic adjustment. Review of human and animal research. In Keene, et al. eds. Proceedings of third annual current topics in chiropractic: Reviews of the literature. Sunnyvale, CA: Palmer College of Chiropractic-West, 1986.

40. Schafer RC, ed. Basic chiropractic procedural manual. Arlington, VA: American Chiropractic Association, 1984.

41. Lewit K. Manipulative therapy in rehabilitation of the locomotor system. London: Butterworth, 1985.

42. Janda V. Muscle function testing. London: Butterworth, 1983.

33

"WORK HARDENING" USING WORK FOR REHABILITATION

Rowlin L. Lichter

Until the last decade, bed rest, passive physical therapy, and medication have been the mainstays of conservative back care. Now we have learned that not only is bed rest ineffective for back care but, when prolonged, it may be a serious error in therapy and may perpetuate disability. Classic pain-oriented passive physical therapy programs fail to address the basic functional deficit of the chronic low back pain patient. The proper use of work simulation ("work hardening") prevents and corrects these therapeutic errors and effectively reduces back pain disability.

This approach is based upon the author's experience with over 12,000 chronic low back pain patients treated at CHART rehabilitation facilities. It has restored or improved work status in 60% of essentially unselected patients in a 1982 study (1) and over 70% of these patients in a 1988 study (2).

HISTORY

Work performance has certainly been used to restore function since people began to work. The formal application of this rehabilitation modality, however, has been quite recent. The earliest attempts were recorded in 1838 and until 1918 appeared to be morally inspired by religious groups who pitied and employed the impaired in sheltered workshops. The first workshops were created mostly for the blind. Later, the mentally ill and hearing disabled received some help. These efforts were aimed at work as a tool to restore dignity and relieve boredom without regard to productivity and value of the work produced (3).

The Society of St. Vincent de Paul preceded the Salvation Army (1879) and Goodwill Industries (1902) in teaching the handicapped to refurbish used items (4). As sheltered work sites matured, they were encouraged by the influx of war casualties and legislation to benefit all types of disability. Provisions were made to allow a substandard employee to work at reduced productivity and/or with inappropriate work behavior. Emphasis was on fitting and restructuring the job to the employee rather than the reverse. With few exceptions, these operations proved expensive, unprofitable, and largely segregated. The employee was rarely returned to a normal socioeconomic milieu. The environment was modified to suit the impairment (5).

Using the activity of normal work instead of crafts as therapy probably began in the 1930s when mental hospital inpatients were drafted into performing routine hospital work (3, 6). World War I had added many more disabled veterans to the U.S. economy and necessitated restoring the economic potential of these injured citizens. This gave further impetus to work rehabilitation. Later, this expertise was applied to injured workers and evolved into "curative workshops." The workshops continued therapy beyond the hospital in an effort to return the client to mainstream work. The focus was on restoring function to the injured body part.

371

An early example of a curative workshop was the Rochester Rehabilitation center directed by A.L. Stevens, an occupational therapist. He sought to match stable patients with available jobs after maximizing their abilities in basic work functions.

The advent of workers' compensation, which became nationwide in 1940, placed socioeconomic emphasis on the rehabilitation of the injured worker. Efforts began to focus on the most costly of all work-related complaints—low back pain. The coinage by Mixter and Barr of the term "ruptured disc," which seems to imply an injury, has added fuel to the fire. This emphasis and the law have helped to bring us to the current levels of concern for back disability and its rehabilitation, now a virtual Western epidemic (7).

L. Wegg, as cited by Mathesson and colleagues (6), was perhaps before his time when he noted in the 1950s that work simulation could duplicate job stresses to estimate the patient's ability. He also felt work could be used as an exercise form to develop proper working habits, confidence, endurance, strength, flexibility, coordination and dexterity. Familiar work situations and clearly set goals, he thought, were psychologically advantageous. The worker used familiar tools to increase speed and skill under graded, progressively stressful conditions.

The growth of sports medicine in the 1960s gave birth to the concept of sport specificity in rehabilitation of the injured athlete. It rapidly became clear that a similar approach could be helpful in rehabilitation of the injured worker. As a result, in the late 1970s a move to utilize these principles began under the guise of work hardening in Downey, California (6) and work simulation in Honolulu, Hawaii (1).

In the 1980s, many facilities opened throughout the United States that used work activities as part of their rehabilitation programs. Although the concepts have often been similar, the cost, patient mix, therapeutic emphasis, and result have differed from group to group.

With the propagation of facilities, there has been growing confusion in the terminology of work rehabilitation. "Work hardening" has been one of the most popular, confused, and loosely used terms perhaps because it communicates an emotion rather than a process.

What Is "Work Hardening"?

Depending upon the point of view, work hardening has been commonly confused with, and thought to be similar to, back school, work simulation, work capacity evaluation, sheltered workshops, and functional restoration. A comprehensive definition is provided by Blankenship:

> A systematic program of gradually progressive work-related activities performed with perfect body mechanics, which recondition the person's musculoskeletal, cardiorespiratory, and psychomotor systems to prepare that person for return to work (8).

Mathesson offers an all-inclusive definition of work hardening. It is a portion of work capacity evaluation that is "a systematic process of measuring and developing an individual's capacity to dependably sustain performance in response to broadly defined work demands [that] includes work conditioning (for tolerance and rate), pain coping, work adaptation devices, and behavior modification regarding work habits and confidence" (9). Elsewhere he states that it encompasses job modification to improve strength, flexibility, endurance, and function through effective adaptive behaviors and to decrease impairment in "societal roles" (6).

Even back school has been defined by some authors in such a way as to include functional activities of work, such as work hardening (10, 11). The American Occupational Therapy Association recognizes the term and describes the benefits but does not clearly define the program. Oregon has defined work hardening by statute (OAR 436-10-005) (9).

The Commission on Accreditation of Rehabilitation Facilities (CARF) defines work hardening as

> Programs, which are interdisciplinary in nature, [and] use conditioning tasks that are graded to progressively improve the biomechanical, neuromuscular, cardiovascular/metabolic, and psychosocial functions of the person in conjunction with real or simulated work activities. Work Hardening provides a transition between acute care and return to work while addressing the issues of productivity, safety, physical tolerances, and worker behaviors. Work Hardening is a highly structured, goal-oriented, individualized treatment program designed to maximize the person's ability to return to work (12).

The confusion in naming the process of restoration of function through work is exemplified by this statement of one of the leading proponents of this method of rehabilitation: "If (among other conservative measures) work hardening and work simulation programs have been unsuccessful ... consider referring [the patient] to a functional restoration program" (13).

For purposes of this chapter, a *back school* is an educational instrument or facility solely for training clients in the proper function and use of the spine and the avoidance of back pain and injury. Further, we will reserve the term *work capacity evaluation* for the evaluation of a patient's ability to perform work tasks when tested according to a prearranged protocol. This may be general and exploratory or focused on a specific occupational classification. The tests may be performed over a period of several hours or be extended as needed to several days. It is a logical extension of work simulation training.

Active Rehabilitation with Work Simulation

The originators agree that there are strong differences in each of their programs. Nonetheless, the work-oriented programs are even more closely linked by their similarities. All of these sports medicine derived therapies have the common feature of being "active"—requiring the patient to participate fully in voluntary activity. This lends sharp contrast to the traditional occupational therapy approach and the classic physical therapy approach that is passive, thermal, mechanical, and electrotherapeutic. Perhaps a more descriptive, if general, term for these rehabilitation methods is *active rehabilitation with work simulation*. It is particularly appropriate and encompasses all of the disciplines described to date.

The components of active rehabilitation programs such as CHART are based on sports medicine principles of integrating basic exercises with work-specific activity. They include work simulation or duplication, back schools and other educational programs, work capacity evaluation, and work endurance. They share having functional, usually work-oriented, goals. Many offer provisions for increasing the patient's strength, endurance, and flexibility by more formal, less specific means such as free

weights, swimming and isotonic or isokinetic machines. Some programs also incorporate psychologic and vocational support.

Work Simulation

When employed to its fullest potential, work simulation is the use of actual or simulated work activities under reproducibly controlled conditions of physical and psychologic stress to evaluate and restore the functional capacity of an injured and/or deconditioned patient. It is only one part of a larger, more complete active rehabilitation program based on a psychophysical approach. Work simulation is goal oriented toward return to work by restoration of previous work performance abilities or maximal function. In the controlled environment, the stresses placed on the patient are gradually and reproducibly increased as his mental and physical capacities improve. Ergonomic aids and job modification supplement this therapy.

Work simulation affords concurrent evaluation of ability to work as a natural consequence of the process. However, it may be used for evaluation alone (8).

Duplication of Environmental Factors

A strong effort is made to duplicate those critical environmental factors that the patient may face on return to work. This includes the physical, social, and psychologic stresses as well as the rewards for compliance and achievement. The ability to function well as an employee must be developed, tested, and restored under physical conditions as similar as possible to actual employment. This should include attention to ambient working temperature, humidity, lighting, work posture in crawl spaces and during ceiling work, protective clothing, cramped areas, footing, terrain, and other work site factors.

Other environmental factors are more psychologic. These include noise, confusion, deadlines or quotas, work-rest patterns, and a host of other stressors that a clever therapist may duplicate. Often these very factors are the truly disabling ones and the physical impairment only the facade. Addressing these psychologic problems may uncover an unknown problem or desensitize the patient to a known one.

PSYCHOSOCIAL FACTORS

To encourage and reassure the patient, offering the social rewards of working is helpful. Recognition of the milestone of accepting job-like responsibility is important. The praise and encouragement when the patient arrives on time for therapy simulates and stimulates the need to arrive at work on time. A time clock may be used to sign in. Completion of appropriate assigned work activities must also be recognized. The comradeship of fellow workers is duplicated by keeping the patients on similar treatment timetables. Fellow patients begin to recognize each other and enjoy each other's company.

DETAIL IS IMPORTANT

The use of an organizational logo in small rewards, such as visors and T-shirts, for achievement and compliance heightens the fellowship as well as mimics the bonus system in industry. These rewards offer tangible recognition of important milestones in therapy and positioning for reentry into work. A reward system also adds to the feeling of group effort, of not being alone in efforts to rebuild working ability. The therapist heightens the feeling to increase the patients' support system though emotional bonding.

Work Evaluation through Work Simulation

The ability to work is the psychophysical product of what the worker can do as modified by what the worker believes he or she can do. Not only are the absolute physical capacities of the worker important but also the worker's perception of ability and limitations. The patient's disability is the result of this combination, even though the perception of what is or may be painful is for the most part unreliable (14).

The process of work simulation as practiced at CHART and other centers continually tests the patient's ability to work in the most reliable, accurate and reproducible way yet demonstrated. To date, machine testing reliably duplicates or simulates only a small part of the actual demands of work. Therefore, its reliability for predicting return to work, work ability, and protection from reinjury is limited to the tested function of back flexion and extension

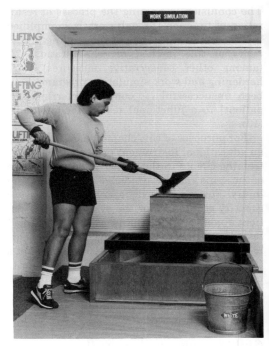

Figure 33.1 Patient shovels real sand in simulated working environment.

under the special circumstances of the individual machine's range, frequency and stress signature (15, 16). Figures 33.1 through 33.4 illustrate work simulations.

WHY WORK?

J.D.G. Troup in his Volvo award address in 1987 said, "When further treatment, investigations, and surgery are deemed futile, the only solution is to encourage the victims of low back pain to confront their pain and resume active bending and heavy work" (14). This truth cannot be denied. Additionally, properly timed work rehabilitation may obviate the need for further treatment, investigations, and surgery (1, 17, 18).

Need for a Broad Range of Work Stresses

Minimally, work-oriented programs focus on straight, vertical lifting ability. Yet the sources of low back pain and deficiencies are protean (15, 18–20). According to Manning and colleagues (21) lifting accounts for fewer than a

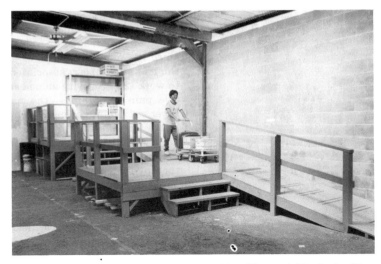

Figure 33.2.   Patient rebuilds physical capacity for material handling activities in familiar work-like setting.

quarter of back injuries. Others agree that it accounts for fewer than half (19). Restoring a single functional deficit, such as the ability to perform a straight, isolated lift, will not logically reduce most back disabilities. Therefore, it is necessary to account for most of the physical stresses of daily living and of the job to be certain that the patient's physical capacity meets the demands expected. This is accomplished through simulating the activities of daily living and work tasks in the laboratory or facility.

USE OF BACK MACHINES

The abstract activity of isokinetic or isotonic lifting using a back machine correlates best with the subject's ability to lift a comparable weight one to three times a minute. Perceived (psychophysical) lifting capacity correlates best with lifting ability at frequencies of three to six times a minute (22). According to sports medicine principles, injured workers should remedy the perception of their ability as well as restore

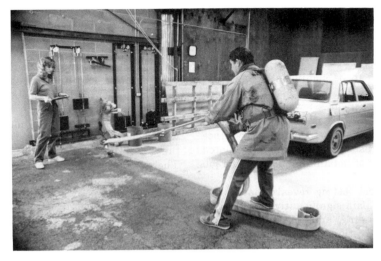

Figure 33.3.   Patient pulls real firehose while wearing breathing apparatus to recreate his workplace demands as closely as possible.

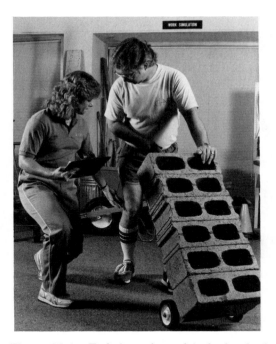

Figure 33.4. Techniques learned in back school are continually reinforced during work simulation.

their capability for return to work using the type and frequency of lifting required at work. Since lifting in industry corresponds more closely to the psychophysical capacity (23), real lifting tasks and actual material handling are used exclusively for work simulation. Progressive lifting capacity tests have been developed using real weighted boxes and shelves and are being used at CHART and other centers.

OVERUSE AND DECONDITIONING

Overuse appears to be significantly related to back injury (7, 19, 23). It has also been shown that stronger workers have fewer injuries. When job demands exceed strength capacity, injuries occur (24). Yet this is not the whole story, since the incidence of back pain is not directly related to the frequency of maximum effort on the job (25).

Psychophysical testing reveals that disuse due to low back pain significantly affects walking, forward bending, and dressing (6). This proves the observation that back pain has a global effect on one's functional abilities.

Patients often feel more disabled than their impairment necessitates. Published studies of

patients who are objectively tested suggest that they are able to do more than they believe (20). This perception appears to be self perpetuating since the mere avoidance of activity increases the fear and anxiety associated with the return to work (26). Activity alone can change subjective pain complaints—the more activity, the fewer complaints of pain (27). Work activity is a tool for equating the patient's perceptions to ability. This would account for the rapid gains in apparent ability in the short-term active therapy systems (26).

Work therapy concurrently rebuilds the strength as well as neuromuscular functions needed for safe return to work. These include motor power, endurance, flexibility, coordination, timing, balance, and other motor skills. All these functions are part of physical conditioning, which maximizes work ability and protects against future back injuries (28, 29). Since back-injured or complaining subjects have weaker back strength than noncomplainers (24, 30, 31), it seems logical to use these proved preventive measures of strengthening as therapy.

Legal Aspects

The Equal Employment Opportunity Commission recommendations require definite work-relatedness of tests on which personnel actions are based (32, 33). Thus, testing and training under circumstances simulating or duplicating the occupational tasks required best fit those needs and should minimize exposure to litigation.

Socioeconomic Aspects

In a great number of jurisdictions, workers' compensation and other no-fault laws entitle disabled patients to periodic benefits until they feel able to work. The length of disability may be unlimited. Thus, the law may favor negative work behavior. This increases the need to impress on the patients their ability to work. There is no better way of doing this than by showing them practically that they can perform each required activity at work safely and repeatedly without untoward consequences.

Maintaining or reestablishing proper work behavior becomes a critical part of rehabilitation. Reestablishing punctuality and responsibility, as well as proper rest and recreation habits to balance work stresses, is important.

The removal of other economic barriers to return to work must be addressed. Some of these, such as child care and role reversal, are eliminated by the return to regular hours required in the rehabilitation program. Other positive factors include the comradeship of fellow patients and the staff, the use of familiar tools and clothing to perform familiar functions associated with work, and the need for transportation to and from the "work site."

Educational Reinforcement

The use of simulated or real work tasks in rehabilitation allows direct observation of the patient's ability to perform work functions. During this time, proper work habits are incorporated into habit patterns. Observed improper function can be repeatedly challenged and immediately corrected.

Using work simulation also allows the therapist to see the effect of changes in motor task ergonomic efficiency. These changes are to be monitored and tailored as the patient's ability dictates. Ergonomic aids can be developed for individual tasks and their effectiveness can be evaluated. If problems in their use arise, these are to be corrected immediately.

Safety

The controlled stresses of the facility with the presence of professional aides increase the safety factor. The psychophysical evaluation of a work task is highly useful, inexpensive and, most importantly, safe. Maximum strength values derived from isokinetic machines are greater than psychophysically acceptable values (24, 34). In some cases the psychophysically acceptable stress is as small as 25% of the machine-derived values. Since changes in psychophysical measures of lifting ability more closely correlate with the presence of low back pain than machine measurements (14), exceeding these psychophysical limits may cause pain and simulate, if not cause, injury.

Quite logically, extreme confidence is needed to propose to an injured patient that his or her perception of limited ability is only a quarter of real ability and then ask the patient to prove it! The safer psychophysical lifting tests (14, 18) are as sensitive as tests of maximal isometric lifting strength (14). Since they are also less expensive to administer than isokinetic strength

tests, they have an obvious application as an outcome measure for therapeutic trials (14).

Practical Application of Therapeutic Emphasis

The multiple factors of back disability and back pain make rehabilitation beyond minimal restoration of work ability or activities of daily living function important. *Change what can be changed and accommodate for the unalterable.* The therapist, physician, employer and the patient must address those conditions and perceptions that can be altered by global physical and behavioral rehabilitation as well as those that require external aids or work modification.

Back injuries vary with perceived and actual work load. There are more injuries in workers who function at heavy physical demands than in those performing at light demands (35). As long as the worker thinks the job is heavy and beyond his capability, he or she will be more likely to have back complaints (36, 37). Perception and ability can both be modified in work simulation.

Factors related to back disability, such as lack of physical fitness, poor posture, and obesity (28), can be modified. Obesity is approachable through exercise as well as diet. Lack of conditioning or fitness can be reversed by exercise. Backache due to postural stress can be reduced through back school and work simulation.

Other aspects of disability cannot readily be changed. Workers who have had back problems are more likely to have more problems. Tallness and the long back, age, prolonged duration of prior complaints, presence of residual leg pain, and multiple back operations also predict recurrence or persistence of low back pain (17, 20, 37). In these cases, aids and adjustment of work conditions are needed. Further, this suggests that a basic failure rate of return to work is currently immutable.

Reality Therapy

Perhaps the most important of the more subtle aspects of work simulation is the absence of the hospital or "sick environment." Work therapy is best carried out in a storeroom, garage, warehouse, out of doors, or in an office setting, as is appropriate for the patient's occupation. Providing treatment within the "natural environment" by getting away from the medical setting appears to have a more durable effect on relief of pain and promotion of activity (38).

The cost effectiveness of work rehabilitation is measured by the application of the patient's renewed skills on the job, the actual return to work. Improvement of the patient's perception of his or her condition without the practical benefit of restoring productivity is of little value to society and of even less to industry. Rehabilitating through work focuses on both of these needs.

WHO BENEFITS?

Because it is a practical, concrete, real-time, real-stress therapy, work simulation provides the patient with immediate and direct feedback as to stage and rate of recovery. No interpretation of graphs or numbers is needed.

The employer knows which work functions the employee can and cannot perform. This aids in planning return to work and interim coverage.

The doctor can recognize quite readily whether the patient is progressing or plateauing, and tailor medication and other therapies more effectively.

The insurer can be more objective and reserve the necessary funds more accurately knowing the patient's status in the return-to-work program. With more current, precise, and readily available information about the patient's changing level of disability, a more rapid and sensitive response should be forthcoming from both the attorney and insurer.

Perhaps the greatest benefit accrues to the vocational rehabilitation specialist who knows exactly the patient's current physical abilities without interpretation. A closer match to available jobs is possible than is available through physician "guesstimates." Feasibility for return to work is relieved of guesswork.

Qualifications of a Work Simulation Therapist

Current curricula of occupational therapy schools prepare students for the technicalities anticipated in the application of work therapy. There is now greater emphasis on the overlapping disciplines of biomechanics, ergonomics, and occupation assessment. However, more

training is needed in behavioral psychology, especially related to pain, tension, anxiety, anger and depression, communication skills, teaching, and interpersonal relationships. The therapist must be able to consult effectively with other professionals such as the physical therapist, ergonomist, and the vocational rehabilitation specialist. The therapist also must work well with the employer and employer's representatives. Above all the therapist must be creative and skilled in use of real work as an exercise and evaluative tool.

PRACTICAL APPLICATION OF WORK TO REHABILITATION

The following description of work simulation therapy is derived from the author's experience as National Medical Director of CHART (Comprehensive Health and Active Rehabilitation Training) facilities. This is a national active physical rehabilitation organization currently serving 14 communities in seven states.

Integrated Program

Work rehabilitation is the major portion of an integrated program that is most effective when combined with fully directed and supervised back school, strengthening exercises, and stretching and endurance programs.

By Prescription

All programs must be prescribed by a physician. A reasonably accurate diagnosis is important. The possibility of injuring a patient whose diagnosis and limitations are poorly understood makes this step mandatory. The functional diagnosis of the physical therapist supplements this step.

Medical Director

Because of the fragility of patients whose disabilities may be profound and significantly complicated, a physician must be easily accessible to the therapists. All work simulation programs should have the involvement, support, and direction of a physician who is knowledgeable and skilled in the care of the injured back. This medical director is not expected to see or be personally involved with the patient, but should be consulted in all cases where progress is not as expected or therapy is significantly different from the usual. The medical director is there to solve problems and assure quality.

Appropriate Patient Selection

There is no reason for a feasibility screen. Current screens are so inaccurate they select out many appropriate patients. Inappropriate patients are rare. If the patient is sent by a physician, is disabled from work, and is willing to participate in the program, he or she should not be denied treatment. A proven 70% rate of success at CHART in returning patients to work or improving their employment status, regardless of duration of disability, is justification enough for a trial of work therapy (1, 2).

Team Approach

The therapeutic approach involves a team with a minimum of two members: the work therapist, who is a specially trained occupational therapist, and a physical therapist trained in active rehabilitation. Where possible, a third member is added whose training and interests are in the field of exercise and sports—an exercise therapist. Other professionals, including psychiatrists, psychologists, vocational specialists, and rehabilitation nurses are involved as needed.

Patient Evaluation and Baseline Studies

The first effort is to understand the patient and delineate the patient's functional deficits. This process is divided into the evaluations of physical impairment and of functional impairment or psychophysical dysfunction. The work therapist consults the physical therapist and the physician to obtain the organic diagnoses and their view of the patient's physical limitations. This includes the duration of symptoms, stability, previous therapy and response, absolute limitations in range and stress, and a medical assurance that the patient may be safely stressed to the targeted physical demand level.

The patient is then evaluated for basic levels of strength, endurance, and flexibility. Cardiac reserve is estimated as well as any other absolute or relative contraindications to exercise.

The evaluation by the work therapist includes an evaluation of activities of daily living by questionnaire and by observation of standard activities. This is followed by a gross functional assessment in multiple areas of stress, including range of motion under load for lifting both straight and diagonally, pushing and pulling on the level and up and down ramps, carrying, climbing, and general mobility.

OCCUPATIONAL DESCRIPTION

After the physical assessment is complete, the occupation goal must be clarified. Two references, the *Dictionary of Occupational Titles* (33) and *Classification of Jobs* (32), are helpful for broad description and for reference or cataloging. Where possible, the employer is contacted for a job description. A vocational rehabilitation specialist can be an excellent resource for this information. On occasion, a job site visit may be needed. The patient is consulted to determine any further specifications.

JOB ANALYSIS

The specific tasks required of the worker are determined. For example: a painter drives a truck, erects and disassembles scaffolding, loads it on and off a truck at the work site and at the warehouse, removes forms, sweeps the shop, unloads and loads a compressor and 10-gallon paint cans, carries and spreads canvas, climbs ladders with tools and supplies, and also paints. These job demands are recorded on an activity card.

MATCHING PATIENT CAPACITIES

The job demands are compared with the patient's capabilities in 16 basic functions: lifting, carrying, standing, sitting, walking, pushing, pulling, twisting, reaching, squatting, stooping, bending, kneeling, crawling, manipulation, and balancing. By observation, these functions are matched to the patient's capabilities. Where deficiencies exist, they are noted.

IDENTIFYING CRITICAL ACTIVITIES

The therapist identifies and assigns priorities to each occupational activity. The most important activites are compared to the patient's current functional abilities and deficits. Those activities essential to the safe, efficient performance of the job, which the patient is currently incapable of performing satisfactorily, are noted.

ESTABLISHING THERAPEUTIC FOCUS AND STRATEGY

The critical activities in which the patient is deficient become the therapeutic focus. These activities will be further analyzed for the source of the functional impairment to develop a therapeutic strategy. The help of the team physical therapist is enlisted to determine if the deficit is related to an anatomic defect, pathologic loss of function, a psychologic dysfunction, deconditioning, poor body mechanics, or some combination of factors. The possibility of changing these factors is also assessed. Factors not readily altered require different strategies for adaptive behavior.

The patient's psychosocial status is explored by the team in order to understand the economic and social pressures affecting the patient's motivation.

Order of Progression

Part of the therapeutic strategy involves the order of progression of stress. A determination, based on the patient's deficits, is made as to whether the therapist should initially emphasize strength, speed, coordination, endurance, repetitions, flexibility, or some other factor or combination of factors. The priority levels of such factors are also established at this point.

WORK PERFORMANCE TREATMENT PLAN

Entry Level Activities

Combining critical activities around the therapeutic focus, the therapist develops entry level tasks such as lifting a weight from knee to waist level, carrying weighted bags or boxes, and climbing a ladder. These tasks are joined into a meaningful activity appropriate for the anticipated occupation such as building a wall or painting pipes. These activities may last for about 15 to 20 minutes. The program may be extended or several programs can be linked to form an average 50-minute activity program. Activities are individually tailored and work-specific. They are not the classical, standardized work stations. The reality of the activity is emphasized to give meaning and purpose to the procedure. The process is intended to reassure the patient in his or her ability to perform the work activities needed on return to work.

Through review of the patient's physical capabilities developed through self-limited, submaximal testing, the proper and safe levels of submaximal stress can be applied and the prescription initiated.

Establishing Stress-related Requirements

Quantifiable values are set for each activity in terms of distance, height, weight, number of repetitions, frequencies or speed, rate, duration of the activity, and productivity requirements. The working environment is outlined and noise, obstacles, terrain, and other factors established.

GOAL SETTING AND CONTRACTS

Attainable, work-specific, realistic goals are developed. By agreement, the patient contracts to perform toward clearly outlined short- and long-term goals, which are recorded and confirmed. Progress toward the contracted goals is continuously monitored by the ongoing performance of work-specific tasks. The patient's progress, or the lack of it, is immediately apparent. Periodically, as appropriate, these goals are reviewed with the patient.

Failure to attain a goal is cause for concern. If goals prove unrealistic on a physiologic and pyschologic basis, they are modified. However, if proper goals are not reached, the therapeutic approach may have to be changed. If this is ineffective, the problem is referred to a review board or conference for resolution.

BALANCING AND SEQUENCING STRESSES

The order in which activities are performed can properly or adversely affect progress. Fatigue must be avoided before the maximally stressful activity of the session. On balance, however, the therapist must arrange the activities to provide maximal interest and minimal boredom. This may prove challenging, since occupational boredom is a frequent fact of life and our goal is to duplicate that occupation as faithfully as possible—even the boredom!

It is essential to balance exercise demands in an integrated program. As the patient gets nearer to discharge, the therapeutic emphasis on work simulation increases and emphasis on general nonspecific exercise diminishes.

Monitoring Progress

Weekly team conferences discuss the patient's progress and problems and coordinate his concurrent nonwork therapy. These essential activities include flexibility exercises, strengthening programs to supplement the work activities, endurance activities and specific therapeutic programs such as temporomandibular joint therapy, muscle stimulation, and manipulation. Coordination of effort avoids duplication of stresses and overuse through fatigue.

Goal setting is an ongoing process. Goals are modified as the patient attains or fails them. Modification is based on the work therapist's evaluation, the physical therapist's examination and history, and input from the patient. As each goal is passed, a new one is set in the same fashion.

Rate and Duration of Therapy

The basic program design is three sessions a week, each lasting about 2 hours. This is continued until all goals have been met or progress plateaus short of required physical demand levels. Duration and frequency can be varied upward to a 5-day-a-week 8-hour-a-day program. The rate of progress and the duration of therapy is related to the cause of the disability, and the source and the extent of the impairment.

If psychopathology is the basic disability, a shorter, more aggressive therapeutic plan is developed to demonstrate to the patient his or her capabilities and restore confidence in the ability to work. The more intensive programs may not allow for physiologic rest and repair. These programs are most effective for psychophysical reeducation with minimal physical reconditioning.

If significant biologic adaptation is required, the particular tissue's response to stress guides the rehabilitation. For example, muscle weakness due to deconditioning can be restored in a matter of a few weeks; restoration of strength

from muscle destruction due to trauma or surgery may require a month or so; and strengthening and/or stretching collagenous tissues such as ligaments and tendons may take still longer. On the average, a physically impaired back patient disabled 3 or more months requires 11 to 12 weeks of therapy to reach maximum function (1).

The Exceptional Patient

Not too rarely, a patient is encountered who is highly motivated and must be restrained from self-injury. Careful limits are set and maximum, not minimum, goals are established. As these goals are reached, the patient is observed for signs of fatigue, postactivity soreness, knowledge and use of body mechanics, and progress toward a long-term employment goal. The therapist and patient then agree on a revised rate of progress and new maximum goals.

Records

A work activity card is designed for recording the patient's activities in quantifiable terms. The less esoteric the terminology, the better, since many of the people concerned with the patient's progress will not understand foot pounds, newtons, and torque. This calls for practical terms such as "repetitions per time period" rather than frequency, and "load over distance" rather than work, wherever possible.

Patient Support Conferences

If goals are not timely met, if therapeutic problems develop, or if duration of treatment exceeds the average 12 weeks, a conference is held to guide further therapy. At CHART, we call the procedure outlined below a *patient support conference*.

The importance of this function must be emphasized. The conference acts as a quality control measure, an educational tool, and a safety device. This mechanism protects the patient from premature discharge and monitors potential abusers of the system. The group opinion dilutes medicolegal liability and bears proof of the facility's study and concern for all involved.

Those present should include all of the therapy team: the work therapist, the physical therapist, and the exercise therapist who supervises the supplemental, non–work-related programs.

The facility's medical director is present as a medical resource knowledgeable in spine pathology. A patient advocate balances the group and represents the socioeconomic and human side of the conference. This role is usually filled by an administrator in the facility.

Two other members are essential for proper balance. They are independent, nonaligned professionals: a second medical specialist such as an orthopaedist, neurosurgeon, or neurologist and a psychologist or psychiatrist. These members add new dimension and prevent inbred opinion.

Others invited are the referring physician, the employer or insurer, a vocational rehabilitation counselor or nurse, and the patient's attorney when it's appropriate. It is important that the patient not be at this meeting.

Before the conference, a report of the patient's background gathered from the physician, the patient, and any other reliable sources is prepared. At the conference, the patient's progress and problems are outlined. Further information or help might be requested and suggestions are made for change of therapy. These are communicated to the treating physician for decision and action.

Follow-up at 3 Months

No program is complete without knowledge of its successes or failures. For this reason, it is essential that all discharged patients be followed to determine the effect of the program. There is no more appropriate measure of success of a work-oriented program than return to work or improvement in work status (28). A success rate of 50% or more is expected. Less than this suggests inappropriate procedures.

Analysis of Failures

A periodic review of failures helps to reduce future problems and avoid pitfalls. This should be a separate educational activity at each facility. Each case should be analyzed to determine if anything could have been done by the facility to avoid or salvage the failure.

SUMMARY

Work simulation or work hardening has become an essential and effective therapeutic rehabilitative tool. With this method of back care, even the most difficult chronic back pain problem may be successfully addressed. The therapy is simple, direct, and without mystery. The expertise is readily available. The process can be adapted to a moderate-sized rehabilitation facility with reasonable ease. All facets of the socioeconomic chain benefit from its use. Although in its infancy, this therapeutic tool has great promise for the present as well as the future.

References

1. Lichter RL, Hewson JK, Radke SJ, Blum M. Treatment of chronic back pain: A community-based comprehensive return-to-work physical rehabilitation program. Clin Orthop 1984; 190:115–123.
2. Lichter RL, Corrigan KH, Fujita G. Unpublished data.
3. Harvey-Krefting L. The concept of work in occupational therapy: A historical review. Am J Occup Ther 1985; 39:301–307.
4. Gardner KA. The private work-oriented rehabilitation facility. Ann Rev Rehab 1981, 2:173–191.
5. Vash CJ. Sheltered industrial employment. Ann Rev Rehab 1980; 1:80–120.
6. Mathesson LN, Ogden LD, Violette K, Schultz K. Work hardening: Occupational therapy in industrial rehabilitation. Am J Occup Ther 1985; 39:314–321.
7. Waddel G. A new clinical model for the treatment of low-back pain. Spine 1987; 12:632–644.
8. Blankenship KL. Work capacity and industrial consultation. Course manual. Macon, GA: American Therapeutics, 1984.
9. Mathesson LN. Work capacity evaluation manual. Anaheim, CA: M & A Press, 1986.
10. Hayne CR. Back schools and total back care: A review. Physiotherapy 1984; 70:14–17.
11. Snook SH, White AH. In Pope MH, Frymoyer JW, Andersson G eds. Occupational low back pain. Philadelphia: Praeger, 1984; 233–244.
12. 1990 Standards Manual for Organizations Serving People with Disabilities. Commission on Accreditation of Rehabilitation Facilities, Tucson, AZ.
13. Deyo RA, Mayer TG, Pedinoff S, Pinals RS, Schwartz SA, Spengler DM. The painful low back: Keep it moving. Patient Care October 30, 1987; 47–59.
14. Troup JDG, Foreman TK, Baxter CE, Brown D. The perception of back pain and the role of psychophysical tests of lifting capacity. Spine 1987; 12:645–657.
15. Hazard RG, Reid S, Fenwick J, Reeves V. Isokinetic trunk and lifting strength measurements:

Variability as an indicator of effort. Spine 1988; 13:54–57.

16. Kamon E et al. Dynamic and static muscular strength of steel worker. Am Ind Hyg Assoc J 1982; 43:853–857.

17. Frymoyer JW, Cats-Baril W. Predictors of low back pain disability. Clin Orthop 1987; 221:89–98.

18. Snook SH, Campanelli RR, Hart JW. A study of three preventative approaches to low back injury. J Occup Med 1978; 20:478–481.

19. Klein BP, Jensen RC, Sanderson LM. Assessment of workers' compensation claims for back sprains/strains. J Occup Med 1984; 26:443–448.

20. Troup JDG. Causes, prediction and prevention of back pain at work. Scand J Work Environ Health 1984; 10:419–428.

21. Manning DP, Mitchell RG, Blanchfield LP. Body movements and events contributing to accidental and non-accidental back injuries. Spine 1984; 7:734–739.

22. Mital D, Channaveeraiah C, Fard HF, Khaledi H. Reliability of repetitive dynamic strengths as a screening tool for manual lifting tasks. Clin Biomechan 1986; 1:125–129.

23. Nordin M, Ortengren R, Andersson GBJ. Measurements of trunk movements during work. Spine 1984; 9:465–469.

24. Griffin AB, Troup JD, Lloyd DCEF. Tests of lifting and handling capacity. Their repeatability and relationship to back symptoms. Ergonomics 1984; 27:305–320.

25. Chaffin DB, Herrin GD, Keyserling WM. Preemployment strength testing: An updated position. J Occup Med 1978; 20:403–408.

26. Linton SJ. The relationship between activity and chronic back pain. Pain 1985; 21:289–294.

27. Fordyce W, McMahon G, Rainwater S, Jackins S et al. Pain complaint—Exercise performance relationship in chronic pain. Pain 1981; 10:311–321.

28. Cady LD, Bischoff DP, O'Connell ER, Thomas PC, Allan JH. Strength and fitness and subsequent back injuries in firefighters. J Occup Med 1979; 21:269–272.

29. Keyserling MW, Herrin GD, Chaffin DB. Isometric strength testing as a means of controlling medical incidents on strenuous jobs. J Occ Med 1980; 22:232–236.

30. Karvonen MJ, Viitasalo JT, Komi PV, Nummi J, Jarvinen T. Back and leg complaints in relation to muscle strength in young men. Scand J Rehab Med 1980; 12:53–59.

31. Nummi J, Jarvinen T, Stambej V, Wickstrom G. Diminished dynamic performance capacity of back and abdominal muscle in concrete reenforcement workers. Scand J Work Environ Health 1978; 4(Suppl 1):40–44.

32. Dictionary of occupational titles. U.S. Employment Service, Employment and Training Administration, U.S. Dept of Labor, 1977. Washington, D.C.

33. Field TF, Field JE. Classification of jobs according to worker trait factors (rev ed). Athens, GA: VDARE Service Bureau, Inc. 1984.

34. Nordin M, Frankel VH. Evaluation of the workplace: An introduction. Clin Orthop 1987; 221:95.

35. Anderson GBJ. Epidemiologic aspects of low back pain in industry. Spine 1981; 6:53–60.

36. Frymoyer JW, Pope MH, Costanza MC et al. Epidemiologic studies of low-back pain. Spine 1980; 5:419–423.

37. Bergenudd H, Neilsson B. Back pain in middle age; Occupational workload and psychologic factors: An epidemiologic survey. Spine 1988; 13:58–60.

38. Cairns D, Mooney V, Crane P. Spinal rehabilitation: Inpatient and outpatient treatment results and development of predictors of outcome. Spine 1984; 9:91–95.

34

FUNCTIONAL RESTORATION OF THE INJURED WORKER

Roy A. Slack

This chapter will reflect the essence of my experience and philosophy, fact and premise, about functional restoration. My position is that of a clinician rather than of a research scientist. My practice has been dedicated, exclusively, to spine and functional restoration for the past 6 years. During that time, I have been privileged to work with a growing team of superb, concerned colleagues. The method of treatment we have developed to effect functional restoration works. There is a strong need for clinicians to reevaluate their treatment, as well as their perception of how spine injuries should be dealt with. New developments in attitudes and methods have made spine care one of the most dynamic, exciting, and evolving areas in medicine.

Somehow, the worker with a low back injury has become a medical enigma, after seen only reluctantly by the physician. It is not unusual for spine specialists either not to see these patients, or to limit the number they will take. This, I believe, is the result of the frustration we have all experienced in having to face an unsatisfactory therapeutic outcome.

The injured worker is the type of patient who has experienced an injury to the spine while performing job-related activities. All of us are aware of the multifaceted challenge this opportunity presents for treatment. The longer the time after injury, the more convoluted the labyrinth from the patient's initial evaluation to return to work. We must recognize in our evaluation that many of these patients are genuinely and with reason burdened with frustration, fear or even terror, and anxiety and are

becoming disillusioned because we "healers" have not been able to heal them.

Functional restoration, in this chapter, refers, quite simply, to the body regaining the ability to satisfactorily perform physically within normal parameters of range of motion, strength, and endurance with safety and stability resulting in the patient's ability to function productively in gainful employment.

Work hardening has been discussed in a previous chapter. Here, the term signifies therapeutic simulation of the physical activities relating to a job.

GOALS

To maximize effectiveness in the functional restorative process, goals must be set and achieved by all concerned. Evaluation of the patient implies comprehensive and accurate physical diagnosis by the physician and the physical therapist. It also must be utilized (according to plan) as the beginning of solid rapport with the patient, emphasizing both diagnostic and therapeutic authoritative concern and competence. Genuinely putting patient needs first in restoring function and creating an atmosphere where the patient is not afraid or embarrassed to ask any question of the physician is vital. Special attention during the history and physical must be paid to ascertaining their level of function or dysfunction in areas such as work ability, activities of daily living, sleep, sex, personal hygiene, recreation, and exercise.

The goal of treatment is to help the patient become physically capable of performing work and thereby capable of providing for himself or herself and family. This can best be accomplished by teaching (intellectually, emotionally, and physically) the patient how to take and gain control of his or her physical problem. Successful realization of this process instills in patients the necessary confidence to get back into life with the knowledge that they can handle ups and downs appropriately. They control their symptoms and their problems.

In this chapter, it is my intent to provide practical information that can be implemented in daily practice. I also strive to raise questions in minds much keener than mine that will result in the continued evolution of our knowledge and the development of increasingly effective methods of treatment. We must more effectively serve the patients to whom we have dedicated our professional lives.

There are numerous sources for statistical data that enumerate the staggering challenge to address this problem more effectively (1, 2).

PHILOSOPHY OF TREATMENT

The primary focus of treatment is on function, rather than on pain or the perception of pain. This treatment direction is most completely described by Mayer (3). Our approach to treatment differs greatly from the traditional medical model. Rehabilitation of these patients has, historically, been ineffective (hence the current statistics). Consequently, until recently, many of the specialists (medical and surgical) have been conditioned through negative experience not to utilize rehabilitation as an important resource in their therapeutic armamentarium. This situation is understandable, but outdated. Functional restorative therapy, utilizing sports medicine techniques applied to the injured spine under the supervision of physical therapists and physicians, has proved to be reliable and provide consistent success. Recently, spine surgeons who have access to this type of therapy consistently utilized it during the diagnostic process, preoperatively, in nonsurgical patients, and postoperatively.

In our clinic, we have not found it necessary to use a multidiscipline approach to treat the majority of our patients successfully, and have tried to reduce treatment to the simplest yet most effective format. Let me add that the majority of patients in our experience have suffered the chronic failed back. Even with this compli-

cated chronic patient, our experience is that a lean, focused approach has been extremely successful. The treatment team consists of patient, physical therapist, physician, and office manager, all playing a vital role. Close supervision by the physical therapist and physician during evaluation, as well as treatment in the clinic, is crucial. We have tried to minimize patient's time, necessary staff, equipment, and modalities, to arrive at a concentrated, focused formula resulting in optimal functional restoration.

Equipment selection requires careful analysis to result in hardware that will not only promote patient safety and encourage us, but that will also actually produce the results expected from the biomechanical standpoint.

Passive physical therapy modalities, i.e., ice, heat, ultrasound, electrostimulation, and soft tissue techniques, provide a valuable adjunct to the core of therapeutic exercise and, when used effectively, enable patients to cross barriers in performance both initially and during their progress in rehabilitation.

DYNAMIC STABILIZATION

Dynamic stabilization is the primary goal of therapy. Its achievement will precede functional restoration. Gracovetsky and Farfan described a "privileged stable zone" in which stress applied to the spine is equalized (4).

Optimal stability of the spine in multiple planes while performing movement is obtained when range of motion is regained, ligamentous integrity is restored, and muscular strength developed so that throughout the normal range of motion symmetrical strength and stability are provided by the muscle-ligament-disc-joint complex. This is the foundation of functional restoration.

Instability of the spine is probably the most common cause of back dysfunction (5–9). To date, most of the attention paid to this condition has been from the surgical perspective. It is my opinion that the symptoms of instability are present with consequent dysfunction well before they are objectively identified and are the result of muscular atrophy and ligamentous laxity. Much work is needed to identify the role of the muscles in this condition. They have been ignored too long. For example, most slides of the functional spinal unit at conference presentations do not include the muscles.

EVALUATION OF THE PATIENT

Initial and reevaluation of the patient must focus on his or her functional ability or degree of dysfunction in addition to parameters normally covered in a routine medical history and physical or physical therapy evaluation. Look for symptoms of instability at rest (static) or during movement (dynamic) and address them in therapy. Range of motion measurements are critical to an accurate functional assessment (10). Equipment includes the Cybex EDI 320 (approx. $600); fluid filled inclinometer (approx. $80); Ace Hardware construction protractor (approx. $8). Whatever you use, learn to use it well and use it consistently. Comparison of initial data with successive measurements is vital in defining progress or identifying problem areas. Precision in measurement provides reproducibility that is diagnostically and therapeutically valid. Toe touching and fingertips to floor are misleading and should not be used.

Trunk Strength

We are now entering an area of controversy. Experience has shown that equipment to measure trunk strength reliably (flexion, extension, rotation), is very expensive. This equipment is not critical or even necessary to provide good rehabilitation. Criteria for selection are reviewed by Mayer (3) and others. In brief, look for function, i.e., does the instrument actually measure trunk muscle strength, which requires isolation of pelvis to eliminate lower extremity musculature and eliminate upper extremity musculature as well. Does the instrument minimize variables to consistently provide measurement of the same muscle group(s). Check on the software and backup guarantees and if there are new products coming from this company.

Our experience has been with static and/or isometric trunk testing using the Nautilus low back and abdominal tensiometers (Fig. 34.1). We have found this type of equipment very useful and safe in our treatment of these patients, especially in dealing with diagnostic and therapeutic challenges, where these machines provide valuable information as well as help with functional capacity ratings.

In other areas of medicine, increasing precision usually translates into more effective treatment. It is reasonable to assume that such will be the case with trunk testing equipment.

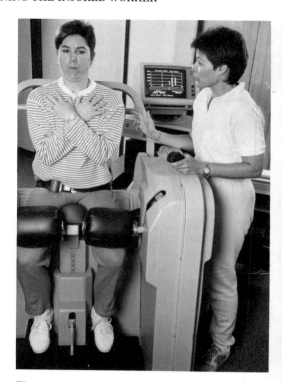

Figure 34.1. Measuring lumbar extensor strength, utilizing the Nautilus Low Back Tensiometer. Test is a series of eight isometric contractions through a 70° range.

There are two major ways to measure: isokinetic and static. Cybex has established a strong position in isokinetic measurement and has developed a large normative database (11, 12). MedX is building a solid reputation with static measurement (13). This is a relatively new area and, as Mayer (3) concludes, we are still learning what we can do with it.

TRUNK TESTING

In our experience, trunk testing has proved to be a useful and appropriate tool. It provides a means of initially evaluating a new patient in a performance-based fashion. This gives a base line of the functional impact of the patient's injury. Normally, we do not test patients who have demonstrated or suspected disc herniations. We do not initially test recent postoperative patients either. However, patients from either of the aforementioned groups will be tested after being treated in the clinic for several visits, depending on their performance and response to therapy.

Careful scrutiny of trunk testing results enables specific modification in a patient's treatment protocol. Periodic retesting (every 3 to 4 weeks) demonstrates progress or problems reliably. The equipment is utilized for therapy as well and allows for specific strengthening of muscles (extensor or flexor) in an area of the curve shown to be particularly deficient.

Trunk testing results are very helpful during a final evaluation, at which point a patient is to be discharged from formal therapy.

Results that conform to our normal values are a reliable indicator of intrinsic functional ability and are included in the patient's final assessment and rating.

Another valuable use of trunk testing equipment is in the evaluation of the efficacy of the patient's maintenance program. Obviously, if strength curves are consistent with exit results, at least one important goal of maintenance is being achieved.

As previously mentioned, this *very costly* trunk testing equipment is not critical for the delivery of good quality rehabilitation. However, in our experience, it can be utilized effectively and efficiently throughout the process of rehabilitation and functional restoration to provide data important to a thorough functional assessment. This controversial aspect of spine rehabilitation has much room for growth and protocols for equipment design and application to clinical use are still being developed.

TREATMENT

Education: Back School

Information presented to the injured worker should be concise, clear, as individually specific as possible, and should conform to the concept of spaced repetition. There should also be a way for the patient to rephrase instruction so that the instructor can be sure of the patient's level of understanding.

Providing information before beginning therapy helps to establish an understanding of what is expected from the patient, as well as to develop a rapport in a nonthreatening environment. Combining education with performance in rehabilitation reinforced by reeducation and performance is most effective.

The primary goals of education are to: 1) create a logical understanding of the structural elements of the spine, of their interaction, and of how their interaction may result in the patient's dysfunction; and 2) provide an informational foundation on which the patient can rebuild the self and restore function. The patient must understand that this rebuilding happens from the inside out. It cannot be done to the patient. The process of helping patients realize that they are controlling their rehabilitation is the cornerstone of long-term success.

Problems are going to arise during treatment. They should be anticipated and means for appropriate response must be prepared. Setting achievable goals of therapy is vital to this process. When a patient is having a significant symptom flare up, often review of these goals can serve as an anchor to help the patient remain focused on improved function and not worry inappropriately about subjective response to pain. This can be a very delicate balance, however, and requires a coordinated effort (and feedback) among the physician, physical therapist, and the patient. Usually, active therapy should continue in spite of symptom flare-ups, with modification of activity. A critical element is to reinforce continued activity in spite of symptoms, rather than to affirm that increased pain necessitates inactivity. The negative feedback cycle must be broken. Improvement can result from careful analysis of the patient's condition, both initial and current, and the design of a progressive functional restoration program. The vital importance of the physician-therapist-patient working relationship must be stressed, thereby allowing for specific activity modification that will maintain range of motion, movement against resistance, and cardiovascular endurance, and promote the healing process.

When this is done within the delicate balance of pushing hard enough to heal but not so hard that symptoms flare up, the patient learns that the road to restored function is through action, not inactivity. The result is that when flare-ups or minor reinjuries occur, the patient knows what to do, how and when, and can continue working with confidence. This is functional restoration.

Attitude

A most critical element is the development in the patient of a positive mental attitude. Consistent effort to develop and maintain this on the part of each member of the treatment team, especially the patient, is essential. Often proven, although sometimes seemingly "corny" methods are available. Be sincere and be creative. Develop and use a reward system. Recognition is a powerful motivator and can easily be utilized. For example, patient photographs on a bulletin board, T-shirts, a round of applause for achievement, gold or silver stars on record, all work! Use them.

Range of Motion

Stretching exercises are a cornerstone of functional restoration. Virtually every patient suffers from severe chronic loss of range of motion. The significance of this has been appreciated by the American Medical Association as seen in their guidelines for disability ratings. Within anatomic or pathologic restrictions imposed by injury, disease, or surgery, we attempt to help our patients regain the maximum range of motion through a closely supervised program of flexibility exercises. Stretching must be progressive, sustained (not ballistic), and repeated. Patients are taught to control discomfort by stretching. This normally is extremely effective. We consider our patients to be athletes and encourage them to stretch before every athletic contest, i.e., vacuuming, mowing the lawn, sleeping, sex, rehabilitation, and working.

Virtually every patient we have seen clinically suffers from weak, tight hamstrings. Proprioceptive neuromuscular facilitation (stretch, contract, relax) is, when used judiciously, probably the most rapid method for regaining range of motion (Fig. 34.2).

From the first day of treatment, the patient is trained with reinforcement that stretching must be performed twice daily—forever. It works. In follow-up, range-of-motion measurements are a reliable indicator of how consistently a patient is adhering to the maintenance program. This is one of the most important tools for short-term relief and long-term survival our patients learn.

Strength

Muscular strength is a major element in dynamic stabilization. Stability throughout the range of motion of a joint complex is the product of muscular strength, and of integrity of the ligaments and capsular elements which maintain the appropriate relationship of the joint surfaces. In the spine, the complexity of the ligamentous network is striking. The role played by the intervertebral disc also provides a challenge to understanding function versus dysfunction.

Increasing strength conservatively is one of the easier variables to improve. Results can be impressive. Methods for and effects of increasing muscular strength have been studied and reported extensively (14–16). Functionally, the

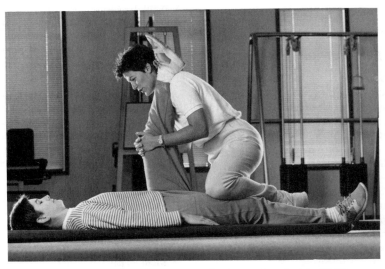

Figure 34.2.   Stretch-contract-relax hamstring stretch (PNF).

spine reacts like any other musculoligamentous articular complex. Restoring a balance of increased range of motion, improved strength, and increased endurance results in increased function and a decrease of symptoms. This can be accomplished with a variety of formats.

Equipment

Nautilus and Eagle are two industry leaders. However, everyone has a favorite. Virtually any type of strength-training equipment will work if used properly. In general, look for ease of use, biomechanical validity, affordability, guarantee, maintenance needs, and manufacturer's track record in responding to problems.

We use a combination of brands, including free weights, in an effort to provide resistance exercises with body part isolation or integration, as desired. A closely supervised (by physical therapist and physician) program of progressive resistance including isotonic and isometric as well as manually resisted exercises is designed for each patient. Depending on the patient's abilities and needs, repetitions will vary from six to twenty, sets from one to three, with exercises performed on an every-other-day schedule. Advances are made through a combination of increasing weights and maintaining reps, maintaining weight and increasing reps, decreasing weights and increasing reps, and increasing weights and decreasing reps. Additionally, the number of sets is also modified. In concert with therapeutic exercises, passive modalities (i.e., ice, ultrasound), are added to maximize performance and minimize complaints and or symptoms.

The typical patient in this setting suffers from a chronic injury and exemplifies the "deconditioning syndrome." Our initial focus is thus on muscle groups isolated from the injured area, beginning with a general approach and subsequently progressing to a specific focus. When the patient performs therapeutic exercises and works up a sweat, endorphin release is promoted, which contributes to helping the patient break through the "invalid psychosis" and begin to develop a sense of physical ability and well-being. We all feel better immediately after exercising, so therapy is reinforced with feeling better, which lends support to the patient's hope that maybe this treatment program will be effective.

This process of strengthening is one of the most challenging parts of the functional restorative process. It is vital to success, yet is widely misunderstood and typically not respected by physicians. Usually, it is regarded with the same attitude as PE class or a health club. That is like comparing a dime store periscope to a fiber optic arthroscope. Moreover, if strengthening is regarded superficially, it will be boring to the therapy staff, who will not realize significant professional challenge or growth; the patient will lose. Therapeutic strengthening should be viewed as, and understood to be, a highly skilled application of diagnostic and therapeutic ability. This attitude will translate into maximum patient benefit as well as professional stimulation and gratification with neverending challenges and rewards.

Imperative in this area is providing the patient with a system of progressive successes and self-generated feedback supported by the medical staff in a secure and positive environment. Many of the subtleties that result in obstacles to successful therapeutic outcomes stem from deep-seated frustration, fears, anxieties, low self-esteem, and insecurities, all of which are natural for the injured worker to feel. A very effective way of dealing with these feelings is to put patients in an active setting where they are guided to gain control of their situation by doing something physical. Teach them to get better with physical therapy or sports medicine in a secure environment. Give them a ladder to climb with clear goals, success indicators, and rewards. They will walk, run, and then soar. Professionally, we as clinicians also need and deserve the rewards of helping our patients make a strongly positive impact on their lives.

Stabilization is the foundation of this entire process. Initially, the patient must be taught to stabilize the spine to minimize symptoms. As therapeutic progress is accomplished, dynamic stabilization predominates. The result is that through the physical process, the patient restores stability to his or her life.

Endurance

Usually, the injured worker needs to return to an 8-hour per day (at least) job. Being strong for 1 or 2 hours, then collapsing for the rest of the shift is not good enough. Increasing muscular strength enhances muscular endurance. Increasing cardiovascular endurance enhances sustained muscular performance (17–19). A useful therapeutic tool for this is the Schwinn Airdyne bicycle ergometer. It is less boring than many stationary cycles and the breeze is enjoyable to the rider. Aerobically, it has been proven to be very effective.

Maintenance—Step·down

There is life after rehab! The protected environment created for our patients must provide a means for transition back to the real world, as well as a system for maintenance and follow-up.

Partly this means helping the patient develop a program of exercise consistent with his or her personality, lifestyle, and real needs, a program that we can realistically expect the patient to practice faithfully. If behavioral changes must be made, they should be minimal. We should not expect our patients to completely change their lifestyles.

Some patients will make the transition into a health club setting, others will invest in extensive home exercise equipment. Most patients will do much less. Functional restoration is a lifelong process, not a finite goal that, when achieved, can be assumed to be complete. In our experience, twice-daily stretching is the minimum that a patient can do and expect good results. This means performing vigorous stretching exercises for 20 to 40 minutes at each of two daily sessions. The patient should be taught how to incorporate the stretching exercises into a normal routine, as during relaxation, while watching TV, on the job during break time, and while on the phone. We have struggled to come up with a program that will at least maintain and possibly continue to increase new-found trunk strength. At present, we are using a Roman chair and a system of latex tubing and plastic handles called "Lifeline" to develop a home program. This is an evolution, however. For an investment of $250 to $300 a patient can have the means to continue therapeutic exercises at home in a way that can realistically be expected to provide the desired results. Depending on the case, we will progressively taper treatments in the clinic so as to wean the patient from a medically supervised setting to independance. Vital to this process are regular follow-up evaluations, with range-of-motion measurements and, if possible, measurements of trunk strength. Such follow-up is normally accomplished with visits at intervals of 3 weeks to 2 months for 6 months to 1 year, or longer, if indicated. Spine-related dysfunction in this regard more closely approximates hypertension or diabetes than appendicitis.

SUMMARY

Functional restoration of the injured worker is a multifaceted challenge, which, when accomplished, provides tremendous rewards. In the typical chronic patient, the level of intensity applied to treatment is crucial to successful results. The spine responds to vigorous efforts at physical rehabilitation and should be treated carefully, but intensively. Open communication among the patient, physical therapist, and physician **must** occur continuously and in an atmosphere of trust, confidence, and mutual respect. Traditional approaches have for the most part failed and should not cloud the thinking of clinicians.

Our focus in therapy is to restore, as fully as possible, the body's ability to function with stability within the limits of its design and thereby to regain the physical integrity to function at the job site, doing not only routine tasks, but also being physically capable of withstanding the unusual events (accidents, falls) that most often result in injuries. In order to completely fulfill the expectations of a work hardening prescription, we must closely evaluate reality. What actually happened to precipitate this patient's injury? Not only the incident, but the self-inflicted lifestyle disease of deconditioning that may have set the stage for injury must be considered.

What methods of evaluation are going to provide a clear insight into the patient's physical condition when there is not a clear-cut surgical diagnosis? What methods of treatment are going to be the most effective in actually helping the patient in the transition from injured worker to functionally restored worker? How can we not only effect this transition, but maintain it?

We are driven by these questions. As clinicians, our focus must be on keeping both our feet on the ground and helping our patients do the same. Action yields results. Our skill in providing our patients with a course of action through which they can achieve the desired results of functional integrity will be rewarded by the positive result we will effect.

References

1. Frymoyer JW et al. Functional restoration with behavioral support. Spine 1989; 14(2):157–161.
2. Bigos J et al. Back injuries in industry: A retrospective study. Spine 1986; 11(3):241–251.
3. Mayer T, Gatchel R, Febinger L. Functional restoration for spinal disorders: The sports medicine approach. 1988
4. Gracovetsky S, Farfan H. The optimum spine. Spine 1986; 11(6):543–573.
5. Kirkaldy-Willis WH. Presidential symposium on instability of the lumbar spine. Spine 1985; 10(3):254.
6. Kirkaldy-Willis WH. Radiologic diagnosis of degenerative instability. Spine 1985; 10(3):262–276.
7. Gertzbein SD et al. Centrode patterns and segmental instability in degenerative disc disease. Spine 1985; 10(3):257–261.
8. Paris SV. Physical signs of instability. Spine 1985; 10(3):277–279.
9. Nachemson A. Lumbar spine instability. Spine 1985; 10(3):290–291.
10. Mayer T. Using physical measurements to assess low back pain. J Musc Med 1985; 2(6):44–59.
11. Mayer TG, Mooney V, Gatchell RJ, Smith SS et al. Quantification of lumbar function, Part I and Part II. Spine 1985; 10(8):757–772.
12. Mayer TG, Mooney V, Gatchell RJ et al. 1985 Volvo award in clinical sciences, objective assessment of spine function following industrial injury. Spine 1985; 10(6):482–493.
13. Pollock ML et al. Effective resistance training on lumbar extension strength. Submitted for publication: Am J Sports Med.
14. Berger RA. Comparative effects of three weight-training programs. Res Q 1963; 35:396–398.
15. Hickson RC, Rosenkoetter MA, Brown MM. Strength training effects on aerobic power and short-term endurance. Med Sci Sports Exerc 1980; 12:336–339.
16. Fleck SJ, Falkel JE. Value of resistance training for the reduction of sports injuries. Sports Med 1986; 3:61–68.
17. Stone MH, Wilson GD, Blessing D, Rozenek R. Cardiovascular responses to short-term Olympic style weight training in young men. Can J Appl Sports Sci 1983; 8:134–139.
18. Stone MH, Pierce K, Godsen R et al. Weight training: A scientific approach. Minneapolis: Burgess International, 1987.
19. Rodahl K, Astrand P. Textbook of work physiology. New York: McGraw-Hill, 1970.

35

FUNCTIONAL AND WORK CAPACITY EVALUATION

Patrick P. Venditti

PRESENT NEED FOR CAPACITY ASSESSMENTS

You have been treating Eugene Davies of the A. Z. Smith Co. The employee sustained a severe lumbosacral sprain/strain because of a lifting injury at work. His improvement through your treatment regimen has progressed slowly but positively. He has been off work for approximately 2 months. In your best judgement as his physician, you feel he is ready to return to work. Because of his 2-month layoff, you send him back to work with a note to place him on restricted duty. You anticipate that this restricted duty may last 2 to 4 weeks and then the employee should be able to return to regular duty work. Your responsibilities as a treating physician have been met.

If this were 1980, the above scenario would have been readily accepted by the employer and the workers' compensation carrier as standard operating procedure. Your recommendation would have been reluctantly accepted, but further demands for substantiation or documentation would in all likelihood not have been made. Today, this picture is rapidly changing. With the cost of workers' compensation claims steadily rising each year and a larger portion of that cost nipping away at a company's bottom line, companies and insurance carriers are taking a more aggressive and active role in the monitoring and tracking of their employee injuries. To this end, more and more companies that pay the bill for medical treatment, diagnosis, and rehabilitation are questioning the opinions of the physicians. The days of carte

blanche acceptance are fading. Physicians are being asked and, in some instances, required to substantiate their recommendations and findings. Functional and work capacity testing is rapidly becoming a requested procedure both for preemployment and return-to-work assessments.

DEFINITION

Functional capacity in its simplest sense is the testing and assessment of a person to determine ability to perform certain predetermined functions. In the broadest definition, these functions would incorporate activities that occur both on and off the job. The ability to perform activities of daily living is often incorporated in a functional capacity assessment.

Work capacity evaluation is a specific subset of functional capacity assessment. In this instance, a person is tested for ability to perform those functions that are required by the job. In preemployment, this means determining whether or not a person has the physical and mental ability to perform a job function adequately and safely without risk of incurring an injury. For return to work, it is the postinjury assessment of whether the worker can return to his regular job without risk of reinjury.

Companies that have experienced increased costs from injuries of new hirees or recurring injuries of returning workers are anticipating the benefits and advantages that functional and work capacity assessments will provide. The hope is that they will reduce costs by screening out people with greater risk for injury and determine whether a returning worker can meet the physical demands of the job.

REQUIREMENTS

There are several criteria that should be met in performing any quantitative tests for functional and work capacity. These were defined by Chaffin (1, 2) and outlined in the NIOSH Work Practices Guide (3). The results from functional and work capacity testing affect the selection process—hiring, placement, or rehabilitation.

1. Safety of administration—Any procedure or test used to quantify functional or work capacity should be safe and pose no hazard to the subject.
2. Relationship to job requirements—Current federal legislation (4, 5) concerning equal employment opportunity requires that any test for employment including but not limited to hiring, promotion, demotion, membership, referral, retention, licensing and certification, and selection for training or transfer be related to the job.
3. Reliability—Tests used to determine capacity should be reproducible. A common measure of this is the coefficient of variation of the repeated tests, which is the standard deviation of the repeated values divided by their mean value. The coefficients of variation should range from between 5 to 15% (6–8).
4. Prediction of future illness or injury—The ultimate test of any medical selection or testing system is its ability to predict which people are at the highest risk of becoming injured. Functional and work capacity assessments in turn should be able to adequately predict the range of performance a person is capable of withstanding without risk of injury.
5. Practicality—The tests should require minimum hardware expense, be capable of simulating different job conditions, require minimum time to administer, and require minimum instruction and learning time.

Before performing an assessment on any person, the physical demand of the job should be determined. It would be nice if we could just contact the place of employment and ask for a physical demand schedule of all the jobs in the facility or at least of this patient's particular job. Alas, as welcome as this information would be, it is often not readily available. Many companies don't know what the specific physical demands of their jobs are. Health care professionals with a good background in biomechanics may be able to assist a company by visiting the site and performing an analysis of the particular job in question.

Site visits not only enhance communication efforts with industry but give the health care provider firsthand knowledge of the physical demands imposed upon the patient. The practitioner will have a better idea of which tests would establish the patient's ability to return to work. In addition, a tour of the facility might also enable the health care professional to observe other job tasks with lesser physical demands. These might well suit the patient's present functional capacity and permit a quicker return to a productive role in society.

Figure 35.1 shows a form that can be used to determine the physical demands of the job. It takes approximately 10 minutes to make a good estimate of the job's physical demand requirements by careful observation of the various tasks involved.

Visiting the job site, however, may not be possible for most health care professionals. They must depend upon the perception of their patients to determine their job's physical demand. Figure 35.2 is a form that should be sent to the employer and simultaneously filled out by the patient at the beginning of the treatment regimen. When the physician or therapist has a good idea of the physical demands of the job, functional capacity testing can proceed.

JOB-SPECIFIC TESTING CRITERIA

The primary purpose of functional capacity assessments is to determine the ability to return to work. Therefore, the test parameters must be designed to incorporate relevant work activities and functional tasks representative of the stresses on the job.

Our initial example, Eugene, has recovered from a back injury. He has reached a point of medical maximum improvement. His job requirements, which were ascertained from his form as well as from information supplied by his employer, define the physical demands shown in Table 35.1.

From the description given of the physical demands of the job we could classify it as "heavy work." From the ergonomics guide of the

WORKSITE ANALYSIS SURVEY FORM

Department [   ]   Date [   ]

Job [   ]

Task [   ]

General Description of Job:

Work Hours: Start _____Finish_____ Average Hours [   ] Days[   ]

Hourly ☐ Piecework ☐ Number of Shifts_____ Breaks per shift_____Length_____

Production schedule: #[   ] per hour ☐ per shift ☐   Overtime per week [   ]
How often?

	Physical Demands				
1	1° Static some Dynamic	1° Dynamic some Static		Static then Dynamic	
2	Standing	none	< 25% (shift)	25-50%(shift)	>50% (shift)
3	Walking	none	< 25% (shift)	25-50%(shift)	>50% (shift)
4	Sitting	none	< 25% (shift)	25-50%(shift)	>50% (shift)
5	Twisting☐ Bending ☐	none	< 25% (shift)	25-50%(shift)	>50% (shift)
	Flexion ☐ Extension ☐	none	< 25% (shift)	25-50%(shift)	>50% (shift)
	Lateral ☐ R☐ L☐	none	< 25% (shift)	25-50%(shift)	>50% (shift)
6	Pushing	none	< 25% (shift)	25-50%(shift)	>50% (shift)
7	Pulling	none	< 25% (shift)	25-50%(shift)	>50% (shift)
8	Reaching above shoulder Hgt.	none	< 25% (shift)	25-50%(shift)	>50% (shift)
	Forward ☐ Right ☐				
	Side ☐ Left ☐				
9	Reaching at shoulder height	none	< 25% (shift)	25-50%(shift)	>50% (shift)
	Forward ☐ Right ☐				
	Side ☐ Left ☐				
10	Reaching below shoulder Hgt.	none	< 25% (shift)	25-50%(shift)	>50% (shift)
	Forward ☐ Right ☐				
	Side ☐ Left ☐				
11	Head/Neck position				
	Extension	none	< 25% (shift)	25-50%(shift)	>50% (shift)
	Flexion	none	< 25% (shift)	25-50%(shift)	>50% (shift)
	Lateral flexion R ☐ L☐	none	< 25% (shift)	25-50%(shift)	>50% (shift)
	Rotation R ☐ L☐	none	< 25% (shift)	25-50%(shift)	>50% (shift)

© 1985 P. Venditti, D.C.

Figure 35.1 Worksite Analysis Survey Form.

American Industrial Hygiene Association (9; see Table 35.2), we would expect the total energy expenditure to be about 7.5–10.0 kcal/min with heart rate ranging from 125 to 150 beats per minute.

Upon questioning Mr. Davies further, we find out that rest breaks are given every 2 hours for 15 minutes. There are essentially no substantial pauses during the work shift. The time cycles spent in loading vary according to the work demands. Some days workers load a full 8 hours; on other days, they may only spend 2

12	Right Shoulder motion	Flexion	Extension	Abd.	Add.
		Int. Rot.	Ext. Rot.		
	frequency	none	< 5 min	5-20 min.	> 20 min.
	duration	none	< 5 min	5-20 min.	> 20 min.
13	Left Shoulder motion	Flexion	Extension	Abd.	Add.
		Int. Rot.	Ext. Rot.		
	frequency	none	< 5 min	5-20 min.	> 20 min.
	duration	none	< 5 min	5-20 min.	> 20 min.
14	Left Forearm motion	Flexion	Extension	Pron.	Supin.
	frequency	none	< 5 min	5-20 min.	> 20 min.
	duration	none	< 5 min	5-20 min.	> 20 min.
15	Right Forearm motion	Flexion	Extension	Pron.	Supin.
	frequency	none	< 5 min	5-20 min.	> 20 min.
	duration	none	< 5 min	5-20 min.	> 20 min.
16	Right Hand/wrist motion	Dorsiflex.	Palmar	Ulnar	Radial
	frequency	none	< 5 min	5-20 min.	> 20 min.
	duration	none	< 5 min	5-20 min.	> 20 min.
17	Left Hand/wrist motion	Dorsiflex.	Palmar	Ulnar	Radial
	frequency	none	< 5 min	5-20 min.	> 20 min.
	duration	none	< 5 min	5-20 min.	> 20 min.
18	Finger Manipulations	none	pressing	holding	picking
	frequency	none	< 5 min	5-20 min.	> 20 min.
	duration	none	< 5 min	5-20 min.	> 20 min.
19	Lifting- one ☐ two ☐ hand	none	< 10 #	10-25-50#	> 50#
	frequency	none	< 5 min	5-20 min.	> 20 min.
	duration	none	< 5 min	5-20 min.	> 20 min.
	distance	none	< 10 feet	10-30 feet	> 30 feet
20	Carry - one ☐ two ☐ hand	none	< 10 #	10-25-50#	> 50#
	frequency	none	< 5 min	5-20 min.	> 20 min.
	duration	none	< 5 min	5-20 min.	> 20 min.
	distance	none	< 10 feet	10-30 feet	> 30 feet
21	Grip Strength RO☐ LO☐	insignificant	< 25 #	25-50#	> 50#
	frequency	none	< 5 min	5-20 min.	> 20 min.
	duration	none	< 5 min	5-20 min.	> 20 min.
22	Pinch Strength RO☐ LO☐	insignificant	< 10 #	10-25#	>25#
	frequency	none	< 5 min	5-20 min.	> 20 min.
	duration	none	< 5 min	5-20 min.	> 20 min.
23	Tools used	none			
24	Vehicles used	none			

Figure 35.1. (continued)

hours loading and unloading, with the rest of the time spent in various physically easier warehouse tasks.

Most traditional medical examination procedures won't help you render an opinion as to Mr. Davies' fitness to return to his normal work duties. These procedures are designed to determine freedom from symptomatology or freedom of motion without exacerbation of symptoms. In order to make a work-fitness determination, other performance factors must be assessed. Several characteristics have been previously se-

Job Description

1. Job Title _____

2. Brief Description of Tasks Performed _____

    _____

    _____

3. Shift Hours: _____ Hours per day _____

4. Production Schedule _____

5. Rate of Pay: ____ Hourly   _____ Incentive (Piecework)

    _____

    _____

Figure 35.2. Job Description Form.

Table 35.1

Physical Demands	
Job Title:	Warehouse Operator
Employee:	Eugene Davies
Standing	greater than 50% of his workshift
Carrying	greater than 50% of his workshift weight between 50–70#, 5 times a minute, for a distance of 10–30 feet.
Walking	greater than 50% of his workshift
Lifting	waist level and from waist to above shoulder height, greater than 50% of the workshift.
Reaching Bilateral	Forward from below to above the shoulder height, greater than 50% of the workshift, 5 times a minute, arms fully extended with weights 50–70 lbs

Table 35.2

Class of activity	Range for class	
	Energy expenditure kcal/min	Heart rate beats/min
Rest, sitting	1.5	60–70
Very light work	1.6–2.5	65–75
Light work	2.5–5.0	75–100
Moderate work	5.0–7.5	100–125
Heavy work	7.5–10.0*	125–150
Very heavy work	10.0–12.5*	150–180
Unduly heavy work	over 12.5*	180+

*rest pauses are necessary
Note: This was devised for reasonably fit men. Corresponding rates for women are 10–15 beats higher.

How much time during the workshift is spent:

	NONE	<2 HRS	2-4 HRS	4-6 HRS	>6 HRS
6. STANDING	_____	_____	_____	_____	_____
7. SITTING	_____	_____	_____	_____	_____
8. WALKING	_____	_____	_____	_____	_____
9. LIFTING	_____	_____	_____	_____	_____

a) Heaviest weight lifted? _____

b) Most frequently lifted weight? _____

c) Types of materials lifted? _____

d) Where materials are lifted from? Floor ____ Pallet ___ Shelf ____

    Box/Bin _____   Other _____

e) How many boxes, etc. are picked up per minute? _____

Figure 35.2.   (continued)

lected as representative of the spectrum of physical performance factors thought to be job related (1, 2, 10–15; see Table 35.3). We can now design an assessment that will enable us to determine the capacity of the employee to return to work without the risk of injury.

DESIGN OF THE FUNCTIONAL CAPACITY EVALUATION

The design of the functional and work capacity evaluation should be tailored to suit the capabilities required to perform a job task successfully. In addition to the physical performance factors listed in Table 35.3, a psychological measurement of the employee's capacities is advocated.

Perception of Functional Capacity and Disability

In the case of an employee who is returning to work after a substantial time off work (6 weeks or longer), an estimate of the person's perception of both disability and capacity is important. All the quantitative data collected to substantiate a person's capacity for work will not be predictive if that person's own perception is

		NONE	2 hrs.	2-4 hrs.	4-6 hrs.	6 hrs.
10.	Carrying	_____	_____	_____	_____	_____

    a) How far are materials carried? < 10 ft. ____ 10-30 ft. ____ > 30 ft. ____

    b) How much weight is normally carried? _____

11.	BENDING/					
12.	TWISTING	_____	_____	_____	_____	_____
13.	PUSHING	_____	_____	_____	_____	_____
14.	PULLING	_____	_____	_____	_____	_____

15.   Do you reach above your shoulder during your job? _____

16.   What is your head/neck position? looking up ___ down ___ straight ahead ___

17.   Do you do repetitive motion tasks with your hands? _____

18.   Do you do tasks which require finger manipulations? _____

19.   Do you do jobs which require you to use grip strength? _____

20.   Do you do jobs which require pinch strength? _____

Figure 35.2. (continued)

of limited capabilities and an exacerbation of pain and restriction in the performance of certain tasks.

The Oswestry Low back Pain Disability Questionnaire (16) is an excellent tool in determining a person's perceived functional capacity and disability. This questionnaire is divided into ten sections designed to assess limitations of various activities of daily living. Each section has six statements from which the one statement that most closely describes the problem must be selected. Each section is scored from 0 to 5.

All ten scores are then added up, divided by the total possible score and then multiplied by 100 to give a per cent. The higher the score, the higher the disability. Because this questionnaire is an attempt to quantify a patient's sub-

21. Do you use any tools? ____   What are they? _____

_____

22. Do you use any vehicles? _____ What are they? _____

23. Briefly describe what physical demands do you feel your job places on your

body?

_____

_____

_____

_____   _____

Patient Signature   Date

Figure 35.2. (continued)

jective perception of ability, it should not be used in isolation but as a guide to the individual's placement and future treatment and rehabilitation goals. There are other psychological measurements that can be utilized as an aid in assessing an individual disability and capacity profile. The pain chart (17), Visual Analog Scale, and Hendler's screen for chronic low back pain are just a few examples.

Table 35.3
Physical Performance Factors.

Static strength
Dynamic strength
Endurance
   a) cardiopulmonary
   b) muscular
Range of motion
   a) Muscular
   b) Joint
Work speed
Coordination
Balance
Safety

STRENGTH

When we think of functional capacity we usually think of the strength required to complete a task. How much can a person lift or pull or push or carry? It has been determined that people without the basic strengths required for their jobs have a higher potential for injury (6, 18, 19). The problem in functional capacity is how to assess this strength.

The type of strength utilized in job tasks is isotonic. This incorporates variable speeds and torque output. Isometric testing can give us values equivalent to an individual's maximum voluntary contraction (MVC) and isokinetic testing can provide torque values. Neither is directly correlated with realistic dynamic strengths.

Static Strength

Static strength testing was originally utilized by Chaffin and colleagues as a method for determining employee selection procedures. As Chaffin describes it, isometric strength testing

FUNCTIONAL AND WORK CAPACITY ASSESSMENT

SYNOPSIS

DATE: AUGUST 23, 1988

NAME: EUGENE DAVIES

COMPANY: A. Z. SMITH CO.

JOB TITLE: WAREHOUSE OPERATOR

DATE OF INJURY: JUNE 12, 1988

TYPE OF INJURY: LIFTING SPRAIN/STRAIN

DIAGNOSIS: LUMBOSACRAL SPRAIN/STRAIN

REFERRING PHYSICIAN: DR. J. HOULDEN

TOTAL TIME OFF WORK: 9 WEEKS

APPLICABLE SURGERY: N/A

PRIOR TREATMENT: N/A

CURRENT MEDICATIONS: NAPROSYN, prn

Figure 35.3. Sample Assessment Forms.

involves the exertion of a force in a given posture against a fixed resistance (1, 2). He further defines it as "the maximal force muscles can exert isometrically in a single voluntary effort" (24). Isometric strength testing was chosen because it was determined to be a safe procedure and fit the criteria originally developed by Chaffin and detailed above.

Dynamic testing (such as lifting a totebox filled with steel shot) was not utilized because

PATIENT REPORT

PAIN AND DISABILITY ASSESSMENT

PAIN CHART

Patient indicates sharp pain across the low back with numbness and tingling radiating into posterior thigh and buttocks. Pain does not cross the knee. Anatomic representation is good. No excessive or exaggerated remarks are indicated in the pain drawing.

Visual Analog Scale

3.4 out of 10

Oswestry Low Back Pain Questionnaire

16% — indicates minimal impairment

The patient exhibits episodic pain and discomfort in his low back which he attributes to "overdoing it". The parameters used to assess his perception of his pain and disability indicate a "Mild Impairment". If his physical capacities meet job demands this is not expected to restrict a full return to work status.

Figure 35.3.   (continued)

it was felt that it would expose the individual to the hazards of dropping the object and the dynamic stresses imposed by the motion imparted to the object. In studies conducted using static strength testing versus other, more traditional medical criteria (e.g., age, gender, somatotype, muscular atrophy, skeletal anomalies, clinical impressions, and radiologic findings), static strength testing predicted three times the incidence of reported injuries (6, 18, 19). Studies done since 1974 have given us substantial data. Equipment for this type of testing is currently becoming available to the health care profession. Many of these instruments incorporate

PHYSICAL CAPACITIES ASSESSMENT

___XXX___   STATIC STRENGTH

                   Six lifting parameters as outlined by NIOSH were
                   performed on a Dynatron 2000 Static Strength Testing
                   Device. Coefficient-of-Variation ranged between 2.2 and
                   8.3%. Test results indicate patient has static strength
                   within the physical requirements of his job.

___XXX___   DYNAMIC STRENGTH

                   A simulated task was performed for a duration of fifteen
                   minutes. 50# sacks were lifted from a pallet to a shelf
                   fifteen feet away. Rate was 12 sacks per minute. Patient
                   ranged from 14 to 8 sacks a minute with a mean of 10.
                   patient did not complain of pain or fatigue through the
                   test procedure.

___XXX___   ENDURANCE

                   A)HEART RATE

                   A Vitalog Heart Rate recording monitor was used during
                   the simulated task. Heart rate peaked at 130 beats per
                   minute with an average of 110. This indicates a level
                   within the demands of his job.

Figure 35.3. (continued)

the NIOSH standards both for testing procedure as well as interpretation of data. In addition, some offer computerized analysis of coefficient of variation to make the validity of test-retest attempts easier to calculate.

Static strength testing is only one test parameter that has been demonstrated to meet requirements for functional and work capacity testing. Since it does not adequately simulate realistic job requirements, it has, and will continue to, come under criticism (25). Until a testing procedure is developed, studied, and deter-

XXX

B) MUSCULAR

Static Torso strength (MVC) done prior to simulated task was recorded as 180 lbs. Recorded immediately after the task it was 165 with a coefficient-of-variation between two tests of 3.7%. This is 91% of his MVC and within expected norms.

___XXX___

RANGE OF MOTION

All ranges of motion taken with a Leighton Inclinometer were within normal limits for lumbar spine as established by the American Academy of Orthopedic Surgeons.

___XXX___

WORK SPEED

During the simulated tasks, the patient had an average rate of 10 sacks per minute. This is 2 sacks per minute less than the job requirement. JOB CONDITIONING SHOULD BE A PART OF THIS EMPLOYEE'S RETURN-TO-WORK.

___XXX___

COORDINATION & BALANCE

Moberg's Pick-up and the Minnesota Pegboard tests were done for manual dexterity. Performance was within normal limits. Tests for balance were not performed.

Figure 35.3. **(continued)**

mined to fit the criteria of realistic job simulation, static strength testing will remain a valid and safe strength measurement procedure for functional and work capacity where lifting is the physical demand.

Dynamic Strength

Several attempts have been made to develop dynamic lifting tests, since dynamic lifting rep-resents a better simulation of the actual job requirements (10, 11). Sophisticated machinery for testing dynamic strength (isotonic, isoki-netic, and isodynamic) has been on the market for some time. Unfortunately, there have been no studies to date showing the effectiveness of dynamic strength testing as a predictive mea-sure for workplace injuries (20). However, com-parisons of isokinetic and isometric tests indicate consistencies and reproducible rela-

XXX   SAFETY

Lifting and safety procedures were observed during the
simulated task. During the beginning of the lifting the
patient exhibited caution and lifting behavior which
would serve to protect the lumbar spine. As the task
progressed, especially when the he was below the
established rate, his techniques involved more twisting
and jerking motions. Job training on protective lifting
procedures should be established.

FINAL STATUS: FULL RETURN TO WORK.

TWO WEEK CONDITIONING PERIOD WHERE THE RATE IS DECREASED
TO 8 SACKS PER MINUTE AND THEN INCREASED UNTIL HE IS AT
THE PRODUCTION RATE OF 12 PER MINUTE WITHIN TWO WEEKS.
SINCE THE WAREHOUSE OPERATION IS NOT MACHINE REGULATED
THIS REQUIREMENT SHOULD NOT BE DIFFICULT TO MEET.

JOB TRAINING IN PROTECTIVE LIFTING PROCEDURES.

Figure 35.3. (continued)

tionships between the two tests (21). This area of testing holds significant promise for the future.

ENDURANCE

Cardiopulmonary

Physical work capacity has also been defined by Kamon and Ayoub as the physiological mechanisms that underlie the performance, using large muscle groups in rhythmic contractions (22).

An assessment then of work capacity could be based upon aerobic capacity (VO_2 max). As work load increases, the demand for oxygen consumption also increases. With moderate to heavy work, this increase in oxygen consumption has a linear relationship with heart rate. Job demand classifications have been devised based upon these demands (9; see Table 35.2).

Tests to determine oxygen consumption are somewhat difficult to perform in an office or at the job itself. Other methods based upon heart rate have been found that correlate with VO_2 consumption. The heart rate accompanying performance of work is a function of individual physical fitness, demands of the work, and overlying environmental stresses. A continually increasing rate over the course of a shift while the same task is being performed is usually accompanied by development of symptoms of fatigue (22).

The meaning of a particular heart rate in terms of relative strain for an individual is quite consistent (9, 22). Thus, if a worker after being tested exhibits a heart rate of 150 beats per minute, the work done may be classified as moderately heavy or heavy for this worker, even if the level of work is classified as light for a fit person.

Systems for making such predictions have been developed by Astrand and others (23). In addition, the heart rate of a man or woman who is physically fit may be used to rate the relative physical demands of a particular job. Several instruments are available for testing in offices, including the cycle ergometer, the motor-driven treadmill, and the stepping stool. Standards have been adopted in the use of ergometers in testing (22).

The bicycle ergometer is most effective when resistance to pedaling instead of speed is changed. The standard testing range for pedaling speed is 50 to 60 rpm while the standard resistance expressed in watts is 100. The Aerobicycle by Universal has a built-in computerized fitness test that compares the results with a 10,000-person database compiled by the YMCA. Other ergometers can supply similar data. The motor-driven treadmill can be adjusted either for speed or for incline. The optimal walking speeds are 4.8 km/hr (3 mph) for females and 5.6 km/hr (3.5 mph) for males. The incline can be changed when change in workload is desired. An angle up to 25% is acceptable. The height of a stepping stool should be between 15 and 20 cm (6–8 in) and the stepping frequency between 12 and 30 steps per minute. Most tests range from 8 to 10 minutes. The heart rate will usually plateau during that time and can be used as a measurement of fitness.

Although an aerobic capacity test will provide information regarding the overall fitness level, it will not indicate the ability to perform the specific requirements of the job. It is necessary to measure the heart rate either on the job or in a simulated task. For example, Eugene is placed in a job simulation task where he picks up 50-lb sacks from floor height and carries them 15 feet to a shelf at shoulder height. His heart rate is 180 beats per minute. This would classify him as performing very heavy work. A job analysis of the company where Eugene works shows that workers with the same job classification had heart rates during this task of 110 to 150. So it is a safe assumption that Eugene has lost some aerobic capacity to perform his normal duties and needs additional conditioning before returning to full work status.

Muscular

In most jobs where the frequency of the task is part of the requirement, known as repetitive motion tasks, muscular endurance plays an important role. As muscles tire they are less able to perform. The worker will compensate for this fatigue by incorporating other muscle groups and various altered postures and motions to complete the assigned task. This puts stress on other structural systems and could lead to eventual injury. The measurement of aerobic capacity is usually a good indicator of endurance.

Another test parameter under consideration and based upon physiological considerations is pre- and postactivity static strength measurement (4). For example, a worker who demonstrates a static strength torso lift of 150 lbs is asked to perform a job simulation task of lifting 50-lb bags for 10 minutes at ten contractions per minute. Immediately upon completion, the worker is retested for static strength capacity. Studies have indicated that this person should maintain at least 80% of MVC (26–28). Since 50-lb bags are only ⅓ of tested MVC, we would expect the worker to be within 80% of the original 150 lbs, or at 120 lbs. The retest gives us a static strength of 85 lbs. As this is only 56% of original MVC, we could conclude, therefore, that after only 10 minutes of work, muscular endurance decreased by 44%.

If would be safe to assume that this worker lacks the muscular endurance to safely perform the intended task. No studies have yet been established to determine the predictability of this type of testing and caution must always be exercised when dynamic work tasks are being simulated.

Range of Motion

Range of motion usually indicates the level of flexibility an individual possesses. Although this is one parameter that is the primary focus for impairment rating through the AMA and the American Academy of Orthopedic Surgeons, it has not been shown to be a good predictor of job performance or injury occurrence. However, the key to using information gathered from range of motion testing is its relationship to job demands. For example, the job demands require a worker to bend forward at the waist in order to reach a specific object. This forward bending is about 45°. If the range of motion for trunk forward bending indicates a restriction motion to only 25°, this worker lacks the capacity to perform this aspect of the job. If the job demands can be changed to meet the functional aspects of the employee, then the employee can return to work. Range-of-motion testing also suffers from reliability of procedures. Studies have indicated questionable inter- and intrarater reliability when hand-held devices like goniometers and tapes are used. New computerized devices that may improve this are coming on the market.

Work Speed

The speed at which an individual works is often determined by the job. In some assembly line work, the pace is set by the speed of the machine or line. In some jobs, incentive systems motivate employees to work at speeds that may compromise their musculoskeletal systems. In order to test for work pace, the physical demands of this pace must be ascertained from the employee or the employer. A simulated job task can be established and the pace measured and compared to that required on the job. For example, an employee is required to pick up sacks from a conveyor belt and place them on a pallet at a pace of 10 to 12 sacks per minute. If a simulated test procedure for 15 minutes indicates an average rate of 8 sacks a minute, then this worker is not able to perform the task successfully.

Coordination and Balance

Functional capacity testing should incorporate tests for manual dexterity. Most jobs require some level of hand coordination. Good hand coordination helps in lifting as well as makes an employee suitable for other job tasks if injury prevents return to more demanding lifting jobs. Possession of transferable skills is important for return to productive capacity. Functional

capacity assessment should document this. Tests for manual dexterity include the Moberg Pick-up test and the Minnesota pegboard test.

The Moberg pick-up test is actually two tests. A box containing nine household objects (safety pin, cottonball, key, screw, piece of felt, piece of sponge, paper clip, coin, nail) is placed in front of the subject who, with eyes closed, picks up each object and tries to identify it. This portion of the test determines stereognosis, the ability to discern objects through sensation. This may be important for placement in a job where search and detection procedures are required. The second part of the test measures the time it takes to pick up the objects from the box one at a time and place them in a designated spot on the table. This is done twice—once with eyes open and then with eyes closed. The procedure is timed and compared between hands. Moberg suggested a time of 10 seconds as normal with eyes open. We have been using a time of 25–30 seconds for the eyes closed portion as a normal cut-off. However, each hand is compared to the other to determine percentage deficit between hands.

In the Minnesota pegboard test, a number of pegs must be removed from the board and then replaced. Each hand is tested separately. The procedure is timed and compared against a norm. The pegboard test is more representative than the Moberg of some repetitive motion tasks and can assess capacity for this type of job.

Other instruments standardized by Valpar can also simulate repetitive motion hand tasks and can be utilized to determine specific work capacities. In many instances, simulated tasks can be custom-made out of easy-to-find parts from the local hardware store.

Balance is a skill involving the back, lower extremities, cervical spine, and cerebellar and vestibular function. When a worker has a musculoskeletal injury the proprioceptive mechanisms in the muscles, tendons, ligaments, and joints may be impaired. A person with balance problems may be more likely to sustain an injury. Emphasis should be placed upon establishing balance capacity, especially if the job requires it in order to be performed safely. For example, a construction worker returning to the job after a back injury who is required to work at varying heights and on narrow walkways. The assessment of balance capabilities would be essential before placement back on the job.

Safety

Before an employee can return to work it must also be demonstrated that he or she can perform the job in a manner that would not cause harm to self or others. If, during a testing procedure, a patient exhibits behavior that would potentiate an injury it should be documented and noted. Before returning this worker to the job, the physician should ask the company for further training for this worker in safety procedures. This is a moral and ethical question for the health care professional. A therapist should not recommend placement for a worker who demonstrates unsafe work practices even if all other physical demand requirements are met.

REPORT OF FINDINGS

The role of the health care professional in functional and work capacity testing is to document and report the actual findings as determined by the testing procedure. The report should indicate fitness to return to work or to be placed in a job based upon the known physical demands of that job. In addition, information should be provided to the employer that denotes the types of activities the individual has demonstrated a capacity for. This will assist the employer or agency in returning a worker to a job that fits his or her capacities.

It would be beneficial to include a cover sheet that summarizes the types of tests performed and provides a scaled grading system. The rest of the report can be in a form of a narrative that describes the testing procedure and the results and contains evaluator comments.

SUMMARY

Functional and work capacity evaluation is a valuable tool that the trained health care professional can use in the office to better quantify the abilities of patient or employee to perform certain functional tasks without the risk of injury or reinjury. No one predetermined format is possible since job demands will differ from employer to employer and from job to job. The ability to delineate the types of abilities an employee possesses permits the employer to place a worker in a job setting that matches his or her abilities and to return a worker to the job site sooner. This should reduce the number of injuries and the amount of time lost because of injuries, and improve the mental condition of injured workers by returning them to a productive lifestyle in alternative job settings that meet their capabilities.

It is important that those health care professionals who wish to incorporate functional and work capacity testing in their office become familiar with their surrounding industries; stay informed about the latest studies on valid and reliable testing procedures and instruments; and be willing to share ideas on new procedures and work within the guidelines established by NIOSH, AIHA, and the EEOC in implementing functional and work capacity testing. Information from future studies will serve to augment and possibly change some of the information presented here, thus insuring our ability to provide quality service to our patients and the companies who employ them.

References

1. Chaffin DB. Ergonomics guide for the assessment of human static strength. Am Indus Hyg Assoc J 36:505–510, 1975.
2. Chaffin DB. Functional assessment for heavy physical labor. Occup Health Saf, 1981 (January)
3. NIOSH work practices guide for manual lifting. Cincinnati: US Department of Health and Human Services, 1981.
4. Adoption by four agencies of uniform guidelines on employee selection procedures. Federal Register Vol. 43, No. 166—Friday August 25, 1978.
5. The Equal Employment Opportunity Act of 1972. Washington, DC: Bureau of National Affairs, 1973.
6. Keyserling WM. Isometric strength testing in selecting workers for strenuous jobs, PhD Dissertation, University of Michigan. Ann Arbor: University Microfilms, 1979.
7. Keyserling WM, Herrin GD, Chaffin DB. Isometric strength testing as a means of controlling medical incidents on strenuous jobs. J Occup Med 1980; 22:50, 333.
8. Chaffin DB, Herrin GD, Keyserling WM. Preemployment strength testing—an updated position. J Occup Med 1978; 20:403–408.
9. Ergonomics guide to assessment of metabolic and cardiac costs of physical work, Am Indus Hyg Assoc J 1971; 32:560–564.
10. Bernauer EM, Bonanno J. Development of physical profiles for specific jobs. J Occup Med 1975; 17:27–33.
11. Kamon E, Kiser D, Pytel JL. Dynamic and static lifting capacity and musculoskeletal strength of steelmill workers. Am Indus Hyg Assoc J 1980; 43:730.

12. Kroemer KHE. Testing individual capability to lift material: Repeatability of a dynamic test compared with static testing. J Safety Res 1985; 16:1.

13. Biering-Sorenson F. Physical measurements as risk indicators for low-back trouble over a one-year period. Spine 1984; 9:106.

14. Cady LD, Bischoff DP, O'Connell ER et al. Strength and fitness and subsequent back injuries in firefighters. J Occup Med 1979; 21:269.

15. Nicolaisen T, Jorgensen K. Trunk strength, back muscle endurance and low back trouble. Scand J Rehab Med 1985; 17:121.

16. Fairbank JCT, Davies JB, Couper J, O'Brien JP. The Oswestry low back pain disability questionnaire. Physiotherapy 1980; 66:271–273.

17. Ransford AO, Cairns D, Mooney V. The pain drawing as an aid to the psychologic evaluation of patients with low back pain. Spine 1976; 1:127.

18. Chaffin DB, Herrin GD, Keyserling WM, Foulke JA. Preemployment strength testing in selecting workers for materials handling jobs. Cincinnati; NIOSH Physiology and Ergonomics Branch, Contract No. CDC-99-74-62, 1977.

19. Chaffin DB. Functional assessment for heavy physical labor. In Alderman MH, ed. Clinical medicine for the occupational physician. New York: Marcel Dekker, 1979.

20. Snook SH. Approaches to the control of back pain in industry: Job design, job placement and education training. In Deyo RA, ed. Spine: Occupational back pain. Philadelphia: Hanley and Belfus, Inc. 1987; 48.

21. Kishino N, Mayer T, Gatcher R et al. Quantification of lumbar function. IV. Isometric and isokinetic lifting simulation in normal subjects and low back dysfunction patients. Spine 1985; 10:921–927.

22. Kamon E, Ayoub M. Ergonomics guide to assessment of physical work capacity. Am Indus Hyg Assoc J 1976;

23. Astrand PO, Radahl K. Textbook of work physiology: Physiological bases for exercise, 3rd ed. St. Louis: McGraw-Hill, 1986.

24. Roebuck JA, Kroemer KHE, Thompson WG. Engineering anthropometry methods. New York: John Wiley and Sons, 1975.

25. Ayoub MM et al. Modeling of lifting capacity as a function of operator and task variables. In Drury CG ed. Safety in manual materials handling. Cincinnati: DHEW (NIOSH) Publication No. 78-185, 1978.

26. Molbech S. Average percentage force at reported maximal isometric muscle contractions at different frequencies. Communications from the Testing and Observations Institute of the Danish National Association for Infantile Paralysis: 1963; No. 16.

27. Asmussen E, Hansen O, Lammert O. The relation between isometric and dynamic muscle strength in man. Communications from the Testing and Observations Institute of the Danish National Association for Infantile Paralysis. 1965; No. 20.

28. Asmussen E. Growth in muscular strength and power. In Ranck GL. (ed.), Physical activity human growth and development. New York: Academic Press, 1973; 60.

36

SCIENTIFIC BASIS OF FUNCTIONAL ASSESSMENT OF THE LUMBAR SPINE PATIENT

Mark J. Sontag

This chapter will analyze current technologies utilized in evaluating lumbar trunk strength, which will be placed in context of a host of other variables that affect low back injury and recovery. Medical practitioners are exposed to numerous isometric, isokinetic, and isoinertial technologies that all report to be the most reproducible and efficient methods of evaluating strength and predicting injury. The following review of the scientific literature related to trunk strength evaluating technologies will hopefully clarify the above claims.

NECESSITY OF FUNCTIONAL ASSESSMENT OF THE LUMBAR SPINE PATIENT

Low back pain affects approximately 85% of all persons in the western world at some point during their lives (1). Low back pain is second only to upper respiratory infections as the most frequent reason people seek medical attention. It is the most frequent cause of activity limitation and disability in persons under age 45 years and the third most frequent cause in the 45 to 64 year age group (2).

Approximately 2% of all workers injure their backs annually (3). Although the majority of low back pain sufferers improve within 3 months, the costs still exceed $16 billion each year (4). Incredibly, 10% of the injuries require 80% of the total costs (5). It is estimated that 50% of those people who are disabled because of low back pain have absolutely no objective findings (6, 7).

Exorbitant amounts of American health care money are spent on a small percentage of low back sufferers who have very few objective abnormalities. The economic magnitude of this problem has prompted investigators to try to objectify spinal function and dysfunction in an attempt to quantitate true abnormalities. Because of the complexity of the spinal unit and the large discrepancies among actual spinal diagnoses, practicing clinicians often completely rely on a patient's subjective complaints. Recently, an attempt has been made to evaluate low back patients functionally rather than subjectively. The current cerebrovascular scales, for instance, concentrate on function and not subjective complaints of pain. James Evans and Abbott Kagan (8) have developed a functional rating scale for chronic low back patients that quantifies the patient's level of activity and relative personal independence. Richard Deyo recently reviewed current functional status measurement techniques and their usefulness (9).

POTENTIAL BENEFITS OF FUNCTIONAL ASSESSMENT

It is clear that, in the current medical-legal climate of industrial and personal injury back claims, inordinate importance is placed on subjective complaints and not on objective findings or functional parameters. The benefits of functional assessment of the lumbar spine would include objective analysis of a patient's condition and subsequent recovery. By objectively analyzing the spinal unit, one can determine deficits and conceivably correct them more rapidly. Also, through assessment of the multiple aspects of spinal function, our biomechanical and psychological understanding of the spine will increase. Functional assessment of the spine conceivably would legitimize the qualified injured worker and identify the malingerer or individual concerned with secondary gain issues. Actual functional testing should reassure the worker of capability of performing the job task before returning to the actual job site. Once normative data have been obtained and the predictiveness of the testing has been established, preplacement screening can be instituted to prevent injuries.

METHODOLOGIES TO REDUCE INDUSTRIAL BACK INJURIES

Historically, preemployment histories and physical examinations were used to screen potential employees (10). Although it is established that a previous history of low back pain predisposes to additional low back pain (11), prospective employees can distort their own history to facilitate employment. Rowe estimates that only 7 to 8% of individuals prone to developing low back pain can be screened via the preemployment history and physical examination (12). However, Chaffin (13) and Snook (14) were unable to identify susceptible workers using preplacement examinations.

In the 1950s and 1960s, preplacement radiographs of the lumbar spine had gained acceptance (15–17). However, other studies have concluded that preemployment radiographs alone are not predictive of future low back injury (18–21). Recently, Frymoyer has demonstrated an association between low back pain and radiographic L4-5 disc space narrowing and spurs (22, 23). Current research is investigating the relationship between lumbar spinal canal diameter and the likelihood of low back pain (24). Jeff Saal has demonstrated that those with herniated nucleus pulposus who do not respond to nonoperative conservative care programs are likely to have spinal stenosis (25). Thus, although plain radiographs are not predictive of low back injury, it is possible that spinal canal diameter might be a predictive factor.

Anthropometric measurements such as height, weight, or body frame have not been predictive of subsequent low back injury (11, 18,

26). Psychological factors certainly play a role in low back injury recovery, but they also are not by themselves good predictors of the development of low back pain.

The three current approaches to managing low back injuries in the work place include 1) ergonomic changes, 2) preplacement or preselection screening, and 3) education and training for employees. Stover Snook defined ergonomics as "designing the job to fit the capabilities and limitations of the worker" (27). Snook analyzed the above three approaches and found that only ergonomic change in the work place was actually successful in reducing injuries, while preplacement screening and education were not successful (14). Ergonomic changes, however, are often cumbersome and expensive to incorporate into the work place.

Preplacement screening is currently very appealing to employers. Rather than designing the work site for the worker, employers attempt to select workers who can be productive at a given work site. The preselection process is often based on determination of strength. The various techniques of evaluating strength will be discussed later in this chapter.

The most common technique used in the attempt to reduce injuries in the work place is education and training. The education often consists of inhouse instruction in proper lifting and bending techniques. A scientific review of these inhouse programs has not demonstrated a preventive value (14, 28).

Biomechanical studies have offered great insight into the stress and torque placed on the lumbar spine during manual material handling (29). Gunnar Andersson has demonstrated that the distance an object is away from the body influences the stress on the back more than the actual method used to lift (30). Physiologic studies have evaluated cardiovascular stress and muscular fatigue in relationship to low back injury (29). Additional prospective studies are needed to evaluate the efficacy of biomechanical and physiologic methodologies.

BACK PAIN IN INDUSTRY

To successfully analyze and objectively measure spinal function, one must understand the multifactorial nature of low back injury. For clarity, low back injury will be analyzed on the basis of both physical and psychosocial factors. To emphasize one at the expense of the other would trivialize the actual problem. It is simplistic to try to isolate one or even a few variables that control low back pain and its recovery.

Epidemiologically, lifting is one physical factor that correlates with over 33% of low back injuries (31). Lifting places a compressive load on the intervertebral disc. Augustus White relates that workers whose spines are exposed to compression greater than 6000 newtons have an eight times higher incidence of low back injuries than those individuals whose spines are exposed to a compression of 3500 newtons (32). The frequency of lifting is also related to low back injury. Those who lift the most frequently are most likely to be injured, followed by those who rarely lift; those who lift occasionally seem to have less risk of injury (6). The amount of weight actually lifted also appears to correlate with the development of low back pain (26, 33, 34). Jobs requiring lifting loads greater than 25 pounds are associated with increased risk of low back injury (35, 36). There appears to be a definite relationship between the development of low back pain and the amount of lifting required in a specific occupation. Heavy industry workers, nurses, and truck drivers all must do significant lifting and these are the professions with the highest prevalence of low back pain (37).

Alexander Magora correlated sudden maximum physical efforts characterized by their unexpectedness as related to the development of low back pain (38). Magora hypothesizes that an unexpected sudden maximum motion is more likely to injure the spine than a controlled, rehearsed motion. Improper lifting is the most frequent cause of low back injury (39). Vibrational exposure and static work postures are also correlated with the development of low back pain (22).

The determinants of lifting and bending are also multifactorial. Successful lifting requires coordination, propioception, pulmonary fitness, training, experience, intelligence, flexibility of the extremities and spine, strength of the extremities and trunk and, finally, endurance.

Psychosocial factors play a tremendous role in low back injury and recovery. The classic retrospective Boeing Aircraft Employee Study found a correlation between the incidents of back injury and poor employee appraisal rating performed by the employee supervisor 6 months prior to the injury (40). Magora demonstrated that employees not satisfied with their occupation, place of employment, or social status had a higher incidence of low back pain than controls. He also demonstrated that people who perceive a high degree of responsibility and mental concentration requirement at work, resulting in a feeling of tenseness and fatigue, were also more likely to develop low back pain (41). Richard Deyo reports that psychosocial and demographic features such as education, number of prior episodes of back pain, and whether or not a patient "always feels sick" correlated with low back pain outcome better than physical parameters such as presenting physical examination or the type of physical therapy undergone (42).

Programs directed at altering management's perspective of the injured worker have been extremely successful in reducing low back injury costs. The Chelsea Back Program consisted of structural, technological, and attitudinal changes of management and resulted in a 75% reduction in the total cost per back injury claim (43). David Wood compared a management attitudinal program with a back school program in back injury prevention. Interestingly, the management attitudinal program was successful in reducing injuries while the back school program had no effect (44).

It is quite apparent that there are multiple variables that affect the development of pain and the outcome. The amount and frequency of lifting is an important physical variable that affects the development of low back pain. The functional task of lifting consists of multiple components, one of which includes strength (45). Increased abdominal and trunk strength has been correlated with improved outcome following low back injury (46–49). In the remainder of this chapter we will evaluate techniques of quantifying lumbar trunk strength and their relationship to the prediction of low back pain. Table 36.1 summarizes the multiple factors affecting the manual materials handling activities.

TECHNIQUES OF EVALUATING STRENGTH

There are three common methods of evaluating strength: isometric, isokinetic, and isoinertial (psychophysical). Isometric strength is defined as the static measure of maximum voluntary contraction with the muscle at a fixed length.

Table 36.1.
Factors Affecting Manual Materials Handling Activities

Work variables	Task variables	Environmental variables
Physical Factors: age, sex, anthropometry strength, etc.	The Load: mass, size, shape, stability, coupling, etc.	Heat Load
Physiological Factors: aerobic power, anaerobic power, endurance, etc.	The Work Place: space, obstacles, etc.	Noise
Psychological Factors: attitudes towards work, job satisfaction, etc.	Temporal Aspects	Vibration
Training and Experience	Complexity	Work Surface: geometry, stability, traction, etc.

Isokinetic strength is defined as a dynamic measure with body segments moving at a constant rate of speed. Isoinertial (psychophysical) strength is defined as a dynamic measure of maximum weight moved through a range. The following six criteria will be used to evaluate the above methods.

1. Safe to administer,
2. Reliable and reproducible,
3. Practical to administer,
4. Predictive of capability and/or risk,
5. Specific to the requirements of the job,
6. Ethically and legally defensible (50).

ISOMETRIC STRENGTH TESTING

There are two current basic techniques used in evaluating isometric strength. Technique 1 will be described as a low-technology approach using a simple strain gauge, while the high-technology approach uses computerized instrumentation such as Cybex, Kincom, Biodex, or LIDO. The low-tech strain gauge apparatus (Fig. 36.1) costs approximately $300, while the high-tech computerized equipment generally runs over $50,000 per unit.

The reliability and reproducibility of isometric strength instrumentation has been established (51). One major concern with isometric testing is the safety of the actual procedure. Hansson, using biomechanical analysis, has calculated compressive loads on the L3 vertebral body ranging from 5,000 to 11,000 newtons during squat and torso lifting in isometric testing (52). These loads in vitro have caused structural failure in the vertebral endplates. Hansson noted, however, that isometric testing of trunk flexors and extensors caused significantly

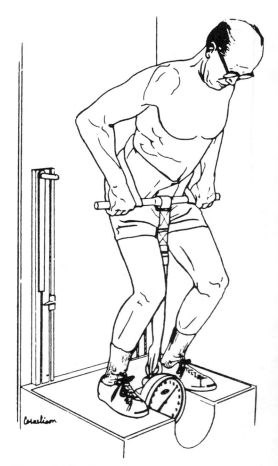

Figure 36.1. Low-tech isometric strength testing device. (Reproduced by permission from Cady LD, Bischott DP, O'Connell ER et al. Strength and fitness and subsequent back injuries in firefighters. J Occup Med 1979; 21(4):271. © Am. College of Occupational Medicine.)

less load on the L3 vertebral body. Zeh analyzed over 1,000 volunteers testing isometric strength (53). Approximately 5% of the subjects could not continue testing because of pain and 0.5% actually developed an injury. Zeh's recommendation was to reduce the number of exertions, which substantially reduced the probability of injury and still provided accurate assessment of isometric strength. Overall, isometric techniques, particularly using the strain gauge device, are quite simple and practical to administer.

Don Chaffin is a pioneer in isometric strength testing. In a series of elegant papers, Chaffin first demonstrated that the incidence rate of low back pain is correlated with increased lifting strength requirements (11). In a following study, he demonstrated that the incidence of back pain increased when loads exceeded a subject's isometric lifting capability (11, 54, 55). Finally, in a classic study, Chaffin actually reduced low back injuries by selecting workers on the basis of their isometric strength and placing them in jobs where their strength exceeded their lifting requirements (50, 57). However, Battie and Bigos have found no correlation between isometric strength and injury, yet they did not match job demands with strength (58). Considering there is no demonstrated significant difference in static back extensor strength among workers performing a wide variety of physically demanding jobs (45), isometric strength testing might be a useful tool in preplacing workers. Currently, no scientific study demonstrates that isokinetic or isoinertial technologies are predictive of subsequent back injury (59).

ISOKINETIC STRENGTH TESTING

There are four popular, commercially available isokinetic testing devices. Cybex provides a sagittal strength device as well as a torsional strength device. Kincom provides an attachment to its extremity dynamometer so that it can be used as a back testing device. Biodex also provides an attachment to the existing extremity system. Finally, LIDO provides a sagittal strength tester similar to the Cybex unit, but theirs allows subjects to sit or stand. (See Figure 36.2, the LIDO isokinetic trunk tester.) Tom Mayer and Robert Gatchel provide an excellent review of the above manufacturers' equipment (60).

The allure of isokinetic trunk testing is that dynamic testing theoretically would more closely re-create functional lifting than would static testing. This premise, however, has not been proven scientifically. Also, individuals do not actually lift items isokinetically, but rather isoinertially. Isokinetic testing, however, has been proven to be safe and the data are reproducible and reliable (61–67).

Another popular aspect of isokinetic testing is curve analysis. The hypothesis is that curve variability distinguishes submaximal from maximal efforts in isokinetic trunk and lift testing. The hope is that through computerizing strength testing, it would be possible to distinguish a malingering patient from an injured one, or one who is not providing full effort from one who is. Certainly this would be a tremendous help in the medicolegal arena. Rowland Hazard and co-workers evaluated the variability of isokinetic curves as an indicator of effort. Their conclusion is that clinical observation of the subject using the isokinetic equipment is more accurate than analyzing curve variability. It was extremely difficult to discriminate between submaximal effort secondary to pain, malingering, or fatigue (Fig. 36.3).

Although isokinetic technology is safe and provides repeatable, reproducible data, it is extremely costly. It also has not been scientifically shown to have greater inferential capacity than the available isometric technologies described above. It is also not specifically job-related, as people do not lift isokinetically. It does appear, however, that quantifying trunk strength using isokinetic technologies facilitates recovery from low back injuries.

ISOINERTIAL STRENGTH TESTING

There are two basic approaches to isoinertial strength testing—a low-technology and a high-technology approach. Stover Snook introduced the first strength evaluation using a low-technological isoinertial approach (69). This involved lifting boxes filled with lead shot or bricks. More recently, Thomas Mayer has introduced progressive isoinertial lifting evaluation *(PILE)* (70, 71). In the high-technological arena, Isotechnologies has introduced a computerized isoinertial testing device.

The data from the low-tech and high-tech approaches are repeatable and reproducible (72). The technology is safe to administer and relatively easy to use, particularly with the low-technological approach. The cost for Snooks' or

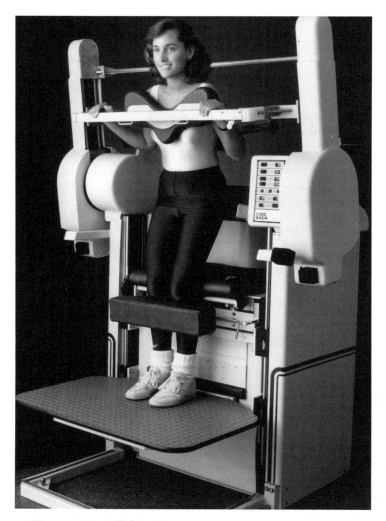

Figure 36.2.   LIDO back isokinetic system. Courtesy of Loredan.

Mayer's low-technological approaches is minimal, while the cost for Isotechnologies' equipment exceeds $50,000 per machine. Although isoinertial techniques are job-related, as a multiaxial, uncontrolled speed evaluation most closely replicates motion of the spine (73), they are poor predictors of future low back pain (74).

It has been demonstrated that using high tech isoinertial testing can reduce low back disability time (75). It is likely that the reduced disability time associated with using both isokinetic and isoinertial high-technological approaches is related to the actual objectification of function. By objectifying function, the patient has a direct feedback about recovery, which most likely serves as a motivator.

Table 36.2 is a summary slide of the six criteria that isometric, isokinetic, and isoinertial testing devices have been judged by. It is clear that all of the devices are relatively safe, easy to use, and provide reproducible data (76). The costs for the high-tech isokinetic and isoinertial equipment appear prohibitive. The costs for isometric and low-tech isoinertial devices are quite reasonable. Only isometric and isoinertial techniques are actually job-related. Most importantly, only isometric strength testing has been proven to be predictive of future low back injury.

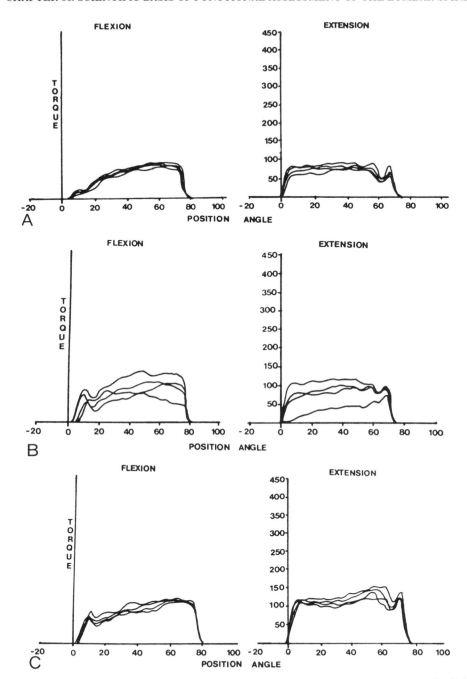

Figure 36.3. Cybex trunk extension/flexion curves. **A,** consistent curves; **B,** variant curves; **C,** slightly variable curves. (Reproduced by permission from Hazard R, Reid S et al. Isokinetic trunk and lifting strength measurements: Variability as an indicator of effort. Spine 1988; 13(1):55.)

Table 36.2.
Status of Whole Body Strength Testing

Criterion	Isometric	Isokinetic	Isoinertial
Repeatable	Excellent	Excellent	Excellent
Safe	Good	Excellent	Excellent
Easy to Use	Excellent	Excellent	Good
Cost	Medium	High	Low
Job-Related	Good	?	Good for Lifting
Predictive	Good	?	?

STRENGTH VERSUS ENDURANCE

One major question in the scientific literature is whether low back pain sufferers have weaker trunk muscles or if muscles become weak once pain develops. Multiple scientific studies have demonstrated that low back pain sufferers have less isometrically tested strength of the trunk muscles (77–80). There is also abundant literature reporting that low back pain sufferers have weaker trunk muscles as tested dynamically (68, 81–83). However, Berkson and Nachemson report that there is no difference in isometric abdominal or trunk strength in those individuals with low back pain and age-matched controls (84, 85).

Biering-Sorensen has published two studies stating that trunk strength alone is a poor predictor of low back pain (86, 87). However Biering-Sorensen has demonstrated that isometric back endurance is significant for predicting the first back pain occurrence in men (87). Nicolaisen and Jorgensen found no difference in abdominal and back strength in back pain patients and normals. However, they did find decreased endurance of the trunk muscles in low back pain sufferers (88, 89). Reduced endurance in the trunk musculature might force the spine to perform functional activities in an uncoupled, unprotected manner, making injuries more likely.

It is quite obvious that there is extensive controversy about the relationship between trunk strength and low back injury. After this critical review of the literature, Chaffin's concept of matching the strength of workers to the strength demands of their jobs based on pure isometric strength testing still carries tremendous merit. Additional investigation in isometric strength versus isometric endurance needs to be explored in light of Biering-Sorensen's, Nicolaisen's, and Jorgensen's recent studies.

MEDICOLEGAL ASPECTS OF EVALUATIONS

In the state of California, discriminative hiring based on latent or potential disability is against the law. To reject a job applicant legally on the basis of a potential back problem, the employer must meet the following criteria: 1) The applicant is unable to do the specific job; 2) all or substantially all of the excluded people are unable to safely and efficiently perform the job; and 3) there is an identifiable and substantial immediate danger imposing a substantial degree of risk. Currently, preemployment screening is illegal in the state of California because it is deemed discriminatory based on a latent or potential disability. However, preplacement screening, once a person is hired, is legal. Chaffin's techniques using isometric strength testing and matching a worker's job to actual lifting capabilities once the worker is hired is legally defensible.

FUTURE APPLICATIONS OF FUNCTIONAL ASSESSMENT

Lee Cady's classic description of firefighters demonstrated that the most physically fit individuals had the least number of low back injuries. The prospective measurements included flexibility, isometric lifting strength, bicycle ergometer exercise measurements of 2-minute recovery of heart rate, diastolic blood pressure at a heart rate of 60 beats per minute and watts of effort required to sutsain heart rate at 160 beats per minute (90). In a follow-up study, Cady demonstrated that after a 14-year program promoting health and physical fitness, there was a 16% increase in the physical work capacity, a slight increase in spinal flexibility, no clear increase in muscle strength, a decrease in smoking, a decrease in disabling injuries, and a 25% decrease in workers' compensation costs (91). Cady's demonstration of decreased workers' compensation costs as a result of a physical fitness program, Chaffin's demonstration of reduced injuries using isometric testing, and management approaches described previously all suggest that there are active ways that modern industry can reduce the incidents of low back pain and subsequent compensation.

In summary, evaluating low back injury is a complicated problem affected by a myriad of physical, psychosocial, and legal issues. To focus on only one variable, such as strength, results in a gross simplification of this challenging problem. It is quite apparent that industry requires uniformity in testing of the multitude of variables. It also appears that emphasis placed on objective parameters appears to facilitate recovery from a low back injury. Ergonomic changes, preselection of the worker, and a more informed management appear to be the prerequisites for reducing low back pain in industry. Generally improved fitness also appears to be very promising. Certainly, additional research and standardization is required in all of these areas.

References

1. Beals RK, Hickman NW. Industrial injuries of the back and extremities. J Bone Joint Surg 1972; 54A:1593–1611.
2. Andersson GBJ. Symposium: Low-back pain in industry. Spine 1981; 6(1):53–56.
3. Bond MB. Low back injuries in industry. Indust Med Surg 1970; 39:28–32.
4. Snook SH, Jensen RC. Cost. In Pope MH, Frymoyer JW, Andersson G eds. Occupational low back pain. New York: Praeger, 1984; 115–121.
5. Spengler DM. Back injuries in industry: A retrospective study. Spine 1986; 11(3):241–245.
6. Vallfors B. Acute, subacute and chronic LBP: Clinical symptoms, absenteeism, and working environment. Scand J Rehab Med 11 (Suppl) 1, 1985.
7. Nachemson A. Work for all. Clin Orthop 1983; (179):77–82.
8. Evans JH. The development of a functional rating scale to measure the treatment outcome of chronic spinal patients. Spine 1986; 11(3):277–281.
9. Deyo RA. Measuring the functional status of patients with low back pain. Arch Phys Med Rehab 1988; 69(12):1044–1053.
10. Ayoub MA. Control of manual lifting hazards: III. Preemployment screening. J Occup Med 1982; 24(10):751–761.
11. Chaffin DB, Park KS. A longitudinal study of low-back pain as associated with occupational weight lifting factors. AIHA J 1973; 34:513–525.
12. Rowe ML. Backache at work. Fairport, NY: Perinton Press, 1983.
13. Chaffin DB, Herrin GD, Keyserling WM. Pre-employment strength testing in selecting workers for materials handling jobs. U.S. Dept Health Educ Welfare (NIOSH) CDC-99-74-62, 1976.
14. Snook SH, Campanelli RA, Hart JW. A study of three preventive approaches to low back injury. J Occup Med 1978; 20(7):478–481.
15. Bond MB. Low-back x-rays. J Occup Med 1964; 6(9):373–380.
16. McGill CM. Industrial back problems: A control program. J Occup Med 1968; 10(4):174–178.
17. Hurley WJ. Lost time back injuries: Their relationship to heavy work and preplacement back x-rays. J Occup Med 1972; 14(8):611–614.
18. Rowe LM. Low-back pain in industry—A position paper. J Occup Med 1969; 11(4):161–169.
19. LaRocca H, MacNab I. Value of pre-employment radiographic assessment of the lumbar spine. Can Med Assoc J 1969; 101(7):49–54.
20. Redfield VT. The low-back x-ray as a pre-employment screening tool in the forest products industry. J Occup Med 1971; 13(5):219.
21. Montgomery CH. Preemployment back x-rays. J Occup Med, 1976; 18(7):495–498.
22. Frymoyer JW et al. Risk factors in low-back pain. J Bone Joint Surg 1983; 65A(2):213–217.
23. Frymoyer VW, Newberg A, Pope MH et al. Spine radiographs in patients with low back pain. J Bone Joint Surg 1984; 66(7):1048–1055.
24. Porter RW, Hibbert C, Wellman P. Backache and the lumbar spinal canal. Spine 1980; 5(2):99–105.
25. Saal JA, Saal JS. Nonoperative treatment of herniated lumbar intervertebral disc with radiculopathy. Spine 1989; 14(4):431–437.
26. Hult L. Cervical, dorsal, and lumbar spinal syndromes. Acta Orthop Scand 1954; 17(Suppl):1–102.
27. Snook SH. Approaches to the control of back pain in industry: Job design, job placement, and education/training. In Deyo R. Occupational back pain. Spine, State of the Art Reviews. 1987; 2(1):49–54.
28. Dedobbeleer N, German P. Safety practices in construction industry. J Occup Med 29(11):863–868.
29. Chaffin DB. Manual materials handling: The cause of over-exertion injury and illness in industry. J Environ Path Toxicol 1979; 2(5):31–66.
30. Andersson GBJ. Quantitative studies of back loads in lifting. Spine 1976; 1(3):178–185.
31. Kelsey J et al. An epidemiologic study of lifting and twisting on the job and risk for acute prolapsed lumbar intervertebral disc. J Orthop Res 1984; 2(1):61–66.
32. White AA, Gordon SL. Synopsis: Workshop on idiopathic low-back pain. Spine 1982; 7(2):141–149.
33. Rowe ML. Low back disability in industry: Updated position. J Occup Med 1969; 13(10):476–478.
34. Wickstrom G. Effect of work on degenerative back disease: A review. Scand J Work Environ Health 1978; 4 (Suppl 1):1–12.
35. Adams MA, Hutton WC. Prolapsed intervertebral disc. A hyperflexion injury. Spine 1982; 7(3):184–191.

36. Adams MA, Hutton WC. The relevance of torsion to the mechanical derangement of the lumbar spine. Spine 1981; 6:241–248.

37. Jensen RC. Epidemiology of work-related back pain. *Topics in acute care and trauma rehabilitation.* Indus Back Injuries Part 1 1988; 2(3):1–17.

38. Magora A. Investigation of the relation between low back pain and occupation. Scand J Rehab Med 1973; 5:186–190.

39. Bigos SJ et al. Back injuries in industry: A retrospective study: II. Injury factors. Spine 1986; 11(3):246–251.

40. Bigos SJ et al. Back injuries in industry: A retrospective study: III. Employee-related factors. Spine 1986; 11(3):252–256.

41. Magora A. Investigation of the relation between low-back pain and occupation. Scand J Rehab Med 1973; 5:186–190.

42. Deyo RA, Diehl AK. Predicting disability in patients with low back pain. Clin Res 1986; 34(2):814A.

43. Fitzler SL. Attitudinal change: The Chelsea Back Program. Occup Health Safety 1982; 51(2):24–26.

44. Wood DJ. Design and evaluation of a back injury prevention program within a geriatric hospital. Spine 1987; 12(2):77–82.

45. Kamon E, and Goldfuss AJ. In-plant evaluation of the muscle strength of workers. Am Ind Hyg Assoc J 1978; 39(10):801–807.

46. Kendall HP, Jenkins JM. Exercises for backache: A double-blind controlled trial. Physiotherapy 1968; 53:154–159.

47. Lidstrom A, Zachrisson M. Physical therapy on low back pain and sciatica. Scand J Rehab Med 1970; 2:37–42.

48. Kraus H, Nagler W. Evaluation of an exercise program for back pain. Am Fam Phys 1983; 28(3):153–158.

49. Manniche C, Bentzen L et al. Lancet 1988; Dec 24–31:1473.

50. Chaffin DB. Ergonomics guide for the assessment of human static strength. Am Ind Hyg Assoc J 1975; 36(7):505–511.

51. Kroemer KHE. Testing individual capability to lift material: Repeatability of a dynamic test compared with static testing. J Safety Res 1985; 16:1–7.

52. Hansson TH et al. The load on the lumbar spine during isometric strength testing. Spine 1984; 9(7):720–724.

53. Zeh J et al. Isometric strength testing: Recommendations based on a statistical analysis of the procedure. Spine 1986; 11(1):43–44.

54. Chaffin DB. Human strength capability and low-back pain. J Occup Med 1974; 16(4):248–254.

55. Chaffin DB. Preemployment strength testing: An updated position. J Occup Med 1978; 20(6):403–408.

56. Keyserling WM. Isometric strength testing as a means of controlling medical incidents on strenuous jobs. J Occup Med 1980; 22(5):332–336.

57. Keyserling WM. Establishing an industrial strength testing program. Am Ind Hyg Assoc J 1980; 41(10):730–736.

58. Battie MC et al. Isometric lifting strength as a predictor of industrial back pain reports. Spine 1989; 14(8):851–856.

59. Rothstein JM, Lamb RL, Mayhew TP. Clinical uses of isokinetic measurements. Phys Ther 1987; 67(12):1840–1844.

60. Mayer T, Gatchel R. Functional restoration for spinal disorders: The sports medicine approach. Philadelphia: Lea and Febiger, 1988.

61. Thistle HG et al. Isokinetic contraction: A new concept of resistive exercise. Arch Phys Med Rehab 1967; 48:279–282.

62. Elliott J. Assessing muscle strength isokinetically. JAMA 1978; 240(22):2408, 2410.

63. Davies GJ. Trunk testing using a prototype Cybex II isokinetic dynamometer stabilization system. J Orthop Sports Phys Ther 1982; 3:164–170.

64. Langranada NA, Lee CK. Isokinetic evaluation of trunk muscles. Spine 1984; 9(2):171–175.

65. Langranada NA et al. Quantitative assessment of back strength using isokinetic testing. Spine 1984; 9(3):287–290.

66. Smith SS et al. Quantification of lumbar function. Part I: Isometric and multispeed isokinetic trunk strength measures in sagittal and axial planes in normal subjects. Spine 1985; 10(8):757–764.

67. Hazard R, Reid S et al. Isokinetic trunk and lifting strength measurements: Variability as an indicator of effort. Spine 1988; 13(1):54–57.

68. Mayer TG et al. Objective assessment of spine function following industrial injury: A prospective study with comparison group and one-year follow-up. Spine 1985; 10(6):482–493.

69. National Institute for Occupational Safety and Health. Work practices guide for manual lifting (Pub 81-122). Cincinnati: NIOSH, U.S. Public Health Service, 1981.

70. Mayer TG, Barnes D et al. Progressive isoinertial lifting evaluation: I. A standardized protocol and normative database. Spine 1988; 13(9):993.

71. Mayer TG, Barnes D et al. Progressive isoinertial lifting evaluation: II. A comparison with isokinetic lifting in a disabled chronic low-back pain industrial population. Spine 1988; 13(9):998.

72. Parnianpour M, Li F et al. A database of isoinertial trunk strength tests against three resistance levels. Spine 1989; 14(4):409.

73. Parnianpour M, Nordin M et al. The triaxial coupling of torque generation of trunk muscles during isometric exertions and the effect of fatiguing

isoinertial movements on the motor output and movement patterns. Spine 1988; 13(9):982.

74. Troup JDG et al. The perception of back pain and the role of psychophysical tests of lifting capacity. Spine 1987; 12(7):645–657.

75. Seeds RH et al. Electronic equipment provides accuracy in back injury analysis. Occ Health Safety 1988; 1(1):38–42.

76. Beimborn D, Morrissey M. A review of the literature related to trunk muscle performance. 1988; 13(6):655–660.

77. Alston W et al. A quantitative study of muscle factors in the chronic low back syndrome. J Am Geriatr Soc 1966; 14(10):1041–1047.

78. Karvonen MJ et al. Back and leg complaints in relation to muscle strength in young men. Scand J Rehab Med 1980; 12:53–59.

79. McNeill T et al. Trunk strength in attempted flexion, extension, and lateral bending in healthy subjects and patients with low-back disorders. Spine 1980; 5(6):529–538.

80. Kishino ND et al. Quantification of lumbar function: Part 4: Isometric and isokinetic lifting simulation in normal subjects and low-back dysfunction patients. Spine 1985; 10(10):921–927.

81. Nummi J et al. Diminished dynamic performance capacity of back and abdominal muscles in concrete reinforcement workers. Scand J Work Environ Health 1978; 4(Suppl 1):39–46.

82. Smidt G et al. Assessment of abdominal and back extensor function: A quantitative approach and results for chronic low-back patients. Spine 1983; 8(2):211–219.

83. Mayer TG. Quantification of lumbar function. Part 2. Sagittal plane trunk strength in chronic low-back pain patients. Spine 1985; 10(8):765–772.

84. Berkson M, Schultz A, Nachemson A, Andersson G. Voluntary strengths of male adults with acute low back syndromes. Clin Orthop Rel Res 1977; 129:84–94.

85. Nachemson A, Lindh M. Measurement of abdominal and back muscle strength with and without low back pain. Scand J Rehab Med 1969; I:60–65.

86. Biering-Sorensen F. Low back trouble in a general population of 30, 40, 50 and 60 year old men and women. Don Med Bull 1982; 29(6):289–299.

87. Biering-Sorensen F. Physical measurements as risk indicators for low-back trouble over a one-year period. Spine 1984; 9(2):106–109.

88. Nicolaisen T, Jorgensen K. Trunk strength, back muscle endurance and low-back trouble. Scand J Rehab Med 1985; 17:121–127.

89. Jorgensen K, Nicolaisen T. Trunk extensor endurance: Determination and relation to low-back trouble. Ergonomics 1987; 30(2):259–267.

90. Cady LD, Bischoff DP et al. Strength and fitness and subsequent back injuries in firefighters. J Occup Med 1979; 21(4):269–272.

91. Cady LD et al. Program for increasing health and physical fitness of fire fighters. J Occup Med 1985; 27(2):110–114.

Section IX

CHALLENGE OF LOW BACK PAIN

37

LEARNED SPINE SOCIETIES AND MEETINGS

Scott Haldeman

The spine and its diseases have become one of the most difficult and challenging areas to understand. Unlike any other organ, it does not consist primarily of a single tissue type and does not serve a single primary function. The spine is an intricate relationship of both central and peripheral neural elements surrounded by a complex bony structure connected by both a cartilaginous disc with unique qualities and diarthrodial joints. It then is acted on and held together by a large number of ligaments and muscles that can be affected by both biomechanical and psychological factors. Finally, its primary symptom is pain, one of the most complex and poorly understood neural functions.

Symptoms arising from the spine have been treated by perhaps the widest group of clinicians to respond to any disease. Apart from the traditional back pain medical specialties of neurology, physiatry, radiology, orthopaedic surgery, and neurosurgery, patients with back pain are commonly seen by family physicians, rheumatologists, psychiatrists, and occupational medicine specialists. A large number of patients with spinal symptoms are treated by chiropractors and osteopaths and are often referred to physical and occupational therapists as well as psychologists. This organ, in addition, has been studied by anatomists, physiologists, and mechanical engineers.

This diversity of scientists and clinicians involved in the investigation and treatment of spinal problems has led in the past to a fractionalization of the scientific and clinical literature. Disputes have often arisen between chiropractors and medical doctors, conservative and surgical specialties and, at times, between different groups of surgeons or conservative care physicians. These disputes have often been ex-

pressed without any interaction or discussion. Different groups of clinicians often read only journals and articles published in their own fields and attended only meetings, often technical rather than scientific, within their own profession or specialty. The basic scientists were commonly ignored or simply unknown to the spine clinicians. This situation began changing in the 1970s and the change accelerated in the 80s. There was a realization that no single profession or specialty had all the answers and the skills to treat all patients with back pain. This notion has continued to grow so that today there appears to be an excess of multidisciplinary spine societies, meetings, and journals and it is becoming very difficult to sort out the names of the societies and their goals and objectives.

This chapter will attempt to sort out some of the major learned spine societies and educational meetings. It is impossible to mention all of the meetings and societies as well as the multiple courses for specific techniques of evaluation and treatment methods. Below, however, is one method of classification.

PROFESSIONAL ASSOCIATION SPONSORED MEETINGS

Virtually every profession that investigates and treats the spine has regular and routine inhouse educational courses or meetings. Societies such as the American Academy of Neurology and the American Academy of Orthopaedic Surgery have courses in conjunction with their annual conferences. These courses tend to be only one of multiple subspecialty courses sponsored by the various academies and classically draw speakers primarily from association members.

Research papers on the spine are commonly intermixed with research papers of other topics in the field and, in many of the specialty societies, such papers are sporadic. The American Academy of Orthopaedics has put a day aside for presentation of the best research from the interprofession National Spine Associations and these papers have been well received at the meetings and tend to widen the scope of presentations. Other societies, such as the Foundation for Chiropractic Education and Research, sponsor specific research meetings and present only formal papers that are accepted from other professions and researchers.

Many of these courses offered by professional associations are purely technical and are of very little interest to other groups. Thus it appears unlikely that a physical therapist would want to attend a course for neurosurgeons on a specific spinal operation or that a psychiatrist would want to learn the latest techniques of spinal manipulation. Other purely scientific courses on, for example, conservative management, biomechanics, or anatomy may be of interest to multiple professions. This is particularly true of the meetings sponsored by an international society. Thus, at a recent course by the International League Against Rheumatism (ILAR), the major international society for rheumatologists, speakers from a number of other professions were invited to present a course on the management of back pain.

SYMPOSIA BY GOVERNMENT AGENCIES AND FOUNDATIONS

Periodically, a government or private agency such as an institute within the National Institutes of Health or an academy or foundation will sponsor a major conference, workshop, or commission of enquiry to establish the state of the art or make recommendations concerning a specific topic. These meetings are usually by invitation only but often allow observers. The publications that result from such meetings or commissions can be of major importance as they may set political or scientific policy. Examples of these proceedings include "The Research Status of Spinal Manipulative Therapy," edited by M. Goldstein, NINCDS (1979); "The Quebec Task Force on Spinal Disorders" chaired by W.O. Spitzer (Spine 12:75, 1987);

and the New Zealand "Commission of Enquiry into Chiropractic" by Inglis et al. (1979).

MAJOR INTERNATIONAL SOCIETIES

These societies draw members from many countries and multiple specialties and often from other scientific professions with a similar interest. They tend to hold a single meeting every 1 to 3 years for the presentation of scientific papers and their discussion. They are extremely important as they allow for the dissemination of ideas and information among countries. The most prominent of these societies are described below.

International Society for the Study of the Lumbar Spine (ISSLS)

This society was founded in 1974 and had its first meeting when Dr. Harry Farfan called on leading spine researchers and clinicians to come together and form a society. Its list of initial members and subsequent presidents reads like a Who's Who in spine research. The society has a membership now limited to 200 in order to allow for intimate and intense discussion of research and ideas. Membership is by application supported by two sponsors who are members, the presentation of a paper at a meeting, and a bibliography demonstrating active independent research on the lumbar spine. The society consists of members from all the clinical specialty groups as well as anatomists, biomechanical engineers, and biochemists. It includes leading researchers from North America, Europe, Australia, Africa, and Singapore and Israel. In order to remain a member one must present a paper every 5 years and not miss three meetings in a row. Thus, this society remains somewhat exclusive. Its meetings, however, are among the most interesting and informative available. Nonmembers may attend at the invitation of a member or by having a paper accepted for presentation.

Cervical Spine Society (CSS)

This society had its beginnings in 1973 in New York (Pierce DS, Spine, 11:647, 1986). The meetings initially were small, devoted to the presentation of scientific papers and discussion. Like ISSLS, its membership consists of orthopaedic surgeons, neurosurgeons, neurologists, radiologists, engineers, and anatomists. It has presented symposia and is responsible for two textbooks on the state of the art in the understanding of cervical spine mechanics, diagnosis, and treatment. Its membership is international and its meetings are held globally. It is a growing society beginning to exert influence through participation in committees of various specialty societies. Its meetings are open to members and guests.

The Scoliosis Research Society (SRS)

The Scoliosis Research Society was formed in 1966 when Dr. John Moe called a group of surgeons interested in this problem to study together. It has a single meeting each year for presentation of research papers, which are as much on spine deformities as on scoliosis. The membership consists primarily of orthopaedic surgeons and biomechanical engineers. Members may bring a guest, and the program committee will review papers submitted by both members and nonmembers.

International Back Pain Society (IBPS)

This is a somewhat smaller and less well-known society than the three described above. It is, however, open to both researchers and to clinicians who are not active in research. The primary organizer of this society is Professor Malcolm Jayson of Manchester University, England. It organizes a single meeting each year, usually in Europe, but has had one meeting in Hong Kong. The meetings consist of an education symposium of invited guest lecturers and workshops as well as the presentation of research papers. Its meetings are advertised and open to any clinician who wishes to attend.

International Federation for Manual Medicine (FIMM)

This society is the international arm of at least 21 national societies for manual or manipulative medicine. There is no direct membership, but the members of individual societies that make up the federation are automatically members of the federation. It holds one meeting every 3 years, usually in Europe, which includes both invited speakers and research papers. It is responsible for the journal *Manual Medicine* in German and English.

NORTH AMERICAN SOCIETIES

There are numerous societies in North America with direct or indirect interest in the spine. Only three will be mentioned.

North American Spine Society (NASS)

The North American Spine Society was formed in 1984 by the amalgamation of two other societies that had functioned briefly to promote scientific investigation of the spine and the advancement of clinical skills and training. This society has grown rapidly and within a few years has become one of the largest and most influential of the spine societies. Its membership requires either board certification in an AMA recognized specialty board or a Ph.D. That means that all members have at least four years of full-time postprofessional degree training. Its membership is open to such specialties as orthopaedic surgery, neurosurgery, radiology, neurology, and physiatry as well as basic scientists, some of whom have their professional training in chiropractic, osteopathy, or physical therapy. It holds a single meeting each year for the presentation of submitted research papers. The society has active committees in such fields as nomenclature, residency certification, and standards of practice. It already has liaison with the Academy of Orthopaedic Surgery and the Academy of Neurology and is seeking liaison with other academies and associations.

American Back Society (ABS)

The American Back Society was established to fill a gap caused by the major international research societies. Unlike those societies and NASS, this society is open to anyone who treats the spine. It includes large numbers of orthopaedic surgeons, neurosurgeons, neurologists, and physiatrists as well as growing numbers of chiropractors, physical therapists, and nurse practitioners. Membership is by application only and meetings are open to anyone who wishes to attend. The meetings are held twice a year, once on the East Coast and once on the West Coast. The meeting consists of discussion and presentation of ideas and research from across the health professions. Symposia and workshops at the same meeting will include technical hands-on teaching of specific surgical techniques, presentation of chiropractic manipulation techniques, the most popular myofascial physiotherapy techniques, radiology presentations, and neurodiagnostic procedures. It has numerous committees, which are just beginning to be active. Its initial formation was the idea of Dr. Aubrey Swartz but the support of Dr. René Caillet and Dr. Kirkaldy-Willis as its first two presidents has greatly enhanced its prestige.

North American Academy of Musculoskeletal Medicine (NAAMM)

This is perhaps one of the oldest of the independent medical spine societies. For many years, it was known as the North American Academy of Manipulative Medicine. It is the recognized North American member of FIMM. Initially organized by prominent medical practitioners of manipulation such as Dr. John Mennell and Dr. Janet Travell in the early 1960s, it has maintained a small but dedicated membership with annual meetings and courses. It opened its doors to osteopathic physicians as full members and physical therapists as associate members. The change of name to the North American Academy of Musculoskeletal Medicine is an attempt to broaden its scope and interests.

YEARLY INDEPENDENT MEETINGS

There are too many courses and meetings held each year to even begin mentioning them. Two such independent courses have stood the test of time and consistently draw large audiences.

Challenge of the Lumbar Spine

This is an independent corporation headquartered in San Antonio. Its only goal is the organization of a yearly meeting of the highest quality. The meeting draws perhaps the largest and most qualified speakers of any course in the country. By spending virtually all profits on the speakers' pool, it has been able to draw clinicians and scientists from virtually every profes-

sion and from around the world. Meetings consist of formal presentations and workshops and each year are held in a different, but always beautiful, setting. Established in 1978, it appears to grow in popularity each year.

Annual Occupational Low Back Pain Conference

This conference held its first meeting in 1979 when a group of highly respected clinicians and basic scientists whose primary interest was occupational back pain came together to present the latest information on the topic of their special interests. It has held a single meeting once a year in different resorts around the country and has been drawing increasingly larger audiences. This conference has concentrated on the causes of occupational back injuries, ways industry can modify the work place to avoid back injuries, optimum management of the injured worker, and determination of disability. It has no formal office or address. The sponsors of this meeting are the institutions in which the chairperson of a meeting holds a faculty or clinical position.

SUMMARY

Any clinician or scientist interested in spinal pain will find it increasingly difficult to keep up with the rapidly expanding research and knowledge concerning the spine. It is no longer possible to be knowledgeable about the latest theories and clinical techniques for the understanding and management of patients with spinal pain solely by attending the meetings within a specific profession or specialty. There are available, however, multiple societies and meetings that present a broad spectrum of ideas and research. Clinicians and scientists can now pick a society or meeting that best fits their needs and, if necessary, move from one meeting or society to another as interest changes. The results of these meetings and societies is to spread knowledge and understanding; break down barriers between professions, specialties, and basic sciences; and produce a higher standard of care for the large portion of society suffering from spinal pain and other spine disorders.

38

THE CHALLENGE OF CONSERVATIVE CARE

Authur H. White
Robert Anderson

The lumbar spine has offered a challenge to physicians for centuries, stretching deeply into antiquity. By the early 1930s, it seemed that the challenge of back pain would eventually be met through developing surgical techniques. Several decades of increasing surgical excess was the result. However, by the 1970s it was clear that, yes, surgery could work seeming miracles for some patients but, no, not for most.

Perhaps 99% of all low-back-pain and sciatic patients should not be operated upon. Other methods of a conservative nature would have to accomplish what the scalpel could not achieve. Yet conservative methods themselves were still stuck in an unremarkable past that had endured to the near present. The 1970s, then, required a retreat from excessive surgery by applying more rigorous diagnostic methods to screen out those who were poor candidates. The 1970s also date the onset of a growing acceleration and intensification of efforts to perfect conservative, nonsurgical methods.

Within medicine, the perfectable healing potential of conservative care first became apparent when it was discovered that many people got better from back school programs. Education had a curative effect, but it also could work to prevent future back pain in individuals at risk. For this reason, the challenge of back care was early thought of as the need to develop and test back school programs.

The idea of back school offers so much inherent appeal that one needs to be reminded that it was by no means obvious to those who treated back pain earlier in the century. Where did the idea come from? Apparently, it emerged independently in several parts of the world at about the same time.

Alfred L. Kroeber, an anthropologist, once drew our attention to major inventions and discoveries in history that emerged at about the same time and yet more or less independently of each other. He referred to them as simultaneous inventions, and the most interesting one in medicine took place within a 3-month period in 1900, when the Hollander De Vries, the German Correns, and the Austrian Tschermak simultaneously rediscovered the basic principles of genetic inheritance that Gregor Mendel had identified in what is now Czechoslovakia more than thirty years earlier (1).

Were Kroeber alive today, he might add back school to his list of simultaneous inventions. One place in which it emerged was California. Arthur White, looking for alternatives to surgery, spent a year and a half visiting spine centers in various parts of North America and Europe. Not one was impressive in the realm of conservative care. Back in San Francisco, he spent time personally tutoring his individual spine patients on biomechanics, posture, and movement; drawing stick figures on the paper that rolled over the examination table; spending time teaching that might have been spent in the operating room. Lynne White recalls chiding him for taking so much time with each patient. Working with Bill Mattmiller, a physical therapist, Lynne started what turned into several years of developing demonstration slides and teaching aids to free the surgeon up for other things.

That search for better conservative methods at one point brought White to Southern California, where he encountered the first program he knew of that trained and educated back pain patients. It was a private enterprise called Postural Therapeutics. Shortly after, in a 1974 meeting in Los Angeles, he met Alf Nachemson, a Swedish orthopaedist, and learned that a program named "back school" had been developed in the Volvo automobile factory in the late 1960s. Still later, White encountered another orthopaedic surgeon, Harry Fahrni, who had developed a back education program in Canada. Thus, when the Whites developed the California Back School in the 1970s, it was a product of early independent experimentation enlarged by lessions from Southern California, Sweden, and Canada.

The concept is still evolving as skilled individuals in various parts of the world work with it. Elizabeth Kirkaldy-Willis in Canada, for example, developed a way to reduce the costs of such programs through the use of volunteers. Patricia Kunse, in association with the San Francisco Spine Institute, is currently experimenting with techniques for introducing prevention techniques to school children. Sandra Dutro and Lindsay Wheeler, as well as Sigmund Miller, are active in promoting the back school concept within the chiropractic profession.

Back schools provide elementary training in posture and movement that, in the last couple of decades, has led to more elaborate programs to help people to help themselves—what we have termed patient-active approaches. Again, simultaneous inventions and overlapping concepts took place.

One of the most profoundly important developments was the practice of teaching patients to stabilize their spines in a neutral position. The roots of this technique are complex. A physical therapist, Eileen Vollowitz, contributed importantly. Vollowitz undertook postgraduate training in Oslo, where she studied with Olaf Evjenth. Evjenth recognized that low back pathologies cannot be resolved until the spine is maintained in nonstressed positions. He developed exercises for patients to increase their strength and flexibility. Vollowitz also attended "back parties" in which patients got together to exercise in a mutually supportive atmosphere. In this stimulating context, trial and error produced exercises that could be performed by holding the spine in positions that were not painful. When White first learned of these practices in 1978, maintaining a neutral lumbosacral posture was referred to as the pelvic tilt. Later, Michael Moore introduced the

term stabilization, which tended to supplant the earlier designation.

Michael Moore, originally a student of Vollowitz, went beyond teaching his patients to stabilize in a pain-free position. He developed ways to train them to stay stabilized while they exercised in supine, prone, kneeling, and standing positions. He developed many instructional techniques, including such practical tasks as passing heavy river rocks from patient to patient while maintaining the neutral stabilized position. As the concept spread within physical therapy, others also helped to perfect and adapt it. Gregory Johnson and Vicky Saliba, for example, are especially known for their work in dynamic stabilization, which they identify as the lumbar protective mechanism. (On the patient-passive side of conservative care, Johnson and Saliba are equally appreciated for their innovations in soft tissue mobilization.)

From centers all over the world, ideas flowed in for exercise and stabilization, and from the perspective of many involved, it seemed that conservative approaches to the treatment of back and neck pain were evolving in the hands of many physical therapists and a few venturesome orthopaedic surgeons. In fact, similar concepts were emerging more or less independently in the work of physiatrists and others in the new field of sports medicine.

For athletes to recover from sports injuries, they must learn to modify their body mechanics and, if the back is injured, they must be stabilized by methods first encountered, at least in the experience of Jeffrey Saal, in the practice of T'ai Chi and other Asian martial arts.

With the effectiveness of modern transportation and communication, it becomes fruitless to attempt to say who was first in designing and applying many of the contributions in exercise and stabilization technique. One man can be identified, however, who uniquely elaborated techniques of posture and exercise for the treatment and prevention of mechanical back and neck pain. Robin McKenzie is a New Zealand physical therapist. McKenzie recalls that he first became known in the United States when White invited him to see patients in a spine center in San Francisco and later wrote an introduction to his definitive textbook (3). More recently, Ronald Donelson became a leading American advocate of the McKenzie method. Donelson is an orthopaedic surgeon who feels that he does better with his patients by practicing the McKenzie method than he did when he brought them in for spinal surgery.

In meeting the challenge of conservative care, how open should one be to practices that exist outside mainstream medicine? We take the view that every approach should be judged entirely on merit, and we do not care that Rolfing was developed by a biochemist, the Alexander method by an actor, the Feldenkreis method by a physicist, or Aston Patterning by a dancer. The only question is, can they contribute to back care? Brian Miller, a physical therapist who has had extensive training in several of these difficult methodologies, believes that they can. He refers to them as alternative somatic therapies. The efficacy of these methods is not substantiated by research, which is a priority now for those who advocate their use.

The challenge of the lumbar spine includes a willingness cautiously to explore unorthodox medical methods, as well as those outside mainstream medicine. We are frankly skeptical of the value of sclerosing injections (prolotherapy) in the treatment of low back pain. However, based upon relevant research and experience, Thomas Dorman, an orthopaedic surgeon, argues persuasively that proliferative injections can be beneficial in selected cases and physicians who treat back pain need to be aware of his work.

Epidural blocks, facet injections, and other ways of locally injecting analgesics and steroids are better known as diagnostic techniques, but they can also be employed for palliation. Richard Derby, an anesthesiologist whose practice is entirely limited to spinal injection procedures, has done more than 10,000 in the lumbar spine alone. He and his associate Garrett Kine find that in some instances, long-term relief is achieved. Commonly, patients respond to a regimen of injections repeated at intervals of months to years. More commonly, blocks provide short-term relief that is valuable because pain control permits the patient to participate in conservative treatment activities not otherwise possible.

For the lumbar spine, perhaps no other field of patient care offers a greater challenge to be openminded than manual medicine and the allied professions in which the practice of spinal mobilization and manipulation is prominent or central.

Manual medicine, also known as orthopaedic medicine, manipulative medicine, or musculoskeletal medicine, and far better known in Continental Europe and the United Kingdom than in North America, often raises the query, what is it? Although is emergence out of bonesetting can be traced to the second half of the nineteenth century in England, it grew in prominence as a medical speciality after World War II and especially during the 1970s as a patient-passive component of the international search for effective methods of conservative care (4–6).

Practitioners of manual medicine may exercise a wide variety of treatment options, but they are most known for utilizing techniques of spinal manipulative therapy (SMT). Because manual medicine relies solely upon conservative measures, and above all because SMT defines the field, even though it does not delimit it, the specialty of manual medicine may be virtually indistinguishable from the specializations of certain osteopathic physicians, of most chiropractors, and of a minority of physical therapists who have undergone advanced training in manual therapy.

During the first part of the twentieth century, it was possible to identify approaches to SMT that distinguished one profession from another. Above all, osteopathic manipulative therapy was characterized by the application of long-lever manipulations of low velocity, in contrast with chiropractic techniques based upon the use of short-lever but high-velocity spinal adjustments (manipulations). Among medical doctors who practice manipulation, it is difficult to identify what is heritable from bonesetters. The current methods of medical manipulators, although variable and, in some ways, unique, appear to reflect a large osteopathic influence, as seen, for example, in the work of J.F. Bourdillon (7).

Osteopathic physicians are still known for versions of the original high-amplitude/low-velocity manipulation, but an osteopathic physician such as Philip Greenman, based upon his structural diagnosis, may draw upon other techniques that have been perfected by osteopaths. He might employ craniosacral techniques first introduced by W.G. Sutherland and currently taught by John Upledger, among others (8). Similarly, drawing upon the work of H.W. Hoover and C.H. Bowles, he might invoke a functional indirect technique. Or, muscle energy techniques introduced by Fred L. Mitchell, Sr. might be utilized.

Chiropractors such as Kelli Pearson and Tammy DeKoekkoek utilize combined high- and low-velocity moves as well as short and long levers in the widely used Diversified Technique. Even so, the low-amplitude/high-velocity technique remains a highly valued method that is still more used by chiropractors than by others, although any nonchiropractic practitioner of SMT may use it at times. A very large number of other techniques round out the armamentarium of the chiropractor. To mention just one, a chiropractic version of the craniosacral technique is taught in chiropractic seminars as the Sacro-Occipital Technique (S.O.T.) of M.B. DeJarnette (9).

Some chiropractic techniques are more widely employed than others. James Cox singlehandedly converted chiropractors to the use of his flexion-distraction technique. The Cox method is thoroughly chiropractic, yet an openness across professions is evident in his work. His father was an osteopath, and his treatment table is decended from the old osteopathic McMannis table, which he refined and perfected. More, Cox evaluates his work in terms consistent with the tenets of medical science.

Physical therapists, the most recent profession to take on SMT, often rely upon the nonmanipulative methods of Robin McKenzie. Many also employ manipulative methods devised by another physical therapist, G.D. Maitland. In the Maitland technique, the emphasis is upon mobilization, with relatively little use of the manipulative thrust so widely prized in orthopaedic medicine, osteopathy, and chiropractic (10). Physical therapists throughout North America and in many places abroad have adopted refinements of concept and technique devised and taught by Stanley Paris. Thus, newness in this field has not limited the inventiveness of therapists.

It should be noted that some physical therapists also at times apply chiropractic-like adjustive thrusts, and that much that they do is taken from the work of osteopathic and medical physicians. This would include a version of the osteopathic muscle-energy technique that they call the contract-relax technique. The contract-relax technique is not simply an offshoot of osteopathy, however. Margaret Knott of the Kaiser Rehabilitation Center in Vallejo, California, elaborating the work of Herman Kabat, M.D., developed an approach akin to the muscle-energy technique when she introduced proprioceptive neuromuscular facilitation for the rehabilitation of stroke victims (2).

In summary, then, each profession has contributed to the development of SMT. Mutual sharing and cross-disciplinary stimulation make it at this time a highly complex area of growth in innovative approaches to the conservative treatment of low back pain. No form of treatment utilized in the care of low back pain, whether surgical or nonsurgical, is more thoroughly researched than is the efficacy of SMT. It is clear from a number of randomized, controlled clinical trials that spinal manipulation can help some patients get well faster. It has never been demonstrated that SMT in and of itself changes the long-term course of the disease, however.

More research on the efficacy of SMT is under way, including a metaanalysis of previous clinical trials that we are doing with two scientist chiropractors, William Meeker and Robert Mootz, as a collaborative effort involving the San Francisco Spine Institute, the Palmer College of Chiropractic-West, the Los Angeles College of Chiropractic, and the Pacific Consortium for Chiropractic Research.

Scott Haldeman, a neurologist/neurophysiologist who began his career as a chiropractor, is currently involved in at least two collaborative trials. He has written extensively on the efficacy of SMT (11–13). Haldeman has also been an active participant in nearly every professional association dedicated to the nonsurgical treatment of low back pain, both in North America and abroad. He has served as the elected president of several.

John Triano reflects a consensus among ourselves, Meeker, Mootz, Pearson, DeKoekkoek, Greenman, Paris, Haldeman and many others that SMT has a valuable role to play as part of what can be offered in the treatment and prevention of back and neck pain. All the same, Triano also reflects a consensus of current opinion that SMT is merely one among many options in the conservative care of low back pain, and that time frames for manipulative treatment need to be respected. After a reasonable trial of SMT, whether administered by a medical or osteopathic physician, a chiropractor, or a physical therapist, it should be discontinued if the patient is not progressing.

Equally as challenging as the place of manual medicine in the management of low back pain is the role of psychiatry and psychology.

Traditionally, the psychologist administered and evaluated psychological tests and the psychiatrist did therapy. Their roles no longer can be so neatly distinguished. Either may serve as therapist in back pain cases. Reliance upon psychological testing is in a state of critical reevaluation. Psychiatrists such as David Anderson and Michael Moskowitz and psychologists such as Ross Goldstein and Richard Hunt currently conclude that testing has only limited value, although testing is still done. They take a broad view of what enters into a mental health assessment. Peter Polatin, a psychiatrist, notes that physical findings and the medical history need to be correlated with demographic and environmental factors, personal habits, and family situations, as well as with other lifestyle realities, if complex spinal patients are to be cured or rehabilitated. Anderson, Moskowitz, Goldstein, and Hunt agree. They see the clinical interview as a highly skilled clinical art that allows them to play a critical role if success is to be achieved for difficult patients.

Because it is difficult to evaluate mental states, it is difficult to evaluate the techniques of psychiatrists and psychologists. Moskowitz finds hypnotism highly valuable in his work with low back pain patients, but can one really be so sure that it makes a significant difference? Anderson finds it useful to apply anthropological theory as well as the contributions of Carl Jung as he guides patients through the health-seeking process. We find his application of the concept of disabling back pain as a rite of passage to be one of the most stimulating concepts in the field of conservative care today. Yet, until subject to authenticating clinical trials, it must be acknowledged as provocative, but not as proven.

It is not difficult to identify many other challenges of the lumbar spine. Jerome Schofferman is an internist who has elaborated one approach to making pain clinics work. In chronic pain programs, difficult issues are involved that overlap those of medicine, physical therapy, and psychiatry. How do you help chronic pain patients break their dependency upon narcotic medications? How do you teach them to live with their pain? Can they reduce their pain by adopting a more active lifestyle when all therapeutic measures have failed? Is it not true that if you involve them in psychotherapy combined with detoxification and physical reconditioning, their pain will lose its control over them even if it cannot be eliminated? Short-term benefits can be documented. However, more studies are needed to determine if the considerable expense involved is warranted by long-term benefits.

But what of the patient who cannot be managed straightforwardly as a back pain patient because of the coexistence of some other incapacity, such as diabetes or heart disease? Physiatrists such as Gerald Keane encounter this type of patient regularly. Keane assures us that while these can be extremely difficult cases, they are not hopeless. One can usually find a window of opportunity even in the complexities of severe multiple pathologies.

The challenges of curative approaches are enormous. Are they any the less if we shift our attention to prevention? We have already noted that success still eludes us in attempting to teach habits for healthy backs to school children, although we continue to try. We are more sanguine of opportunities in the work place. Nikki Burrous, a specialist in risk management, reminds us that preemployment screening involves legal, social, and medical complications that make it difficult if not impossible to identify and select out many of those in danger of injury on jobs for which they have applied. Properly done, however, screening can play a role.

Once in a job, the challenge is to change the work situation and to train the worker. Back schools can be adapted to workplaces. The Whites did this early in the history of the California Back School. Sigmund Miller and others are still doing it. This involves not only teaching spinal anatomy and biomechanics, as is done by many, including two chiropractor-scientists with extensive research expertise, John Triano and Gregory Cramer. It involves not only teaching ergonomics. It also involves engineering evaluation, design, and implementation. One of the most experienced in this complex area is an engineering professor from Stanford University, David Thompson. When the work site is set up so that stress on the spine and mind is minimized, then a Duane Saunders can assess the workers for strength, flexibility, and fitness and tailor an exercise program for them that offers the promise of fewer injuries, fewer expenses, happier workers, and higher production to the industry whose risk management philosophy made it possible.

The reality is that the incidence of back injuries in industry is high. One enormous challenge is to recondition and rehabilitate injured workers. This begins with the onset of injury. The acute patient of today, though soon well again just by the natural history of the diesase, is by the very fact of the first injury subsequently at greater risk for chronic disease. The first responsibility of the physician, then, is to get the acute patient well again faster than will happen if one just waits for nature to take its course. Out there in the world of health care, many still treat these patients much as they were treated a century ago, prescribing bed rest, analgesics, and muscle relaxants.

Robert Mootz is one among many, now, who specialize in back pain and who recognize the need for a comprehensive approach to these patients. One needs to adapt the treatment process to the different treatment needs presented by successive stages in the physiologic response characteristic of traumatic insult.

It is still only recently in the history of health care that some chiropractors such as Mootz, and some physiatrists specializing in sports medicine such as Jeffrey Saal, Joel Saal, and other back pain clinicians of whatever professional backgrounds, approach both acute and chronic patients in these terms. Bed rest, if recommended, is for a very limited initial period only. Otherwise, it is counterproductive. With few exceptions, only nonnarcotic analgesics are recommended, and their purpose is not so much palliation for its own sake, but palliation to permit the patient to commit to rigorously designed exercises carried out with good stabilization. Saal and Saal have demonstrated that even patients considered to be surgical candidates because of disc herniations with radiculopathy that proved to be unresponsive to other conservative care can be treated successfully with aggressive, nonoperative methods if they are patient-active rather than patient-passive.

Getting injured workers back to work after they have become chronic is one of the greatest of treatment challenges. Roy Slack is among those who have successfully used exercise equipment to recondition individuals unable to work because of back pain. Mark Sontag would remind us, as would many other physicians and therapists, that very expensive computerized equipment has not been demonstrated clearly to accomplish the job of evaluation and rehabilitation any more effectively than the use of simple, inexpensive equipment.

Whatever the nature of the conditioning equipment, the key to success in reconditioning individuals with severe chronicity appears to be to expand the early back school lessions of training patients in exercises and stabilization. What began in back school as a few simple demonstrations with a few hours of supervised practice, needs to be expanded, for selected patients, into programs that simulate the work situation of the individual employee, and train that person by supervising laboratory-based daily work until patients have learned to practice good body mechanics even when they are fatigued and heavily engaged in work tasks. It should be possible, in many cases, even for a fire fighter or a coal miner to return to work, as Rowlin Lichter has found in his experience with work hardening and work simulation.

We should say, *sometimes* return to work, because still another specialization is that of evaluating what the impaired individual can still do if a return to the original kind of employment is no longer physically or psychologically possible. Patrick Venditti is a chiropractor. Mark Sontag is a physiatrist. Duane Saunders is a physical therapist. Yet each has specialized in this aspect of identifying the remaining functional and occupational capabilities of chronic back pain patients who otherwise would live out their lives in pain, misery, and poverty. No one would claim to have final answers here. No one believes that the American political and legal structure is good in this area. But for the present, at least, more is done now than was even thought of in 1970.

What, then, is the challenge of conservative care? It is still surgical, to be sure. Far more, however, in terms of the number of patients, the number of clinicians, and the potential for success, the big challenge is to develop and apply conservative methods of prevention and treatment.

At every point in the history of medicine, at least during the last century or two, it has been tempting for medical writers to review the field of spinal disorders as known to them in their time, and to conclude that much progress had been accomplished; that the effectiveness of the physician had greatly improved. We are no different. In our time, we have learned some important lessons and have witnessed the development of some effective methods. Not the least, we have recognized the value of collaboration that cuts across disciplines in order to take advantage of the many special techniques that no one individual or profession alone can bring to the difficult back pain case.

In our time, however, we also see each area of expertise as still in need of improvement. In our various professions, we are distant, still, from the goal of being able to say that health issues relating to the spine are under control. We do not expect, in our lifetimes, to write a book on the accomplishment of lumbar spine control. We expect, in interprofessional collaboration with outstanding colleagues such as those discussed above, and many others, to continue to struggle in this fight against pain and dysfunction, to overcome disappointments in the future as in the past, and above all to enjoy the excitement and joy of trying harder and of being a part of a worldwide effort to increase our effectiveness and the success of our patients. That, truly, is the challenge of conservative care.

References

1. Kroeber AL. *Anthropology.* New York: Harcourt, Brace and Co., 1948.
2. Knott M, Voss DE. *Proprioceptive neuromuscular facilitation: Patterns and techniques.* New York: Harper and Row, 1956.
3. McKenzie RA. *The lumbar spine: Mechanical diagnosis and therapy.* Waikanae, New Zealand: Spinal Publications, 1981.
4. Cyriax J. *Textbook of orthopaedic medicine.* 2 vols. 7th ed. London: Ballière-Tindall, 1978.
5. Lewit K. *Manipulative therapy in rehabilitation of the motor system.* London: Butterworth, 1985.
6. Maigne R. *Orthopedic medicine: A new approach to vertebral manipulations.* Springfield, IL: Charles C Thomas, 1972.
7. Bourdillon JF. *Spinal manipulation.* 3d ed. New York: Appleton-Century-Crofts, 1982.
8. Upledger JE, Vredevoogd JD. *Craniosacral therapy.* Chicago: Eastland Press, 1983.
9. DeJarnette MB. *Sacro occipital technic of chiropractic.* Nebraska City NE, privately published, 1952.
10. Maitland GD. *Vertebral manipulation.* London: Butterworth, 1964.
11. Greenland SLS, Reisbord S, Haldeman S, Buerger AA. Controlled clinical trials of manipulation: A review and a proposal. *Occup Med* 1980; 22(10):670–676.
12. Haldeman, Scott. Spinal manipulative therapy: A status report. *Clin Orthop* 1983; 179:62–70.
13. Haldeman, Scott. Spinal manipulative therapy in sports medicine. *Clin Sports Med* 1986; 5(2):277–293.

INDEX

Page numbers in *italics* denote figures; those followed by "t" denote tables.